Natural Cancer Science

The Evidence for Diets, Herbs, Superfoods, and
Other Natural Strategies that Fight Cancer

By Case Adams, PhD

Natural Cancer Science: The Evidence for Diets, Herbs, Superfoods, and Other
    Natural Strategies that Fight Cancer
Copyright © 2020 Case Adams
LOGICAL BOOKS
Wilmington, Delaware
https://www.logicalbooks.org
All rights reserved.
Printed in USA

Publishers Cataloging in Publication Data
Adams, Case
        Cancer: The Holistic Approach
First Edition
1. Medicine. 2. Health.
Bibliography and References; Index

ISBN-13: 978-1-936251-54-4

Other Books by the Author:

THE CONSCIOUS ANATOMY: Healing the Real You

THE GLUTEN CURE: Scientifically Proven Natural Solutions to Celiac Disease and Gluten Sensitivities

THE LIVING CLEANSE: Detoxification and Cleansing Using Living Foods and Safe Natural Strategies

THE MEANING OF DREAMS: The Science of Why We Dream, How to Interpret Them and How to Steer Them

THE SCIENCE OF LEAKY GUT SYNDROME: Intestinal Permeability and Digestive Health

TOTAL HARMONIC: The Healing Power of Nature's Elements

YOUR PLAN FOR LIFE: Personal Strategic Planning for Humans

Table of Contents

Introduction

Everyone has cancer. Yes, every body is attacked by cancer every day. But for most of us, the body is also eliminating those cancer cells.

Through a strong immune system and with a minor cancer challenge, most of our bodies will remove the tumor-causing cells and their developing support structures. The immune system will either short-circuit the cell with a kill order or shut down the supply system that services the potential tumor.

That is, if the immune system is strong enough – and as long as the cancer cause is not pervasive and out of control.

Cancer is currently killing more humans than any other condition. Why?

And why is cancer killing more people in modern times than ever before? Yes, cancer deaths have gone down a tad over the past few years because of better treatment methods. But the risk of contracting cancer is still higher than ever before. Why is this? What are we doing to ourselves?

The current state of affairs is that we eat whatever we want and expose our bodies to whatever we want and not worry about cancer until it strikes. Then, after the body revolts with cancerous tumors, the proposed solution is a novel treatment that will magically kill all the cancer in our bodies.

Some have compared this attempt to find a cure for cancer to the moon shot of the 60s.

Yes, we can applaud this moon shot-effort to cure those who are currently fighting cancer. The task certainly has merit, and new immunotherapy strategies do look promising.

But to ignore the real solution – of how nature fights cancer – is to miss the real opportunity. As we will find in this book, scientists have been finding more and more natural compounds – from natural foods and herbs – that inhibit the growth of cancer and inhibit tumor growth.

Now if this were one isolated case we could appreciate that it was a lucky hit. But as we'll find in this book, there are so many natural foods, herbs and compounds that inhibit cancer.

Approximately 75 percent of anti-tumor medicines used by conventional medicine today are natural products or analogues. And of the 140 anticancer medicines that have been approved over the past half-century, more than 60 percent were derived from a natural product. Of those 126 molecular agents used for cancer treatment, 67 percent are natural in origin (Cragg and Newman 2005).

Paclitaxel (sold under the brand name Taxol) for example, is one of the most used chemotherapy treatments for all types of cancer. Taxol is produced by plants and fungi. It is used for the treatment of ovarian cancer lung cancer, prostate cancer, melanoma, oral cancers, breast cancers and many other cancers. Even up to 1993, paclitaxel was derived from the bark of the Pacific yew tree (*Taxus brevifolia*).

Today, most paclitaxel is produced through a semi-synthetic process.

Nature works to not only combat cancer as it is developing. It also prevents most cancers before they happen.

1

In other words, nature has already accomplished the moonshot of beating cancer. We just have to get on board the mission.

This isn't just my opinion, mind you. Over the past two decades, numerous medical scientists have become focused upon relationships between our diets and different forms of cancer. They aren't studying this to pass the time. They are discovering that there are so many things are causing cancer in our modern lifestyles. Many things that we can avoid.

That is what we will investigate in this book.

We will investigate research that shows that certain diets and certain foods help prevent cancer.

Then there are certain natural herbs, roots and foods that specifically inhibit the growth of cancer in our body. Some of these can even help the immune system shut down a growing case of cancer according to the research.

Yes, nature does have mechanisms in place that halt the growth of tumors, in the form of certain compounds and mechanisms that work in tandem with our immune system.

Part of this text discusses the effect of toxins on our risk of cancer. Our bodies continue to absorb toxins at an ever-increasing rate. This rate parallels with the rate of cancer over the past few decades.

We will discuss how to maintain a regular cleansing program to help clean toxins from the system.

Is this book a cure for cancer? Sorry. What this book presents, however, is scientific proof that nature can prevent cancer and cure cancer if given the chance.

What about conventional treatments for cancer?

Most of today's conventional treatments for cancer have been developed alongside a significant amount of trial and error, and research proving their effectiveness. And yes, many of these are based upon naturally-produced compounds.

But this book does not deny or contradict the role of these treatments for helping people recover from cancer.

Rather, this book is about nature's role in helping to prevent cancer and help the body fight cancer. The key is that nature works with the body to stimulate the body's defenses.

What this book won't deliver is a host of anecdotal discussions of herbal products reputed to treat cancer. This text will focus strictly on peer-reviewed scientific evidence.

Finally, a warning: If you have been diagnosed with cancer we suggest that you discuss any changes or additions you want to make with your doctor before making them.

Furthermore, the reader with any other health issues or on any medications should discuss any changes with their health professional prior to implementation.

Chapter One

How Our Body Fights Cancer

Cancer grows within our bodies every day. And a majority of our cells can become transformed into cancer cells.

This means that each of us has cancer to some degree.

How does Cancer Develop?

Cancer cells develop through a change in the DNA of a cell. This change in DNA is called a mutation. A typical cell can have as many as 100,000 DNA mutations each and every day.

This means that every DNA mutation will not cause cancer. Most of these mutations are immediately repaired. A string of DNA may have a slight mutation of a pair of chromosomes, and the cell will immediately fix that mutation. Or it will destroy the DNA strand and purge it.

But if the cell doesn't repair the DNA damage, the cell may become re-modeled. This remodeling means the cell develops a new character.

This character changes from being a working part of an organ or tissue system into being a heretic cell.

Once this heretic cell develops, the cell's previous chromosomal system that aims to divide and support a tissue system in the body. The cancer cell begins to divide faster to quickly produce more like-minded cancer cells. This develops into a tumor.

In addition, other cells can be corrupted and enterprised into the expanding tissue system. This is sometimes termed a clonal evolution. The evolution process happens as healthy cells are corrupted by the cancer cells.

Eventually, this growing tissue system converts into a type of organ – a survival system for a rapidly expanding system of carcinogenic cells.

This means the tumor will develop its own delivery system. It may enlist current lymph channels and blood vessels. Or it may develop its own channels for bringing in nutrients.

All of these tendencies of developing tumors come from cancer cells that collectively lock down the capacity to align with the body's organs.

They can lock down the body's processes for controlling growth, for example. This means the cancer cells can grow outside the controls of the body. They can also bypass inhibitions for the entry into other organs and tissues.

Cells that were controlled in terms of their abilities are unlocked when they become cancerous: They can expand in ways the original cells were prevented from.

This means they can invade other cells, organs and tissue systems.

An expanding cancer cell may also lock down the typical kill switch – the p53 switch that allows the immune system to kill the cell. By locking off this switch, the cancer cell system can grow far outside the body's ability to control it.

Can the mutation be stopped?

Let's back up for a moment. Most oncologists focus upon the DNA mutation event – also often called an epimutation.

But epimutations happen all the time in every cell. Some of these mutations are driven by the cell itself or its immediate environment.

The cells' typically have their own DNA repair system. They can also halt DNA mutation before it progresses into uncontrolled cancer cells.

But if there is a deficiency in the DNA repair system in the cells – called DNA repair deficiency – the cell may not be able to repair every mutation. Especially if there is a swarm of mutations.

Some mutations are the result of outside triggers.

There are a number of elements that can promote the mutation of DNA within a cell.

Yes, there are heredity factors and there are genetic sequencing errors. But these make up a minority of cancerous DNA mutations. The majority of cancerous DNA mutations are caused by a build up of free radicals that damage the cell or its membrane.

Reactive Oxygen Species

Reactive oxygen species production is implicated in various types of cancers, even when lipids are not involved. Even the initiation process of the lipid peroxidation is started by a reactive oxygen species (ROS). What is ROS?

This is also often called a free radical. A free radical is an unstable molecule or ion that forms during a chemical reaction. In other words, the molecule or ion needs another atom, ion or molecule to stabilize it. Once it is stable, it is not reactive.

While a free radical is unstable, it can damage any number of elements it meets. These include the cells, organs and tissues of the body.

What Causes Free Radicals?

A number of external and internal relationships in the body produce free radicals. These can range from radiation to a variety of toxins that get into the body through ingestion.

Free radicals can be formed as a result of a number of unnatural and natural biochemicals within the body. These include hydrolysis, oxidation, alkylation, methylation and a number of other biochemical reactions include base mismatches.

Free radicals are basically unstable compounds. They need other compounds in order to make them stable. That means they will steal atomic structures from tissues and cells in order to become stable.

That 'stealing' will damage cells – producing mutations in the DNA.

Yes, radiation from the sun and other types of radiation-producing sources produce free radicals within the skin, which can in turn damage cells.

But consuming toxins through breathing, drinking or eating is a large cause of free radical production. As compounds unnatural to the body find their way in, they can turn into free radicals.

How do our Bodies Remove Free Radicals?

Once free radicals develop, our body's detoxification processes have the ability to neutralize them. That is, unless our detoxification processes are overwhelmed with many free radicals.

One of the primary free radical clearing system is the liver's production of glutathione. The critical component in this mystery is glutathione peroxidase—an enzyme produced in the liver. Glutathione peroxidase is the leading enzyme responsible for the breakdown and removal of one of the most dangerous types of ROS—lipid hydroperoxides.

Nature produces many, many free radicals. However, nature typically accompanies radicals with the molecules, atoms or ions that stabilize the radical. In the atmosphere, for example, radicals become stabilized by ozone and other elements.

In plants, radicals become stabilized by antioxidants from nutrients derived from the sun, soil and oxygen. In the body, radicals are stabilized by antioxidizing enzymes, nutrients and other elements.

Another anti-oxidation process within the body utilizes the *superoxide dismutase* (SOD) enzyme. The SOD enzyme is typically available within the cytoplasm of most cells. Here SOD is complexed by either copper and zinc, or manganese—similar to the way selenium is complexed with the glutathione peroxidase enzyme.

Several types of SOD enzymes reside within the body—some in the mitochondria and some in the intercellular tissue fluids. SOD neutralizes superoxides before they can damage the inside and outside of the cell—assuming the body is healthy, with substantial amounts of SOD. The immune system produces superoxides as part of its strategy to attack microorganisms and toxins.

Another broad anti-oxidation process utilizes *catalase*. Here the body provides an enzyme bound by iron to neutralize peroxides to oxygen and water. It is a standard component of many metabolic reactions within the body.

Yet another enzyme utilized for radical reduction is *glutathione reductase*. This enzyme works with NADP in the cell to stabilize hydrogen peroxide oxidized radicals before they can damage the cell.

Notice that all of these antioxidizing enzymes require minerals. We have seen either selenium, copper, zinc, manganese or iron as necessary to keep these enzymes in good supply. Many other minerals and trace elements are used by other antioxidant and detoxifying enzyme processes. These minerals, and many of the enzymes themselves, are supplied by various foods and supplements, as we'll discuss further.

Another tool that the healthy body utilizes to stabilize radicals are the antioxidants supplied by plant foods. Plants produce antioxidants to protect their own cells from radical damage. Thus, their plant material contains a host of these oxidation stabilizers, which our bodies use to neutralize radicals.

What is Lipid Hydroperoxidation?

Let's take a closer look at lipid hydroperoxidation, or lipid peroxidation. Lipid peroxidation means the fats (lipids) in our cell membranes are being robbed of electrons. This 'robbery' results in an unstable cell membrane. Let's take a closer look at the process of lipid peroxidation.

The first step takes place with the entry of a reactive oxygen species into the proximity of the cell. Reactive oxygen species are elements that require an electron—such as hydrogen (H+)—in order to become stable.

Fatty acids that make up the membranes of cells are the likely candidates for hydroperoxidation. The name "lipid" refers to a fatty acid. Fatty acids include saturated fats, polyunsaturates, monounsaturates, and so on (see fatty acid discussions later on).

Several types of lipids make up cell membranes. Fatty acids will combine with other molecules to make phospholipids, cholesterols and glycolipids. Saturates and polyunsaturates are typical, but there are several species of polyunsaturates.

These range from long chain versions to short versions. They also include the cis-fats and the trans-fats. Cell membranes that utilize predominantly cis- versions with long chains are the most durable. Those cell membranes with trans- configurations can be highly unstable, and irregularly porous. This is one reason why trans fats are unhealthy. The other reason is that trans fats easily become peroxidized.

Cell membranes with more long chain fatty acids are more stable and are less subject to peroxidation. Shorter chains that provide more double bonds are less stable, because these are more easily broken. Also, monounsaturated fatty acids such as GLA are more stable.

Once the fatty acid is degraded by an oxygen species, it becomes a fatty acid radical. The fatty acid will usually become oxidized, making it a peroxyl-fatty acid radical. This radical will react with other fatty acids, forming a cyclic process involving radicals called cyclic peroxides.

Lipid hydroperoxides are one of the most damaging molecules within the body. They are responsible for many cancer cases. Research has confirmed that lipid peroxides, *"participate in chain reactions that amplify damage to biomolecules including DNA. DNA attack gives rise to mutations that may involve tumor suppressor genes or oncogenes, and this is an oncogenic mechanism."* (Cejas *et al.* 2004)

When lipid hydroperoxides accumulate and damage our cells, they can also short-circuit the mechanisms that shut off cancer. These are the tumor suppressor genes discussed above.

The damage from lipid hydroperoxides typically stimulates an inflammatory response. Researchers have called the initial signal from the cell that initiates this inflammatory response *lipid peroxidation/LOOH-mediated stress signaling*. In other words, the cells are stressed by lipid peroxidation, and this initiates a distress signal to the immune system.

The liver produces one of the best facilities to remove lipid hydroperoxides, in the form of glutathione peroxidase. We'll discuss this further in the section on the liver.

But the liver's glutathione production is an example of how the immune system naturally combats and prevents the growth of cancer.

Nature has provided our bodies with not only an adaptive immune system, but a series of active combatants to swarm and overwhelm cancer cells as they develop in our body.

These warriors also include our antibodies, our immune cells and our probiotics, working in conjunction with each other to take down cancer cells as they develop.

In other words, inflammation is simply a defense measure by an immune system that is overwhelmed.

Barriers to Toxins

Before cancer-causing toxins can intrude the body they must first get through the body's outside barriers. These are designed not unlike the moat systems used in medieval castles throughout Western Europe centuries ago.

Our immune system utilizes a network of tissue and biochemical barriers that work synergistically to prevent cancer-causing agents from getting into the body.

The barrier structures include the ability of the body to shut down its orifices. We can close our eyes, mouths, noses and ears to prevent invaders or toxins from entering the body. Within these lie further defensive structures: Nose hairs, eyelashes, lips, tonsils, ear hair, pubic hair and hair in general are all designed to help screen out and filter invaders.

Most of the body's passageways are also equipped with tiny cilia, which assist the body evacuate invaders by brushing them out. These cilia move rhythmically, sweeping back and forth, working caught pathogens outward with their undulations.

The surfaces of most of the body's orifices are also covered with a mucous membrane. This thin liquid membrane film contains a combination of biochemicals and cells that prevent invaders from penetrating any further. These mucous membranes lining the passageways accomplish this with a combination of immune cells, immunoglobulins and colonies of probiotics.

The digestive tract is equipped with another type of sophisticated defense technology. Should any foreigners get through the lips, teeth, tongue, hairs, mucous membranes, cilia and sneak down the esophagus, they then must contend with the digestive fire of the stomach. The gastrin, peptic acid and hydrochloric acid within a healthy stomach keep a pH of around two.

This is typically enough acidity to kill or significantly damage many bacteria. However, a person can mistakenly weaken this protective acid by taking antacids or acid-blockers. In this case, the stomach's ability to neutralize pathogens will be handicapped. In addition, a number of microorganisms are accustomed to acidic environments, and still others can tuck away into clumps of food—especially food that has not been chewed well enough.

Respiratory cancer protection

Many cancer causing agents may penetrate our oral protection system and get into the lungs. At the same time, our lungs provide one of the body's most effective means of filtering and screening out toxins.

With every breath, we purge the body of toxins. The epithelial cells of our airways house sub-mucosal ducts that push toxins out to the mucous membranes. As we breathe out and as our mucous is channeled out, we send these toxins out.

In addition, the lungs filter and prevent the body from inheriting more toxins. As air moves through the nostrils through to the *pharynx*, the *larynx* and the *trachea*, it passes over a mucous membrane lined with tiny hairs called *cilia*. These cilia capture foreign particles with a web of sticky mucous. After being stuck, the particles are gathered up within the mucous. The tiny cilia hairs will undulate the mucous and foreign particles towards exit points like the throat, nostrils and mouth. At these points, the particles can be sneezed or coughed out as phlegm, blown out through the nose, or swallowed down into the acidic abyss of the stomach.

More offensive particles like bacteria and viruses are attacked by the macrophages and probiotics that line the mucous membranes. They break down the foreigners and escort their parts out of the body. These may travel out with the mucous, or be absorbed into the lymph or blood and pushed out through urine, sweat or the colon.

About 97% of our incoming oxygen is delivered to the cells by hemoglobin molecules. After being escorted through the micro-capillaries to the cells, the oxygen disassociates from the hemoglobin. Only about 20% of oxygen disassociates from hemoglobin while we rest. More disassociates as needed. The rest stays in the bloodstream, on standby. This standby oxygen effectively alkalizes the blood, inhibiting oxidative radicals with the presence of O_2.

Should exhalation not be able to deplete this acidic environment in the blood, one of the first locations of damage will be to the walls of the blood vessels and alveoli. The acidic radicals look for stability as they borrow atomic elements from the molecules making up these tissues. This leaves these tissues damaged and in need of repair.

This later process of energy production in the absence of oxygen (oxygen debt) produces many more acids than does the Krebs cycle. The result is a bloodstream subject to acidosis, which corresponds to overexertion.

The bottom line is that better and more complete breathing helps detoxify the bloodstream and keep the blood in more of a radical-free alkaline state.

Cilia

The bronchial epithelial cells of the airway passages are also equipped with microscopic hairs called cilia (see previous and next drawing). The cilia act like tiny brooms: They undulate towards the exits—the sinuses, mouth and pharynx. The little hairs "sweep" out the mucous, together with toxins and dead cell parts caught in the mucous membrane.

The ciliary hairs lining the airways beat rhythmically with the expansion and release of the lungs. This expansion and contraction increases the mucous surfactant as well.

Should toxin particles remain airborne, they will also likely be moved out through breathing and rhythmic ciliary hair undulations in healthy airways.

The membrane and ciliary hair move in slow waves—very similar to what we see among kelp beds as they move with undulating ocean waves. This wave-like action of the ciliary hairs acts as an effective transport system.

This transport mechanism—the clearing of toxins and cell parts out of the area by the cilia—is called the *mucociliary clearance apparatus*. This is a self-cleaning system of the airways: Should these 'automatic sweepers' become caught in the thick mucous of a toxin-rich and/or ionically imbalanced mucous membrane—they become ineffective.

The mucociliary clearance apparatus explains how we will gather an accumulation of phlegm within the throat and sinuses. Most of us clear our throats or blow our noses without a second thought. Little do we realize that much of that phlegm is the result of the cilias' self-cleaning undulations that sweep out toxins and mucous. This sweeping mechanism also helps prevent polluted air and particles from being absorbed into our blood. Those particles not tossed out with the breath or mucous get phagotized (broken down) and swept out. Or they may be transported to the blood or lymph and escorted out of the body through the colon, urinary tract or sweat glands.

However, should the mucosal fluid not be healthy and ionically balanced, thickened mucous will build up within the mucosal membrane. This will overwhelm and in effect *drown* the ciliary hairs—making them far less effective for removing toxins and toxin-rich mucous.

The cilia are stabilized by being seated in a thin pool of thicker mucous, with another layer of thinner mucous on top. The thinner mucous towards the surface of the mucous membrane allows the hairs to undulate faster near and at the surface of the mucous membrane.

It is essential that these cilia are healthy, vibrant, and free of toxin-debris. This is why, as we'll explain, that tar and soot from smoking and pollution can wreck such havoc on the lungs. The tops of the cilia—and mucous—become jammed up in this gummy residue.

Mucosal Membranes

Mucous membranes cover just about every region of epithelial cells, including our skin, nose, throat, mouth, airways, digestive tract, urinary tract, vagina and other surfaces. Some surfaces, such as the skin, have very thin mucosal membranes. Other surfaces, such as the digestive tract and airways, have thick mucosal membranes.

The mucosal membrane is a thin layer of glycoproteins (mucin), mucopolysaccharides, special enzymes, probiotics, immune cells and ionic fluid. The ionic fluid provides a transporter medium, which escorts a host of elements back and forth between the epithelial cells and the surface of the mucosal membrane. These elements include chloride ions, sodium ions, oxygen, nitrogen, carbon dioxide, hydrogen carbonate and others.

Some of these—such as the sodium, bicarbonate and chloride ions—provide the transport mechanisms into the cells and tissues of the skin surfaces. These travel through openings or pores among the cells, attached to nutrients, oxygen and other elements—transporting them in, in other words.

Certainly, the body is choosy about what kinds of elements it will allow into the epithelial cells and tissues. There are countless toxins, microorganisms, debris allergens and other foreigners that the body wants kept out.

We might compare this to how oil lubricates and protects an engine from overheating and dirt. In a well-maintained car, good motor oil will be circulated through the rods and cylinders. The oil doesn't just allow the steel parts to move with minimal friction: The motor oil also helps keep the engine clean, and prevents dirt and other contaminants from clogging up the system. Imagine what would happen if a car were to run without oil for a few miles? The engine would surely seize up, and likely would break down completely. While this is a crude example, there are several elements that are consistent.

So just how does the body keep these invaders from penetrating the body's internal and external surfaces? The short answer is the mucosal membranes. This is why these membranes contain a host of immune cells. These include immunoglobulins such as IgA, B-cells, T-cells and others that are looking to trap foreigners before get any further. Once they find a foreigner, they will take it apart using a one of many immune system strategies.

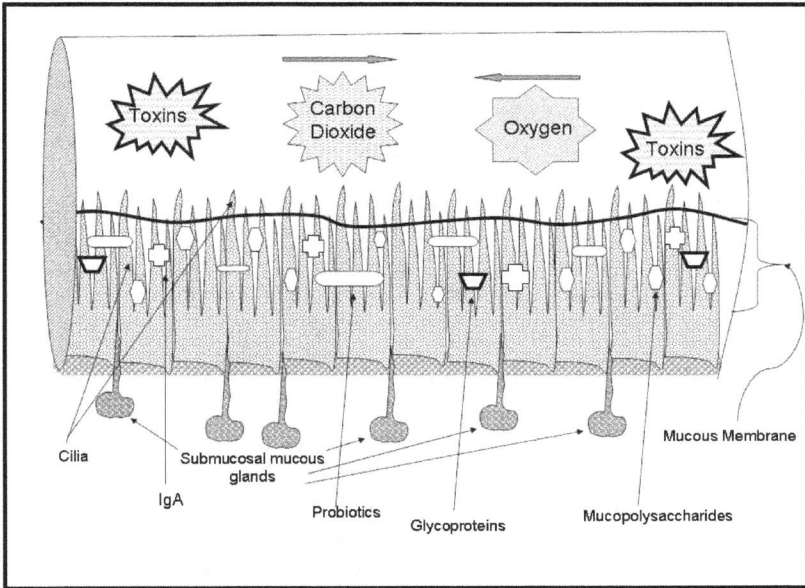

Airway Mucosal Membranes and Cilia

The mucous membranes are living structures. Probiotics populate our mucosal membranes, and are an important part of the "wall" of protection provided by these membranes. Tiny protective probiotic bacteria will inhabit all healthy mucosal membranes, including the skin. Like the immune system, these bacteria are trained to protect their territory. If an invading microorganism enters the mucosal membrane, the probiotics will lead an attack on them, with the immune cells in close pursuit.

The chemistry of the mucosal membrane also buffers and calms immune response. The mucosal membrane will help transport components such as corticosteroids from the adrenals to squelch inflammatory immune responses among our epithelial tissues. In other words, a healthy mucosal membrane is *calming* to our digestive tract, airways, skin and so on.

Other than our skin, which has been covered by placenta fluid, our mucosal membranes are raw and not well developed at birth. Gradually, as probiotics begin to colonize the sinuses, mouth and intestines—the mucosal membranes begin to mature. This maturity, as we'll discuss in detail, requires a host of nutrients as well as strong probiotic populations in order to populate the mucosal membranes. As this colonization occurs, the body's epithelial cells and mucous glands provide their balance of chemistry and protective attributes.

This is the basis for the hygiene theory, a product of many studies showing that infants and children that are allowed to roam the floors, parks, soils, and those among larger families have stronger immune systems. This is be-

11

cause all that roaming allows our bodies to collect a variety of probiotic species, which eventually colonize and territorialize our mucosal membranes.

Then there is the transporter mechanism. The mucous membranes utilizes this surfactant quality and ionic capabilities to transport nutrients among the epithelial cells, allowing them to function efficiently. It also transports toxins out of the area—assuming a healthy mucosal membrane.

Should this transport mechanism not be functioning properly, the region can become laden with a thickened, toxic mucous. Instead of the mucous membranes keeping these surfaces clean, the mucous itself becomes toxic.

This thickened mucous membrane is typical in hyperactive airway responses among COPD, asthma, and hay fever conditions. In the intestines, the condition produces irritable bowel syndrome, colitis, Crohn's and other intestinal issues. In the lower esophagus and stomach, weakened mucosal membranes produces ulcers and acid reflux. And weakened skin mucosal membranes produce eczema, dermatitis, hives and other skin irritations.

Mucous is secreted by tiny mucous glands that lie within goblet cells scattered throughout these epithelia surfaces. They are called goblets because they are shaped like little goblet glasses, except their upper surface extends through the (internal) surfaces in tiny fingers. In the intestines and airways, they are called microvilli. On skin and other surfaces, they are become pores. They function almost identically with respect to their production of mucous.

The goblet cells and their end points both produce mucin through a process of contraction and glycosylation within the Golgi apparatus of the cells. This glycosylation of proteins produces the glycoproteins that are the mainstay in mucin.

The mucosal goblet cells of the respiratory tract are also similar to the gastric cells of the stomach and duodenum. The difference here is that these produce mucous fed by the pyloric glands in addition to the highly acidic gastrin. As we'll be discussing more at length throughout the remainder of the text, this similarity between the goblet cells, the villi and the gastric/pyloric cells facilitates an understanding of the mystery of GERD-related respiratory disorders.

The mucous membrane fluids can also become dehydrated if the ions that open the pores are blocked. Here the pores may be blocked due to an imbalance of ion chemistry in the sub-mucosal membrane. Tests have shown that chlorine and bicarbonate anions stimulate the opening of the pores that bring liquids into the mucous membrane.

The mucin proteins produced by the submucosal membrane glands have to be diluted with these ion fluids to give the mucous membrane the right balance of stickiness and fluidity.

Among dehydrated mucosal membranes, the mucous is thickened and not fluid enough to provide its surfactant and transport functions.

In addition, exposure to toxins, pathogenic microorganisms, cold air and any number of other triggers can stimulate the production of mucous by the goblet cells. In a healthy body, this stimulates the quick removal of the toxin or invader, as the excess mucous is swept out by the cilia or other drainage facilities of the surface.

However, should the body be immunosuppressed or otherwise overwhelmed by the invasion, the goblet cells will over-produce mucous, which can swamp the epithelial surfaces with dead cell parts and toxins. When these surfaces are drowning in mucous, the removal process is deficient. The lack of mucous transport, combined with the need to remove toxins, produces inflammation as the immune system must engage to remove the toxins.

Humoral Defense

The immune response to a cancerous cell involves a highly technical strategic attack. This first identifies a cancer cell as it develops, followed by a precise and immediate offensive attack to exploit the weaknesses of the cell. This is often called humoral immunity.

More than a billion different types of antibodies, macrophages and other immune cells mobilize and execute specific attack plans upon cancer cells. As an immune cell scans a particular cancer cell, it may recognize a particular biomolecular or behavioral weakness within the cell.

Upon recognizing this weakness, the immune system will devise a unique plan to exploit this weakness. It may launch a variety of possible attacks, using a combination of specialized B-cells (or *B-lymphocytes*) in conjunction with specialized antibodies to destroy the cell.

Cruising through the blood and lymph systems, the antibodies and/or B-cells can quickly sense and size up invading microbes. Often this will mean the antibody will lock onto or bind to the invader to extract critical molecular information.

This process will often draw upon databases held within certain helper B-cells that memorize vulnerabilities. The specific vulnerability is often revealed by molecular structures of pathogenic cell membranes. Each pathogen will be identified by these unique structures or antigens.

The B-cell then reproduces a specific antibody designed to record and communicate that information to other B-cells through biochemical transception. This allows for a constant tracking of the location and development of pathogens, allowing B-cells to manage and constantly assess the response.

Cell-Mediated Immunity

Another anticancer process used by the immune system is the cell-mediated immune response. This also incorporates a collection of smart white blood cells, called T-cells. T-cells and their surrogates wander the body scanning the body's own cells. They are seeking cells that have become infected or otherwise damaged by microbes or toxic free radicals.

Infected cells are typically identified by special marker molecules (antigens) that sit atop their cell membranes.

These antigens have particular molecular arrangements that signal roving T-cells of the damage that has occurred within the cell. Once a damaged cell has been recognized, the cell-mediated immune system will launch an inflammatory response against the cell.

This response will typically utilize a variety of cytotoxic (cell-killing) cells and helper T-cells. These types of immune cells will often insert a kill-switch into the cancer cell. Or it may directly kill the damaged cell by inserting toxic chemicals into it. Alternatively, the T-cell might send signals into the damaged cell, switching on a self-destruct mechanism within the cancer cell.

The immune system produces at least five different types of white blood cells. Each is designed to identify and target specific types of pathogens and potential cancer-causing agents.

Once they identify an intruder or toxin, they will either initiate an attack with other components, or directly begin their attack. The main types are lymphocytes, neutrophils, basophils, monocytes and macrophages. Each plays an important role in the pathogen-identification and inflammatory process. Lymphocytes are the body's self-specific immune response team.

The primary lymphocytes are the T-cells (thymus cells) or B-cells (bone marrow cells). These cells and their specialized proteins work together to strategically attack and remove invaders. Then they memorize the strategy in preparation for a future invasion.

Consider this in the case of lipid peroxidation. The damage by lipid free radicals starts a chain reaction that results in the cell membrane becoming completely destroyed and dysfunctional. The dysfunction then stimulates a genetic mutation, which changes the nature of the cell.

These changes are communicated to the immune system, indicating that the cell is compromised and has become malignant.

The T-cell immune response will often initiate the cell's self-destruct switch: TNF—tumor necrosis factor.

Alternatively, the cell may be directly destroyed by cytotoxic T-cells. The combined process stimulates inflammation. As these cells are killed or self-destruct, they are purged from the system—provoking increased mucous formation.

The immune system responds by initializing a state called *systemic inflammation*. As we discussed earlier, during systemic inflammation, the immune system launches an ongoing supply of eosinophils, neutrophils and mast cells, which release granulocytes that inflame the airways.

During ongoing peroxidation, the immune system is on a hair-trigger. Imagine a person at work who is stressed from being buried in work and a myriad of problems. You walk into their office and they immediately react: "And what do *you* want?" they ask.

If they were not overloaded with work, problems and deadlines, your coming into their office would probably be met without such a frantic response. But since they were overloaded, they reacted (hyper reacted is a better word) more defensively than needed, *because they thought you were going to add to their workload.*

All white blood cells are initially assembled by stem cells in the bone marrow. Following their release, T-cells undergo further differentiation and programming in the thymus gland. B-cells undergo a similar process of maturity before release from the spleen. Both T-cells and B-cells circulate via lymph nodes, the bloodstream and among tissue fluids. Both also have a number of special types, including memory cells and helper cells to identify and memorize invaders.

B-cells look for foreign or potentially harmful pathogens moving freely. These might include toxins or microbes. Once identified, B-cells will stimulate the production of a particular type of antibody protein, which is designed to destroy or break apart the foreigner. There are several different types of B-cells. Most are monoclonal, which means they will adjust to the specific type of invader.

Some B-cells are investigative and surveillance oriented. They are focused on roaming pathogens. Once activated, they can then damage these invading pathogens using a variety of biochemical secretions or physical activities. B-cells that circulate and surveil the bloodstream are often called plasma B-cells. Others—like memory B-cells—record previous invasions for future attacks.

T-cells, on the other hand, are oriented toward the body's own cells. They are focused upon internal cellular problems, toxin absorption, or those pathogens that have invaded cells.

There are different types of T-cells. Each is programmed in the thymus to look for a different type of problem, and each has the capability of destroying different types of cells and infections.

Many T-cells simply respond to a pathogen that has invaded the cell by destroying the cell itself—this is the *killer* T-cell. It does this by inserting special chemicals into the cell or submitting instructions for the cell to kill itself. Cell death is called apoptosis, and T-cells capable of killing our cells are called cytotoxic T-cells and natural killer T-cells.

T-cells work through a communication system of cytokines to relay instructions and information amongst the various T-cells. Prominent cytokine communications thus take place between helper T-cells, natural killer cells and cytotoxic T-cells.

The initial scanning of an infected cell by a helper T-cell utilizes electromagnetic scanning just as the B-cells do. The T-cell's support network also includes delta-gamma T-cells. Delta-gamma T-cells are stimulated by specific molecular receptors on cell membranes. In general, helper T-cells communicate previous immune responses, memorize current ones, and pass on strategic information on the progress of pending attack plans.

The helper T-cell scan surveys the cell's membrane for indications of either microbial infection or some sort of genetic mutation due to a virus or toxin. This antigen scan might reveal invasions of chemical toxins, protozoa, worms, fungi, bacteria and viruses that have intruded or deranged the cell. The scanning helper T-cell immediately communicates the information by releasing their tiny coded protein cytokines. These disseminate the information needed to coordinate macrophages, NK-cells and cytotoxic T-cells for attack.

Most cells contain tumor necrosis factor or TNF—a sort of self-destruct switch. When signaled from the outside by a T-cell, TNF will initiate a self-destruct and the cell will die.

Under some circumstances, entire groups of cells or tissue systems may be damaged. Macrophages may be signaled to cut off the blood supply to kill these deranged or infected cells.

The two primary helper T-cell types are the Th1 and the Th2. The Th1 T-cell focuses on the elimination of bacteria, fungi, parasites, viruses, and similar types of invaders. The Th2 cells, on the other hand, are focused upon allergic and antibody responses. The Th2 is thus explicitly involved in the responses of inflammation and allergic reaction.

This is important to note, because research has revealed that stress, chemical toxins, poor dietary habits and lack of sleep tend to suppress Th1 levels and increase Th2 levels. With an abundance of Th2 cells in the system, the body is prone to respond more strongly to allergens and toxins, causing problems like hay fever and allergies. This is why we sometimes see people who are under physical or emotional stress overreacting with hives, psoriasis and other allergic-type responses.

Neutrophils are white blood cells that circulate within the blood stream, looking for abnormal behavior among various cells and tissues. Once they identify a problem, they will signal a mass assembly and begin the process of cleaning the area. This typically involves inflammation, as they work to break down and remove debris.

Cytokine Inhibition

Cytokines are communication devices that allow different immune cells to communicate. This is especially important in situations where a cell has become cancerous or is at risk of becoming so.

Cytokines have complex names like interleukin (IL), transforming growth factor (TGF), leukemia inhibitory factor (LIF), and tumor necrosis factor (TNF). There are five basic types of cell communication: intracrine, autocrine, endocrine, juxtacrine and paracrine.

Autocrine communication takes place between two different types of cells. This message can be a biochemical exchange or an electromagnetic signal. The other cell in turn may respond automatically by producing a particular biochemical or electromagnetic message. We might compare this to leaving a voicemail on someone's message machine.

Once we leave the message, the machine signals that the message has been received and will be delivered. Later the machine will replay the message. The immune system uses this type of autocrine message recording process to activate T-cells. Once the message is relayed, the T-cell will respond specifically with the instructed activity.

A paracrine communication takes place between neighboring cells of the same type, to pass on a message that comes from outside of the tissue system. Tiny protein antennas will sit on cell membranes, allowing one cell to communicate with another. This allows cells within the same tissue system to respond in a coordinated manner.

Juxtacrine communications take place via smart biomolecular structures. We might call these structures relay stations. They absorb messages and pass them on. An example of this is the passing of inflammatory messages via immune cell cytokines.

An intracrine communication takes place within the cell. First, an external message may be communicated into the cell through an antenna sitting on the cell's membrane. Once inside the cell, the message will be communicated around cell's organelles to initiate internal metabolic responses.

The endocrine message takes place between endocrine glands and individual cells. The endocrine glands include the pineal gland, the pituitary gland, the pancreas, adrenals, thyroid, ovary and testes. These glands produce endocrine biochemicals, which relay messages directly to cells.

Their messages stimulate a variety of metabolic functions within the body. These include growth, temperature, sexual behavior, sleep, glucose utilization, stress response and so many others.

One of the functions of the endocrine glands relevant to disease is the production of inflammatory co-factors such as cortisol, adrenaline and norepinephrine. These coordinate and initiate instructions that stimulate inflammatory processes to help remove malignant cancer cells.

Antibody Defense

Antibodies are also called immunoglobulins. These are proteins programmed for a particular type of response. They initiate immune responses to different pathogens that can have varying degrees of cancer-producing agency. In other words, antibodies can help our bodies protect against all types of agents that can produce the free radicals that cause cancer.

IgA immunoglobulins line the mouth and digestive tract, scanning for pathogens that might infect the body. IgDs sense infections and activate B-cells. IgEs attach to foreign substances and launch histamine responses—typically associated with allergic responses. IgGs cross through membranes, responding to growing pathogens that have already invaded the body. IgMs are focused on new intrusions that have yet to grow enough to garner the attention of the IgGs.

Each of these general antibodies contain numerous sub-types geared to different types of pathogens and responses.

One aspect of antibodies is the CD glycogen-protein complex. CD stands for cluster of differentiation. CDs are molecules that sit on top of immune cells to navigate and steer their behavior. They will sit atop T-cells, B-cells, NK-cells, granulocytes and monocytes, identifying pathogens and infected cells. They often negotiate and bind to pathogens. This allows the lymphocyte to proceed to attack the pathogen, often by inserting a toxic chemical that destroys the pathogen or the cell hosting it.

CDs are identified by their molecular structure: This is also referred to as a ligand. The specific molecular arrangement (or CD number) will also match a specific type of receptor at the membrane of the cell or pathogen. Each CD number will produce a bonding relationship with a certain receptor structure on the cell to allow the accompanying immunoglobulin or lymphocyte to have interactivity with the pathogen. This gives the immunoglobulin or lymphocyte an access point from which to attack the pathogen.

Lymphatic Cancer Prevention

One of the most important players in the body's purging of cancer-causing toxins is the body's lymphatic system. The lymphatic system is a network of channels that flow through the body just as blood flows through the body.

But instead of blood, the lymphatic system pumps an immune cell and anti-inflammatory-rich lymph fluid throughout the body. And instead of a centrally-located pump called the heart, the lymphatic system pumps lymph using our muscular system. When our muscles flex, it pumps our lymphatic system to flow lymph throughout the body.

This is one reason why exercise is so important for immunity. When we exercise we increase the pumping action of the lymphatic system. That distributes anti-cancer lymph through the bodies organs and tissue systems.

One of the central features of the lymphatic system is thymus gland. The thymus gland is located in the center of the chest, behind the sternum. The thymus is one of the more critical organs of the lymphatic system. Some have compared the thymus gland of the lymphatic system to the heart of the circulatory system.

The thymus gland is not a pump, however. The thymus activates T-cells and various hormones that modulate and stimulate the immune and autoimmune processes. The thymus converts a type of lymphocyte called the thymocyte into T-cells or natural killer cells. These activated T-cells are released into the lymph and bloodstream ready to protect and serve. Within the thymus, the T-cells are infused with CD surface markers—which identify particular types of problematic cells or invading organisms. The CD markers define their mission.

In other words, the thymus codes the T-cells with receptors that will bind to particular toxins and the cells that have been invaded or damaged by toxins. The types of cells or toxins they bind to or identify are determined by the major histocompatibility complex, or MHC determinant.

During the process of converting thymocytes to T-cells, their receptors are programmed with MHC combinations. This allows them to tolerate particular frailties within the body while attacking what the body considers to be true invaders (Kazansky 2008).

Therefore, it is the MHC that gives the T-cell the ability to identify the difference between *self* and *non-self* parts of the body. A non-self identification will produce an immunogen—a factor that stimulates an immune response. Once the immunogen is processed, it stimulates the inflammatory cascade.

The thymus gland develops and enlarges from birth. It is most productive and at its largest during puberty. From that point on, depending upon our diet, stress and lifestyle, our thymus gland will shrink over the years.

By forty, an immunosuppressed person will often have a tiny thymus gland. In elderly persons, the thymus gland is often barely recognizable. For some, the thymus is practically non-functional.

Throughout its productive life, the thymus gland processes T-cells with the appropriate MHC programming. If the thymus gland is functioning, it will continue to produce T-cells with MHC programming that reflects the body's current status. The revised programming will accommodate the various genetic changes that can happen to different cells around the body as we age and adapt to our changing environment.

With a shrunken and non-functioning thymus, however, its ability to reprogram T-cells with a new MHC—enabling them to identify the body's cells that have adapted—is damaged. The T-cells will have to keep working off the old MHC programming. This means the T-cells will not be able to properly identify self versus non-self.

The Liver Cleanup

The liver is the body's most important detoxifying organ. The liver is a blood filtering mechanism, where it screens out many toxins. The liver also produces numerous enzymes and proteins that break down and otherwise metabolize toxins.

This ability to filter and remove toxins, and its ability to neutralize free radicals before they damage our cells makes the liver critically important to cancer prevention.

Yet increasingly we are finding more and more people are suffering from liver damage and cirrhosis. This is the result of an increasing burden of environmental and dietary toxins combined with alcohol abuse and the overuse of pharmaceutical medicines.

As we will discuss, this combination has crippled the liver's ability to prevent cancerous mutations caused by toxins.

The liver sits just below the lungs on the right side under the diaphragm. Partially protected by the ribs, it attaches to the abdominal wall with the falciform ligament. The ligamentum teres within the falciform is the remnant of the umbilical cord that once brought us blood from mama's placenta. As the body develops, the liver continues to filter, purify and enrich our blood. Should the liver shut down, the body would die within hours.

Into the liver drains nutrition-rich venous blood through the hepatic portal vein together with some oxygenated blood through the hepatic artery. A healthy liver will process almost a half-gallon of blood per minute. The blood is commingled within well cavities called sinusoids, where blood is staged through stacked sheets of the liver's primary cells—called hepatocytes. Here blood is also met by interspersed immune cells called kupffers.

These kupffer cells attack and break apart bacteria and toxins. Nutrients coming in from the digestive tract are filtered and converted to molecules the body's cells can utilize. The liver also converts old red blood cells to bilirubin to be shipped out of the body. Filtered and purified blood is jettisoned through hepatic veins out the inferior vena cava and back into circulation.

The liver's filtration/purification mechanisms protect our body from various infectious diseases and chemical toxins. After hepatocytes and kupffer cells break down toxins, the waste is disposed through the gall bladder and kidneys. The gall bladder channels bile from the liver to the intestines. Recycled bile acids combine with bilirubin, phospholipids, calcium and cholesterol to make bile. Bile is concentrated and pumped through the bile duct to the intestines. Here bile acids help digest fats, and broken down toxins are (hopefully) excreted through our feces. Assuming we have healthy probiotic colonies within the intestines.

The liver produces over a thousand biochemicals the body requires for healthy functioning. The liver maintains blood sugar balance by monitoring glucose levels and producing glucose metabolites. It manufactures albumin to maintain plasma pressure. It produces cholesterol, urea, inflammatory biochemicals, blood-clotting molecules, and many others.

Interspersed within the liver are functional fat factories called stellates. These cells store and process lipids, fat-soluble vitamins such as vitamin A, and secrete structural biomolecules like collagen, laminin and glycans. These are used to build some of the body's toughest tissue systems.

We know that our livers become burdened from the avalanche of toxins pelting our bodies. Today our diets, water and air are full of plasticizers, formaldehyde, heavy metals, hydrocarbons, DDT, dioxin, VOCs, asbestos, preservatives, artificial flavors, food dyes, propellants, synthetic fragrances and more. Every single chemical requires the liver to work harder.

Frankly, most livers are now overloaded and beyond their natural capacity. What happens then? Generally, two things. First, the hepatocytes collapse from overtoxification, causing genetic mutation, cell death, and liver exhaustion. Secondly, their weakened condition opens hepatocytes to diseases from infectious agents such as viral hepatitis.

Liver disease—where one or more lobes begin to malfunction—can result in a life-threatening emergency. Cirrhosis is a common diagnosis for liver disease, often caused by years of drinking alcohol or taking prescription medications.

During its downfall into cirrhosis, the sub-functioning liver can also cause jaundice, high cholesterol, gallstones, encephalopathy, kidney disease, clotting problems, heart conditions, hormone imbalances and many others. As cirrhosis proceeds, it results in the liver cells' massive die-off and subsequent scarring, causing the liver to begin to shutdown.

While most of us have heard about the damage alcohol can have on the liver, many do not realize that pharmaceuticals and even some supplements can also be extremely toxic to the liver. The liver must find a way to break down these foreign chemicals. Many pharmaceuticals require a Herculean effort simply because the liver's various purification processes were not designed for these foreign molecules. As liver cells weaken and die their enzymes leak into the bloodstream. Blood tests for AST and ALT enzymes can reveal this weakening of the liver.

We must therefore closely monitor the quantity and types of chemicals we put into our body. Eliminating preservatives, food dyes and pesticides in our foods can be done easily by eating whole organic foods. We can eliminate exposures to many environmental toxins mentioned above by simply replacing them with natural alternatives.

A number of herbs help detoxify and strengthen the liver. These include goldenseal, dandelion, milk thistle and others.

Intestinal Immunity

Cancers of the gastrointestinal tract are a leading form of cancer. Stomach cancer, intestinal cancer and colon cancer take hundreds of thousands of lives a year.

Furthermore, a weakened intestinal barrier increases the likelihood of cancer-causing toxins entering the blood stream. Thus healthy intestines are critical to preventing cancer.

When intestinal villi and their junctions are damaged, endotoxins (the poop and byproducts of pathogenic bacteria) and other toxins can get into the bloodstream—overloading the immune system and producing systemic inflammation.

The intestines utilize non-specific, humoral, cell-mediated and probiotic immunity to protect intestinal tissues from larger peptides, toxins and invading microorganisms.

This is all packaged nicely into what is referred to as the *intestinal brush barrier*. The intestinal brush barrier is a complex mucosal layer of mucin, enzymes, probiotics and ionic fluid—sealed by villi separated by tight junctions.

The intestinal mucosal membrane forms a protective surface medium over the intestinal epithelium. It also provides an active nutrient transport mechanism for nutrients and toxins. This mucosal layer is stabilized by the grooves of the intestinal microvilli. It contains glycoproteins, mucopolysaccharides and other ionic transporters, which attach to amino acids, minerals, vitamins, glucose and fatty acids—carrying them across intestinal membranes.

This mucosal layer is policed by billions of probiotic colonies, which help process and identify incoming food molecules; excrete various nutrients; and control toxins and pathogens.

The breakdown of the mucosal membrane causes it to thin. This depletes the protection rendered by the mucopolysaccharides and glycoproteins, probiotics, immune IgA cells, enzymes and bile. This thinning allows toxins and macromolecules that would have been screened out by the mucosal membrane to be presented to the intestinal cells.

In its entirety, the brush barrier is a triple-filter that screens for molecule size, ionic nature and nutrition quality. Much of this is performed via four screening mechanisms existing between the intestinal microvilli: tight junctions, adherens junctions, desmosomes, and colonies of probiotics.

The tight functions form a bilayer interface between cells, controlling permeability. Desmosomes are points of interface between the tight junctions, and adherens junctions keep the cell membranes adhesive enough to stabilize the junctions. These junction mechanisms together regulate permeability at the intestinal wall.

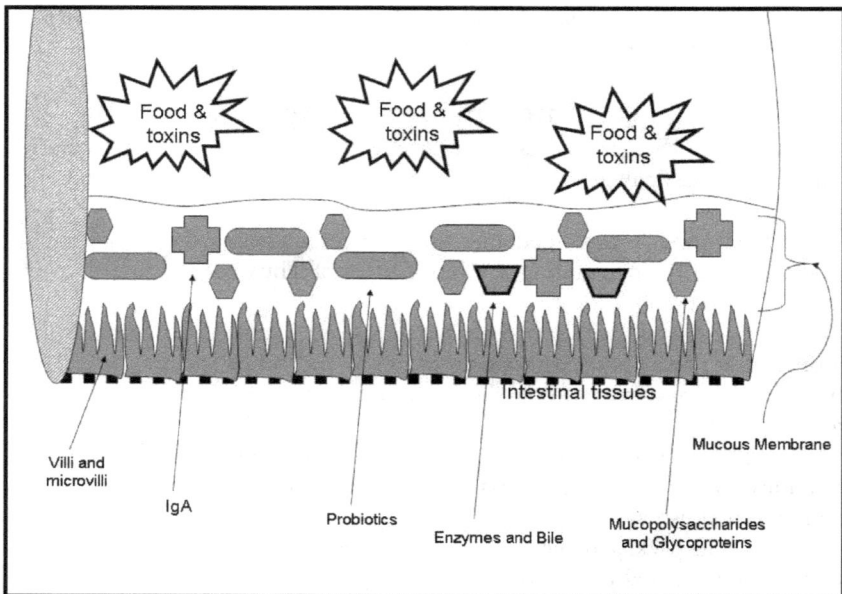

The Healthy Intestinal Wall

This mucosal brush barrier creates the boundary between intestinal contents and our bloodstream. Should the mucosal layer chemistry become altered, its protective and ionic transport mechanisms become weakened, allowing toxic or larger molecules to be presented to the microvilli junctions. This contact can irritate the microvilli, causing a subsequent inflammatory response. Research illustrates that this is a contributing cause of irritable bowel syndrome (IBS).

Should the mucous membrane thin, these mechanisms become irritated, producing an inflammatory immune response that causes the desmosomes and tight junctions to open. These gaps allow toxins and food macromolecules to enter the blood, where they can become allergens and contribute to systemic inflammation. Scientists call this condition *increased intestinal permeability*.

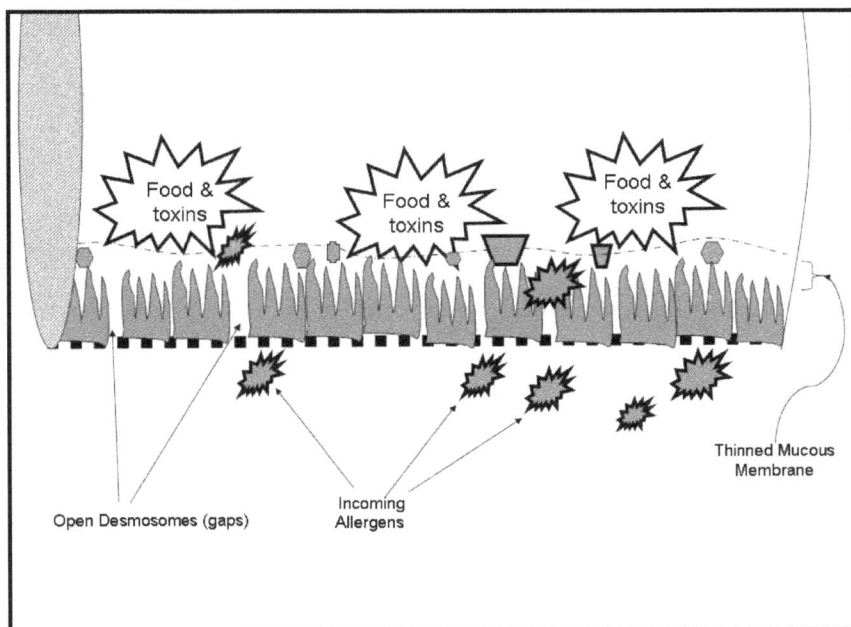

The Unhealthy Intestinal Wall

The Intestinal Permeability Index

How do scientists and physicians test for increased intestinal permeability? Intestinal permeability is typically measured by giving the patient indigestible substances with different molecular sizes. Urine samples then show relative levels of these, illustrating degrees of intestinal permeability. For example, alcohol-sugar combinations such as lactulose and mannitol are often used. These indicate intestinal permeability because of their different molecular sizes. A few (typically 5-6) hours after ingestion, the patient's urine is tested to measure the quantities of these two molecules in the urine.

Because lactulose is a larger molecule than mannitol, greater permeability will be indicated by high lactulose levels in the urine relative to mannitol levels. Intestines with normal permeability will have less lactulose absorption.

These relative levels create a ratio between lactulose and mannitol, which scientists call the L/M ratio. This L/M ratio is used to quantify intestinal permeability. When the lactulose-to-mannitol ratio is higher, more permeability exists. When it is lower, less (more normal) intestinal permeability exists. Higher levels are compared using what many researchers call the *Intestinal Permeability Index.*

Other molecule substances are also sometimes used to detect intestinal permeability using the same protocol of measuring recovery in the urine over a period of time. These other substances include polyethylene glycols of various molecular weights, horseradish peroxidase, EDTA (ethylenediaminetetraacetic acid), CrEDTA, rhamnose, lactulose, and cellobiose. Because these substances are not readily metabolized in the intestine or blood, and have varying molecular sizes, they can also give accurate readings on the relative intestinal permeability.

Inflammation and Cancer

Our anticancer immunity utilizes a reactive process called inflammation. Inflammation has a bad reputation. But inflammation actually provides the body with a defense system that rids the body of many toxins before they can provoke cancer in cells.

Inflammation is identified with various symptoms, including swelling, redness, pain, lack of motion and more.

Inflammation means the immune system is working. When there is a major threat to the body the immune system must use this extreme mechanism to protect the body. The inflammatory process is utilized by the immune system to channel immune cells and repair mechanisms to the site while it seals off cells and tissue systems.

At the same time, inflammation is used by the body to inform us of a problem. This can also mean we are dealing with pain. But without pain, we might continue doing something that continues the problem or makes the problem worse. So pain, like inflammation, might not feel good but they are important factors in our immune response.

Inflammation involves reactive oxygen species. Indications of this during systemic inflammation include higher levels of superoxide anions and thiobarbituric acid-reactive products (TBARs), as well as hydrogen peroxide. This is because one of the main inflammatory byproducts of superoxide reactions is hydrogen peroxide (H_2O_2).

Research has illustrated that those with inflammatory conditions generate more hydrogen peroxide when they breathe out than normal people. In one study, asthmatics breathed out 26 times the levels of hydrogen peroxide as healthy subjects did. They also found that TBAR levels among asthmatics were 18 times the levels of healthy subjects (Antczak *et al.* 1997).

Inflammatory eosinophils—evidenced by higher eosinophil cationic protein (ECP) levels—are also significantly higher in inflammatory conditions. ECP can damage microorganisms such as viruses and bacteria, along with our body's cells. ECP damages cells by forming pores in the cell membranes, which produce a type of cell membrane damage called *permeability alteration.*

Research has indicated that ECP builds up in the airways and epithelial tissues in an inflammatory condition. While ECP is a defense measure in the case of infection, an overload of ECP damages the epithelial cells.

The build-up of ECP is simply part of an inflammatory process that occurs as part of an immune response: A deranged immune response that medical researchers call hyperreactivity.

Our body's immune system launches inflammatory cells and factors that heal injury sites and prevent bleed-outs. This process is often stimulated by leukotrienes and prostaglandins.

Leukotrienes are molecules that identify problems and stimulate the immune system. They pinpoint and isolate areas of the body that require repair. Once they pinpoint the site of repair, one type of leukotriene will initiate inflammation, and others will assist in maintaining the process. Once the repair process proceeds to a point of maturity, another type of leukotriene will begin slowing down the process of inflammation.

This smart signaling process takes place through the biochemical bonding formations of these molecules. Leukotrienes are paracrines and autocrines. They are paracrine in that they initiate messages that travel from one cell to another. They are autocrine in that they initiate messages that encourage an automatic and immediate response—notably among T-cells, engaging them to remove bad cells. They also help transmit messages that initiate the process of repair through the clotting of blood and the patching of damaged tissues.

Leukotrienes are produced from the conversion of essential fatty acids (EFAs) by an enzyme produced by the body called arachidonate-5-lipoxygenase (sometimes called LOX). The central fatty acids of this process are arachidonic acid (AA), gamma-linolenic acid (GLA), and eicosapentaenoic acid (EPA). Lipoxygenase enzymes produce different types of leukotrienes, depending upon the initial fatty acid.

The important point of this is that the leukotrienes produced by arachidonic acid stimulate inflammation, while the leukotrienes produced by EPA halt inflammation. The leukotrienes produced by GLA, on the other hand, block the conversion process of polyunsaturated fatty acids to arachidonic acid.

Prostaglandins are also produced through an enzyme conversion from fatty acids. Like leukotrienes, prostaglandins are messengers that transmit particular messages to immune cells. Their messaging is either paracrine or autocrine. Prostaglandins are critical parts of the process of injury repair. They also initiate a number of protective sequences in the body, including the transmission of pain and the clotting of blood.

Prostaglandins are produced by the oxidation of fatty acids by an enzyme produced in the body called cyclooxygenase—also called prostaglandin-endoperoxide synthase (PTGS) or COX. There are three types of COX, and each convert fatty acids to different types of prostaglandins. The central fatty acid that causes inflammation again is arachidonic acid. COX-1 converts AA to the PGE2 type of prostaglandin. COX-2, on the other hand, converts AA into the PGI2 type of prostaglandin.

The central messages that prostaglandins transmit depend upon the type of prostaglandin. Prostaglandin I2 (also PGI2) stimulates the widening of blood vessels and bronchial passages, and pain sensation within the nervous system. In other words, along with stimulating blood clotting, PGI2 signals a range of responses to assist the body's wound healing at the site of injury.

Prostaglandin E2, or PGE2, is altogether different from PGI2. PGE2 stimulates the secretion of mucus within the stomach, intestines, mouth and esophagus. It also decreases the production of gastric acid in the stomach. This combination of increasing mucus and lowering acid production keeps healthy stomach cells from being damaged by our gastric acids and the acidic content of our foods. This is one of the central reasons NSAID pharmaceuticals cause gastrointestinal problems: They interrupt the secretion of this protective mucus in the stomach.

This means that the COX-1 enzyme instigates the process of protecting the stomach, while the COX-2 enzyme instigates the process of inflammation and repair within the body. In the case of autoimmune disease, the COX-2 process often lies at the root of pain and swelling.

Cyclooxygenase also converts ALA/DHA and GLA to prostaglandins. Just as lipoxygenase converts ALA/DHA and GLA to anti-inflammation leukotrienes, the conversion of ALA/DHA and GLA by cyclooxygenase produces prostaglandins that either block the inflammatory process or reverse it. This means that a healthy diet with plenty of GLA and ALA/DHA fats will balance inflammation response. ALA is found in walnuts, soybeans, flax, canola, pumpkin seeds and chia seeds. The purest form of DHA is found in certain algae, and the body produces EPA from DHA. Fish and krill also get their DHA up the food chain from algae. GLA is found in borage, primrose oil and spirulina.

The body's two adrenal glands supply elements of the inflammation system. The outer cortex is stimulated by master hormones from the hypothalamus and pituitary gland, while the inner medulla is stimulated directly with nerves. The adrenals produce an array of hormones, many of which are related to inflammation and/or stress.

For example, the medulla produces epinephrine and norepinephrine, and other catecholamines. Epinephrine (as well as norepinephrine) relaxes the smooth muscles of the airways and constricts the blood vessels, increases the heart rate, increases metabolism, dilates the pupils and halts digestive activity, all in an effort to reduce inflammation and respond to inflammation and stress.

This multi-organ adrenal response might seem beneficial, but it also comes with a double-edged sword: Epinephrine and norepinephrine also significantly slow the rate of mucous secretion by submucosal glands that feed the mucous membranes.

This effect can be quite dangerous to the highly-stressed individual, because the decreased mucous membranes also leave our lungs and digestive tracts open to irritation from toxins and environmental changes.

The adrenal glands also produce important steroids. Two of the most critical are cortisol and aldosterone.

Aldosterone and other mineralocorticoids are produced by the outer shell, or cortex, of the adrenal gland. Aldosterone and other mineralocorticoids adjust and balance the body's levels of sodium, potassium and other minerals; as well as alter sodium ion channels among various cells.

These are critical to the acid/alkaline status of the blood and body fluids, and the body's ability to remove toxins through the kidneys, sweat glands and colon. Aldosterone is a critical player in maintaining blood pressure as well, and this affects the performance of respiration.

Aldosterone also balances the use and availability of cortisol and cortisone, because many aldosterone receptors also bind with cortisol. This means that a balanced production of these two steroids (cortisol is a glucocorticoid) by the adrenals is critical to the detoxification efforts of the body—along with the body's ability to balance inflammation with efforts to heal the body.

This means that adrenal glands stimulated by stress and inflammation repeatedly for long periods begin to wear down. As mentioned earlier, this is called adrenal exhaustion. When this happens, the adrenal glands produce inconsistently deficient levels of theses critical steroids and catecholamines.

This creates drastic imbalances within the body, affecting the body's ability to respond to toxins, inflammation and stress. Signs of adrenal exhaustion include being easily fatigued, overstressed and over-reactive to toxins and environmental changes. Adrenal exhaustion is typical in an immune system over-responding with hyper-inflammation.

The progression of inflammation also stimulates an activation of neutrophils, phagocytes, immunoglobulins, leukotrienes and prostaglandins. Should cells become damaged or mutated, they will signal the immune system using paracrines located on their cell membranes.

Once the intrusion and strategy is determined, B-cells will surround the cancerous cells while T-cells attack any mutating cells. Natural killer T-cells may secrete chemicals into cancerous cells, initiating the death of the cell.

Leukotrienes immediately gather in the region of toxicity or cancerous mutation, and signal to T-cells to coordinate efforts in the process of killing.

Prostaglandins initiate the widening of blood vessels to bring more T-cells and other repair factors (such as plasminogen and fibrin) to the site. Histamine opens the blood vessel walls to allow all these healing agents access to the injury site to clean it up.

Prostaglandins also stimulate substance P within the nerve cells, initiating the sensation of pain. At the same time, thromboxanes, along with fibrin, drive the process of clotting and coagulation in the blood, while constricting certain blood vessels to decrease the risk of bleeding.

Depending upon the toxin or invader, the inflammation response will also accompany an H1-histamine response. As mentioned earlier, histamine is primarily produced by the mast cells, basophils and neutrophils after being stimulated by IgE antibodies. This opens blood vessels to tissues, which stimulates the processes of sneezing, watering of the eyes and coughing.

These measures, though sometimes considered irritating, are all stimulated in an effort to remove the toxin and prevent its re-entry into the body. As histamine binds with receptors, one of the resulting physiological responses is alertness (also why antihistamines cause drowsiness). These are natural responses to help the body and mind remain vigilant in order to avoid further toxin intake.

At the height of the repair process, swelling, redness and pain are at their peak. The T-cells, macrophages, neutrophils, fibrin and plasmin all work together to purge the allergen from the body and repair the damage.

As macrophages continue the clean up, the other immune cells begin to retreat. Antioxidants like glutathione will attach to and transport the byproducts—broken down toxins and cell parts—out of the body. As this proceeds, prostaglandins, histamines and leukotrienes are signaled to reverse the inflammation and pain process.

One of the central features of the normalization process is the production of bradykinin. Bradykinin slows clotting and opens blood vessels, allowing the cleanup process to accelerate. A key signaling factor is the production of nitric oxide (NO).

NO slows inflammation by promoting the detachment of lymphocytes to the site of infection or toxification, and reduces tissue swelling. NO also accelerates the clearing out of debris with its interaction with the superoxide anion. NO was originally described by researchers as endothelium-derived relaxing factor (or EDRF)—because of its role in relaxing blood vessel walls.

The body produces more nitric oxide in the presence of good nutrition and lower stress. Probiotics also play a big role in nitric oxide production in a healthy body. Lactobacilli such as *L. plantarum* have in fact been shown to remove the harmful nitrate molecule and use it to produce nitric oxide (Bengmark *et al.* 1998). This is beneficial to not only reducing inflammation: NO production also creates a balanced environment for increased tolerance.

Low nitric oxide levels also happen to be associated with a plethora of conditions, including diabetes, heart failure, high cholesterol, ulcerative colitis, premature aging, and many types of cancers. Low or abnormal NO production is also seen among lifestyle factors such as smoking, obesity, and environmental air pollution.

In cases of toxicity from air pollutants, the cough reflex may be enlisted to help clear toxins. Irritated sites in the airways and lungs stimulate coughing, but this is also attenuated by a neural cough center located within the brainstem and within the cerebral cortex, where coughing is often initiated, suppressed or modified by consciousness. The cough reflex is, as put by Dr. John Christopher, *"a result of nature's effort to expectorate mucous from the lungs, after which breathing becomes easier."*

Typical associations with inflammation include artery damage and plaque build-up, obesity, diabetes, a sedentary lifestyle, and a diet high in saturated fats and/or fried foods. High blood pressure and fast or irregular heart rate, especially in persons over 40 years old, are also strong markers.

Along with these associations come higher levels of total cholesterol, low-density lipoprotein (LDL) and very low-density lipoprotein (VLDL) cholesterol, and total triglycerides are also key markers. The link between small LDL particle size and atherosclerosis is a key factor, and the oxidation of LDL particles is the match that lights the fuse. These involve hyperperoxides, as they readily form oxidative radicals. The cascade towards LDL oxidation also seems to be accelerated by lipooxygenases like 15-LOX-2 along with cyclooxygenases. The process as a whole is lipid peroxidation.

In addition to launching systemic inflammation due to widespread cell damage, the body also produces processes that attempt to halt the peroxidation cycle. One of these components is the glutathione peroxidase enzyme discussed earlier, formed by the body using selenium as a substrate. Depending upon the rate of lipid peroxidation, however, this could be like trying to blow out a forest fire. There is simply too much fire spreading too quickly.

C-reactive Protein

High C-reactive protein levels are linked to cardiovascular inflammation. Research has confirmed that higher C-reactive protein levels are also linked to greater cancer risk. This is because inflammation failure will often produce a high degree of mutation among cells.

For example, a 2017 metastudy (Li *et al.*) analyzed hs-CRP levels and cancer deaths. The researchers investigated 14 studies that followed 83,995 people, comparing high and low levels of CRP. The research found that higher levels of CRP was linked to a 25 percent greater incidence of dying from cancer.

Systemic inflammation

We discussed how lipid free radicals can damage cells, causing the immune system to initiate systemic inflammation.

Localized inflammation is often caused by physical injuries like broken bones or tissue damage. But systemic inflammation is typically caused by the bombardment and overload of toxins or pathological microorganisms.

Systemic inflammation indicates that the immune system is overburdened. The extent or combination of the elements mentioned simply overwhelms the immune system. Typically, the immune system can resolve most of these problems when it is presented with a small amount or a few of them at a time. But when an avalanche of them becomes too great, the immune system goes on alert, resulting in systemic inflammation.

Systemic inflammation is the immune system's version of all-out war. The immune system begins to launch the nukes. These can include fever, vomiting, diarrhea, swelling and pain.

The rest of this chapter will more specifically discuss lifestyle choices that produce or worsen systemic inflammation within the body. In other words, these are all *contributing causes*. This means that just one of these factors may not in itself cause systemic inflammation. But any one of these, in addition to others, can overwhelm the immune system—producing systemic inflammation.

Systemic Inflammation Factors

While toxin overload is the primary condition, the following list summarizes conditions that collectively contribute to systemic inflammation:

1) *Toxemia:* An overload of toxins that produce radicals.
2) *Infections:* Infection with microorganisms that produce mutagenicity, toxins and radicals: viruses, bacteria, yeasts and parasites.
3) *Antioxidant enzyme deficiencies:* An undersupply of antioxidizing enzymes that stabilize radicals, including glutathione peroxidase, glutathione reductase, catalase and superoxide dismutase.
4) *Dietary antioxidant deficiencies:* An undersupply of antioxidants from our foods to help stabilize radicals.
5) *Barriers to detoxification:* Lifestyle or physiological factors that block our body's ability to rid waste products and toxins. Detoxification requires exercise, fresh air, sweating, sunshine and so on.
6) *Poor dietary choices:* A poor diet burdens the body with toxins, unstable fatty acids, refined sugars and overly processed foods.
7) *Immunosuppression:* A burdened or defective immune system.

The Microbiome Defense

Another critical and powerful element of our cancer-prevention system takes place among the body's probiotics. This is the backbone of the living immune system, because our probiotics drive many of our immune processes.

The human body can house more than 32 billion beneficial and harmful bacteria and fungi at any particular time. When beneficial bacteria are in the majority, they constitute up to 70-80% of the body's immune response. This takes place both in an isolated manner and in conjunction with the rest of the immune system.

Probiotic colonies work with the body's internal immune system to organize strategies that prevent toxins and pathogenic microorganisms from harming the body. Probiotics will communicate and cooperate with the immune system to organize cooperative strategies. They will stimulate the body's immune cells, activating the cell-mediated response, the humoral response, and indirectly, the body's exterior barrier mechanisms through immunoglobulin stimulation.

As we will see in the research, they stimulate T-cells, B-cells, macrophages and NK-cells with smart messages that promote specific immune responses. They also activate cytokines and phagocytic cells directly to coordinate their intelligent immune response.

Probiotics can also quickly identify harmful bacteria or fungal overgrowths and work directly to eradicate them. This process may not directly involve the rest of the immune system. Even still, the immune system will be notified of any probiotic offensives. The immune system will support the process by breaking up and escorting dead pathogens out of the body.

Probiotics also produce chemical substances that coordinate with our immune system. Because probiotics are extremely intelligent and want to survive, they have developed various strategies to defend their territory. When they sense cells acting out, they produce a variety of substances that alert the immune system.

As we will find, bacteria sometimes provoke mutations that produce cancerous cells. Probiotics produce antimicrobial biochemicals that manage, damage or kill pathogenic microorganisms.

In some cases, they will simply overcrowd the invaders with biochemistry and populations to limit their growth.

In other cases, they will secrete chemicals into the fluid environment to eradicate large populations. In still other cases, they will insert specific chemicals into the invaders, which will directly kill them. Probiotic mechanisms are quite complex and variegated to say the least.

Probiotics also help prevent an environment in the gut that can lead to intestinal or gastric cancer. The lactic acid produced by *Lactobacillus* and *Bifidobacteria* species sets up the ultimate pH control in the gut.

Lactic acids are not alike, however. There are different lactic acid molecular structures, and combinations with other chemicals. For example, some

31

probiotics produce an L(+) form of lactic acid and other probiotics may produce the D(-) from. Many probiotic strains also produce a molecular combination with hydrogen peroxide called lactoperoxidase.

Probiotics also produce acetic acids, formic acids, special lipopolysaccharides, peptidoglycans, superantigens, heat shock proteins and bacterial DNA—all in precise portions to nourish each other, inhibit challengers and/or benefit the host.

Precision and proportion is the key. For example, some bifidobacteria secrete a 3:2 proportion of acetic acid to lactic acid in order to barricade certain pathogenic microbes.

Probiotics also secrete a number of key nutrients crucial to its host's (our body) immune system and metabolism, including B vitamins pantothenic acid, pyridoxine, niacin, folic acid, cobalamin and biotin, and crucial antioxidants such as vitamin K.

Probiotics also produce antimicrobial molecules called bacteriocins. *Lactobacillus plantarum* produces lactolin. *Lactobacillus bulgaricus* secretes bulgarican. *Lactobacillus acidophilus* can produce acidophilin, acidolin, bacterlocin and lactocidin.

These and other antimicrobial substances equip probiotic species with territorial mechanisms to combat and reduce pathologies related to *Shigella, Coliform, Pseudomonas, Klebsiella, Staphylococcus, Clostridium, Escherichia* and other infective genera. Furthermore, antifungal biochemicals from the likes of *L. acidophilus, B. bifidum, E. faecium* and others also significantly reduce fungal outbreaks caused by *Candida albicans* (Shahani *et al.* 2005).

These types of antimicrobial tools give probiotics the ability to counter the mighty *H. pylori* bacterium—known to be at the root of a majority of stomach cancers. *H. pylori* inhibition has been observed in studies on *L. acidophilus* DDS-1, *L. rhamnosus* GG, *L. rhamnosus* Lc705, *Propionibacterium freudenreichii* and *Bifidobacterium breve Bb99*, as we will see later.

Furthermore, probiotics will specifically stimulate the body's own immune system to attack pathogens. For example, scientists from Finland's University of Turku (Pessi *et al.* 2000) gave nine atopic dermatitis children *Lactobacillus rhamnosus* GG for four weeks. They found that serum cytokine IL-10 levels specific to the infection increased following probiotic consumption.

Whatever the strategy, smart probiotic microorganisms work collectively and synergistically with the other three components of our immune system. Our probiotic system works within the non-specific immune system to help protect the body from invasions.

Probiotics live within the oral cavity, the nasal cavity, the esophagus, around the gums, and in pockets of our pleural cavity (surrounding our lungs).

They dwell within our stomach, within our intestines, within the vagina and around the rectum, and amongst other pockets of tissues. This means that for microbes to invade the bloodstream, they must first get through legions of probiotic bacteria that populate those entry channels—assuming a healthy body of course.

Probiotics also play a large role in helping protect our liver. As mentioned above, the liver is essential for producing enzymes like glutathione that remove oxidized free radicals that produce the mutations that trigger cancer cells.

When pathogenic bacteria get out of control in the intestines, they can overload the liver with endotoxins—their waste products. The bombardment of endotoxins onto the liver produces a result similar to alcohol or pharmaceuticals: When complex proteins (such as found in animal products) are putrefied by pathogenic bacteria, one of the metabolites is excessive ammonia. Ammonia is toxic to the liver.

In addition, urea is metabolized by pathogenic bacteria such as *Clostridium* spp., resulting in ammonia and carbon dioxide. Liver cells are damaged by this onslaught of endotoxins and metabolites produced by pathogenic bacteria.

In a study from scientists at the G.B. Pant Hospital in New Delhi (Sharma *et al.* 2008), 190 cirrhosis patients were given a combination of probiotics for one month. The probiotic group experienced a 51.6% improvement in symptoms, as measured by psychometric testing and blood ammonia levels.

Probiotics participate deeply in immune activity. In one study, the probiotic organism *Bifidobacterium lactis* HN019 or a placebo was given to 30 healthy elderly volunteers (average age 69 years old) for nine weeks. The probiotic group had significant increases among total T-cells, helper T-cells (CD4+), activated (CD25+) T-cells, and natural killer T-cells. Cytotoxic capacity among mononuclear and polymorphonuclear phagocytes and tumor-cell killing activity among natural killer cells also increased among the probiotic group (Gill *et al.* 2001).

Neutrophils are also coordinated by probiotics. Researchers from the Liver Failure Group and The Institute of Hepatology at the University College London's Medical School (Stadlbauer *et al.* 2008) found in a study of 20 liver failure patients that neutrophil function and cytokines were significantly modulated by the probiotic *Lactobacillus casei* Shirota.

Starting neutrophil phagocytic capacity was significantly lower than healthy controls (73% versus 98%) before probiotic treatment. Neutrophil phagocytic capacity after probiotic treatments were equal between the cirrhosis patients and the healthy volunteers at the end of the study—while the placebo group's neutrophil capacity did not change. In addition, endotoxin-stimulated TNF-receptors 1 and 2 and interleukin-10 (IL-10) levels were significantly lower among the probiotic group.

The scientists concluded:

"Our data provide a proof-of-concept that probiotics restore neutrophil phagocytic capacity in cirrhosis, possibly by changing IL10 secretion and TLR4 expression."

33

Monocytes are like the neolithic ancestors of the attack soldiers. After being produced in the marrow, monocytes differentiate into either macrophages or dendrite cells. The macrophages are particularly good at engulfing and breaking apart pathogens.

Dendritic cells are interactive cells that stimulate certain responses. They may, for example, isolate and present a pathogen to the T-cells. Dendritic cells also stimulate the production of those special inter-white blood cell communication proteins called cytokines.

Probiotics modulate the inflammatory Th1/Th2 system. Illustrating this, yogurt with *Bifidobacterium longum* BB536 or plain yogurt was given to 40 patients with Japanese cedar pollinosis for 14 weeks. Peripheral blood mononuclear cells from the patients indicated that *B. fragilis* microorganisms induced significantly more helper TH cell type2 cytokines such as interleukin [IL]-6, and fewer Th1 cytokines such as IL-12 and interferon (Odamaki *et al.* 2007).

Probiotics utilize cytokine communications to transmit intelligent information to the body's network of white blood cells. Illustrating this, Scientists from the Slovak Institute of Cardiovascular Diseases (Hlivak *et al.* 2005) gave a placebo or probiotic *Enterococcus faecium* M-74 to human volunteers for 60 weeks. Peripheral blood analysis indicated significant decreases in cytokines sICAM-1, CD54 on monocytes, and CD11b on lymphocytes after one-year. These are related to anti-adhesion strategies following inflammatory responses to artery damage.

In order to better understand the relationship between probiotics and our immune system, let's discuss the other players among the body's immune system and their interaction with our probiotic populations.

Probiotics, on the other hand, stimulate a healthy thymus gland. Illustrating this, medical researchers from the University of Bari (Indrio *et al.* 2007) gave a placebo or a probiotic combination of *Bifidobacterium breve* C50 and *Streptococcus thermophilus* 065 to 60 newborns in a randomized, placebo-controlled study on thymus size. Thymus size was significantly larger in the probiotic group compared to the standard formula (placebo) group after the probiotic treatment period.

Probiotics utilize these systems to communicate with the body's various cells. They utilize paracrine and juxtacrine communications to pass on messages about the location, type and weaknesses of invading organisms. These messages are then compared with the programmed history within helper T-cells and helper B-cells. This creates a coordinated response. For example, the immune system might launch phagocytic cells to help attack the pathogens a probiotic colony may be battling.

Scientists from the Nagoya University Graduate School of Medicine's Department of Surgery (Sugawara *et al.* 2006) found in a study of 101 patients that supplementation with probiotics increased NK activity and lymphocyte counts. Pro-inflammatory IL-6 cytokines decreased significantly among the probiotic group. Serum IL-6, white blood cell counts, and C-reactive protein also significantly decreased among the probiotic group.

Furthermore, probiotics have the ability to *uniquely modify* cytokines depending upon the condition and disease of the person. Illustrating this, a probiotic drink with either placebo or a probiotic combination of *Lactobacillus paracasei* Lpc-37, *Lactobacillus acidophilus* 74-2 and *Bifidobacterium animalis* subsp. *lactis* DGCC 420 (*B. lactis* 420) was given to 15 healthy adults and 15 adults with atopic dermatitis. After 8 weeks, CD57(+) cytokines levels increased significantly among the healthy group taking probiotics, while CD4(+)CD54(+) cytokines decreased significantly among the AD patients who were taking the probiotics, compared with the placebo group and compared to the levels at the beginning of the trial (Roessler *et al.* 2008).

Immunoglobulins and CDs are also tools probiotics utilize to define or influence appropriate responses for the immune system. Probiotics stimulate IgAs through CDs, for example, when they discover a pathogen has invaded parts of the body's entry passageways.

CDs are also utilized by our body's probiotics to define the cells and tissue systems that have been damaged by toxins, bacteria, or viruses. Probiotics will respond appropriately, signaling back and forth with the immune system. This signaling often stimulates particular inflammatory and injury-healing responses.

Illustrating this, Finnish scientists (Ouwehand *et al.* 2009) gave healthy elderly volunteers lactitol (a milk sugar) with *Lactobacillus acidophilus* or a placebo. The group given the probiotics showed a significant modification of pro-inflammatory IgA and PGE2 levels.

The researchers also noticed that levels of bifidobacteria in the stool of the elderly subjects were similar to those of a young person—as usually bifidobacteria colonies are reduced among the elderly. They also observed improved spermidine levels—an enzyme involved in DNA synthesis. These improvements suggested increased mucosal and intestinal immunity and probiotic content among the probiotic group.

In a study of 105 pregnant women, University of Western Australia scientists (Prescott *et al.* 2008) found that *Lactobacillus rhamnosus* and *Bifidobacterium lactis* stimulated higher levels of cytokine IFN-gamma, higher levels of TGF-beta1, and higher levels of breast milk IgA. Plasma of their babies had lower CD14 levels, and greater CB IFN-gamma levels. These indicated improvements in immune response stimulated by the probiotics.

In another example, researchers from the Turku University Central Hospital in Finland (Rinne *et al.* 2005) gave 96 mothers either a placebo or *Lactobacillus rhamnosus* GG before delivery and continued the supplementation in their infants after delivery. At three months of age, immunoglobulin IgG-secreting cells among breastfed infants supplemented with probiotics were significantly higher than the breastfed infants who received the placebo. In addition, IgM-, IgA-, and IgG-secreting cell counts at 12 months were significantly higher among the breastfed infants who supplemented with probiotics, compared to breastfed infants receiving the placebo.

In yet another example, researchers from the Teikyo University School of Medicine in Japan (Araki *et al.* 1999) gave *Bifidobacterium breve* YIT4064 or placebo to 19 infants for 28 days. Rotavirus shedding in the feces of the probiotic group was significantly reduced compared to the placebo group. IgA levels also significantly changed among the probiotic group.

All this means is that our body's probiotics stimulate our immune system and our ability to protect itself against cancer.

During the same period where our society has reduced our probiotic populations through the widespread use of antibiotics, we have had a dramatic growth in the incidence of cancer. Is this a coincidence?

Chapter Two

Toxins and Cancer

Do Toxins Cause Cancer?

In the last chapter we discussed how cancer is caused by DNA mutations. We also discussed how these mutations are linked to damage to the cells and their membranes from free radicals like lipid hydroperoxides. We illustrated the evidence showing how these free radicals are directly associated with normal cells turning cancerous.

There were some publications funded by commercial interests a couple of decades ago that proposed environmental chemicals have not increased the rate or risk of cancer. The hypothesis was based upon data showing that cancer typically occurs later in life. Yes, the data did show that cancer rates were higher in first world countries where environmental toxin exposures were higher.

But their hypothesis was that these countries also had higher average lifespans, which drove the cancer rates higher among these older populations. Their suggestion was that if increased longevity was removed from the equation, cancer rates have not gone up.

Well, since then there has been a lot more targeted research directly connecting chemical exposure to higher cancer rates. These studies are undeniable. Population studies that try to link trends with age and lifestyle are difficult to pinpoint when it comes to determining whether there is a relationship not included in the study – such as environmental toxins.

But when the study isolates the exposure to specific chemical toxins and tracks the rates of cancer among those study populations, this provides a more reliable answer to whether the exposure to chemical toxins causes cancer.

The Silent Spring Institute (Rodgers *et al.* 2018) conducted a meta-review of 158 studies that tested the link between specific chemicals and breast cancer. The studies tested 134 different chemicals.

The researchers identified a number of chemicals that were linked to breast cancer. These included dioxins, dichlorodiphenyltrichloroethane (DDT), perfluorooctane-sulfonamide (PFOSA), and air pollution. The increased risks associated from these chemicals ranged from over twice the risk 214 percent to 500 percent.

The study also found that the exposure to solvents at work and gasoline compounds also increased the risk, ranging from 42 percent to 331 percent.

So the research does definitely link breast cancer to chemical toxins.

The 2007 study from Silent Spring Institute (Rudel *et al.*) found 216 different chemicals were associated with mammary gland tumors. These included industrial chemicals, chlorinated solvents, products of combustion, pesticides, dyes, radiation, drinking water disinfection byproducts, pharmaceuticals and hormones, natural products, and research chemicals.

Of these 216 chemicals, 29 are produced in the United States at volumes greater than one million pounds per year. And 35 of the 216 are air pollutants. 25 of the 216 are exposed to more than 5,000 women a year, and 73 are food contaminants. The researchers also found most of the chemicals caused DNA mutations and produced cancer cells and tumors in multiple organs in the body.

Researchers from the University at Albany (Carpenter and Bushkin-Bedient 2013) conducted a review of research and found that the exposure to chemical toxins early in life resulted in significant cancer risk later on. The researchers wrote:

"Many chemical carcinogens persist in the body for decades and increase risk for all types of cancers. Carcinogens may act via mutagenic, nonmutagenic, or epigenetic mechanisms and may also result from disruption of endocrine systems. The problem is magnified by the fact that many chemical carcinogens have become an integral part of our food and water supply and are in air and the general environment."

As mentioned, these are reviews of research. This means each represents many specific studies that tested specific chemicals with specific types of cancers.

Pervasive Chemical Toxins

Now that we understand that chemical toxins cause cancer, and we know they produce oxidative free radicals, let's take a look at some of the sources of chemical toxins in our environment.

Not every chemical covered in this chapter has been proven in research studies to cause cancer. But most of them have. And those that have no link to cancer are linked to other conditions. And those conditions are in turn linked to cancer.

Over the past century, humankind has opened a Pandora's box of chemical manipulation. The inventive efforts of chemists combined with the brilliant marketing efforts of chemical manufacturers convinced us that synthetic chemicals made life easier, more productive and healthier. Not only did they get this wrong, but we all bought in to it.

Now we are paying the price.

Much of our drinking supplies are now laced with mercury, arsenic, DDT, PCB, nitrates, HTMs, plasticizers, pharmaceuticals and hundreds of other dangerous toxins. Much of the non-organic food we eat is now to full of various pesticide residues. We are gradually discovering that agribusiness' use of chemical fertilizers and pesticides is slowly poisoning our bodies. The toxins are building up in our cells—mutating DNA and suffocating our immune systems.

Most of the furnishings we purchase now are filled with formaldehydes, synthetic materials and preservatives. Most office buildings and many houses still contain hazards like asbestos and other components that cause toxicity. Our entire environment is laced with synthetic chemistry. If the human race stopped chemical production today, we still would have done so much damage over the past fifty years that it will take centuries for the earth's detoxification systems to purify herself.

Today we are building mountains of synthetic chemistry loading up our dumps, landfills, lakes, rivers, and oceans with toxic brews.

A perfect example of this is perfluorooctanoic acid (PFOA) and perfluorooctane sulfonic acid (PFOS) – together with similar compounds called perfluorinated compounds (PFCs).

These chemicals were sold to the public in the form of frying pans and other non-stick applications such as rain gear and plastic coatings.

Now we find our drinking waters contaminated with PFC chemicals. A 2013 study of New Jersey drinking waters found that 57 percent of 23 New Jersey public drinking water systems had levels of PFOA at maximum levels of 100 ng/L. Other locations had multiple PFCs. Some that were near industrial production centers had up to 330 ng/L levels of PFCs.

Worse, perfluorinated compounds have a tremendously long half-life. They have thus been called "forever chemicals" by many scientists.

Not only will they remain in the environment for long periods. They will also accumulate in our bodies, with half lives that range from three to five years depending upon the PFC (Li *et al.* 2018).

A number of cancers have been linked to PFCs. These include breast cancer (Mancini *et al.* 2020), prostate cancer (Hardell *et al.* 2014) and bladder cancer (Steenland *et al.* 2015).

In addition, PWCs have been linked to low birth weight among children, thyroid hormone disruption and damage to our immunity.

These mountains are decomposing very slowly—outgassing and breaking down into potent poisons. *Time Magazine* reported on June 25, 2007 that Americans generated 1,643 pounds of trash per person in 2005. A mere 32% of it was recycled.

Much of this waste is plastic. The problem with plastic is reflective of its benefit—it lasts far longer than do natural materials. While a plastic bag might not tear and rip as fast as a paper bag as we walk from the grocery store, a plastic bag will have as much a 500-year half-life—depending upon its material. That is a long time. Whet happens to the bag while nature works to biodegrade it? It clogs our soils and waters. For this reason our lands, waters, and bodies are steadily becoming laced with polymers and plasticizers.

Plastics are made through reactions between monomers (small molecules) and plasticizers to create longer-chain molecules. Monomers are typically hydrocarbons such as petroleum. Combining ethane monomers and plasticizers forms polyethylene. Combining styrene monomers and plasticizers renders polystyrene. Combining vinyl chloride monomers and plasticizers results in polyvinyl chloride, or PVC. Combining propylene monomers and plasticizers gives us polypropylene. As these plastic combinations are broken down, guess what gets released into the environment?

Nature produces its own types of natural polymers such as rubber from rubber trees. But this isn't enough for our hungry appetite for luxury. In an attempt to improve upon nature, the 1855 lab of Alexander Parkes mixed pyroxylin from cellulose with alcohol and camphor to form the first type of plastic.

This clear, hard plastic was 'improved' by Dr. Leo Baekeland decades later with a polymer process using phenol and formaldehyde in early 1900s. "Bakelite" became a wildly successful product as it effectively replaced shellac and rubber as a general sheathing material. Because it was heat-resistant and moisture-proof, it quickly became the insulator of choice for engines, appliances, and electronics. Dr. Baekeland eventually sold his General Bakelite Company to Union Carbide in 1939 and retired a very wealthy man to Florida. His life was made easy through the 'miracle' of chemistry.

Nylon was an invention of DuPont researchers in the late 1930s. It was made initially with benzene from coal. The introduction of polypropylene as a synthetic rubber followed shortly thereafter. Polypropylene was an accidental discovery by a couple of researchers vying to convert natural gas for Phillips Petroleum.

The American industrial complex gearing up for World War II focused its attention on this synthetic version due to a shortage of natural rubber. Thanks to synthetic rubber, each soldier was able to wear 32 pounds of rubber in clothing and equipment. A tank needed about a ton. America's military might was as likely due to its synthetic rubber as were its bombs. Again, chemistry was seemingly making our lives easier.

The synthetic polymer revolution surged after the Second World War. The plastic revolution raged, as both consumers and manufacturers bonded to replace anything natural with synthetic polymers.

A polychlorinated biphenyl is a grouping of chlorine atoms bonded together with biphenyl. Biphenyl is a molecule composed of two phenyl rings. It is an aromatic hydrocarbon occurring naturally in coal and petroleum. When synthetically combined with chlorine—another naturally occurring element—the result is highly toxic. PCB was banned in the early 1970s when biologists studied a population of dead seabirds and found they died of a toxic dose of PCBs. For more than forty years, PCBs have been used in paints, pesticides, paper, adhesives, flame-retardants, surgical implants, lubricating oil and electrical equipment.

Referred innocently as "phenols" for many years, the PCB ban followed suspicion of toxicity for over a decade. Massive PCB contamination in the Hudson River was found caused by local electrical manufacturing plants. Some two hundred miles of the river was eventually designated a toxic *superfund site*. This woke us up to PCB toxicity. PCBs break down slowly and bioaccumulate in living organisms.

When PCBs get into our waterways, they build up in the smallest organisms and work their way up the food chain, eventually reaching humans.

Today the ban on PCBs does not include many applications considered "closed," such as capacitors and vacuum pump fluids. This means there are still considerable PCBs in our buildings and electrical equipment. PCB poisoning can cause immediate liver damage. Symptoms can include fever, rashes, nausea, and more.

One might argue that that combining earth-borne commodities like hydrocarbons cannot be so unnatural. After all, hydrocarbons are produced by the earth as part of her own recycling process. However, the process of converting nature's hydrocarbon monomers into polymers of our design requires various catalysts—*plasticizers*—to complete.

Plasticizers are used in plastic production to give the long polymer chain its flexibility. Without plasticizers inserted between the polymer chains, plastics would have no flexibility. Without plasticizers, polymers are clear, hard substances: rock-like. The gradations of flex added to polymer chains give the resulting plastic its particular usefulness. A plasticizer adds strength to this flexibility, making the new material difficult to tear or break.

Most plasticizers are *phthalates*. Phthalates are derived from phthalic acid, an aromatic ringed carbon molecule also referred to as dicarboxylic acid. Originally synthesized in 1836 through the oxidation of naphthalene tetrachloride, phthalic acid can also be synthesized from hydrocarbons and sulfuric acid with a mercury catalyst.

Common phthalates are di(2-ethylhexyl) phthalate (DEHP), dibutyl phthalate (DBP), and bisphenyl A (BPA), among others.

Biphenyl A, for example, is used in many types of containers, including baby bottles. BPA can easily leach into food or formula when the bottle is exposed to heat or sunlight. A 2000 Centers of Disease Control study found 75% of those tested had phthalates in their urine, and subsequent studies have found some 95% of the U.S. population has detectable levels of biphenyl A within body fluids. Biphenyls are considered endocrine system disruptors. Long-term effects as their residues build up in our cells, organs and tissue systems are largely unknown.

Scientists from the University of Michigan (Meeker and Ferguson 2011) confirmed that common phthalate plasticizers DEHP, DBP and BPA all disrupt human thyroid hormones—linked to increasing the incidence of thyroid diseases. The research compared and analyzed the metabolites from urine and serum thyroid levels of 1,346 adults and 329 adolescents.

Higher DEHP, DBP, and BPA levels were found to be associated with lower levels of the thyroid hormone metabolites of T4, free T3, total T3 and thyroglobin. Higher DEHP levels were associated with higher TSH levels, while higher BPA levels were associated with lower T3 and TSH levels. This means that the more plasticizers in the bloodstream, the more deranged the hormone levels. The researchers found that lower T4 metabolite levels has the strongest association with higher phthalates. High DEHP levels were associated strongly with lower TSH levels, while BPA was associated with lower T4 and TSH levels.

The study, published in the scientific journal, *Environmental Health Perspectives,* is the first national human study confirming that BPA and other common plasticizers definitely disrupt hormones. Over the past decade, the chemical industry has been disputing the link between BPA and hormone disruption as coincidental.

This large study confirmed previous research that led to the suspicion that these plasticizers, common among food packaging, water bottles, can linings and other consumer goods, disrupt hormone levels.

University of Michigan assistant professor and lead researcher, Dr. John Meeker, commented that the highest 20% of DEHP exposures had as high as 10% decreased thyroid hormones.

Most aromatic carbon rings like the phenyl ring or the benzyl ring used for these polymers have otherwise proven to be hazardous to our environment and well-being. Note there are a number of aromatic carbon rings produced in nature. These, however, do not affect hormone levels, turning males to females, as has been found among fish.

Today there are hundreds of different plasticizers used to produce plastics. Most are variations of aromatic carbons or similarly hazardous compounds. When plasticizers from plastic polymers break down in the environment, these aromatic carbons are released. Our backyards, landfills and oceans—our entire environment for that matter—are silently being inundated by these insidious compounds.

Benzene, for example, is a popular phenyl plasticizer. Benzene has been classified as a volatile organic compound and a carcinogen by the Natural Institutes of Health's National Toxicology Program.

Benzene is among the top twenty most used industrial chemicals. It is used to make adhesives, paint, pharmaceuticals, printed materials, photographic chemicals, synthetic rubber, dyes, detergents, paint and even food processing equipment. As a result, benzene is found throughout our environment—notably in our air and water—and has been implicated in numerous types of cancers.

The problems of synthetic chemicals are pervasive. About 80,000 chemicals have been approved for commercialization over the past fifty years. The *Toxic Substances Control Act of 1976* was set up to evaluate chemicals being introduced. Yet only about 65,000 have been reviewed.

However only a small percentage of these chemicals have been carefully analyzed for their environmental and health effects.

The Environmental Working Group's *Human Toxome Project* has revealed some frightening statistics regarding the poisoning of our bodies by chemicals. In one study of nine adult participants, blood and urine contained 171 of the 214 toxic chemicals in the screen. These included industrial compounds and pollutants like alkylphenols, inorganic arsenic, organophosphates, phthalates, polychlorinated biphenyls (PCBs), volatile and semi-volatile organic compounds and chlorinated dioxins and furans.

In another study, the EWG found 287 of the 413 chemicals screened in the umbilical cord blood of ten mothers after giving birth. These included the chemical types mentioned above and more, including fifty different poly-chlorinated naphthalene compounds (EWG 2007).

By some accounts there are nearly nine hundred different pesticides be-ing used in the United States. Of those, at least thirty-seven contain organo-phosphates—one of our more toxic chemical combinations.

Organophosphates kill insects through nervous system disruption. These neurotoxins are also toxic to humans' nervous systems. The nerve gases Serin and VX are organophosphates, for example.

Organophosphates block cholinesterase—a key neuro-enzyme—from working properly within the body. With cholinesterase blocked, acetylcholine is not regulated. Unregulated acetylcholine causes an over-stimulation of nerve activity, resulting in nerve damage, paralysis, and muscle weakness.

Organophosphates are spreading through ground water, air and through dermal contact. They are exposing us through our breathing, skin contact, swimming, and consumption. Initial symptoms can include nausea, vomiting, shortness of breath, confusion, and muscle spasms. Some of the more com-mon organophosphates include Malathion, Parathion, Diazinon, Phosmet, Clorpyrifos, Dursban and others.

The EPA actually banned Diazinon and Dursban in a phase-out begin-ning in March of 2001, to last through December 2003. Curiously, both Diaz-inon and Dursban are still in use today. Phased bans like this theoretically take several years to allow companies to run out their inventories. Also since these bans were aimed at consumer products, organophosphates are still used profusely in commercial agriculture—our food production.

In a 2003 study done by the Centers for Disease Control and Prevention, thousands of people were tested for 116 chemicals. Thirty-four of these were pesticides such as organophosphates, organochlorines, and carbamates. Nine-teen of the thirty-four were found in either the blood or urine.

The use of pesticides on agricultural land, playgrounds, parks, home lawns, and gardens throughout the United States has growing by staggering proportions. In 1964, approximately 233 million pounds of pesticide active ingredients were used. By 1982, this amount tripled to 612 million pounds. In 1999, the U.S. Environmental Protection Agency reported that some five *billion* pounds of these chemicals were used per year throughout America's crops, forests, parks, and lawns.

One of the fastest growing of these pesticides has been imidacloprid, a neonicotinoid. Introduced by Bayer in 1994, imidacloprid is used against aphids and similar insects on over 140 different crops. Touted as a chemical with a fairly short half-life of thirty days in water and twenty-seven days in anaerobic soil, imidacloprid's half-life is about 997 days in aerobic soil. While it has a lower immediate toxicity compared with hazards like DDT, imidacloprid's use is now widespread. It is rated by the EPA and WHO as *"moderately toxic"* in small doses. Larger doses can disrupt liver and thyroid function. While this pesticide does well at killing off increasingly resistant pests, it also can decimate bee populations.

Chlorinated dioxins are also pervasive in today's environment. Significant sources include cigarettes, pesticides, coal-burning factories, diesel exhaust, and sewage sludge.

Dioxins are also byproducts of the manufacturing of a number of products, including many resins, glues, plastics, and chlorine-treated products.

Dioxins also bio-accumulate in fatty tissues and can take years to fully degrade. Dioxins are known endocrine disruptors. They have also been linked to liver toxicity and birth defects.

Thanks to the chemical industrial complex, there are now thousands of *volatile organic compounds* in our environment. A VOC is classified as such if it has a relatively high vapor pressure, allowing it to vaporize quickly and enter the atmosphere.

Gasoline, paint thinners, cleaning solvents, ketones, and aldehydes are a few of the chemicals considered sources of VOCs. Methane-forming VOCs like benzene and toluene are also carcinogens. VOCs are often used as preservatives for pressed wood and other building materials. As a result, many buildings contain VOCs locked within its building materials.

Once soaked in or inborn with the fabrication, VOCs are trapped within the material, causing them to outgas over time. This outgassing process is speeded up when the building is demolished or taken apart. As the building materials are broken up, VOCs can be released at toxic exposure levels.

VOCs will form ozone as they interact with sunlight and heat. VOC poisoning symptoms include nausea; headaches; eye irritation; inflammation of the nose and throat; liver damage; brain fog; and neurotoxic brain damage. Using cleaning or painting solvents indoors is a common cause of VOC poisoning.

In a series of studies led by Dr. Sarah Janssen (*et al.* 2017), *The Collaborative on Health and the Environment,* more than two hundred diseases are attributable to exposure to industrial chemicals. The diseases listed are some of the most prevalent diseases of our society—including several types of cancers.

The researchers found that over 120 diseases have been specifically linked by research to exposure to specific industrial chemicals. For another thirty-three diseases, the evidence for linking to specific chemicals was considered "good." For the rest of the diseases, research indicated a definite link but the evidence was considered "limited."

Toxin Overload

Hypersensitivities are linked with a depressed immune system, and depressed immunity decreases our bodies ability to combat cancer formation.

Clinical research by Professor John G Ionescu, Ph.D. (2009) concluded that environmental pollution is clearly associated with the development of hypersensitivities. Dr. Ionescu's research indicated that environmental noxious agents, including many chemicals, contribute to the total immune burden, producing increased susceptibility for intolerances due to inflammation.

According to Dr. Ionescu, toxic inputs such as formaldehyde, smog, industrial waste, wood preservatives, microbial toxins, alcohol, pesticides, processed foods, nicotine, solvents and amalgam-heavy metals have been observed to be mediating toxins that produce the physical susceptibilities for toxin sensitization and subsequent inflammation.

This is also consistent with findings of other scientists—as discussed—that chemicals overload the immune system and cause inflammation.

Chemical toxins such as DDT, PBDEs, dioxin, formaldehyde, benzene, butane and chlorinated chemicals tend to accumulate within the body's tissues. This is because many of these are fat-soluble. Other compounds, such as phthalate plasticizers and parabens tend to clear the body faster because they are not fat soluble. Still, these can also cause toxicity issues if they are regularly presented to the body.

The compounding of these synthetics contributes to the body-wide status of systemic inflammation. As the immune system gears up to overdrive due to the overloading of multiple toxins, it becomes weaker and hypersensitive. This can cause a host of issues, including allergies, irritable bowel syndrome and many others.

This is a gigantic discussion, so here we will summarize the major categories and sources of toxic chemicals that add to our immune system burden:

Plasticizers and Parabens

Today, plasticizers and parabens are common amongst many of our medications, toys, foods packaged in plastic and other consumer items. Phthalates are also found in many household items.

While phthalates have shorter half-lives than some toxins, they have been implicated in systemic inflammatory issues, hormone disruption, cancers and other conditions. Many cosmetics and antiperspirants contain parabens. They are thus readily absorbed into the skin where they can provoke inflammatory responses (Crinnion 2010).

A study from the University of California at Berkeley (Pan *et al.* 2016) found that parabens stimulate breast cancer cell proliferation by engaging in ligand cross-talk.

Heavy Metals

Heavy metals are metal elements that exist naturally in trace quantities within our soils, waters and foods. However, extraordinary levels of heavy metals such as cadmium, lead and mercury are produced by humanity's industrial complex in the manufacturing of various consumer items.

We can cite many studies that have associated heavy metal exposure to immunosuppression. Mercury is one of these.

For example, in multicenter research from the Department of Medicine from the Lavoro Medical Center in Bari, Italy (Soleo *et al.* 2002), researchers studied the effects of low levels of inorganic mercury exposure on 117 workers. They compared these with 172 general population subjects.

They found no difference in the white blood cell count between the two groups. However, the worker group exposed to mercury had increased levels of CD4+ and CD8+ cytokines, and CD4+ levels were particularly high. These indicated a state of systemic inflammation. In addition, significantly lower levels of interleukin (IL-8) occurred among the exposed workers—indicating immunosuppression.

This research concluded that even low levels of environmental exposure to mercury and other heavy metals (beyond the trace levels normally found in nature) suppresses the immune system and stimulates inflammation.

Cadmium is another heavy metal bombarding us. Among consumer products, cadmium is used in a number of metal coatings, batteries and colorings. Most cigarettes also contain cadmium.

Cadmium has been linked to cancer tumors in the kidneys, breasts, prostate and lungs (Hartwig 2012). A 2013 review of research since 1984 found that cadmium is linked to bladder cancer (Feki-Tounsi and Hamza-Chaffai 2014).

Consumer Toxins

In conjunction with a mandate to lower toxin levels among the state's residents, in 2010 the Minnesota Department of Health compiled and released a list of the most toxic chemicals used in consumer products, building materials, pesticides, hair dyes, detergents, aerosols, cosmetics, furniture polish, herbicides, paints, cleaning solutions and many other common sources. The list also referenced research connecting the toxins to disease conditions. They were labeled *"chemicals of high concern."*

The list contained 1,755 chemicals.

Here is an excerpt from the paper (bold added):

(e) "Chemical of high concern" means a chemical identified on the basis of credible scientific evidence by a state, federal, or international agency as being known or suspected with a high degree of probability to:

(1) harm the normal development of a fetus or child or cause other developmental toxicity;

(2) cause cancer, genetic damage, or reproductive harm;

(3) disrupt the endocrine or hormone system;

(4) damage the nervous system, immune system, or organs, or cause other systemic toxicity;

(5) be persistent, bioaccumulative, and toxic; or

(6) be very persistent and very bioaccumulative.

Taken in total, we might compare this to moving dirt. A small handful of dirt can be carried around easily, and dispersed without much effort. However, a truckload of dirt is another matter completely. What can we do with a truckload of dirt? If we dumped a truckload of dirt on our lawn, we'd have a hill of dirt that would bury the access to our front door and annihilate our lawn and/or garden.

This is a useful comparison because while our bodies can handle a small amount of toxins quite easily, modern society is increasingly dumping toxic 'dirt' into our atmosphere, water and foods, effectively inundating our bodies 'by the truckload.'

With this increased burden, the research shows that the body's defenses are lowered. The mucosal membrane is weakened. The immune system is on alert. Systemic inflammation becomes evident. In this immunosuppressed state, the body is more likely to succumb to a variety of disease conditions.

Water Pollutants

Our industrial society has been dumping massive amounts of synthetic chemistry into our waters for many decades, and we are paying the price. Water contamination comes from manufacturing, wastewater streams from houses, air pollution, ship and boat waste streams and pollutants, run-off from farms and the gutters and streets. All of these to one degree or another end up in our drinking water supplies.

While municipalities have extensive chlorination systems in place to clear microbiological content, removal systems for chemical pollutants are still in various stages of development. As a result, our drinking water supplies have numerous contaminants.

Even some of the cleaning agents used in some municipal water supplies are toxic. This includes trichloroethylene. Trichloroethylene is a chlorinated hydrocarbon used to separate oil from water. The solvent was popularized in the dry cleaning business, and is a common cleansing agent in many local water municipalities.

In a 2013 study from the National Institutes of Health (Karami *et al.*), researchers analyzed data comparing cancer rates to the occupational exposure to trichloroethylene. The researchers found that trichloroethylene was significantly linked to non-Hodgkin's lymphoma.

Pharmaceutical medicines in our water supplies make for a perfect example. In 2007, researchers from Finland's Abo Akademi University (Vieno *et al.*) released a study showing that pharmaceutical beta-blockers, antiepileptic drugs, lipid regulators, anti-inflammatory drugs and fluoroquinolone drugs were all found in river waters.

The concentrations of these were well above drinking water limits. The researchers also found that water treatment only eliminated an average of 13% of the concentration of these pharmaceuticals. This means that 87% of these pharmaceutical medicines remained in the drinking water, ready to dose each and every person drinking that water with prescription medication.

Other pollutants that are commonly found in our drinking water supplies include PCBs, and other biphenol compounds, dioxin, chlorine metabolites, pesticides, herbicides, petroleum byproducts, nitrates, and many others.

Agricultural runoff is a huge source of drinking water contamination. In addition, nitrogen-rich fertilizers choke rivers and oceans with extra nitrogen, causing abnormal blooms of algae. These massive algal blooms cut off oxygen supplies and lead to the die-offs of many species of marine life. *Dead zones* have been reportedly growing in many of the world's waterways, as we will discuss shortly. The cause is the massive use of nitrogen-based synthetic fertilizers.

The use of pesticides on agricultural land, playgrounds, parks, home lawns, and gardens throughout the United States is staggering, and it is growing. In 1964, approximately 233 million pounds of pesticides were applied in the U.S. By 1982, this amount tripled to 612 million pounds. In 2006 and 2007, the U.S. Environmental Protection Agency reported that some five *billion* pounds of these chemicals were applied per year throughout America's crops, forests, parks, and lawns.

A 2013 study from Spain's University of Almería (Parron *et al.*) studied nearly two million people between 1998 and 2005. They found that people living in areas with higher pesticide use had up to three-and-a-half times the risk of cancer.

One of the more increasingly popular pesticides is imidacloprid, a neonicotinoid. Introduced by Bayer in 1994, imidacloprid is used against aphids and similar insects on over 140 different crops. Touted as a chemical with a fairly short half-life of thirty days in water and twenty-seven days in anaerobic soil, imidacloprid's half-life is about 997 days in aerobic soil.

While it has a lower immediate toxicity compared with hazards like DDT, imidacloprid's use is now widespread. It is rated by the EPA and WHO as *"moderately toxic"* in small doses. Larger doses can disrupt liver and thyroid function. While this pesticide does well at killing off increasingly resistant pests, it has also been shown to decimate bee populations.

Cleaning agents are used with or rinsed by water. They will thus immediately enter our greywater systems. According to the U.S. Poison Control Centers, about ten percent of all toxin exposure is caused by cleaning products, with almost two-thirds involving children under six years old.

We might be shocked to find a child toying with a bottle of drain cleaner containing sulfuric acid, hydrochloric acid and lye. But we do not think twice about dumping this same product into our waterways. We wear gloves to protect our skin from the harmful affects of ammonia and bleach while we do our cleaning but assume they disappear once poured down the sink.

An example of this is 1,4-dioxane, a common ingredient in many shampoos and other cleaning products. The California EPA documented that 1,4-

dioxane is a carcinogen that can also damage kidneys, nerves and lungs. It biodegrades very slowly and is becoming a threat to drinking water supplies. This is but one of many.

In a 2002 U.S. Geological Survey report on stream water contaminants, 69% of stream samples revealed non-biodegradable detergents, and 66% of the samples contained disinfectant chemicals. Phosphates—central ingredients in many commercial laundry soaps—have been banned for dumping in over eleven states in the U.S. because of their dangerous effects upon the environment. Yet many people still use these soaps without any consideration of their effects upon our waters.

Biphenyls are considered *xenoestrogens,* or endocrine system disruptors. Long-term effects as their residues build up in the tissues of aquatic species, and bio-accumulate up the ladder to our cells, organs and tissue systems. Research has found that biphenyls have produced sexual re-orientation of fish in some water supplies.

Our waters are filling up with plastic particles. As plastics break down into smaller particles, they are absorbed by filtering marine plants and aquatics and passed up the food chain. Research led by Captain Charles Moore of the *Algalita Marine Research Foundation* (2001; 2002; 2008) found an astounding six-to-one ratio of plastic particles-to-plankton in some areas.

This means that for every pound of algae—the key nutrient for nearly all marine life—there are six pounds of plastic in the oceans. This also means that our marine life is eating plastic particles with their meals: and so are humans who eat fish.

Captain Moore was first alerted to the plastic problem in 1997 when he sailed through a region of the Pacific Ocean between Hawaii and California called the *North Pacific Gyre.* He came upon a large area of floating garbage, consisting primarily of plastic debris. The *Great Pacific Garbage Patch* is now documented from a number of studies, the earliest from a 1988 National Oceanic and Atmospheric Administration paper.

Requiring some 500 years to breakdown, plastics are known to disrupt hormones and accumulate hydrocarbons as mentioned earlier. It is estimated that about twenty percent of the plastic polluting our waters comes from discarded plastic pellets used to make plastic by manufacturers. These pellets are being swept or blown into the water from careless manufacturers and transport companies. The other eighty percent of the ocean's plastics is estimated to come from daily consumer use and the careless littering of waterways and runoffs.

These combined factors are increasingly problematic to a human population seeking to sustain life on the planet. Research by Slovenian researchers Tatjana Tisler and Jana Zagorc-Koncan (2003) has shown that we are drastically underestimating the effects of toxic industrial waste. Our typical method for toxicity research has been to study each individual chemical and its possible toxicity. What we are missing with this type of research is the combined effects of the thousands of chemicals we are putting into our waters. As these chemicals mix, they create a toxic soup of new chemical combinations. Some of these are combinations are exponentially more toxic than the individual chemicals.

Cancer and Microorganisms

Some microorganisms and their endotoxins have been linked to cancer development.

Microorganisms can grow on anything wet—especially mold. Almost any type of sitting water or dampness will grow mold, especially those in dark areas (as many fungi abhor sunlight).

Research has confirmed that infective microorganisms from viruses, bacteria and fungi can stimulate serious systemic inflammation. As we'll discuss later, microorganism infection requires a sharp living immune system—as we'll discuss in the next chapter. While a periodic super-cleanse might be helpful to clear microorganism toxins, a vibrant living immune system will consistently protect the body against infection. Let's talk about the possible microorganism infections we can face.

Bacteria were first discovered in 1673 by Dutch scientist Antony van Leeuwenhoek. Leeuwenhoek began writing letters to the Royal Society of London about the images he was seeing in his newly invented microscope. In 1674, Leeuwenhoek described his microscopic creatures as *"wound serpent-wise and orderly arranged, after the manner of the copper or tin worms."* He described *"many very little living animalcules."*

There are a variety of different

Types of Microbes

Fungi	Yeasts, molds and others; over 100,000 species; live in earth, air, water and damp, moist environments; can infect the body via food, water, air, and skin
Bacteria	Single-celled organisms; live in water, earth, air, on and inside other living organisms; can infect via food, water, air, and skin
Viruses	Non-living; genetic mutation triggers; exist in water, earth, air and skin; infect by altering cellular DNA, and spreading through ongoing cell division and mutation
Mycoplasmas	Ancient slow-moving bacteria; live primarily on earth and water; infect mostly via food, water and touch
Parasites	Tiny organisms that infect and live within another living organism. Includes worms, protozoa and amoeba
Thermophiles	Opportunistic bacteria that can live in very hot environments, such as deserts, boiling water or even in ovens
Psychophiles	Opportunistic bacteria that can live in the very cold,

	such as the artic or in freezers
Nanobacteria	Extremely small bacteria that typically have a hard calcium shell. Are thought to cause some diseases considered autoimmune.

Fungal Infections

A few molds have been linked to cancer. The most well known of these are aflatoxins. Aflatoxins are produced by several types of molds, often as a result of rotting foods and grains.

Aflatoxins are considered mutagens. They are produced by molds including *Aspergillus flavus* and *Aspergillus parasiticus*. The *Aspergillus flavus* mold is where aflatoxin gets its name from.

Aflatoxins grow within the soil, but also in rotting grains or hay. Sometimes they grow in stored foods including rice, chili peppers, millet, peanuts, sesame and sunflower seeds, corn, wheat and various nuts.

Many animals are fed food that has been contaminated with aflatoxin. This will carry aflatoxins into meat and dairy products. Because aflatoxin contamination is prevalent in third world countries, meats and eggs from those countries are more often contaminated with aflatoxins.

U.S. FDA action levels for aflatoxins in foods starts at 20 parts per billion.

The primary cancer caused by aflatoxin is liver cancer. This can follow what is called aflatoxicosis, which is an inflammation of the liver as a result of aflatoxin poisoning.

Viral Infections

Viruses have been implicated in several types of cancers. Many of these are herpesviruses (Moore and Changg 2010):

Epstein-Barr virus (EBV) is also known as herpesvirus 4 or HHV4. This virus has been linked to a number of cancers. These include Most Burkitt's lymphoma and nasopharyngeal cancer, most lymph cancers, Hodgkin's disease and some non-Hodgkin's lymphomas, and some stomach and colon cancers.

Hepatitis C virus (HCV) has been linked to liver cell cancer and some lymphomas.

Hepatitis B virus (HBV) has been linked with some liver cancers.

Kaposi's sarcoma herpesvirus (KSHV) is also known as human herpesvirus 8 (HHV8). It has been linked to Kaposi's sarcoma, primary effusion lymphoma and some Castleman's cancers.

Human T-lymphotropic virus-I (HTLV-I) has been linked to T cell leukemia.

Human papillomaviruses (HPV) such as HPV16 and HPV18 and a few others have been linked to cervical cancer, penile cancers other genital cancers, along with many head and neck cancers.

Merkel cell polyomavirus (MCV) has been linked to Merkel cell cancer.

Certainly, viral infections relate to exposure. But they also relate to a weakened or compromised immune system that cannot combat them. A weakened and compromised immune system has been linked to more severe responses to viral infections.

Cancerous Bacteria

Bacterial infections can cause an overload on the immune system because they produce endotoxins that form radicals in the body. Beyond that, some bacteria have specifically been linked to cancer in different parts of the body.

A few microorganisms linked to cancer:

➢ *Staphylococcus aureus*
➢ *Staphylococcus epidermidis*
➢ *Enterococci faecalis*
➢ *Pneumonococcal aerogenes*
➢ *Escherichia coli*
➢ *Fusobacterium nucleatum*
➢ *Streptococcus mutans*
➢ *H. pylori*

Gastric cancer and H. Pylori

A number of studies over the past 20 years has indicated that H. pylori is linked with cancer. H. pylori isn't as simple as that, but worldwide studies have indicated the link. A 2016 review of the research by Brown University's Dr. Steven Moss concluded:

"Nested case-control studies have shown that H pylori infection increases the risk of gastric cancer significantly, both of the intestinal and diffuse subtypes, and that H pylori is responsible for approximately 90% of the world's burden of noncardia gastric cancer."

Mysteriously, for much of the world's population, H. pylori is a natural part of the digestive tract and isn't linked to any disease. In many populations, H. pylori are perfectly healthy. What is going on here?

The mystery is that Helicobacter pylori, a gram-negative bacterium species typically found in the stomach, has been linked to ulcers, gastritis and gastric cancer – specifically stomach cancer. Yet most of the population of third world countries host *H. pylori*, with extremely low gastric cancer rates.

Some studies have shown that nearly all healthy children host the bacterium throughout the third world, and those countries with the highest H. pylori communities have the lowest rates of gastric cancers.

Furthermore, the host rate of *H. pylori* infection among Americans has been going down dramatically over the past 50 years, and U.S. *H. pylori* rates are now extremely low.

However, those who do harbor the bacteria in America and other western countries have an extremely high risk of contracting stomach cancer. Over 800,000 stomach cancer cases occur each year worldwide.

Aside from these mysteries, the central mystery is why *H. pylori* does not have ill effects – including stomach and duodenal cancers – in over 80% of those populations infected by the bacterium.

A study from Columbia's University del Valle (Bustamante-Rengifo *et al.* 2017) tested 176 patients who were infected with H. pylori. The researchers used a triple antibiotic strategy. The effective treatment rate was close to 75 percent.

However, there was a huge post-treatment infection rate of 64 percent. This means they were growing back fast. But even more important, some strains were growing faster than others.

The strains that were growing back fast had genes recognized as CagA-positive. CagA is a part of the DNA – an oncoprotein secreted by certain species of H. pylori.

As it turns out, the CagA-negative strains of H. pylori were much easier to kill. But these are also the healthy strains of H. pylori. CagA-positive strains of H. pylori tend to carry a genotype called vacA s1. This s1m1 genotype is linked to gastritis and cancer.

Research from the Vanderbilt University School of Medicine (Gaddy *et al.* 2013) put together a big element of the puzzle of H. pylori and stomach/gastric cancer in 2013.

The researchers found that gerbils that hosted H. pylori on a high-salt diet had nearly double the rate of stomach cancer than those infected with the same species of H. pylori who ate a normal diet.

Of those with CagA-positive H. pylori, every gerbil on the high-salt diet contracted stomach cancer – yes, 100% – while only 58% of the normal-diet gerbils contracted the cancer.

This led the researchers to conclude that salt somehow exacerbates stomach cancer in CagA-positive H. pylori infections.

The puzzle came together when the researchers found that those on the high salt diet who did not contract stomach cancer were actually infected with another species of H. pylori. This was the species that does not produce CagA.

None of the gerbils on the high-salt diet with CagA-positive H. pylori contracted stomach cancer.

This meant that not only does CagA-negative H. pylori not cause gastritis and cancer. But a high-salt diet in the presence of a CagA-positive infection of H. pylori does produce stomach cancer – at an extremely high rate.

About 60% of isolated H. pylori species have been found to be CagA-positive among Western countries. But most of the third-world infections are of what is considered the Eastern strain of CagA-negative H. pylori.

This means that the Eastern species of CagA-negative H. pylori is actually not a pathogenic bacteria at all, but rather, a eugenic bacteria – not necessarily harmful or helpful to the host.

And it also means that the widespread infection of these hardy strains of CagA-positive H. pylori together with the highly processed and salty Western diet lies at the root of our high stomach cancer rates among Western countries.

Another study from Vanderbilt University School of Medicine (Epplein *et al.* 2014) found that CagA-positive H. pylori infections and high gastric cancer risk are linked to diets with more red meat.

Other research has found that the infection rates of CagA-positive H. pylori are higher among those countries that eat predominantly a western diet, and infections rates are growing among countries who are increasingly eating a western diet.

Gastritis and ulcers are also associated with CagA-positive H. pylori infections.

The mystery of what causes colon and rectal cancers - also called colorectal cancers - has been pretty much solved. Turns out that colorectal cancers are caused by the overgrowth of certain types of bacteria within the gut. Surprised?

The overgrowth of bad bacteria in the gut have now been linked to a number of conditions around the body. This includes cancer as well as cardiovascular disease, liver disease and many other conditions. Finding that a particular type of bacteria is linked to colon cancer is not such a stretch after all. But now there is science to back up this claim.

Two studies by independent research groups have found that colorectal tumors contain significantly high concentrations of Fusobacterium, an invasive anaerobic bacterium known for causing inflammatory issues around the body.

The first study, by researchers from the BC Cancer Agency and the Michael Smith Genome Sciences Center in Vancouver, Canada (Kostic *et al.* 2011) initially screened 11 colorectal patients together with 11 matched control subjects, and found high levels of *Fusobacterium nucleatum*.

Next the researchers, led by Robert Holt, PhD, validated their results using 88 additional specimens of colorectal cancer tumors. Their testing utilized RNA sequencing techniques to illustrate active (living) bacteria that were replicating DNA.

The second study, this one by researchers from Massachusetts Institute of Technology (MIT) (Castellarin *et al.* 2011) was led by Matthew Meyerson, MD, PhD, also from the Dana-Farber Cancer Institute and Harvard Medical School.

This study utilized DNA sequencing on a total of 95 specimens, again finding that Fusobacteria were active and significantly populating colon cancer tumors. They also visualized the Fusobacteria activity within the tumors, and were able to gain some understanding of the alterations that these bacteria were having upon the gut.

Fusobacteria have been previously associated with a number of intestinal and tissue disorders, including periodontitis (gum disease), pericarditis (heart tissue disease), thrombophlebitis (vein inflammation), and inflammatory bowel disease (IBS). IBS is also known as a high-risk factor and potential precursor for colorectal cancer.

Dr. Meyerson discussed the possible relationship between the bacterium and colon cancer. *"It may be that the bacterium is essential for cancer growth, or that cancer simply provides a hospitable environment for the bacterium. Further research is needed to see what the link is,"* he said.

Both research teams were surprised to find such high populations of the Fusobacteria among the tumors. *Fusobacterium nucleatum* is largely found among bacteria populations in the mouth. For this reason, the researchers noted that this finding was *"largely unexpected, given that it is generally regarded as an oral pathogen."*

Are bacteria invading the breasts of women? Actually, yes and no. Bacteria inhabit all women's breasts – and have been for millions of years.

Hopefully these breast bacteria are the good kind, mind you. Some of the same species of bacteria that also inhabit our guts will inhabit breast tissues. This is why breast milk is such a good source of early oral and gut probiotics for babies.

But now we find that species of bad bacteria can also inhabit the breast tissues of women. And it turns out that breast cancer is linked with these species of bad bacteria.

Are we sure that bacteria are in women's breasts?

Yes. A study from London's Lawson Health Research Institute and Ontario's Western University (Urbaniak *et al.* 2014) analyzed the breast tissues of 81 women. The breast tissues were collected from breast surgeries – either for cancer or for breast augmentation/reduction procedures.

The researchers conducted DNA sequencing on each breast tissue sample to determine the species of bacteria that inhabited the breast tissues. DNA sequencing has previously been used to determine bacteria residing in the digestive tract. These analyses have been contributed to our knowledge of what is now called our microbiome – the genetic makeup of our resident microbes.

After their DNA analysis, the researchers found that the breasts of the Canadian women contained numerous strains and species of bacteria. These included:

- Bacillus (11.4%)
- Acinetobacter (10.0%)
- Enterobacteriaceae (8.3%)
- Pseudomonas (6.5%)
- Staphylococcus (6.5%)

- Propionibacterium (5.8%)
- Comamonadaceae (5.7%)
- Gammaproteobacteria (5.0%)
- Prevotella (5.0%)

Interestingly, the breasts of the Irish women contained a different combination of strains and species. Most abundant were:
- Enterobacteriaceae (30.8%)
- Staphylococcus (12.7%)
- *Listeria welshimeri* (12.1%)
- Propionibacterium (10.1%)
- Pseudomonas (5.3%)

That is a significant difference of species between the two countries. But what all the women had in common was that every breast tissue contained numerous species of bacteria.

Of these, some were probiotic – helpful to the body. Others were pathogenic – disease causing. Still others were eubiotic – neither helpful or harmful, based upon current research to date.

As these same researchers continued to test the breast tissues of the subjects, they also discovered that certain species and strains were in fact, linked to breast cancer.

Another study, published in the Applied and Environmental Microbiology (Urbaniak *et al.* 2016), from Ireland's University College Cork and Canada's Western University, again analyzed the breast tissues from 81 women. This time, they investigated species in relation to breast cancer.

Of the women tested, 58 had breast cancer and 23 were women with no history of breast cancer. Of the 58 women who had breast cancer, 13 had benign tumors.

The researchers found that women who had breast cancer had increased colonies of Escherichia coli and Staphylococcus epidermidis and reduced levels of Lactobacillus and Streptococcus species of bacteria.

The healthy women, on the other hand, had increased colonies of Lactobacillus and Streptococcus species. They also had reduced colonies of Escherichia coli and Staphylococcus epidermidis.

Both *Escherichia coli* and *Staphylococcus epidermidis* bacteria have been implicated in a number of other disease conditions besides cancer. But specific to cancer, they have been shown in studies to injure cellular DNA.

Yes, these bacteria cause double-stranded DNA breaks within cells. Double-stranded breaks have been seen in a number laboratory studies of human cancer cells.

The researchers in the above study wrote:

"Double-strand breaks are the most detrimental type of DNA damage and are caused by genotoxins, reactive oxygen species, and ionizing radiation."

What's a genotoxin? A genotoxin is a substance that causes DNA damage. The result of the DNA damage is a mutation of the DNA. Such a mutation can produce a cancerous cell.

There multiple forms of DNA damage. These can include single- or double-strand breaks. The latter is more serious. Other DNA damage includes cross-link damage and repair blocking issues.

The E. coli and S. epidermidis bacteria may be considered genotoxic, but their primary concern is they produce genotoxic chemicals. And it is these genotoxic chemicals that gain access to the cells' DNA to produce their damage.

As mentioned, *E. coli* and *S. epidermidis* produce other disease conditions within the body. These range from urinary tract and kidney infections to lung and digestive conditions.

Good bacteria, on the other hand, have been symbiotically existing within the human body for millions of years. They promote the body's health and help protect the body from disease.

This is once again proven in this study of breast cancer. When probiotic bacteria such as Lactobacilli and Streptococci are more prominent in the breast tissues, the risk of breast cancer was significantly reduced in the women.

These bacteria modulate the immune system. Among other things, the bacteria will stimulate natural killer cells, which are important for controlling cancer cells. Streptococci species such as S. thermophilus will also produce antioxidants to neutralize reactive oxygen species. These also damage DNA and cause cancer mutations.

Pharmaceuticals

Practically any and every synthetic chemical, even a pharmaceutical can add to our body's total toxin burden. This is because the body must eventually break down any synthetic chemical in order to purge it from the body. The isolated or active chemical within the pharmaceutical may have its biological effect upon the body, but in the end it must be broken down.

If the body's toxin burden is too high because the body is trying to remove chemicals, cancer cells can grow unnoticed by the immune system.

Some pharmaceuticals have been specifically linked to cancer. This includes azathioprine or AZA. AZA is sold as Imuran and other brand names. It is an immunosuppressive medication used for ulcerative colitis, rheumatoid arthritis, Crohn's disease, granulomatosis and systemic lupus.

AZA has been linked to **non-Hodgkin's lymphoma**, squamous cell cancer, liver cancer, and mesenchymal cancer. Research by the International Agency for Research on Cancer has found it to be a Group 1 human cancer risk.

AZA is also listed as a human carcinogen by the National Toxicology Program of U.S. Department of Health and Human Services.

Hormone replacement therapy with estrogen has also been linked to breast cancers. Also estrogen-progestogen oral contraceptives have been linked to breast and other hormone system related cancers.

Here is a list of pharmaceuticals currently on the known land probable carcinogens according to the International Agency for Research on Cancer or the National Toxicology Program of U.S. Department of Health and Human Services (*"possible carcinogens"* are excluded):

- Azathioprine
- Busulfan
- Carbadox
- Chlornapazine
- Chlorambucil
- Ciclosporin
- Cyclophosphamide
- Diethylstilboestrol
- Etoposide
- Melphalan
- Metformin (possible link to pancreatic cancer)
- Methoxsalen
- Tamoxifen
- Thiotepa
- Treosulfan

The body rarely if ever utilizes these chemicals as nutrients, in other words. They are foreigners to the body. Thus, enzymes such as glutathione must break down these chemical molecules into forms that can be excreted in urine, sweat, exhalation or stool.

This breakdown and disposal process requires work by the body's detoxi-fication systems. This means that they further burden or stress a system that must remove many other toxins within the body, including other environ-mental toxins, microorganisms and their endotoxins, inflammatory mediators, broken-down cells and other toxins the body must get rid of. In other words, pharmaceuticals can contribute to, and even become another straw that breaks the camel's back.

This is not to say that pharmaceuticals are not useful in treating cancer. But it must be known that ongoing pharmaceutical use can inhibit the body's ability to prevent the formation of cancer in the first place.

We can add to this discussion particular drugs and drug types that have been shown to be particularly toxic to particular organs, or toxic in general:

Drugs particularly hard on the liver:
- Acetaminophen

- Analgesics (pain-killers)
- Anesthetics (given during surgery)
- Antibiotics
- Anticoagulants
- Antihistamines
- Anti-inflammatory drugs
- Blood pressure drugs
- Chemotherapy drugs
- Cholesterol-lowering drugs
- Diabetes drugs
- Heart disease drugs
- Oral contraceptives
- Parkinson's drugs
- Tuberculosis drugs

Drugs that can stress or damage the kidneys:
- ACE inhibitors
- Acyoclovir
- Allopurinol
- Aminoglycosides
- Amphotericin
- Beta-blockers
- Captopril
- Cephalothin
- Chemotherapy drugs
- Chlorothiazide
- Chlopropamide
- Clofibrate
- Cyclosporine
- Diuretics
- Furosemide
- Isoproterenol
- Lithium
- Macanylamine
- Methotrexate
- Methysergide
- Morphine
- NSAIDs (acetaminophen, aspirin, ibuprofen)
- Penicillins
- Phenytoin
- Piperidine
- Probenecid
- Procaine

- ➤ Quinidine
- ➤ Sulfonamides
- ➤ Tolazoline

There are several conditions that will change the body's ability to metabolize drugs, and different factors that will increase or decrease the drug's effects. This can lead to serious outcomes. The factors include sex, age, race, weight, pregnancy, nursing, illness, alcohol consumption, food, multiple drugs, digestion variation, kidney damage, liver damage, nutritional deficiencies, supplements used, exposure to other toxins, exercise, stress and time of the day.

In particular, a number of drugs are metabolized differently in women than men. These include amitriptyline, benzodiazepines, beta-blockers, chlordiazepoxide, diflunisal, imipramine, methylprednisoline, oxazepam, piroxicam, prednisolone and trazodone.

Some drugs can lead to breast enlargement among men. These include ACE inhibitors, amitryptyline, cimetidine, digoxin, famotidine, ibuprofen, indomethacin, ketoconazole, ketoprofen, methyldopa, naproxen, spironolactone and terfenadine.

A number of drugs can cause intestinal issues and diarrhea. These include antibiotics, antidepressants, antihypertensive drugs, statins and heart drugs like digitalis, quinidine, hydralazine, beta-blockers, and ACE inhibitors.

The liver uses what is called the P-450 enzyme pathway to break down many drugs. However, the P-450 pathway can easily become overloaded by too many drugs, combined with other toxins. This can result in a few dire circumstances:

- ➤ The liver can be seriously damaged
- ➤ The drug's effects can be exaggerated, causing dangerous effects.
- ➤ The drugs can remain in the system longer, causing more side effects
- ➤ The unprocessed metabolites of these drugs can produce fatigue, chemical overload and immunosuppression.

Several drugs can block or overload the liver's P-450 pathway:

- ➤ Antirrhythmic drugs (disopyramide)
- ➤ Antihistamines (terfenadine, astemizole)
- ➤ Benzodiazepines
- ➤ Bromocriptine
- ➤ Caffeine
- ➤ Calcium channel blockers
- ➤ Statins
- ➤ Cimetidine
- ➤ Cisapride
- ➤ Macrolides

- ➢ Antifungals
- ➢ Phenytoin
- ➢ Tacrine
- ➢ Theophyllines
- ➢ Tricyclic antidepressants
- ➢ Warfarin

(Adapted from Mindell and Hopkins 1998)

Air Pollution

Air pollution is linked to lung cancer. The evidence is clear. But few imagined that breathing air polluted air might cause other types of cancer. Yes, we are talking breast cancer, liver cancer, pancreatic cancer, intestinal cancers and others.

Clean air contains about 78% nitrogen, 21% oxygen, .9% argon, .03% carbon dioxide and a host of other trace elements. Depending upon the location and source, outdoor air pollution can contain carbon monoxide, nitrogen dioxide, sulphur dioxide, excess carbon dioxide, ammonia, various particulates, chlorofluorocarbons (CFCs), radon daughters, and a variety of toxic metals and volatile organic compounds (VOCs).

There are several types of air pollution, and most of them can overload the body with toxins. The first is *air particle* pollution—when particulate size ranges from .1 micron to 10 microns. This type of pollution is from soot, typical of automobile exhaust, industrial smoke stack exhaust, fireplace smoke, and smoke from forest fires, barbeques and other combustion. Soot is also called *black carbon* pollution, because the excess carbon burn off from burning fossil fuels is the primary component.

Coal gasification, coal tar distillation and coal-tar pitch have all been linked to multiple types of cancer.

Noxious gases are another type of pollution category. These include gasses such as carbon monoxide, chlorine gas, nitrogen oxide, sulphur dioxide and various other chemical gases and vapors. CFCs are a type of noxious gas.

While these two pollution types are distinct, they are often tough to differentiate. Many pollutants are actually vaporized liquids. Molecules become suspended in vapor, appearing like gases or liquid vapors. They are airborne elements derived from synthetic solid and liquid compounds.

We should also specify a difference between *indoor* and *outdoor* air pollution. There are a number of pollutants specifically pervading building ventilation systems and indoor facilities. To this, we can add outdoor pollution entering the house. Examples of indoor pollutants include formaldehyde emitted by foam, treated wood plastics, and chlorine gas emitted in indoor swimming pools.

According to a *American Lung Association State of the Air* report (2007), 46% or about 136 million Americans live within a county having *"unhealthful"* levels of either ozone or particle-based outdoor pollution. Over 38 million

Americans live in a county with *"unhealthful"* levels of both ozone and particle pollution. A third of Americans live in *"unhealthful"* ozone level counties.

Interestingly, this is substantially better than a 2006 report indicating that almost half of Americans live in ozone-rich areas. It is unlikely that the source of ozone pollution—carbon emissions—went down this much in a year. Most likely—just as the ozone hole has been fluctuating with atmospheric rhythms—there are complicated relationships between weather systems, temperature, pressure and so on.

Meanwhile, more than ninety-three million Americans—about one in three—live in areas seasonally high in short-term particle pollution and about one in five Americans lives in an area of high year-round particle pollution. Unlike the fluctuating ozone levels, the number of high particle pollution areas has steadily increased over the past few years.

A study from the American Cancer Society (Pope *et al.* 2002) and several universities showed clearly that air pollution causes lung cancer. This study followed about 1.2 million people and 500,000 people in metropolitan areas in the United States.

The study found that for every 10-μg/m3 increase in fine particulate air pollution, there was a 4% increase in death, a 6% increase in cardiopulmonary cancer and an 8% increased risk lung cancer deaths.

In 2020, the researchers of this study (Pope *et al.*) updated their findings with data from a number of other studies. They found similar results.

Fine Particulates

Particulate pollution can produce severe toxicity. Fine particulate air pollution is rated by particle measurement (PM). A PM(10-2.5) refers to a particle size from 2.5 micron to 10 micron, and PM(2.5) refers to particle sizes below 2.5 micron. 2.5 micron or less is a *fine particulate,* while less than .1 micron is *ultra-fine.* Ultra-fine particles may also be considered noxious gas pollutants, because their molecular size is small enough to pass through the alveoli into the bloodstream.

Researchers from the UK's University of Birmingham and Taiwan's University of Hong Kong (Wong *et al.* 2016) determined that sustained exposure to air pollution causes deaths from various cancers.

The researchers followed 66,820 people from Hong Kong who were 65 years old or older from 1998-2001 through to 2011. They monitored the people for deaths due to any cancer.

The researchers calculated the subjects' local air pollution through the period. This was based upon the recorded air pollution levels of monitoring stations near their homes. They also utilized satellite data.

Because Hong Kong has different air pollution levels in different parts of the city, it is an ideal place to study the effects of air pollution. Some districts of the city are on the shore, others are up high. And still others are within the industrial parts of the city.

The scientists specifically calculated the annual exposure of air pollution of PM2.5 particulates in micrograms per cubic meter for each person. PM2.5 particulates have an average diameter of 2.5 micrometers or less. PM2.5 has been accepted by many scientists as the most dangerous form of air pollution.

The researchers also eliminated the effects of other possible cancer causes, such as smoking and related conditions. They also eliminated deaths for the first three years of the study.

The researchers found that for each increase of 10 micrograms per cubic meter of PM2.5 air pollution on an annual basis increased deaths from breast cancer by 80 percent.

Each 10 ug/m3 of annual PM2.5 exposure increased deaths from upper digestive tract cancers (e.g. stomach cancers) by 42 percent. And for every 10 ug/m3 in PM2.5 increased deaths from cancer of other digestive organs – such as the gall bladder, bile ducts and pancreas – by 35 percent.

Interestingly, deaths from lung cancer increased 36 percent from PM2.5 exposure. Less than breast cancer and stomach cancers.

Deaths from all cancers increased by 22 percent for every 10 ug/m3 of PM2.5 annual exposure.

Note that the results are in graduated exposure levels. This means, for example, that a person with, say, 50 ug/m3 of PM2.5 annual exposure will have a 110 percent increased risk of any cancer, and a 400 percent increased risk of breast cancer.

Senior researcher Dr. Thuan Quoc Thach from the University of Hong Kong commented on the surprising results, with other cancer deaths outside of the lungs connected with air pollution:

"Long-term exposure to particulate matter has been associated with mortality mainly from cardiopulmonary causes and lung cancer, but there have been few studies showing an association with mortality from other cancers. We suspected that these particulates could have an equivalent effect on cancers elsewhere in the body."

The 50 ug/m3 number I used above might sound pretty aggressive. But it's really not that unreasonable. Yes, it is high in comparison to some cities around the world. But it is lower than some cities too.

The World Health Organization has monitored annual exposure levels (Brauer *et al.* 2016) around the world for several years. The world's average, according to their calculations, was 71 ug/m3 per year. This ranged from 26 to 208 ug/m3 around the world. By region, Africa averaged 78 per year, while Europe averaged 49 per year.

Now consider a sampling of the World Bank's average PM2.5 annual exposure per country around the world for 2013 (in ug/m3)

Afghanistan – 22
Argentina – 9
Bahrain – 44
Bangladesh – 48
Brazil – 16

Chad – 31
Egypt – 36
Germany – 15
India – 47
Israel – 26
Ireland – 8
Mali – 36
Mauritania – 70
Mexico – 12
Saudi Arabia – 54
Seychelles – 7
UK – 11
US – 11
Yemen – 36

I cherry-picked from this list, but you can see all of it here. Note that this is the average for the entire country. That means an average between the most polluted cities and the least polluted rural areas.

What about PM2.5 levels in different cities?

Many cities have high PM2.5 levels. Just consider the some of the average annual concentrations of PM2 from the World Health Organization in the table inserted. You can scroll down among the countries and cities.

Here you'll see that cities in China will spike well over 100 ug/m3. Cities in Chile will be in the 50 to 60 range. India cities will range from 40 to well over 100 ug/m3 – with Delhi at 198, and Ludhiana at an astounding 251 ug/m3. Italy will top 40 in some cities, while France and Germany, and the U.S. and the UK will be in the teens and 20s.

While the average PM2.5 concentration may seem on the low side for many Western cities, this can be deceiving because this is often an average of different parts of the city, or even from one measuring station.

A home that sits on a busy road will yield a much greater concentration of PM2.5 exposure compared to a suburb off the main streets, for example.

This also goes for ones personal exposure. One person might spend more time biking or walking on busy roads, while another might live and work on the seashore, for example.

While industrial plants produce plenty of PM2.5, trucks also produce a considerable amount. Especially diesel trucks.

PM2.5 levels linked to deaths in other research

Analyses by the City of New York estimate that PM2.5 levels in the City caused more than 2,000 deaths per year between 2009 and 2011. It is also related to 4,800 emergency room visits and 1,500 hospitalizations.

A study from Harvard measured the long-term effects of PM2.5 pollution on death. They found that for every increase in 2 ug/m3 PM2.5 levels, there was a 3 percent increase in deaths from all causes. That is for younger and older people.

In areas of lower income and lower home value, the researchers found death increases were higher.

In India and China, hundreds of thousands of deaths per year are attributed to PM2.5 levels.

Harvard researchers studied deaths linked to PM2.5 levels among six U.S. cities (Laden *et al.* 2006). They discovered that every 10 ug/m3 increase in PM2.5 increases the risk of death from heart disease by 28 percent, and deaths from all causes by 16 percent.

Particles above 10 micron in size are usually trapped by the cilia and mucous membranes in the nose, throat, or mouth. As mentioned earlier, these are usually disposed through the movement of mucous or broken down by immune cells.

Fine particulates are small enough to escape this labyrinth and get into our lungs, but they are usually too large to get directly into the bloodstream. These particles can become lodged in the tissues of the lungs and bronchi and slowly break down. As they break down, their toxins become absorbed and dumped into the bloodstream.

This accumulation of toxins can quickly overburden the liver and bloodstream, producing an inflammatory airway response. In other words, the pollution of the air quickly becomes the pollution of our bloodstream and liver—producing systemic inflammation.

The chemical makeup of these toxins depends upon the source of the pollution. Particle pollution caused by automobile exhaust will have various fluorocarbons and nitrate particles, while coal fired power plants will emit large numbers of sulphur dioxide molecules.

Course particulate pollutants are typically caused by mining, construction, or demolition. Building demolition can rain fumes of various dangerous substances a mile or more from the demolition site.

The most blatant illustration of the demolition effect is the World Trade Center bombing of 2001. The collapse of the towers caused such a toxic fume that there are still thousands of people suffering from a slow poisoning of the lungs. Dangerous chemicals like asbestos, formaldehyde and many others were breathed by thousands of people.

This effect was not limited to rescuers and those who escaped from the twin towers. Many others who happened to be in the vicinity are now suffering. Cancer rates have skyrocketed as a result for those who were exposed to the disaster.

Another prevalent disease caused by the disaster has been *sarcoidosis*—a life-threatening inflammation of the lungs. Sarcoidosis is not technically cancer, but it can develop into lung, brain and other forms of cancer as the granulomas spread and mutate.

Sarcoidosis scar tissue affects the elasticity and efficiency of the lungs, causing life-threatening lung collapse. A study released by nine doctors (Izbicki *et al.* 2007) who researched the delayed health effects at Ground Zero reported that firefighters and rescue workers were diagnosed with sarcoidosis at a rate of five times the incidence rate prior to 9/11.

An epidemic of respiratory disorders and lung cancer was also an unfortunate result of the Trade Center bombing. While we know asbestos is toxic to the lungs, it is still a popular building material. Many structural components of new buildings use asbestos as an ingredient. Because it is a cheap fire retardant material, buildings still go up using it. Asbestos has been linked to thyroid cancer and lung cancer in many studies, which caused a number of high profile lawsuits and residential building restrictions.

Another toxin released when buildings collapse or are demolished is benzene. Benzene has been identified as a carcinogen, and certain types of leukemia are associated with benzene exposure. Other toxins thought to be released by building collapse include mercury, lead, cadmium, dioxin, polycyclic aromatic hydrocarbons (PAHs) and polychlorinated biphenyls (PCBs). Many of these components are still used to build buildings. All of them were used in buildings a few decades ago, when many of our current skyscrapers were built.

Besides the more publicized cases of cancer and sarcoidosis, ailments associated with the WTC bombing include reactive-airways syndrome and lung cancer. This is because toxins can build up and reside in lung tissue cells, affecting future lung capacity for many years to come. Studies on firefighters involved in the rescue report an average loss of 300 milliliters of lung capacity (Senior 2003).

It is thus safe to say that exposure to these sorts of particulates may not be symptomatic for years after the exposure. This was certainly the case with those exposed to Agent Orange in Vietnam. Cases of prostate cancer, skin cancer, and chronic lymphocytic leukemia did not appear in some veterans for decades later (Beaulieu and Fessele 2003).

Particulate pollution or soot is the most dangerous form of outdoor pollution. Auto exhaust, aerosols, and chemicals from power plants and wood burning are the major sources.

Air pollution particles themselves are too small to be seen by the naked eye. But they can be seen as a whole in the form of a haze in the sunlight. While the body's cilia hair and mucous membranes in the nose and throat might filter and catch some of these particles, many will make it into the lungs where they can trigger inflammation.

Like any living organism, the earth and its atmosphere have means to cleanse toxins out of the system. The atmosphere conducts a number of self-cleaning currents, which move and break down pollutants. One such mechanism is the hydroxyl radical (OH) molecule. The immediate effect of the hydroxyl radical is to form photo-oxidants like nitric acid, which undergoes a photolysis reaction with nitrous acids. These can be highly toxic.

Ozone

Smog is primarily made up of ozone. There are two forms of ozone: The ozone that naturally makes up part of the stratosphere, often referred to as the ozone hole; and the ozone within the lower atmosphere, or troposphere. This latter ozone is called tropospheric ozone or ozone pollution.

This form of O_3 gas is caused not by a nature's interaction between radiation and the atmosphere, but through the reaction between fuel vapors from automobiles and sunlight. For this reason, smog levels tend to peak during hot weather.

Smog levels are also higher in warmer regions like Southern California and urban areas in the southern U.S., such as Atlanta. Other cities also experience greater smog levels during the summer months. Wherever higher concentrations of vehicles combine with warm sunshine, smog levels go up. The 'perfect storm' of almost constant sunshine, warm weather, and vehicle concentration makes Southern California one of the worst smog and ozone regions in the United States.

Ozone will oxidize on a cellular and internal tissue level when taken into the body. These tissues will be damaged in almost the same way other oxidized radicals damage tissues. Ozone is readily absorbed through the alveoli as a gas. From there it can enter the bloodstream and damage artery walls and tissues. Ozone is also a major lung tissue irritant, causing inflammation and epithelial cell damage. This can result in decreased lung capacity and/or decreased lung growth development among children.

Ozone is directly linked to the incidence and worsening of respiratory conditions such as asthma, bronchitis, and COPD. Research indicates that this mechanism is the oxidation of lung surface lipids that line the cells of the lung. These oxidized lipids stimulate inflammation as the body seeks to mitigate ozone's damaging effects. The oxidation stimulates scavenger macrophages, which bind to the oxidized lipids in an effort to reverse the damage (Postlethwait 2007).

This means that ozone will release unpaired oxygen radicals, which can damage cell membranes and tissues causing cancer as we discussed earlier.

Ozone has some redeeming qualities as well. Ozone therapy is gaining recognition among the alternative medical community. Ozone is used in hot tubs as a purification measure. It is also used as an industrial cleaning and sanitizing substance. Ozone is part of our natural mix of gases in our air as well. Typical levels are between 25 and 75 parts per billion.

However, dangerous ozone levels occur with higher levels of carbon monoxide levels, sulphur dioxide, and other pollutants. Like the canary in the coalmine, high ozone levels provide a good indicator of unhealthy air. When combined with other pollutants, ozone has a worsening detrimental effect upon the body.

The EPA's Air quality index rates 85 parts per billion of ozone as unhealthy for sensitive people, and over 105 ppb as unhealthy for anyone. As ozone levels rise, it can irritate the lungs and throat, increasing the potential for inflammatory throat and lung infections. As a result, indoor ozone generating machines—which have become popular over the last decade—are discouraged by both the EPA and the FDA if they emit levels higher than 50 parts per billion.

Ironically, higher ozone levels in the air reflect its cleansing action upon other pollutants. Ozone is part of the atmosphere's normalizing systems. The very same cleaning and antibacterial effect we have begun to utilize are part of the earth's detoxification mechanisms to clean and break down particulate pollution. This doesn't mean it is healthy to breathe in ozone at these levels, however.

Volatile Organic Compounds (VOCs)

Volatile organic compounds (VOCs) are given off by a number of consumer products. These include:

- Adhesives and glues
- Air fresheners
- Building materials and furnishings
- Cigarettes
- Cleaners
- Disinfectants
- Printers and copy machines
- Dry cleaning fluids
- Hobby and craft supplies
- Moth repellants
- Paints and thinners
- Pesticides
- Solvents
- Wood preservatives

VOCs have been linked to a number of types of cancer (Janfaza *et al.* 2019). These include:

- Breast cancer
- Colon cancer
- Head and neck cancers
- Lung cancer
- Pancreatic cancer
- Prostate cancer

Researchers from the Texas Tech University Health Sciences Center (Arif and Shah 2007) collected data on ten VOCs and 550 adults.

Exposures to VOCs ranged from 0.03 micrograms per cubic meter for trichloroethylene up to 14 microg/m3 for toluene. In other words, the higher

68

the level of toxic inhalation, the higher the incidence of respiratory disorders. This is because VOCs present toxins that are quickly absorbed into the bloodstream through the airways. Once in the bloodstream, the body launches an inflammatory response to remove them.

The researchers also found that as a group, Mexican-Americans experience the highest exposure levels to benzene—averaging 2.38 micrograms per cubic meter—compared with whites—who averaged 1.15 microg/m3—and blacks—who averaged 1.07 microg/m3. This relates to exposure levels that are relative to the type of work being done. In other words, this study indicates that Mexican-Americans are likely doing more work involving the use of VOCs, which in turn expose them to greater levels of benzene.

Benzene, like toluene and other VOCs, is highly disruptive to cells and tissues because of its highly reactive aromatic hydrocarbon structure. It can thus damage practically every cell and tissue system in the body, releasing numerous radicals. Not surprisingly, benzene is also known to be significantly carcinogenic.

Smoking

First-, Second- and Third-Hand Smoke

Tobacco smoke is also an important source of VOCs. The Centers for Disease Control estimates that 480,000 Americans die each year from smoking, most from lung cancer. This includes deaths from secondhand smoking.

The CDC also estimates that over 7,000 lung cancer U.S. deaths are caused by secondhand smoking.

Smoking also causes lots of other cancers. The annual rate of lung cancer deaths between 2005 and 2009 was 127,700 according to the CDC. Meanwhile 36,000 smokers died from other smoking-related cancers a year during that period.

Lung cancer maintains between an eleven and fifteen percent chance of survival beyond five years. It should be noted that the highest rates of global lung cancer occur for both men and women in North America and Europe (Field *et al.* 2006). Of course, these are also countries where indoor smoking rates are the highest.

Research has indicated that not only is second-hand smoke dangerous to non-smokers, but it has more than twice the amount of tar, nicotine and other toxins than the smoker inhales.

The smoker will inhale the smoke through the filtering mechanism provided by the packed tobacco inside the cigarette paper. And many cigarettes also have additional filters to screen out toxins. But the second-hand smoker will breathe all the smoke from the cigarette, cigar or pipe. Second-hand smoke contains five times the amount of carbon monoxide—the lethal gas that de-oxygenates the blood—than the smoker inhales.

Second-hand smoke also contains higher levels of ammonia and cadmium. Its nitrogen dioxide levels are fifty times higher than levels considered harmful, and the concentration of hydrogen cyanide approaches toxic levels.

Constant exposure to second-hand smoke increases the risk of lung cancer by 25%, and increases the risk of heart disease by 10%. Second-hand smoke exposure has also been irrefutably linked to emphysema, chronic bronchitis, asthma and other ailments.

Despite significant educational programs, second-hand and third-hand smoke poisoning is still prevalent in the United States. The Centers for Disease Control's National Health and Nutrition Examination Survey from 1999-2008 (CDC 2010) revealed that between 2007 and 2008, about 88 million American nonsmokers over the age of three were consistently exposed to secondhand smoke.

The good news is that the detectible blood nicotine levels among nonsmokers have declined from 52% between 1999 and 2000 to 40% between 2007 and 2008. Still, 40% is simply not acceptable. It should be noted that rates were the highest among children living in households below federal poverty levels.

There is now research that shows that anti-smoking laws decrease disease rates. Researchers from the Harvard School of Public Health (Dove *et al.* 2011) studied the National Health and Nutrition Examination Survey (NHANES) data—a research program run by the U.S. Centers for Disease Control and Prevention's National Center for Health Statistics (NCHS). NCHS's directive has been a continuous survey method focused on specific diseases among representative samples throughout the United States. About 5,000 persons each year are included in the data, from different counties across the nation.

The Harvard researchers used the 1999-2006 NHANES data to correlate locations that had some semblance of required smoke-free public places with asthma incidence. They found that smoke-free laws significantly reduced the odds of asthmatic symptoms among nonsmoking children and adolescents. Smoke-free laws were also linked to reduced asthma episodes ("attacks"), persistent wheeze, chronic night coughing and asthma medication use.

Smoking and Skin Cancer

Most of us know that smoking is linked to cancers of the lungs, the throat and the oral cavity. This research is well-established.

Surprisingly, skin cancer has been linked to smoking. Smoking and lung cancer has been well-accepted by scientists and the general population. The link is irrefutable. But smoking and skin cancer? Yes, in fact, scientific research has found that smoking significantly increases our risk of developing skin cancer.

Despite many years of decreased smoking, smoking is still a problem with youth according to the U.S. Centers for Disease Control. This can come in the form of tobacco vaping.

Smoking also causes some other surprising things. For example, smoking is also linked to anxiety and depression according to other research.

Researchers from Florida's Moffitt Cancer Center and the University of South Florida (Rollison *et al.* 2011) have discovered that squamous cell skin cancer is linked to cigarette smoking among both men and women. The study was carried out among several cancer clinics, which screened cancer patients for smoking. 383 patients with skin cancer were screened and compared with 315 skin cancer-free volunteers.

All were Caucasian, and fairly evenly divided between men and women. Those who smoked at some point in their lives were twice as likely to have squamous cell skin cancer. Women had the highest risk, with three times the squamous cell skin cancer for smokers. The study also found that smoking more cigarettes per day and smoking for more years increased the incidence of squamous cell skin cancer.

While increased risk of basal cell cancer was considered less significant, men who smoked more than 20 years had a 90% greater risk of basal cell cancer.

Both basal and squamous cell cancers are non-melanomas. Basal cell skin cancer incidence is higher than squamous cell cancer in the U.S. Basal cell cancers take place in the layer under the epidermis, the dermis, while squamous cell cancer grows in the top-most layer of skin, the epidermis.

Basal cell cancers do not readily spread to other organs, while squamous cell cancer often spreads among other organs of the body, and is thus more dangerous of the two. This research points to the effects of the more than 1,000 toxins that many cigarettes contain, in addition to nicotine. Dr. Dana Rollison, the lead researcher in the study, suggested that nicotine may metabolize differently in the presence of greater estrogen, which could explain why women smokers were more vulnerable to squamous cell carcinoma.

After years of blindly blaming the sun for all skin cancers, despite research showing that skin cancer rates are lower among regions with more sun, this research confirms that skin cancer is much more complicated than simply exposure to ultraviolet rays of the sun.

Skin Lotions and Sunscreen

Many of the chemical ingredients in many sunscreens have been identified as carcinogenic. These include benzophenone-3, homosalate, 4-methylbenzylidene camphor, octylmethoxycinnamate, and octyl-dimethyl-PABA. These five, alone or in some combination thereof, are contained in about 90% of today's commercial sunscreens.

All five of these chemicals have showed increased cancer cell proliferation both *in vitro* and *in vivo* in a study conducted at the Institute of Pharmacology and Toxicology at the University of Zurich (Schlumpf *et al.* 2001). This study also showed negative estrogenic and endocrine effects among mice from several of these chemicals.

A study done at the University of Manitoba in Winnipeg (Sarveiya *et al.* 2004) reported that all sunscreen ingredients tested—including octymethoxycinnamate and oxybenzone—significantly penetrate the skin. The penetration of common sunscreens was found to increase the penetration of even more dangerous herbicides—a concern for agricultural workers and non-organic gardeners (Pont *et al.* 2004).

Furthermore, it has been established that some organic sunscreens can cause photo-contact allergies (Maier and Korting 2005). Research from Australia's Skin and Cancer Foundation (Cook and Freeman 2001) reported 21 cases of photo-allergic contact dermatitis caused by oxybenzone, butyl methoxy dibenzoylmethane, methoxycinnamate or benzophenone. The Cook and Freeman research has led to a conclusion that these sunscreen ingredients are the leading cause of photo-allergic contact dermatitis.

Contact dermatitis is actually quite rare amongst the general population. A study at the National Institute of Dermatology in Colombia conducted a study of eighty-two patients with clinical photo-allergic contact dermatitis. Their testing showed that twenty-six of those patients—31.7%—were shown to be positive for sensitivity to one or several of the sunscreen ingredients (Rodriguez *et al.* 2006).

The widespread proliferation of these harmful sunscreen ingredients—an occurrence increasing since the 1960s sunbathing era—is a significant factor in the skin cancer epidemic. Their addition to the epidermis layer create an environment of excessive oxidative radicals, as the sun in the presence of oxygen further oxidizes these synthetic molecules without nature's balancing biomolecules.

At the bare minimum, these chemicals substantially increase the toxic burden within skin cells. This burden minimizes the body's ability to neutralize the oxidizing effects of the sun's radiation—intensifying the oxidizing factor. This intensification would essentially convert normally-healthy sun's rays from therapeutic to a dangerous, cancer-causing radiation.

Prior and concurrent to the prevalent use of sunscreen, sun-worshipers have ceremoniously applied various chemical- and oil-based sun lotions onto the skin. This is done to intensify the sun's tanning effects: to obtain that rich, brown tan to look more attractive.

Many chemicals are/were in these products, including various hydrocarbons, which revert to oxidized radicals when exposed to the sun. In addition to sun lotion, sunbathers also apply various other chemical-based lotions onto the skin to condition, hydrate or treat sunburn. These various moisturizing lotions also contain a variety of synthetic chemicals that can become free radicals.

Furthermore, many sunscreens available today effectively absorb UV-B rays, but let UV-A rays through. Because UV-A rays are quite dangerous out of balance with UV-B to an unhealthy body, the risk of skin cancer using these sunscreens is even higher than without any sunscreen protection.

In a 2007 study from the University of California at San Diego, researchers (Gorham *et al.* 2007) reviewed 17 studies of sunscreen use and melanoma. For those studies performed in latitudes over 40 degrees from the equator where skin types are fairer, there was a more significant correlation between sunscreen use and skin cancer.

Many other skin lotions should also be considered toxic. An example is DEET, or N,N-Diethyl-meta-toluamide. DEET is an effective mosquito repellent, yes. But it also poisons us as well. Research has shown that DEET exposure causes impairments to cognition, mood issues and insomnia. Whatever we put on our skin is absorbed into the epidermal and subdermal tissues, and eventually, into the bloodstream, and in the case of DEET, into our central nervous system.

Other toxic chemicals are used for lubricants, moisturizers, exfoliants and masks. Ingredients to steer clear of include methylisothiazalone, DMDM hydantoin, octenylsuccinate (a neurotoxin), methylchloroisothiazalone and triclosan—an antibacterial ingredient that is suspected to be an endocrine disruptor. Common among most soaps and cleansers are sodium laureth sulfate and ceteareth, which can bond to carcinogen chemicals used in manufacturing, such as ethylen oxide and 1,4-dioxane.

Plastics

Plastics are composed of monomers held together with plasticizers. One of the most prevalent types of plasticizers are called phthalates. Another type of plasticizer is better known: bisphenol A or BPA. Phthalates have been found in drinking waters. This is a problem, because phthalate and bisphenol A plasticizers have been found to interfere with human hormones. Let's examine some of the research.

A 2017 study from Taiwan's National United University (Huang *et al.* 2013) tested 279 adults from Taiwan, along with 79 minors. The researchers tested urine and blood for levels of phthalate metabolites. These included di-2-ethylhexyl phthalate (DEHP) and mono-ethylhexyl phthalate (MEHP).

The researchers found that phthalate levels influenced thyroid function and altered the stability of growth hormones. The researchers concluded:

"Our results are consistent with the hypothesis that exposure to phthalates influences thyroid function and growth hormone homeostasis."

This is the classic scenario for hormone disruption. To disrupt the body's natural flow of hormones means to interfere with hormone production in some way. This may result in increases in some hormones in some cases and decreases in other hormones.

Researchers from the University of Michigan (Meeker *et al.* 2011) confirmed that common phthalate plasticizers DEHP, DBP and BPA disrupt human thyroid hormones associated with thyroid diseases.

The research compared and analyzed the metabolites from urine and serum thyroid levels of 1,346 adults and 329 adolescents. Higher di(2-ethylhexyl) phthalate (DEHP), dibutyl phthalate (DBP), and bisphenyl A (BPA) levels were associated with lower levels of the thyroid hormone metabolites of T4, free T3, total T3 and thyroglobin. Higher DEHP levels were associated with higher TSH levels, while higher BPA levels were associated with lower T3 and TSH levels.

The researchers found that lower T4 metabolite levels has the strongest association with higher phthalates. High DEHP levels were associated strongly with lower TSH levels, while BPA was associated with lower T4 and TSH levels.

This study, published in the scientific journal, *Environmental Health Perspectives*, was the first national human study confirming that BPA and other common plasticizers definitely disrupt hormones.

Chemical industry advocates have been disputing the link between BPA and hormone disruption as coincidental. This research confirms previous research that led to the suspicion that these plasticizers disrupt hormone levels.

University of Michigan assistant professor and lead researcher, Dr. John Meeker, commented that those among the highest 20% of DEHP exposure had as high as 10% lower thyroid hormone levels. DEHP, BPA and DBP are common among food packaging, water bottles, can linings and many other consumer goods.

Plastic packaging is now ubiquitous and glues hold them together. Plasticizers such as Bisphenol A (BPA) get a lot of attention for their potentially harmful effects. But the glues that bind labels to the plastic and hold the plastic pieces together can also have negative health effects.

Isn't there enough bad news about plastic to go around? Not enough, actually. Plastics are ruining our health and environment. Microplastic pieces are polluting our oceans along with our bodies. Just consider for a moment how much plastic we are using. Just about every food is now wrapped in plastic. Even fresh foods are now often wrapped in plastic.

And those that aren't usually have a sticker glued onto them. Plastic typically comes in sheets from plastic manufacturers. From there these sheets are glued together to create the sections that are formed around the product. What are the glues that seal these plastic sheets together. Are they healthy? Certainly not.

The glues used to make plastic containers for food were studied carefully in a new research (Nerín *et al.* 2009) published in the Royal Society of Chemistry's *Journal of Materials Chemistry*. The study was conducted by researchers from Spain's University of Zaragoza.

The researchers, led by Dr. Christina Nerin, examined eleven glue compounds used in acrylic adhesives. Of these eleven, four were found to seep through the packaging onto the food contained within. Of these four, one is considered highly toxic, at the level considered for mercury, asbestos and other toxins. The compound is 2,4,7,9-tetramethyldec-5-yne-4,7-diol, used in many packaging label glues.

The study found that levels of 2,4,7,9-tetramethyldec-5-yne-4,7-diol released into the food from the plastic packaging were higher than levels recommended by the International Life Sciences Institute Europe - a group that creates standards for European food safety.

Asbestos

Asbestos contains a number of compounds that have been linked to cancer. Other compounds known to contain asbestos have also been linked to cancer, such as talc and vermiculite.

Asbestos exposure has become less likely since the *Environmental Protection Agency* passed the *Asbestos Ban and Phase Out Rule* as part of the *Toxic Substances Control Act* in 1989—which was for the most part overturned in 1991 by the U.S. *Fifth Circuit Court of Appeals*. What remain are various specific bans such as those from the *Clean Air Act* and remnants of *Toxic Substances Control Act*, including some continued restrictions supported by Congressional rulings.

The CAA has stimulated various bans since 1973. The bottom line is that although paper- and cardboard-based asbestos has been banned along with certain spray-on versions, many products still contain asbestos. These include cement sheets, clothing, pipe wrap, roofing felt, floor tiles, shingles, millboard, cement pipe, and various automotive parts.

Beyond the banned items, there is no ban preventing manufacturers from using asbestos. The important thing to remember is that the EPA does not monitor manufacturers for their ingredients. In general, asbestos inclusion into today's building materials should be considered a given.

Talcum Powder

Multiple studies have linked talcum powder to ovarian cancer among women who apply it to their genital area. The risk may be more considerable for epithelial ovarian cancer and ovarian cancers among African American women.

Johnson & Johnson has been a staple family brand in homes throughout the U.S. for decades. It has also dominated the talcum powder category.

The multinational manufacturing company founded in 1886 is well-known for its medical device and pharmaceutical endeavors, but the name most likely conjures up mental images of its popular consumer goods. It revolutionized infant product offerings with its baby powder, shower gels, and lotions, a market it has been involved in for the past 125 years.

But, the past few years have brought a dark cloud over the company's reputation. Since 2013, nine court cases have taken place to decide if talcum powder causes ovarian cancer.

This ingredient that's derived from the talc mineral is found in Johnson & Johnson's Baby Powder and Shower-to-Shower products, two staple goods from the company that women have been using for a long time. Now in 2018, over 5,000 women have filed claims that place the blame of their ovarian cancer diagnosis on Johnson & Johnson.

We should note that there are other talcum powders on the market not produced by Johnson & Johnson.

This isn't the first instance of possibly toxic ingredients being found in consumer products. Talcum powder is just one example that is still allowed on U.S. store shelves despite regulatory agencies in other parts of the world completely banning it as an ingredient.

Before you stock up on your hygiene products, here's what you need to know about the ingredient and the products it can be found in.

Talcum powder is made from crushed talc, a clay mineral found in large quantities around the world. In powder form, the mineral is used in a multitude of hygiene products due to its ability to effectively whisk away bodily moisture. It is both odorless and absorbent, and it can also be used as an anti-caking agent in food products such as rice and gum.

Talcum powder was first seen as a health concern back in 1971 when researchers studied ovarian cancer tumors and found that 75% contained talc particles. Since then, a number of studies have shown a link between ovarian cancer and talc use in the genital region.

Harvard University researchers conducted an analysis of over 8,500 ovarian cancer cases compared to nearly 10,000 control subjects in 2013. The study showed that talc applied to the genital region increased the risk of epithelial ovarian cancer by 24 percent.

Serous ovarian cancer risk increased by 20 percent. Endometriod ovarian cancer risk increased by 22 percent. And clear cell tumor risk increased by 24 percent. Furthermore, borderline serous tumor risk increased by 46 percent according to the research.

Another pooled analysis of cases concluded little risk, but this included finding a 12 percent increased risk of ovarian cancer when talc was applied to the genital region.

A 2016 study from the University of Virginia and Duke University studied talc powder use among African American women. This study examined 584 cases of ovarian cancer and 745 control subjects. The researchers found that talc powder use was common in over 62 percent of the women with ovarian cancer.

The research also found that talc powder use in the genital region resulted in a 44 percent increase in ovarian cancer incidence. The study also found a dose-response relationship. This means the more they used the talc, the higher their risk of ovarian cancer.

In addition to ovarian cancer, talcum powder has also sparked concern due to its association with asbestos. Although cosmetic companies are often required to purify talcum powder before they include it in their products, there have been instances where testing has revealed a presence of asbestos.

Because of this contamination, Johnson & Johnson has also been involved in litigation for asbestos in its talc-based products. The lawsuit alleges that this asbestos exposure caused one man to be diagnosed with the rare cancer mesothelioma.

As 2018 progresses, we will likely see further developments of the talcum powder and cancer debate as well as additional litigation pending for the family brand.

What products contain talcum powder?

Despite inconclusive studies, it may be beneficial to avoid the potential cancer risks associated with talcum powder exposure. Take the time to read all product labels to look for the inclusion of talcum powder. Many brands have introduced talc-free products that will clearly say so on the label if you decide to make the switch.

Below is a list of common goods to double-check:
➢ Deodorant
➢ Baby powder
➢ Cosmetic foundation
➢ Blush
➢ Eyeshadow
➢ Shampoo & conditioner
➢ Lotion
➢ Educate yourself on the products you buy

Talcum powder is one of many potential toxins that continues to have a presence on our grocery shelves today. Although both the scientific and legal communities are still debating the legitimacy of talc's connection to cancer, the issue has spurred on a greater conversation surrounding the safety and regulation of consumer goods. Before you purchase any product, make it a priority to educate yourself on what ingredients may be posing a health risk to you and your family.

Arsenic

Toxic arsenic levels are found in many drinking water supplies around the world.

Arsenic is a serious cancer-causing agent. How do we know this? Because scientists have linked high arsenic levels in drinking water and other types of exposures with higher cancer rates. Here we'll discuss a few major studies and how we reduce arsenic exposure. We'll also discuss strategies to eliminate toxic arsenic from the body.

A number of studies have linked arsenic with multiple types of cancer. The most linked cancer types have been skin cancers, lung cancers, and urinary cancers and bladder cancers.

Because squamous cells are particularly sensitive to having their DNA altered by arsenic exposure, any organ or location with squamous cells are at risk of cancer with high arsenic exposure. This means the skin, throat, bladder, mouth, lungs and much of the digestive tract have a higher risk of cancer as a result of arsenic exposure.

Even what was considered safe levels of arsenic in drinking water has now been linked to cancer, skin lesions, nerve and brain impairment and heart diseases according to a 2018 study (Smeester *et al.*).

A 30-year review of research from Cancer Care Ontario and the Dalhousie University in 2014 found that increased arsenic exposure is linked to more kidney cancers and bladder cancers. As the arsenic levels go up in drinking water, kidney and bladder cancer rates also go up.

It is therefore not a coincidence that high arsenic levels in the drinking waters of some areas have also been linked with skin lesions. A 2006 study from India's Jadavpur University found in testing nearly 1,000 people, that nearly 20 percent of the adults had skin lesions in high-arsenic areas of the West Bengal area of the Ganges region. They also found high rates of skin cancer.

Low-level arsenic exposure can also increase the risk of prostate cancer. A 2017 study from the University of Iowa found that people who drank water from wells with 2.07 or more parts per billion of arsenic had between 23 percent and 45 percent increased risk of prostate cancer.

This is considered low-level because drinking water with more than 10 parts per billion is typically considered to be cancer-causing from most of the global research.

Other types of cancers are also linked to arsenic. For example, a 2015 study from China's The Medical College of Qingdao University analyzed research data around the world and found that long-term exposure in drinking water nearly doubled the risk of liver cancer in many parts of the world.

Multiple cancers were also found in 2011 research at the National Health and Environmental Health Effects Research Laboratory. The research studied the interaction of arsenic chemicals with the sulfur within proteins. They also found that arsenic interaction in the body produced free radicals, which damage cell membranes and those tissue systems made of those cells.

Symptoms of immediate arsenic exposure include gastrointestinal pain. They can also include fatality at higher levels.

Lung cancer was a late addition to the list of cancers caused by arsenic. A 2017 study from Taiwan's National Cheng Kung University tested 243 town populations in Taiwan. They measured their arsenic levels in their drinking water against their lung cancer rates.

They found towns with increased arsenic in their water showed a significant increase in lung cancer rates. For every one percent increase, there was a 0.27 per 100,000 incidence of cancer in men and .13 per 100,000 in women.

Confirming the aforementioned, the type of lung cancer most prevalent was squamous cell cancer of the lungs.

Childhood exposure can have significant effects according to the research. Exposure to arsenic during infancy or during the prenatal period has been associated with increased risk of lung cancer along with a myriad of neuropathic and developmental disorders.

Scientists working in conjunction with the U.S. Environmental Protection Agency at the National Health and Environmental Health Effects Research Laboratory (Hughes *et al.* 2011) have found that arsenic exposure may be linked to several types of cancer, particularly skin cancer, bladder cancer and lung cancer.

The research studied the interaction of arsenic chemicals with the sulfur within proteins, as well as arsenic's ability to produce free radicals, which serve to damage cell membranes and those tissue systems made of those cells.

Symptoms of immediate arsenic exposure include gastrointestinal pain. They also include fatality. The researchers illustrated that arsenic is increasingly contaminating our foods, our air, our water and our soils. Compounded arsenic is a common ingredient in pesticides and many processed food products. This is because arsenic is toxic to insects and microorganisms (not to mention humans). It is used in wood preservatives and many building materials. It is consistently a byproduct of industrial plant production and building manufacturing. Arsenic is a typical compound in chemotherapy drugs.

The semiconductors gallium arsenide, aluminum arsenide and others are arsenic alloys. According to U.S. Geological Survey studies leading producers of arsenic for industrial use are China, Chile, Peru and Morocco. China produces nearly half of the world's supply of industrial arsenic. As a result of its widespread use, arsenic is increasingly found in our drinking water, especially those in industrial areas.

Ground water supplies in many parts of the world are now contaminated with arsenic. When introduced to the environment, compounds with arsenic will oxidize to become unstable. The reaction seen most often producing this instability is a process catalyzed by arsenic methyltransferase. This reduces the arsenic compound from pentavalency to trivalency.

This step is followed by the oxidative methylation process, which returns the compound to pentatavalency. During the step to the trivalent version of arsenic, the arsenic has the ability to radically damage cells and tissues. Natural forms of arsenic will metabolize to low-toxicity forms of arsenic through methylation as well.

Natural versus Toxic Arsenic

Natural arsenic is found in trace levels within soils and rocks. As you may know, rock-salt is a healthy source of natural arsenic. The body utilizes natural arsenic in trace amounts for a number of enzymatic and neurotransmitter compounds.

For this reason, natural arsenic, in natural, trace levels, is healthy. The body will also use methylation to reduce arsenic to a harmless compound.

But when arsenic compounds are introduced into through industrial combustion or petrochemicals, they will oxidize and become unstable. The reaction seen most often producing this instability is a process catalyzed by arsenic methyltransferase.

Arsenic methyltransferase reduces the arsenic compound from pentavalency to trivalency. During the step to the trivalent version, the arsenic is a radical that can damage cells and tissues.

In healthy people, the body's oxidative methylation process can return even this form of the less harmless pentatavalency form.

We will discuss how to boost methylation in the body below.

Arsenic is increasingly contaminating our foods, our air, our water and our soils. Compounded arsenic is a common ingredient in pesticides and many processed food products. This is because arsenic is toxic to insects and microorganisms (not to mention humans). It is used in wood preservatives and many building materials. It is consistently a byproduct of industrial plant production and building manufacturing. Arsenic is also often a compound used in chemotherapy drugs.

The semiconductors gallium arsenide, aluminum arsenide and others are arsenic alloys. According to U.S. Geological Survey studies, leading producers of arsenic for industrial use are China, Chile, Peru and Morocco. China produces nearly half of the world's supply of industrial arsenic.

As a result of its widespread use, arsenic is increasingly found in drinking water, especially in groundwater basins within industrial areas.

These wells may be contaminated with arsenic due to local industrial farming or industrial manufacturing of some sort. Especially in areas where there are coal-fired plants, because coal tends to contain a lot of arsenic. Significant auto pollution can also peak airborne arsenic levels.

The first and most urgent means of reducing arsenic exposure is to only drink water that's been filtered through a good water filter that screens out arsenic. Many of today's popular filters are rated to remove significant arsenic levels. For a discussion on the best choices for water filters, consider my book, *"Pure Water."*

Another common source is consuming arsenic in foods. We have discussed arsenic levels in rice, for example. Organic rice has significantly less arsenic according to our findings. Other organic foods will contain less arsenic because of arsenic levels in pesticides and herbicides.

Other foods and even herbs can be contaminated with arsenic, but usually, these sources aren't significant because they will not be eaten as consistently.

Nevertheless, carefully checking the labels of our foods or simply knowing the origin of our foods is critical to avoiding arsenic. Avoiding foods and herbs grown in regions most known to contain arsenic is a good idea.

From arsenic maps, we find that large regions of the world, including the U.S., China and India, are contaminated.

Furthermore, as mentioned above, low-level contamination can also be problematic. And these are not showing up in the map. So become aware of the contaminant levels in your local drinking and bathing water. Most municipality water agencies publish their contamination levels on the internet today. If they don't, contact them and ask them to send you their most recent water testing results. At least in the U.S., they are regulated by the EPA so they have to.

If you are using well-water from a private well, this can be more problematic. You will likely have to pay a testing laboratory to test your water for arsenic (or any other contaminant). Most local water authorities will test your water for a reasonable fee.

I mentioned methylation above. Our body's ability to methylate will help reduce the oxidative free radical forms of arsenic into less harmful compounds. What helps our body's methylation efforts, you may ask?

One of the best facilities for reducing our risk of long-term effects of arsenic is to employ a strong B-vitamin supplementation program. This is because B-vitamins are what we call methyl-donors. They donate the needed methyl groups, which give our body more ammunition to reduce free radicals within the body.

This was confirmed by a 2017 study from the Keck Medical School at UCLA. The researchers tested 418 people with arsenic-related cardiovascular disease from New Hampshire. They found that those with good B-vitamin supplementation had reduced levels of arsenic in their urinary samples.

Good B-vitamin supplementation also should include natural folate consumption. Folates, as documented by researchers from the University of North Carolina, are great strategies for helping the body eliminate toxic arsenic.

Supplementing folic acid is not the same as getting sufficient folate. There are sometimes side effects of folic acid over-supplementation. Research has linked too much folic acid with cancer in women, for example.

Good natural folate sources include leafy green vegetables, broccoli, peas, beans and asparagus.

For intense arsenic exposure, chelation is an option. Chelation using Dimercaptosuccinic acid (DMSA) has been shown successful in clinical use.

A 2013 review by Dr. Michael Kosnett from the University of Colorado Medical School confirms from 70 years of clinical use that DMSA is a useful chelation therapy agent for arsenic. (See a doctor if you are considering chelation therapy.)

Formaldehyde

Formaldehyde is a proven carcinogen. It is classified as a known Group 1 human carcinogen by the Research by the International Agency for Research on Cancer and the National Toxicology Program of U.S. Department of Health and Human Services.

Today so many building materials and furniture are built using formaldehyde. These include pressed wood, draperies, glues, resins, shelving, flooring, and so many other materials. The greatest source of formaldehyde appears to be those materials made using *urea-formaldehyde* resins. These include particleboard, plywood paneling, and medium density fiberboard.

Among these, medium density fiberboard—used to make drawers, cabinets and furniture tops—appears to contain the highest resin-to-wood ratio. Another sort of resin called *phenol-formaldehyde* or PF resin. PF resin apparently emits substantially less formaldehyde than the UF resins.

This PF resin is easily differentiated from UF resin by its darker, red or black color. The incidental *off-gassing* of formaldehyde into the indoor environment from these resins results from sun, heat, sanding and demolition. As the formaldehyde slowly off gasses, it becomes a chemical toxin once in the body.

Many consumer products use formaldehyde these days. We have already reported on formaldehyde in flooring, in hair straighteners, in building materials and in second-hand cigarette smoke.

But clothing sources of formaldehyde exposure can be even more toxic than these sources. Why? Because these make direct contact with our skin. Further, our clothing can become a source of chronic exposure as they gradually out-gas.

Formaldehyde exposure from clothing is real. Recently, for example, I purchased a hooded jacket. When I got it home, I noticed the hood had a very toxic smell. The main fabric panel said the jacket was made of polyester. The hood looks like a wrinkle-free cotton blend. But the smell was unmistakable: Formaldehyde.

Melamine-formaldehyde resin is used for many hard-surface applications such as counter-tops and flooring. But a significant amount of clothing – especially clothing from China – is made with urea-formaldehyde. Why? Some manufacturers believe it is the best way to achieve a wrinkle-free piece of clothing.

Formaldehyde has been used for decades to achieve wrinkle-free clothing. Typically it has been used on cotton fabric or cotton/polyester blends. More recently, fully synthetic fabrics or blends can also contain formaldehyde.

Formaldehyde in Imported Clothing

Because synthetic fabrics don't wrinkle as easily, formaldehyde isn't necessary. Still some manufacturers are using formaldehyde in their synthetic clothing, especially when it is blended. While formaldehyde is being used by clothing manufacturers in other countries, testing has indicated that some Chinese clothing manufacturers in particular are using extremely high levels of formaldehyde.

In 2007, New Zealand's Ministry of Consumer Affairs (Donovan *et al.*) investigated tests funded by a NZ program called Target. The company had some Chinese clothing tested by a third-party laboratory. The fabric tests found that the easy-care fabrics had up to 900 times the levels of formaldehyde considered safe in clothing.

The program director, Candace McNabb, commented on the testing results:

"The laboratory we spoke to was really surprised at the results and actually went back and double-checked that they'd done everything right because our results were so high."

In 2010, the U.S. Government Accountability Office submitted a report to Congress on formaldehyde in clothing.

The research accounted a laboratory test of 180 clothing articles purchased in the U.S. Ten of the articles had formaldehyde levels above the 75 parts per million. Three of the top five formaldehyde-containing articles came from China.

The highest levels were found in a dress shirt (100% cotton) from China – at 206 parts per million.

This was followed by:
- ➢ A hat (100% cotton) from China, at 192 ppm
- ➢ Pillow cases (60-40 cotton/polyester) from Bahrain at 189 ppm
- ➢ Khakis from India at 169 ppm
- ➢ Another dress short from China at 95 ppm

Nine of the top ten items were articles worn by children. Their research also found that 34 percent of clothing purchased in the U.S. was made in China.

Yes, urea-formaldehyde does help achieve wrinkle clothing. It bonds with clothing materials to create a stiff fabric. As for being fire retardant, think again. Yes, when bound with urea it can form a heat-resistant barrier. But formaldehyde is flammable when released as a gas. As urea-formaldehyde off-gasses – you guessed it, formaldehyde gas.

The central issue: Formaldehyde is toxic.

As the U.S. GAO review of the research reported, in the short-term, formaldehyde in clothing is linked with nausea, irritation to the eyes, nose and throat; and asthmatic attacks. In the longer-term, formaldehyde has been linked with cancer. Let's take a look at some of the evidence.

Laboratory studies since the 1970s have been linking formaldehyde with cancer. As this research has matured, the link has become more convincing.

In 2011, the U.S. National Toxicology Program – part of the Department of Health and Human Services, officially classified formaldehyde as a human carcinogen. This is in addition to it causing neurological damage.

In the flooring article, we discussed other evidence showing that formaldehyde is a carcinogen. Calculations by the U.S. Centers for Disease Control showed that airborne formaldehyde causes up to 30 cases of cancer in 100,000 people.

The statistic was developed from meta-analyses of multiple studies. The most prevalent cancers from airborne formaldehyde include leukemia, lung cancer, oral and nose cancers.

Clothing is even more concerning. Yes, urea-formaldehyde can off-gas formaldehyde and is linked with these sorts of cancers.

Contact with formaldehyde is carcinogenic. A study from Italy's University of Eastern Piedmont (Lorenzoni *et al.* 2017) studied tested formaldehyde exposure on human skin cells in the laboratory.

They found that even low concentrations of the chemicals significantly increased the activation of what is called ERK (extracellular signal-regulated kinase) expression. ERK expression has been linked with the development of multiple forms of cancer.

A study from Brazil's University of Sao Paulo (Gostner *et al.* 2016) took skin cell samples from 17 volunteers. They were anatomy students, who had air contact with formaldehyde during their anatomy courses. The researchers found that the students had significantly increased levels of mutagenicity among their skin cells. Cell death also increased.

Mutagenicity means the skin cells showed mutations. Mutations within cells means an increased risk of skin cancer.

Researchers from the Medical University of Innsbruck calculated that airborne exposure of 0.1 to 0.5 ppm (parts per million) for three days can have significant toxicity, and cause increased cell death among skin cells. They also stated:

"Formaldehyde toxicity can affect all organ systems in particular those which get into direct contact. The exerted effects range from carcinogenicity to irritation and allergy and depend from the concentration, the duration and the route of exposure."

The CDC's National Institute for Occupational Safety and Health began studying formaldehyde exposure in garment plants since the early 1980s. They found that garment worker deaths from leukemia were significantly higher than in the rest of the population. They also found leukemia deaths were twice the rest of the population in people with ten or more years of exposure. The researchers concluded:

"Results support a possible relation between formaldehyde exposure and myeloid leukemia mortality."

Numerous other studies have collectively linked formaldehyde exposure to cancer. And with direct contact as in clothing and furniture, formaldehyde produces both a long-term and immediate effect.

Doesn't formaldehyde come out in the wash?

Not necessarily, and not readily. A study from India's Kasturba Medical College (Pinkerton *et al.* 2004) tested 20 pieces of clothing purchased commercially. Of the 20 articles, 11 tested positive for formaldehyde using a chromotropic acid testing procedure. Only the cotton or cotton-polyester blends contained formaldehyde.

The researchers proceeded to wash and dry the formaldehyde-containing clothes. After washing and drying the clothes twice, some of the blends showed reduced formaldehyde. But the researchers found no reduction in formaldehyde content among many articles after washing and drying twice. They wrote:

"Polyester cotton and organdy showed reduced formaldehyde content after washing. The other textiles showed no reduction in the intensity of the red purple to violet color after the first and second washes."

The intensity of the red purple to violet is part of the chromotropic acid test. This result means little or no reduction in formaldehyde.

The San Francisco-based Cardno ChemRisk laboratory (Novick *et al.* 2013) also tested formaldehyde in 20 articles of clothing.

Here, the researchers found that only 3 of the 20 had significant formaldehyde levels. However, two of these three had extremely high formaldehyde concentrations: 3,172 parts per million and 1,391 ppm. These were up to 40 times the limit of international textile regulations.

Then the researchers purchased additional versions of these two articles. They washed and dried them using hand-washing and machine washing methods. They also tested air drying and machine drying methods.

They found that the washing and drying only reduced the formaldehyde levels by between 26 and 72 percent. And the washing or drying method didn't significantly change the reduction of formaldehyde in the clothing.

The researchers also tested whether ironing the clothing would further reduce the formaldehyde levels: It didn't.

Some of the research discussed above illustrate that many types of clothing will not contain formaldehyde. This is particularly true of non-wrinkle-free fully synthetic fabrics like polyester.

However, it is apparent that clothing from China should be approached with caution. Especially if it is labeled as easy-care or wrinkle-free. A whiff-sniff test prior to purchasing could be warranted. A whiff-sniff is when you hold your nose about a foot away and fan in some air next to the article. This avoids sticking your nose right into the questionable article and getting further contaminated.

Such a whiff-sniff test could result in a little formaldehyde exposure. But better to be exposed for a second than for the next few months or more as you wear the article.

Yes, it is certainly best to wash and dry new clothes before wearing them. But from the two studies above we find that washing once may not eliminate the formaldehyde content. Even multiple washings may only reduce the formaldehyde content but not eliminate it. Vinegar and/or baking soda might be a consideration, but there's no evidence these will remove it any faster.

Probably better to not purchase clothing that has a strong chemical smell in the first place. Or, as in my case with the jacket, return it as soon as you can. Regardless of how well it might fit.

Another strategy is to wear recycled clothing. Recycled clothing comes with some additional out-gassing from wearing and washing by the original owner. Plus it's cheaper and better for the environment.

Hair Straighteners and Formaldehyde

Many people use hair straighteners. Are they toxic? There are do-it-yourself hair straighteners and there are those done at the hair salon. Hair straighteners are increasingly popular. Especially among people who have naturally curly hair. This does not mean that hair salon straighteners are necessarily safer. As we will find in the research below, hair straightener safety depends largely upon the brand and the ingredients used in the product. One of these questionable ingredients is formaldehyde.

A study of leading "Brazilian-style" hair straighteners that included 45 manufacturers has found that many brands claiming little or no formaldehyde actually contain significant levels. The study, by the Environmental Working Group, included a review of 47 adverse event reports that have been filed with the United States Food and Drug Administration. The study found that *"15 of 16 companies claim little to no formaldehyde but tests show their products contain substantial amounts."*

Tests concluded that some hair straighteners have up to 11.8% formaldehyde. In addition, salon air fume testing conducted during 2010 found that hair salons often maintain high levels of formaldehyde. The researchers noted that solutions containing over one percent formaldehyde will produce significant air vapor formaldehyde levels. U.S. federal law calls for salons to provide medical monitoring and emergency wash stations if they use formaldehyde solutions over 1%. The EWG petitioned the U.S. FDA to take action on what they cite as hazardous products.

Some hair straightener fans have discovered natural black castor oil, which has been reputed (but not confirmed by research) to be a healthy hair straightener. Black castor oil has also been reputed to stimulate hair growth and yield a healthy scalp.

Polybrominates

Polybrominated diphenyl ethers or PBDEs and polyhalogenated aromatic hydrocarbons or PHAHs provide another cancer risk. These are fire retardants used to make automobiles, polyurethane foams, furniture, electronic goods, textiles, airplanes and of course, building materials.

They have also been linked to thyroid cancer. A 2020 study (Huang *et al.*) followed 1484 people who worked with the U.S. Department of Defense. The study found that those more exposed to polybrominated diphenyl ethers and polybrominated biphenyls had double the risk of thyroid cancer.

This means that the air during any kind of sanding, crushing, fire or demolition should be treated with extreme caution. Using a particle or gas mask is more than a good idea under these circumstances, though it should be noted that most particle masks do not form a tight enough bond with the face to filter much at all. Best is to use a gas filter or a mask with a rubber barrier that fits tightly onto the face.

With regard to off-gassing, prior to bringing in any type of new furniture or wood into the house, it is best to off-gas the product by setting it in the sunshine for a couple of days or at least for a full day. As the sun's resonating waves connect with the material, many of its toxins are disassociated and released. Not such a good thing for the environment, but at least it will disburse outside of our immediate breathing environment. Off-gassing can help us avoid more than a potent toxin.

Fresh paint can also be toxic. This is because paint typically contains VOCs.

Radiation

By far, the biggest source of radiation in our lives is our daily dose from the sun. For thousands of years, humans used the light of the sun as the primary means for observation and lifestyle. Fire, of course, augmented the sun at night. As any candlelight dinner will attest, the light given off by flame is a significantly different experience than today's fluorescent or incandescent lights.

Together, these two energy sources—sun and fire—provided the primary means of light and heat.

But to an increasing degree, we have replaced the sun with synthetic versions: electromagnetically driven electricity, heat, lights and other appliances. Modern humankind has harnessed electromagnetic radiation in the form of alternating current.

Today these have been replaced by an electronic light show with innumerable blinking lights and pulsing electronics. Today's environment is drowning in supercharged alternating currents.

Does the synthetic surging of alternating current cause cancer?

Some have been assumed that, outside of electrocution, alternating current had little or no negative effects upon the body. Then about three decades ago, a sounding alarm was made. A plethora of research and documentation offered the possibility of EMR causing various forms of cancer.

Equally important is to what extent electromagnetic radiation from alternating currents may affect our vitality and general wellness. Does it burden our immune system? Does it deplete our energy? This directly relates to our body's ability to detect and remove cancer cells before they develop into tumors.

Ionizing or Non-ionizing?

There are two basic forms of radiation to consider: *Ionizing radiation* and *non-ionizing radiation*. According to a 2005 report by the National Academy of Sciences on low levels of ionizing radiation, about 82% of America's ionizing radiation comes from natural sources: the earth, sun, space, food and the air. The rest—18%—comes from human origin.

The bulk of this fabricated radiation comes from x-rays and nuclear medicine. This accounts for close to 80% of the 18%. Other elements like consumer goods, toxic water, occupational exposure, and nuclear power account for the rest of the ionizing radiation exposure according to this report.

Ionizing radiation is typically defined as electromagnetic radiation capable of disrupting atomic, molecular or biochemical bonds. This disruption takes place through an interference of waveforms between the ionizing radiation and the waveforms of atomic or molecular orbital bonds. As this interference is likely to cause the atom or molecule to lose electrons, ions are likely to develop as a result.

These ions can often turn to oxidative species or otherwise imbalanced molecular species. Should ionizing radiation with enough intensity impact the physical body, it can result in cell injury or mutagenic damage.

Various natural and synthetic radiation forms are considered ionizing. Natural ionizing radiation includes portions of ultraviolet radiation, x-rays, cosmic rays and gamma rays. Fire can also cause ionizing radiation at high temperatures if the radiation comes close enough.

Synthetic versions of ionizing radiation include electrically produced x-rays, CAT-scans, mass accelerator emissions and a host of other electromagnetic radiation produced through alternating current.

Non-ionizing radiation also can be split into natural and synthetic versions. Natural versions include sound, light and radio waves. Most natural non-ionizing radiation can also be synthetically produced.

For example, sound may be digitally produced through the manipulation of alternating current by stereo receivers and speakers. This effect utilizes electrical semiconduction. Some scientists also categorize radiation from electrical power lines, electricity generating or transfer stations, appliances, cell phones, cell towers and other shielded electricity currents as non-ionizing radiation.

Microwaves are also considered non-ionizing. Most assume that non-ionizing radiation is not harmful. This assumption, however, has undergone debate over the past few decades.

The 2005 National Academy of Sciences report, after a review of most of the available research regarding non-ionizing radiation, concluded that even low doses below 100 milliseiverts were potentially harmful to humans and could cause a number of disorders from solid cancer or leukemia.

This jolted the scientific community, because for many years researchers thought that small doses of non-ionizing radiation were not that harmful.

A rem is one unit of radiation dose in roentgens. An mrem is one thousandth of a rem. One hundred rem equals one sievert. One sievert equals one thousand milliseiverts. Ten sieverts (10,000 mSv) will cause immediate illness and death within a few weeks.

One to ten sieverts will cause severe radiation sickness, and the possibility of death. Above 100 mSv there is a probability of cancer, and 50 mSv is the lowest dose that has been established as cancer causing. Twenty mSv per year has been established as the limit for radiological workers. About one to three mSv per year is the typical background radiation received from natural sources, depending upon our location and surroundings.

About .2 to .7 mSv per year comes from air. Soil sources are responsible for about .8 mSv. Cosmic rays give off about .22 mSv per year. Japanese holocaust victims received .1 Sv to 5 Sv from the bomb.

Our total radiation dose is a thus a combination of natural sources and those emitted by our artificial electromagnetic empire. A report from the Hiroshima International Council for Health Care of the Radiation-Exposed noted that the world's average radiation dose from natural radiation sources is 2.4 mSv.

However, they also noted that Japan's natural radiation average is comparably low at 1.2 mSv. Japan's average radiation dose from medical radiation is higher than average, at 2.4 mSv. This gives Japan a significantly higher radiation average of 3.6 mSv.

UK's National Radiological Protection Board estimates that the national radiation exposure in Britain for the average person is 2.6 mSv, with an estimated 50% coming from radon gas, 11.5% coming from foods and drinks, 14% coming from gamma rays, 10% coming from cosmic rays and 14% originating from appliances—primarily medical equipment.

Research indicates that radiation from medical equipment is increasing. This is primarily driven by the growing use of CT scans, which generate a larger dose of radiation than the more traditional x-rays. About sixty-two million CT scans are now given a year in the U.S., as opposed to about three million per year in 1980. Brenner and Hall (2007) reported in the *New England Journal of Medicine* that a third of CT scans given today are unnecessary. The article also estimated that between one and two percent of all cancers are caused by CT scan radiation exposure.

In contrast, the maximum radiation a nuclear electricity generating plant will emit at the perimeter fence is about .05 mSv per year. A set of dental x-rays will render a dose of about .05-.1 mSv. A CT scan will can render a dose of about 10 mSv—*making a CT scan a hundred to a thousand times the dose of an x-ray*.

A grand electromagnetic human self-experiment is unfolding. Unsuspecting humans and animals are the subjects of this experiment. The findings will be available in a decade or two from now.

Most researchers are quick to say gamma rays—from radon and other natural sources—produce significantly more radiation than do appliances. This might be true for someone with a minimal amount of electrical appliances who rarely visits the hospital and dentist's office.

The question that persists is whether humankind's synthetic "non-ionizing radiation" is as innocuous as is currently assumed.

Do Power Lines Cause Cancer?

The American Physical Society, an association of 43,000 physicists, said in a 1995 National Policy (95.2) statement, "....*no consistent significant link between cancer and power line fields....*" This statement was reaffirmed by the APS council in April of 2005.

Power lines emit electromagnetic radiation at ELF or *extra low frequency* levels. Power lines typically release about 50 hertz of pulsed radiation. As an electric current moves through a wire or appliance, magnetic fields move perpendicular with electricity in a cross pattern.

Electricity fields form from voltage while magnetic fields rise and break away from the electronic waveform's motion. While electricity voltage can shock us or burn the body, magnetic fields have more subtle yet lasting influences upon the body's natural biowave systems—such as brainwaves, neurotransmitter release, hormone production, and so on.

Magnetic influences are difficult to perceive directly, it is apparent they may substantially interrupt our immune systems. Between 1970 and 2000, about fourteen international studies analyzed the potential link between power lines and cancer among children. Eight of those studies showed a link between cancer rates and power line proximity, while four studies associated power lines with leukemia.

One of the U.S. studies to show a positive link in between cancer took place in 1979 in Denver, led by Dr. Nancy Wertheimer and Ed Leeper. This studied showed a more than double likelihood of cancer among children living within forty meters of a high-voltage line.

Another Denver study published in 1988 (Savitz *et al.*) also found a 1.54x odds ratio (OR) positive link in all childhood cancers and high power lines.

A Danish study (Olsen *et al.* 1993) also linked general cancer rates (1.5 OR) with power line proximity.

A study done in Los Angeles (London *et al.* 1991) showed a 2.15 OR rate, a Swedish study (Feychting and Ahlbom 1992) showed a 3.8 OR risk and a Mexican (Fajardo-Gutierrez *et al.* 1993) study showed 2.63 OR increased rate of leukemia cancer rates among children with close proximity to high-voltage power lines.

One Swedish study (Tomenius 1986) showed a 3.7 OR increased risk for central nervous system tumors among children living close to power lines. The Danish study mentioned above also showed a 5.6 OR increased potential of all cancers among children. The other positive link studies showed rates above 1 to 1.5 OR, which are not considered by mainstream science to be statistically significant.

Following the release of these studies, a number of governments took steps to warn housing developers of the potential risks of building close to high frequency power line hubs. In some municipalities across Europe and the U.S., building departments have even taken steps to dissuade or ban developments close to larger power lines.

Adult power line studies have yet to illustrate as large a correlation between power line proximity and cancer rates. Still a few have been significant enough to confirm the need for concern. Werthheimer and Leeper's (1982) studies showed increased rates of all cancers. Still, this 1.28 OR rate was not considered that significant.

However a U.K. study (McDowall 1986) showed a SMR 215 increased rate of lung cancer and a SMR 143 increased risk (SMR 100 or less = no risk) of leukemia. Another study in the U.K (Youngson 1991) showed a statistically insignificant 1.29 OR rate for leukemia and lymphoma and Feychting and Ahlbom's (1992) Swedish study showed a 1.7 OR risk for leukemia subtypes. Another significant study (Schreiber *et al.* 1993) showed a SMR=469 rate for Hodgkin's disease.

It must be noted that these studies are epidemiological. They are population studies where groups living in close-proximity to high frequency power lines are compared with groups living further away. The problems that can occur with these studies focusing on cancer are several.

In cancer pathology, there can be a two to twenty year delay between exposure and cancer diagnosis. While some of the populations involved in these studies might have been living in a particular house for many years, most may have only lived there for a year or two at the most.

In addition, some of the studies limited the disease group population, restricting the usefulness of the information. Cancer is seen primarily in the elderly and middle-aged, where there may be a host of various different types of exposures. These would include smoking, alcohol consumption, job-related exposures, chemical toxins, and so on.

For this reason, these studies can be difficult to weigh against the costs of preventing exposure. The economic issues involving power lines are quite substantial. Relocating schools and families away from high-voltage lines or even relocating power lines comes with a substantial economic cost.

Nonetheless, this is increasingly becoming a problem for both home-owners and utility companies. For example, in the mid-nineties, the New Jersey Assembly enacted legislation requiring disclosure from homebuilders of vicinity transmission lines in excess of 240 kilovolts (kV). Other states have followed with real estate disclosure laws for power lines. Lawsuits have followed on power line proximity issues between schools, buyers, builders and utility companies.

One of the problems existing with some of the power line studies is the comparable limits of the distances between households and power lines. For example, is the effect of a transformer 40 meters away significantly different from one 50 meters away?

Another difficulty with these epidemiological power line studies is that some of the studies measured utility wire codes (wire thickness) and distance, while other studies used spot physical measurements to determine exposure levels. In addition, there has been a variance of controls related to whether the child was born in the house or moved there recently.

With regard to the significance of the leukemia studies, we should consider the incidence of leukemia among the childhood population—close to 1 in 10,000. A 2 or 3 OR among a group, unless the size of the groups are in the millions (most of the studies were significantly smaller—in the thousands), would relate to only a small handful of disease cases over the entire study population. If the study group size was five or ten million, then these numbers might be considered more reliable.

As the increased rates have been smaller (rather than the 4 or 5 OR rate that appears in many study groups) then the size of the disease group is not considered to be a significant factor with which to judge the quality of the study. To this point, D'Arcy Holman, a professor at the University of Western Australia, calculated that the UK studies' worst projections might mean one extra childhood leukemia death in Western Australia every fifty years (Chapman 2001).

Occupational studies regarding exposure to EMR have shown unclear results with regard to leukemia and cancer (Kheifets *et al.* 2008). However, studies have pointed to the increased risk of amyotrophic lateral sclerosis (ALS) due to EMR exposure (Johansen 2004).

Studies on electricians, electric utility line workers and other electrical workers have consistently showed higher rates of leukemia and central nervous system-related cancers. In a 2006 meta-study of fourteen studies by Garcia *et al.* (2008), Alzheimer's disease was associated with chronic occupational EMR exposure.

One of the difficulties with assessing the data on EMR effects is the sheer volume of studies of different types that has been published over the past twenty years. The breadth of variances between the studies of plants, animals, and human response to various degrees of radiation is substantial. Because of this huge base of studies, most researchers have been forced to rely upon various reviews by publications and government agencies to assess the implications of this large base of varying research.

These groups have assessed and compared studies to figure out whether there is a correlation between study results, and whether they are significant.

Government-sponsored reviews have included the United Kingdom's National Radiological Protection Board, the Associated Universities of Oak Ridge, the French National Institute of Health and Medical Research; councils in Denmark, Sweden, Australia and Canada together with U.S. agencies such as the Environmental Protection Agency and the Department of Transportation.

In addition, the U.S. National Council on Radiation Protection and Measurements and the US National Academy of Sciences have also put together major reports on EMR research.

A number of respected journals have published reviews of EMR research as well. While some of these studies have found some epidemiological evidence notable, few found conclusive results, and some have presented skeptical views of any significant positive pathological correlation with non-ionizing EMR exposure. Multiple reviews were also presented (Savitz 1993) in *Environmental Health Perspectives.* No interaction mechanism between power line EMRs and biological organisms was determined.

An electrical field is substantially different a magnetic field. An electrical field is generated when there is a charge differential between two terminating points, regardless of whether current runs between them. An electric light bulb will still generate an electric field even when it is turned off. This electrical field allows alternating current to run between the two points when the switch is eventually turned on.

A magnetic field is created by a current flowing with electricity. The magnetic field will be emitted outward with perpendicular orientation to the electrical field. However, because magnetic fields have a particular polarity or direction, a current flowing in the opposite direction placed next to the current wire will cancel the magnetic field.

Most power cords with double wires (hot and ground for a circuit loop) effectively cancel the magnetic field of the incoming current directly related to the distance between the wires. An increase in this separation increases the strength of the magnetic field. This occurs in power lines, where conductors are typically separated by poles and shields for fire protection.

For these reasons, excessive magnetic fields are considered to have the greatest potential for harm. The level of potential harm are thought to be related directly to the distance from the generating source, the distance between other conductors, the size of the coils on the transformer (if any) and of course the amount of current flowing through the system.

It is generally accepted that the relative magnetic field strength halves with the amount of distance from the line. In other words, a line 100-foot away will have one-quarter of the magnetic field strength of a line 50-feet away.

Li *et al.* (1997), after testing 407 residences in northern Taiwan ranging from 50 meters to 150 meters from high-voltage power lines, found that the magnetic fields at the houses ranged from .93 mG for 50 meters to between

.51 and .55 milliGauss for residences under 149 meters, and .29 mG for residences beyond 149 meters.

This data is somewhat contradicted by a 1993 cohort study from the Netherlands that revealed magnetic field intensities, ranging from 1 to 11 milliGauss from two kilovolt power lines connecting to one transformer substation (Schreiber 1993).

Higher voltage wires are typically thought to be an issue because the voltage and speed is boosted to travel longer distances. With a high-speed voltage line comes an increase in magnetic field. Magnetic fields have been connected with decreased melatonin secretion (Brainard *et al.* 1999). A number of studies have linked lower melatonin levels with higher incidence of a number of types of cancers. It would thus seem probable that since lower melatonin levels are associated with higher voltage, high-speed power lines could well be a mechanism for cancer (Ravindra 2006).

In comparison, a typical house or office will range from .8 to 1 mG in magnetic fields. The magnetic field strength from a kitchen appliance at close range for a person working in the kitchen is significantly greater than the strength coming from power lines 50-100 feet away.

Stepping a few feet away from a microwave oven will dramatically reduce this field strength, while that same relative power line reduction will require a more significant change.

A typical microwave oven might cause a field strength of 1,000 mG, which can be reduced to a minimal 1 mG by stepping a few feet away. Moving ones house further away from a power line obviously requires a significant commitment to the reduction of magnetic field strength, and a few feet will not make a significant difference.

Epidemiological studies involving electrical appliances have been limited. They are more difficult because of the control parameters. Nonetheless, a few appliances have undergone controlled studies over the years. Electric blankets have undergone several studies. Some of these illustrated significantly increased risk factors for postmenopausal cancer (Vena *et al.* 1991), testicular cancer (Verreault 1990), and congenital defects (Dlugosz 1992).

Radio Waves

Radiofrequency waves range from about 3 hertz to 300 gigahertz. This means their waves travel from speeds of 3 cycles per second up to 3,000,000 cycles per second.

Extremely low frequency (ELF=3-30 Hz) and *super low frequency* (SLF=30-300 Hz) broadcasting has primarily been used for submarine communications, as these wavelengths transmit well through the water. This is also the frequency range that sound waves travel.

Ultra low frequency (ULF=300-3000 Hz) has primarily been used in mines, where the waves can penetrate the depths. Above these levels, *very low frequency* and *low frequency* (VLF and LF = 3-300 kHz) have been used by beacons, heart rate monitors, navigation and time signaling.

Medium frequency (300-3000 kHz) radio waves are typically used for AM broadcasts, while *high frequency* (HF = 3-30 MHz) is used primarily for short-wave and amateur radio broadcasting.

Very high frequency (VHF = 30-300 MHz) waves are used for FM radio, television and aircraft communications while *ultra high frequency* (UHF = 300-3000 MHz) waves are used for certain television ranges, but also cell phones, wireless LAN, GPS, Bluetooth and many two-way radios. While often considered outside the radio spectrum, *super high frequency* (SHF = 3-30 GHz) waves are used in microwave devices, some LAN wireless systems and radar.

Extremely high frequency (EHF = 30-300 GHz) is used for long-range systems such as microwave radio and astronomy radio systems. The audio frequencies are primarily ELF through VLF brands, covering 20-20,000 Hz.

Note that EMR wavelengths inversely vary to their frequency. For naturally occurring EMR such as sunlight, the frequency will equal the speed of light divided by the wavelength. Thus, an ULF wave can range from 10,000 and 100,000 kilometers long. An UHF wave will range from one meter to ten millimeters in length, while an ELF wavelength will range from one millimeter and ten millimeters long.

Adulterated radiofrequencies have been utilized by humans for only about the last seventy-five years. Early use was primarily for radio transmission, while during the past few decades, various communication and signaling systems have been developed that utilize radiofrequencies. Radiofrequencies are generated with alternating current fed through an antenna at particular speeds and wavelengths.

Studies on radiofrequency radiation proximity at work have also studied possible reproductive and cardiovascular effects. Many of the reports are inconclusive. But there have been positive correlations between radiofrequency exposure and delayed conception (Larsen *et al.* 1991), spontaneous abortion (Quellet-Hellstrom and Steward 1993; Taskinen *et al.* 1990), stillbirth (Larsen *et al.* 1991), preterm birth after father exposure (Larsen *et al.* 1991), and birth defects (Larson 1991).

However, many of these results have either not been replicated or remain uncorroborated. Three studies examined male military personnel exposure to microwaves and radar (Hjollund *et al.* 1997; Lancranjan *et al.* 1975; Weyandt *et al.* 1996). All three found reductions in sperm density.

A number of animal studies have illustrated adverse health effects from radio waves but doubt has been raised regarding the dose comparison with humans. In one study, GSM phone frequency radio waves caused the cell death of about 2% of rat brains.

Researchers hypothesized that the blood-brain barrier was being penetrated by the radiation (Salford 2003). This was correlated by three earlier studies that reported blood-brain barrier penetration with radio wave exposure (Shivers *et al.* 1987; Prato *et al.* 1990; Schirmacher *et al.* 2000). For several years following the release of this last study, other studies could not replicate the findings, nor could they establish a confirmation of the permeation of the blood-brain-barrier from radiofrequencies (Kuribayashi 2005; others).

However, Shivers and colleagues, and Prato and associates had previously determined the effect of magnetic resonance imaging upon the rat brain. They showed that the exposure to radiofrequencies combined with pulsed and static magnetic fields gave rise to a significant pinocytotic transport of albumin from the capillaries into the brain.

Rates of breast cancer, endometrial cancer, testicular cancer and lung cancer have been studied with close range radiofrequency radiation, primarily in occupational settings. Slightly positive correlations with endometrial cancer (Cantor *et al.* 1995) and male breast cancer (Demers *et al.* 1991) were found.

A potential link between testicular cancer and radiofrequency radiation from traffic radar guns, particularly among a small group of police officers (Davis and Mostofi 1993) was also established. Slightly increased ocular melanoma was established among occupational radiofrequency exposure (Holly *et al.* 1996) in another small group.

French and Canadian utility workers were found to have an increased likelihood of lung cancer (Armstrong *et al.* 1994).

Cell phone tower radiofrequencies are popular concerns. The first cell phones communicated with analog frequencies of 450 or 900 megahertz, for example. By the 1990s, cell phones were using 1800 megahertz, and various modulation systems. Now the Universal Mobile Telecommunication System is adhered to, which uses 1900 to 2200 megahertz.

In 2000, over 80,000 cell tower base stations were in use in the United States. By 2006, this number was estimated at 175,000. CTIA, the International Association for Wireless Telecommunications Industry, estimates that by 2010 there will be about 260,000 towers.

These base stations transmit radio waves using around 100 watts of power. The range of GSM towers is about 40 kilometers, while the CDMA and iDEN technologies offer ranges of 50 to 70 kilometers. This obviously is relative to terrain. In a hilly area, the range can be a few kilometers.

In populated areas, cell base towers are placed from one to two miles apart, while in urban areas they can be as close together as a quarter of a mile. Some cell phone bases are mounted on primary towers, and some are built onto elevated structures such as buildings and hillsides.

A base cell tower antenna is comprised of a transmitter(s), a receiver(s)—often called transceivers—an electrical power source, and various digital signal processors. The circuits will utilize copper, fiber, or microwave connections.

They may be connected to the network via T1, E1, T3 and/or Ethernet connections. They are typically strung together through base station controllers and radio network controllers, typically connected to a switched telephone network system. The radio network controller will connect to the SGSN network.

There has been scant research on the risks of radiofrequency waves from radio stations or television stations. The primary reason for this appears to be that most of these have been located outside of densely populated areas, on high towers enabling greater ranges. Cell towers have created more concern because of their close proximity and relatively lower heights.

Research has suggested that exposure from cell towers is reduced by a factor of one to one hundred times inside of a building, depending upon the building materials and style of the building. However, exposure also increases with height. Upper floors can have substantially greater exposure levels than lower floors (Schuz and Mann 2000). Whether this is a factor of pure height or whether the earth provides a buffering factor is not known.

Exposure levels in regions surrounding cell towers will range from .01 to .1% of ISNIRP (International Commission on Non-Ionizing Radiation Protection) permitted levels for general public exposure directly around the station, to .1 to 1% of ISNIRP permitted levels between 100 meters and 200 meters from the tower.

Beyond the 200-meter level, the exposure returns to the .01 to .1% level and reduces as the range increases. It should be noted also that exposure levels from cell phone towers are not substantially greater than exposure levels of radiofrequencies (RF) emitted by radio broadcasting towers. In one Australian study, the greatest level found was .2% (Henderson 2006).

In a 2006 randomized double-blind study performed at the Institute of Pharmacology and Toxicology at the University of Zurich (Regel *et al.*) in Switzerland, UMTS signals approximating the strength of a cell phone tower emission were tested on 117 healthy human subjects, 33 of which reported themselves as sensitive to cell towers and 84 as non-sensitive.

Physiological analyses included organ-specific tests, cognitive tests, and well-being questionnaires. Apparently, significant negative physiological or cognitive results were not found, although there appeared to be a marginal effect on one of the cognitive tests for each of the two groups. Because the difference was slight, and each group (sensitive versus control) had different results, this effect was considered insignificant.

In 2006, the British medical journal (Rubin *et al.*) reported a study done at the King's College in London, which tested 60 self-reported sensitive people and 60 control subjects with no reported sensitivities.

Six different symptoms such as headaches were tracked, and subjects took questionnaires in an attempt to find whether the sensitive subjects could successfully judge whether a cell tower signal was on or off. While 60% of the sensitive subjects believed the tower signals were on when they were on, 63% believed the tower signals to be on when they were indeed off.

There have also been several international studies done on radiofrequency transmissions from masts. Tests in the United States, Britain, Australia and the Vatican City have shown no or low correlation between RF levels and health effects, rendering these studies for the most part, inconclusive. One study in the Netherlands using simulated mobile phone base station transmissions did conclude, however, that the UMTS-like spectrum of cell transmission might have an adverse affect upon the well-being of questionnaire respondents.

In July of 2007, an independent team of researchers (Eltiti *et al.*) from the University of Essex reported findings from a three-year double-blind study using a special laboratory to test potential cell phone tower effects. The study included 44 people who reported sensitivity to cell phone towers and 114 healthy people who had not. The study measured various physiological factors like skin conductance, blood pressure and heart rate while being exposed (or not) to 3G tower signals.

During periods where the researcher and the subject knew the signals were on, sensitive people reported feeling worse, and their physiological factors were affected negatively. However when neither the subjects nor the researchers knew the cell tower signals were on during a series of tests, there was no difference between either the sensitive or non-sensitive subjects with regard to physiological factors.

Only two of the forty-four sensitive subjects were able to guess the cell tower signals being on correctly while five of the control subjects (non-sensitive) were able to guess correctly. Subjects who reported sensitivities to cell phone towers prior to the study reported negative symptoms more often, regardless of whether the cell tower transmitters were on or off.

Cell Phones

Typically, a digital cell phone operates at a power range of about .25 watts, while the newest digital phones might transmit as low as .09 watts. Analog phones were much higher power transmitters. The exposure level of a cell phone will depend greatly upon the way the phone is designed.

The location of the antenna and the power supply/battery will typically govern the strength of the transmission to the dermal layers of the skin. The further away the antenna is from dermal contact (hand or ear), the less exposure.

The orientation of the power supply will also govern exposure. Some phones have shielding between the power supply and the antenna and earpiece. This is thought to reduce dermal exposure. In other words, the manner of carrying and holding the phone will vary the exposure.

There is another factor called *adaptive power*. When a cell phone is further away from a tower, or in a moving car, it will typically increase its internal transceiver power to send and receive signals. This increases the level of electromagnetic exposure as the phone is boosting power and transmissions.

EMR cell phone exposure is thus typically less out of doors than indoors, because there is less interference from building materials out of doors. In addition, exposure to radio waves is greatest on the side of the head the phone is most used and closest to where the antenna is located (Dimbylow and Mann 1994).

Radiofrequencies from handset use have been confirmed to heat the ear canal. In one controlled study of 30 individuals, 900 MHz and 1800 MHz phones against the ear for more than 35 minutes resulted in an increase of 1.2-1.3 degrees F (Tahvanainen *et al.* 2007). Other studies have confirmed this effect. For this reason there has been a great concern regarding the potential for tumor development either in the brain or in the areas surrounding the ears—referred to as an *acoustic neurinoma.*

Adverse effects of tissue temperature rise are not clear, but it is thought that the body's thermoregulation mechanisms may create an increased immune burden on the body. Lab studies have suggested a one-centigrade temperature rise at the tissue level will have immunosuppressive effects (Goldstein *et al.* 2003).

The International Agency for Research into Cancer has sponsored studies in thirteen countries to study the line between cell phone usage and cancer. So far, Australia, Canada, Denmark, Finland, France, Germany, Israel, Italy, Japan, New Zealand, Norway, Sweden and Britain have participated. Through 2005, the research tracked 6,000 glioma and meningioma cases (brain tumors), 1,000 acoustic neurinoma cases and 600 parotid gland cancers.

Of these, the acoustic neurinoma results, primarily from Sweden, showed a significant link with handset use—from both cell phones and cordless phones. The German study also revealed a significant link between uveal melanoma and unspecified handset use. Other types of tumors had OR levels of around or just above 1 to 1.7 OR. The 2001 Swedish study on all brain tumors found a 2.4 OR link with **ipsilateral cancer**—more prevalent on the same side of primary handset use.

Again, we are faced with the fact that many of these associations are occurring at between 1 and 3 OR. A 2 or 3 level OR risk level creates questions in the minds of meta and review researchers. This should be combined with the fact that the rates of these tumors are so small among the general population (10-15 per 100,000 per year) for malignant brain tumors (Behin *et al.* 2003). Additionally, there is often a ten-year or more delay from exposure to diagnosis. This gives some researchers a myriad of reasons to question even the better correlations between cell phones and cancer.

Other researchers firmly disagree, stating that the weaker evidence is actually enhanced by the cancer diagnosis delay. Research from the Japanese nuclear victims of World War II has shown that many cancers arise ten to twenty years and more after the initial exposure. If we extrapolate this with cell phone use, we estimate that because cell phone use among the general population is still within this twenty-year period, especially for many younger adults (who were barely using cell phones five years ago).

This means we should expect to see higher cancer rates among heavy cell phone users within the next five to ten years from now. Possibly this might be ameliorated somewhat by the improved cell phones being made now, with increased shielding (which begs the question; why did they increase the shielding if there was no danger?). Or not. We will see. The grand experiment with EMR rages on.

Our body's natural waveforms include the shorter waves of the brain and nerves, and the weaker biophoton waveforms of the cells, along with the molecular electromagnetic bonding waveforms within DNA. Should electronically driven waveforms interfere with these natural biowaves, the molecular bonding structures of our genetic information could gradually become deranged.

The effects of this interference should appear on a number of fronts. We should see lower cognition levels and brain fog, as unnatural waveforms interfere with our brainwave mapping system. We should see body temperature interference within the basal cell network.

We should see damage to the blood-brain barrier and damage to nerve and brain cells. These effects should release greater levels of radical species from the imbalanced molecular structures—damaging cells and tissues. All of these effects have been documented in the research.

This waveform interference mechanism is illustrated by a study (Thaker *et al.* 2008) showing that a certain popular brand of MP3 player will interfere with the mechanisms of a pacemaker if held close to the chest for about five seconds. Appliance interference has been directly correlated with waveform interference.

This is one reason why the U.S. Federal Communications Commission closely monitors and licenses bandwidths. When we consider that the body maintains various natural biowave "bandwidths" as it cycles hormones, thermoregulation, cortisol, melatonin and the Krebs energy cycle to name a few, it is not difficult to connect the waveform interference of cell phones and other appliances with the disruption of these natural cycles.

The World Health Organization's International Agency for Research on Cancer (IARC) classified radiofrequency (RF) electromagnetism (EMF) as a Group 2B carcinogen in 2011: *"Possibly carcinogenic to humans."*

This was based upon research showing cell phones connected to an increased risk for glioma, a malignant form of brain cancer. Other types of brain cancer included in the research have been meningioma and schwannoma.

However, the Group 2B classification of carcinogen doesn't mean there is a definite link. This has created significant doubt among many agencies and health officials around the world.

Even with this declaration, a number of agencies around the world have announced that cell phones are not linked to cancer. In light of the WHO's classification, this seems to be a hasty conclusion. Especially in light of some 2017 research.

The reason this is a hasty conclusion relates to the delay in cancer diagnosis from the point of causation. Let's use an example. Many people will smoke cigarettes for 20 years or more without necessarily getting lung cancer.

In fact, the link between smoking and lung cancer is delayed. It is a latent link. It takes decades of tobacco use to typically see the resulting lung cancer. For some it might be only a decade, but for many it might be two or three decades before they will get lung, throat or oral cancer.

Apparently, this latency also occurs between cell phone use and brain cancer, especially among adults. Cell phones have only come into our lifestyles in a big way over the past decade or two. So how could a health agency say with certainty that cell phone use isn't linked to an increased risk of cancer so soon in the game?

In fact, most of the epidemiological studies that were reviewed by most of these agencies were done between 2000 and 2010. That barely offers a decade of use.

Later research confirms this hypothesis.

A study from Sweden's Örebro University (Carlberg *et al.* 2017) brought together an ongoing meta-analysis of brain cancer research since 1965. The researchers also conducted this review study in 2013 (Hardell *et al.*) and 2015 (Hardell *et al.*). This research focused upon studies that investigated long-term cell phone use.

The conclusion from the 2013 study was:

"Based on the Hill criteria, glioma and acoustic neuroma should be considered to be caused by RF-EMF emissions from wireless phones and regarded as carcinogenic to humans, classifying it as group 1 according to the IARC classification. Current guidelines for exposure need to be urgently revised."

The "Hill criteria" refers to the World Health Organization's classification of a cancer link. This is based upon a premise proposed by Dr. Bradford Hill to the British Royal Society of Medicine in 1965. This is where the "Group 2B" classification criteria come from.

A study from INSERM and the University of Toronto (Morgan *et al.* 2015) also indicated a revision of the cancer classification for cell phone use, this one from Group 2B ("Possibly carcinogenic to humans") to Group 2A ("Probably carcinogenic").

The Örebro University study included additional research and calculations, which indicated further evidence of a link between brain cancer and cell phone use. These have suggested the new classification should be to Group 1 ("Carcinogenic to humans").

The Swedish researchers reviewed all the earlier research and recalculated the results using the random-effects model. This is a peer-reviewed form meta-analysis now accepted among epidemiology researchers. This utilizes cumulative measures – in the case of cell phone, total estimated hours of phone use – tied to the particular condition to calculate the risk factor.

When the researchers recalculated the shorter-term risk among earlier studies, they found up to a 90 percent increased risk of brain cancer from long-term cell phone use.

When they utilized data from the cell phone companies on hours of cell phone usage to recalculate the risk from a 2011 study, they found that long-term cell phone use increased the risk of brain cancer among children (aged 7 to 19 years old) by more than double (215 percent) for those who had used cell phones for more than 2.8 years.

The researchers combined research for adults between 20 and 80 years old and recalculated the risk. They found an increased risk overall after 10 years. For 1,640 hours of cell phone use, the researchers found the risk of brain cancer more than doubled (218 percent). This was for brain cancers that occur on the same side of the brain as the cell phone is typically used.

The raw research studies these conclusions are drawn from are significant.

For example, a 2014 study from France's INSERM (Coureau *et al.* 2014) tracked 447 brain cancer cases along with 892 matched control subjects. They found that life-long accumulated use almost tripled the risk of gliomas (289 percent) and meningiomas (257 percent). Temporal tumor risk was even higher, and higher for occupational cell phone risk.

A 2015 study from Sweden followed 1,498 brain cancer cases along with 3,530 control subjects. They found that a latency of more than 25 years produced triple the risk of brain cancer (300 percent).

A study from the University of Oxford's International Agency for Research on Cancer (IARC) (Benson *et al.* 2013) – followed 791,710 middle aged-women for seven years – after they reported their cell phone use in 1999, 2005 and 2009. The research discovered 51,680 invasive cancers and 1,261 central nervous system cancers during the period.

Increased meningioma risk was found for long-term use. In addition to this, compared to non-cell phone users, the long-term (10+ years) use of cell phones increased the risk of acoustic neuroma by two-and-a-half times.

According to the research, these risks also increased as cell phone use increased – making the risk "dose-dependent."

When a risk is dose-dependent, it validates the causation element of the study. It means that the longer a person uses the cell phone, the greater the risk.

With regards to meningioma, a study from Swedish researchers published in the *Environmental Health Journal,* also found minimal increased risk from increased cell phone use.

This study tracked 709 meningioma patients and compared them with 1,368 control subject subjects. They compared mobile phone usage among both groups, and analyzed the data using a latency period – the amount of time from tracked usage – of 25 years.

Here the researchers found, once again, little increased risk – but some. And the risk appeared to increase with increased cell phone use.

Two periods of use – between one and five years and over twenty-five years, showed an increased risk of meningioma by 30% among those who used wireless phones over a 25 year period.

In the highest-use quartile, wireless and mobile phone use resulted in a higher risk of meningioma, by 30% for mobile phones and 40% for wireless phones, and 80% increased risk for cordless phone use.

The increased risks was found to be related primarily to those who used their phones equivalent to about 40 minutes a day for 10 years, equated to 2,376 hours of cumulative use.

The researchers stated that:

"There was a statistically significant trend for increasing cumulative use of 3G mobile phones, cordless phones, phones of the digital type (2G, 3G and/or cordless phone), and wireless phones in total."

They also noted that there was more than a seven times increased risk for high-use 3G cell phone use. But this was considered not significant because it was based on only five users.

And previous studies have also exposed this risk among long-time users. As stated in a 2013 review in the *Journal of Pathophysiology*:

"Studies carried out in Sweden indicate that those who begin using either cordless or mobile phones regularly before age 20 have greater than a fourfold increased risk of ipsilateral glioma."

It only makes sense to consider a headset or using the speaker system available on most new cell phones. These provide an increased distance from the source of the radiation, significantly decreasing the risk.

Radon

Radon is another indoor form of radiation worth consideration as a cancer-causing agent. It is estimated that between 12% and 25% of American cancer deaths from lung cancer are caused by radon exposure (Kim *et al.* 2018).

This study concluded:

"These findings suggest that indoor radon exposure contributes considerably to lung cancer, and that reducing indoor radon concentration would be helpful for decreasing the disease burden from lung cancer deaths."

Radon is caused by various soils and rocks from the earth. Increased radon exposure occurs when a house is not properly ventilated, especially in cold weather.

Cold outside weather combined with an unventilated warm indoor environment creates an energy vacuum, drawing radon into the house and keeping it there. Houses without adequate coverage over ground soils may have greater radon exposure.

Radon 222 comes primarily from the nuclear decay of uranium. This natural process takes place within the earth. As this decay proceeds, radon gas is released, together with decay byproducts, called *radon daughters* or *radon progeny*. These particles are known carcinogens. Should we breathe these particles, they can be caught in the lungs. Breathing radon gas delivers the potential of it continuing to decay inside our bodies. This will effectively deposit the radioactive daughters inside our bodies.

The National Council on Radiation Protection and Measurement has developed a maximum safe dosage of radon to be 200 mrem per year.

The relationship between radon and outdoor power lines has not been clearly established, because in order to measure the interaction, an aerosol component (a pollutant of some sort) must accompany the electromagnetic field. Nonetheless, significant *radon daughters* have been measured (Henshaw *et al.* 1998) among power line fields.

The subsequent dose and tolerance of radon particles in the human body is also in question. In some research, heavy electromagnetic fields have been shown to penetrate with no more than about .0001 of the original field strength of radon emissions. Still this penetration effect alerted researchers to the fact that there might be a radon penetration into the lungs and basal tissues of the body (Fews *et al.* 1999).

The link between radon and lung cancer has become more evident in the research. Lung cancer has been the most prevalent form of cancer worldwide since 1985, and has been responsible for more than one million deaths worldwide. The highest rates of lung cancer occurred in 2002 in North America and Northern or Eastern Europe. Although smoking is widely considered to be the primary etiology of lung cancer, uranium miners—who are exposed to increased levels of radon along with dust—experience higher rates of lung cancer (Tomasek *et al.* 2008). Epidemiological studies on radon-exposure and miners have also revealed that thousands of miners die per year of radon exposure (Field *et al.* 2006).

Research has illustrated that while living outdoors does not increase ones risk of lung cancer, unnatural living or working quarters without enough ventilation can lead to a drawing in and encapsulation of radon radiation. A household with poor ventilation poses a higher risk of radon exposure than a well-ventilated house.

Research has illustrated that ventilation around electromagnetic current exposure is an absolute requirement because of a release of radon daughters into the immediate atmosphere (Karpin 2005).

Darby *et al.* (2005) reported in the *British Medical Journal* on a collaborative analysis of thirteen case studies of 7,148 lung cancer cases together with 14,208 control subjects. This found that increased radon exposure is responsible for about 2% of European cancer deaths. Further research has revealed that most buildings, especially work environments that are full of various power lines and equipment, retain higher levels of radon. Radon levels are additionally increased with unventilated soils, higher air temperatures and higher atmospheric levels. Higher household radon levels are particularly associated with leaking and unventilated soils in the house. This research has caused legislation in many states in the U.S. requiring property sellers to disclose known radon issues.

The majority of our everyday radiation input comes from radon. Natural concentrations of radon are found in some granites, limestones and sandstones. Higher radon levels come from disturbed ground. Disturbing the normal landscape allows more permeability, allowing the release of the normally contained daughters. Once a house is built upon disturbed ground, the radon can come in through cracked foundations and spaces around piping and wiring.

Because radon gas is pulled in through pressure changes within the house created by temperature gradients, it is important that our houses be well ventilated. This is particularly significant during the nighttime and during cold weather, as the warmer temperatures inside with colder temperatures outside cause the most pressure differential—the *Bernoulli effect.*

Ventilation will not only allow the escape of indoor radon gas, but it will release some of this pressure, resulting in a lower draw of radon gas into the house.

Household radon levels tend to increase dramatically during the winter, and decrease substantially during the summer for these reasons. Radon levels also go up dramatically during the nighttime hours, as the outdoor temperature cools. This is when ventilation is most important. Disturbed landscaping ground can also leak increased radon daughters.

The U.S. Environmental Protection Agency has recommended safe levels of radon to be 4 *picocuries of radon per liter* (pCi/L). Levels any higher than this should be remedied by cementing over the exposed ground or sealing cracks in current cement foundations. Ventilation systems have also been known to help. Radon detection kits are quite inexpensive and easy to use.

Magnetic Fields

Nature's magnetic fields surround us, and pose little threat. Many species utilize nature's magnetic fields to navigate migration and nesting. In other words, our cells are tuned to the geomagnetic fields of the sun and the earth.

Synthetic magnetic fields, on the other hand, are dispersed with the distribution of unnatural alternating current. The proliferation of electricity and electrical appliances created by power-generating plants that convert nature's kinetic energy into alternating current has deluged our atmosphere with unnatural magnetism.

Most early research on the health effects of electrical appliances and wires focused on the electrical fields and ignored the magnetic fields given off by appliances. While most electrical fields are shielded by insulators within most appliances, magnetic fields can be more disruptive and insidious to the health of the body. This is because they can directly interfere with the body's internal biowaves. Normally, synchronic and harmonic biowaves—including brainwaves, nerve firings, and so on—travel with synchronicity throughout the body.

A magnetic field surrounding the body can induce an abnormal electrical current flow within the body. In a Swedish study (Wilen *et al.* 2004) of RF operators exposed to high levels of magnetic fields, currents were induced within the body at mean levels of 101 mA and maximum levels of one Amp. During this study, exposure levels correlated positively with the prevalence of fatigue, headaches, warm sensations in the hands, slower heart rates and more bradycardia episodes among the subjects.

In a study done by the Fred Hutchinson Cancer Research Center and the Epidemiology Division of Public Health Services in Seattle, Washington (Davis *et al.* 2001), 203 women aging from 20-74 years with no breast cancer history were studied between 1994 and 1996. Magnetic field and ambient light in the bedroom were measured for a 72-hour period during two seasons of the year. Urine samples were taken on three consecutive nights for each subject. After adjusting for hours of daylight, older age, higher body mass, alcohol use and medication use, those women with higher bedroom levels of magnetic fields had lower concentrations of 6-sulfatoxy-melatonin. It was thus concluded that increased levels of synthetic magnetic fields depress nocturnal melatonin.

While this illustrates how unnatural magnetism can significantly affect the body's biochemical rhythms, reduced melatonin also causes negative effects throughout the body. Over several decades since melatonin was discovered in 1958 by Dr. Aaron Lerner and his Yale colleagues, decreased melatonin levels have been linked to a variety of pathologies and immune function deficiencies.

A three milliGauss magnetic field at 60 Hertz will induce about one-billionth amp per square centimeter of the body. A magnetic field at 120 Hz frequency will have double the current effect the same field will have at 60 Hz. A typical American office building or home—filled with various electrical appliances—will contain magnetic fields at levels between .8 and 1 milliGauss.

In a study done at a Canadian school by Akbar-Khanzadeh in 2000, workers, schoolteachers and administrative staff environments had magnetic field exposure levels ranging from .2 to 7.1 mG.

MilliGauss levels will be substantially higher in instrument-heavy environments. Hood *et al.* (2000) recorded the pilot's cockpits of a Boeing 767 with magnetic field levels of 6.7 milliGauss, while the Boeing 737 recorded at 12.7 mG of magnetic field strength. Nicholas *et al.* (1998) documented a mean magnetic field strength of 17 mG among the cockpits of B737, B757,

DC9 and L1011 planes. Meanwhile, cabin measurements ranged from a high of 8 mG in the forward serving areas to 6 mG in the first class seats and 3 mG in the economy seats.

Rail maintenance workers experience magnetic field levels from 3 to 18 mG (Wenzl 1997). In a study published in the *Journal of the Canadian Dental Association* (Bohay *et al.* 1994), dental operating rooms with various ultrasonic scalars, amalgamators, and x-ray equipment revealed magnetic fields ranging from 1.2 to 2225 mG, with equipment distances from zero to thirty centimeters.

Most of these magnetic field readings were accompanied by lower level radiation frequencies ranging from 25 hertz to 100 hertz (though the airline cockpits research recorded up to 800 hertz).

In a population study of 969 women in San Francisco, miscarriage levels positively correlated with higher magnetic field exposure. Li *et al.* (2002) concluded that fields in the region of 16 mG or higher produced the greatest risk of miscarriage.

While higher levels of magnetic fields have been shown not to significantly affect nervous system biowaves such as cardiac pacemakers (Graham *et al.* 2000), 12 milliGauss magnetic fields operating from radiation frequencies of 60 hertz were shown to block the inhibition of human breast cancer cells by both melatonin and tamoxifen *in vitro*.

Melatonin and Tamoxifen have different mechanisms of retarding cancer growth, it was confirmed by Harland and Liburdy (1997) that synthetic magnetic fields prevented their immunity effects. When we consider that the magnetic fields blocked the immune activities of *both* biochemicals—which work within different mechanisms—the affect of synthetic magnetic fields on the human body illustrates an *immune system magnetic interference* model.

This magnetic field interference model of electromagnetic exposure is further supported by research published in 2002 by Saunders and Jefferys. Brain tissue testing showed that even very low frequency electric and weak magnetic field exposure will induce electric fields and currents inside the body. These fields excited various nerve cells and retinal cells, inducing abnormal metabolic activity.

The immune system magnetic interference model mechanism is further confirmed by a study of magnetic and electric fields on neural cells by Blackman (1993). While magnetic fields stimulated abnormal neurite outgrowth between 22 and 40 mG, increased electric fields did not stimulate the same morphological change.

In contrast, the natural magnetic field strength of the earth ranges from about .2 gauss to .6 gauss (200-600 mG)—often also measured as .05 Tesla (1 Tesla=10,000 gauss). To give some reference with nature's levels, an MRI magnet will range from one to three Tesla, or 10,000 to 30,000 gauss. This is equivalent to 10,000,000-30,000,000 mG.

Appliance Magnetic Fields

Appliance	At 4 Inches	At 1 Foot	At 3 Feet
Blenders	50-220	5.2-1.7	.3-1.1
Can openers	1300-4000	31-280	.5-7.0
Clothes dryers	4.8-110	1.5-29	.1-1
Coffee makers	6-29	.9-1.2	<.1
Crock pots	8-23	.8-1.3	<.1
Electric drills	350-500	22-31	.8-2.0
Electric shavers	14-1600	.8-90	<.1-3.3
Faust blowers	3-120	.25-37	<.1-3.1
Fluorescent desk lamps	100-200	6-20	.2-2.1
Fluorescent fixtures	40-123	2-32	<.1-2.8
Hair dryers	3-1400	<.1-70	<.1-2.8
Irons	12-45	1.2-3.1	.1-.2
Microwave ovens*	39-75	2.7-6	.18-.75
Mixers	58-1400	5-100	.15-2.0
Portable heaters	11-280	1.5-40	.1-2.5
Saber and circular saws	200-2100	8-210	.2-10.0
Televisions	4.8-100	.4-20	<.1-1.5
Toasters	10-60	.6-7.0	<.1-.11
Vacuum cleaners	230-1300	20-180	1.2-18.0

Source: Gauger, 1985 *Gauger 1997 (at 3.6, 10.8 and 25.2 in)

CT Scans

A study published in the *New England Journal of Medicine* from the Columbia University Medical Center (Brenner *et al.* 2007) showed that a third of CT scans are unnecessary. The authors also estimated that between one and two percent of all cancers are caused by CT scan radiation exposure. A CT scan will can render a dose of about 10 mSv—*making a CT scan between a hundred and a thousand times the dose of an x-ray.*

In contrast, the maximum radiation a nuclear electricity generating plant will emit at the perimeter fence is about .05 mSv per year. A set of dental x-rays will render a dose of about .05-.1 mSv.

According to a New York Times article (Bogdanich and McGinty 2011), hospitals ordered two CT scans for 80 percent of their Medicare patients. The average rate of double-CT Scans is typically 1%, according to the report.

Teaching hospitals at medical schools, meanwhile, rarely if ever order double CT scans. The growth in CT scans over the past decades has been astronomical. About sixty-two million CT scans are now given a year in the U.S., as opposed to about three million per year in 1980.

Blue Lights at Night

Light is a form of radiation too. It is part of the visible spectrum of radiation that when it interacts with certain cells of the eyes, produces an image. Within the visible light spectrum there are a number of wavelengths. Some are more healthy than others. One of those spectra – blue light – has been implicated in cancer.

Breast cancer and prostate cancer risk is significantly increased by more exposure to more city lights at night according to scientists. This apparently relates exposure to outdoor blue light from city lights to an increased risk of cancer.

Blue light is part of the spectrum of light that comes from the sun. This form of blue light is healthy for us during the day. These blue light wavelengths boost our cortisol levels and make us more awake and energized.

But during the night, blue light has a downside. Because blue light stimulates cortisol levels, it can negatively affect our ability to relax and sleep at night. Nighttime blue light during sleep hours can reduce our REM-stage sleep, which is critical to our brain function and our hormones.

This is why using a computer late at night can harm our sleep. And using a smartphone late at night can also harm our sleep. Night use of smartphones and using computers at night expose us to significant blue light wavelengths.

Typical light bulbs also produce significant blue light, but LED (light-emitting diodes) lights emit a significantly greater level of blue light wavelengths compared to conventional light bulbs.

This is why city lights expose us to a significant amount of blue light. City lights utilize a lot of LED because it shines brighter, attracting our attention more readily. LED lights also tend to utilize less power for their light emission, which can be a good thing when we consider power consumption.

As blue light enters our eyes, it stimulates our hippocampus and pineal gland. This in turn stimulates the production of cortisol and a reduction of melatonin. Because melatonin balances our body's nighttime hormones, this produces an imbalance of our other hormone levels.

These hormone level imbalances, researchers have found, puts us at a greater risk of breast cancer and prostate cancer.

A study from the Barcelona Institute for Global Health (Garcia-Saenz *et al.* 2018) used data from 23 hospitals in 12 regions of Spain and studied more than 4,000 people. This study effectively included 1,218 cases of breast cancer and 623 prostate cancer cases. The researchers analyzed the behaviors of these patients along with 1,385 women control subjects and 879 male control subjects.

The researchers analyzed their lives with respect to their exposure of light during times that would be considered sleep time. They excluded subjects that worked at night so the study could offer a clear comparison between nighttime sleepers, which most of us are.

The researchers also utilized satellite data to include the exposure to city night lights. City light exposure also emits primarily blue light as discussed above.

The researchers found that greater exposure to outdoor blue light during sleep time hours increased the risk of prostate cancer by more than double.

And those women with greater exposure to outdoor blue light at night had a 1.5 times increased incidence of breast cancer.

Prostate cancer was found to be particularly sensitive to blue light in general. Those men whose bedrooms contained more light had nearly three times (2.8) times the incidence of cancer compared to those with bedrooms that were dark.

For those who live in the countryside, we can readily understand how being in the city at night can change our hormone levels. Going to the city at night will expose our eyes to tremendous levels of very bright LED lights. These include street lights and blinking neon storefront signs. Most of us will immediately sense a feeling of heightened energy and alertness as we walk through a brightly-lit city at night.

As mentioned above, this alertness comes from the eyes and pineal gland being exposed to the intense blue wavelengths of the city lights at night. The exposure will boost our body's levels of cortisol, increasing our energy levels.

But as stated above, the downside is that when cortisol is boosted, melatonin levels are reduced. This also has other effects upon other male hormones, unbalancing androgen levels.

This is confirmed by a study (Yu *et al.* 2018) that found melatonin helps balance levels of testosterone and other androgens in the testes and prostate. The researchers stated:

"Melatonin acts as a local modulator of the endocrine activity in Leydig cells. In Sertoli cells, melatonin influences cellular proliferation and energy metabolism and, consequently, can regulate steroidogenesis."

Melatonin also specifically helps block cancer cells from growing.

In a study from Italy's Research University of Milano (Calastretti *et al.* 2018) medical scientists studied the effects of melatonin on breast cancer cells and prostate cancer cells. The researchers found that melatonin specifically inhibits the growth of cancer cells among both breast and prostate cells.

City lights and bright night light in general will reduce the body's natural production of melatonin. And it is this form of natural melatonin – not necessarily synthetic melatonin – that helps our bodies prevent cancer from growing.

This research is also consistent with other studies that have found that night owls tend to die earlier and tend to have more inflammatory conditions.

This points to the reality that night lights in general increase our risk of cancer and affect our health negatively, related to getting a good night's sleep. Good sleep habits naturally encourage healthy melatonin levels.

The Sun

By far, the predominant form of radiation we all deal with is the sun. Most cancer researchers agree that the sun's radiation can cause some forms of skin cancer. But is this absolute? Are there mitigating factors?

110

Many cases of melanoma occur on skin rarely if ever exposed to the sun. This is despite the chorus of conventional medicine that states that the sun is the primary cause of melanoma.

Furthermore, we find that melanoma rates are often lower in regions where year-round sun exposure is greater. Does this sound like the sun is the primary cause of melanoma?

These points are important because even though sunscreen use has continued to increase every year, people are increasingly dying from melanoma. The incidence of melanoma has increased about one percent per year since 2009 according to a study from the Mount Sinai Icahn School of Medicine (Plitzko *et al.* 2017).

Despite increased sunscreen use, between 2009 and 2016, melanoma incidence grew from 22.2 per 100,000 people to 23.6 per 100,000 people.

Each year in the United States, over 80,000 cases of melanoma are newly diagnosed. And more than 9,000 people die from melanoma every year.

The surprising reality is that the sun reduces the risk of many types of cancer. And the sun's role in skin cancer is not as cut and dried as we might think.

The primary reason given for the risk of cancer is increased UV-B exposure. The research shows just the opposite: That healthy UV-B exposure on the skin is associated with a reduction of many types of cancers – including melanoma.

In the decades following Dr. Palm's reports that children from sunny areas did not contract rickets, doctors have slowly taken notice that those with more sun exposure had lower rates of a variety of cancers.

In 1970, cancer mortality maps revealed that sunnier regions had lower mortality rates from internal cancers than did areas with lower sunlight. In 1980, Johns Hopkins University's Dr. Frank Garland reported an unmistakable distribution gradient attributing sunnier locations to lower mortality rates for colon cancer – the leading fatal cancer.

This prompted Dr. Edward Gorham and associates to study the association between serum vitamin D levels and colon cancer. These studies also showed a strong correlation between colon cancer and reduced vitamin D levels. This prompted a flurry of new studies correlating vitamin D with cancers of various types (Mohr 2009).

In a review of cancer studies from 1970 to 1994, the American Cancer Society's journal, *Cancer* (Grant, 2002) reported that UV-B solar radiation is associated with a reduction of cancers of the breast, colon, ovaries, prostate, bladder, kidney, lung, pancreas, rectum, stomach, uterus, and esophagus. Dr. William Grant, the author of the research, noted that the reduction of some cancers ranged from 30-50% with adequate UV-B sun exposure.

Clinical studies have also indicated a 20-30% increase in breast cancer incidence, and a 10-20% increased fatality rate for breast cancer among vitamin D-deficient women (Nielsen 2007).

In August of 2007, Dr. Cedric Garland and fellow cancer researchers at the Moores Cancer Center/University of California determined through analysis that about 250,000 colorectal cancer cases and 350,000 breast cancer cases worldwide could be prevented with increased vitamin D from sunbathing. It was estimated that a quarter of these cases – 150,000 – could be prevented in the United States alone.

In 2006, Dr. Francis Boscoe and Dr. Maria Schymura from the University of New York at Albany's School of Public Health published a major study that confirmed that ultraviolet sun exposure lowers the risk of many types of cancer.

Dr.s Boscoe and Schymura looked at over three million cancer cases that occurred between 1998 and 2002, and three million deaths from cancer between 1993 and 2002 in the United States.

Patient information was cross-referenced with UV-B levels taken from satellite data in thirty-two regions of the U.S. Low UV-B exposure correlated with greater incidence and more deaths from bladder cancer, Hodgkin's lymphoma, myeloma, biliary cancer, prostate cancer, rectal cancer, stomach cancer, uterine cancer, vulva cancer, breast cancer, kidney cancer, leukemia, non-Hodgkin's lymphoma, pancreatic cancer, gallbladder cancer, and thyroid cancer.

Okay, now let's talk about skin cancer. Certainly the sun causes skin cancer, right?

Interestingly, skin cancer rates have gone up dramatically over the past four decades, at close to the same rates as other cancers have gone up. Does this mean more people have gone out into the sun? What about the increased use of sunblock over the decades? Why haven't skin cancer rates gone down with increased use of sunblock?

Some researchers propose that a suntanning trend began in the 1960s, if we consider this issue in relation to the industrial revolution, over the past century more people are working and living indoors than ever before in history. It's actually the opposite. More people worked outdoors in the decades before the 1960s. As the industrial manufacturing age blossomed during and after the World Wars, indoor factory jobs and desk jobs became more prominent.

Before that, more people worked outdoors. They worked on farms or traveled by horse or uncovered wagons. Yet skin cancer rates were significantly lower.

In a study done in Australia of 1,014 subjects (Holman *et al.* 1986), there was no relationship between melanoma and sun exposure, with the exception of the rare Hutchinson's melanoma.

Research has confirmed lower melanoma rates among dark skinned populations, but they do get skin cancer – despite the fact that few dark-skinned people sunbathe. The increased level of melanin in dark-skinned people's epidermal layers screens or filters more ultraviolet radiation, decreasing skin exposure.

Furthermore, research has confirmed that cancer rates have continued to rise over the past two decades despite a dramatic rise in the use of sun-protective agents like sunscreen and hats; and decreased sunbathing in general. Research has also shown that modern society's awareness of the need for sun protection is at an all-time high.

In one study (Stoebner-Delbarre 2005) of 33,021 French adults, 92% understood the sun increased the risk of skin aging and 89% understood it increased cancer risk. With few alternatives, the study's researchers concluded the continued increases in skin cancer are due to this awareness not translating into action. The other possibility might be that the sun doesn't cause cancer.

There are two basic types of skin cancer: Melanoma and non-melanoma skin cancer. Melanoma grows from dysfunctional melanocytes. Melanoma is the more dangerous of the two, rendering far lower survival rates compared to non-melanoma skin cancer.

Yet true melanoma is also rarer. By far, most of the skin cancers diagnosed – at least in the United States – are non-melanoma-related. According to the American Cancer Society, about 62,190 new melanomas were diagnosed in the U.S. and over one million non-melanoma skin cancers were diagnosed in 2006. The Cancer Society also estimates 10,710 skin cancer deaths occurred in 2006 – with 7,910 of those being melanoma.

There are three basic types of cells in the epidermis layer: the *melanocytes,* the *squamous keratinocytes* and the *basal keratinocytes*. Melanoma is associated with genetic damage occurring in melanocytes, and non-melanoma is associated primarily with genetic damage in the keratinocytes. Non-melanoma is divided into two types; basal cell carcinoma and squamous cell carcinoma.

Both of these non-melanoma types are considered *benign*, however. They both can spread if conditions are right, but in most cases, the spread is either slow or visually obvious. Melanoma is known to spread more quickly, leading to greater fatality rates. It can also easily be excised and stopped if caught early.

Basal cell carcinoma occurs at the deeper basal cell level. A good 70-90% of skin cancer is the basal cell version. As for the squamous cell type, this typically occurs around the face, lips, neck, or ears – yet also interestingly in the genital areas. These may form from actinic keratoses – which some refer to as sunspots. There are a number of other non-melanoma skin cancer types such as Kaposi's sarcoma and Merkel cell carcinoma, but these are rare.

The precise mechanisms for both melanoma and non-melanoma skin cancers are still being debated. It is thought that ultraviolet-B rays penetrate the basal cells deep in the epidermis layer, creating genetic damage.

Research however, has indicated a more complex multi-step scenario. Both the sun's ultraviolet-B (280-315 nanometers) and ultraviolet-A (315-400 nm) rays, especially intense during the mid-day, can produce *reactive oxygen species* (also called *free radicals*) among the tissues in the epidermis.

These reactive oxygen species appear to induce genetic mutations among the DNA in the cells – *if they are not neutralized*. Should these free radicals not be neutralized by the body's protective mechanisms, then DNA damage may occur amongst the kerotinocyte skin cells.

Research presented by the Sydney Cancer Center's Melanoma and Skin Cancer Research Institute at the *Photocarcinogenesis Symposium of the 14th International Congress on Photobiology* (Halliday *et al.* 2005) showed that ultraviolet-A causes a similar amount of gene mutations as does ultraviolet-B. While ultraviolet-B mutations predominated in the upper tumor areas, ultraviolet-A damage predominated at the basal (lower) layers.

But while research has resolved that these ultraviolet rays can create mutagenesis – damaging DNA – the picture is still more complex, as there appears to be a decreased presence of mutation-suppressors and mutation-repair mechanisms available among ultraviolet-damaged tumors (Nishigori *et al.* 2004). Again, we find other factors evident besides simply the impact of ultraviolet radiation onto the skin.

Melanoma has been the fastest growing cancer in America (Fecher 2007). While it was assumed that sun exposure was the causal agent in non-Hodgkin types of melanoma, three studies revealed that the risk of melanoma actually decreased from 25% to 40% with increased recreational sun exposure. One study (Armstrong 2007) indicated that possibly this effect is related to higher-levels of vitamin D intake.

Studies are now illustrating that vitamin D reduces a wide variety of cancers, including prostate, colon and breast cancer (Schwartz 2007). The connection between sun exposure and skin cancer has thus been connected to immunosuppression – deficiencies of the body's immune system and antioxidant levels to regulate and neutralize oxidization and the free radicals that cause damage within the tissues (de Vries *et al.* 2007).

Research at the National Cancer Institute of the National Institutes of Health (Millen, *et al.* 2004) studied 1,607 outpatients from various clinics, including 502 newly diagnosed melanoma patients. Their diets were studied in detail.

Those with diets low in alpha-carotene, beta-carotene, cryptoxanthin, lutein and lycopene – all plant-based food nutrients – had significantly higher levels of risk of melanoma. Alcohol consumption was also significantly associated with higher risk of melanoma. And of course, lower vitamin D levels were also associated with higher melanoma incidence in this study.

This means that eating a good diet of plant-based foods, along with lower alcohol intake and more sunshine decreases ones risk of melanoma.

Other studies have confirmed the link between diet and skin cancer. During the 1980s, several animal studies illustrated that UV-skin cancer occurred more readily with higher dietary fat intake.

Switching back to a low-fat diet following UV-radiation dosing reversed the increased risk. In human research a few years later, 115 actinic keratosis and non-melanoma cancer patients adopted diets of either 20% fat or 40% fat content for two years. Those with the lower fat content had significantly lower levels of keratosis, and significantly fewer cancer lesions (Black 1998).

Other research has indicated that certain types of dietary fats increase the risk of skin cancer. A 2005 study (Harris *et al.* 2005) of 656 people, including 335 squamous cell carcinoma patients at the Arizona Cancer Center reported on the link between fatty acids and cancer risk.

Fourteen different fatty acids were studied and measured from red blood cells. It was determined that increased levels of *arachidonic acid* – a fatty acid prominent in most meats and saturated oils – increased the risk of skin cancer, and palmitic acid and palmtoleic acid decreased the risk of skin cancer.

Palmitic acid is a saturated fat found in palm oils and dairy products, while palmtoleic acid is a monounsaturated fat found in nuts and certain plant foods. Arachidonic acid is also linked to increased risk of inflammation and autoimmune disorders.

Cooked (especially fried) meats also produce carcinogenic cyclic amines. In 2007, researchers (Mohr *et al.*) at the University of California at San Diego reviewed skin cancer research from 107 countries. They found that skin cancer incidence was associated with lower levels of UV-B rays, obesity, and animal diets.

The Department of Radiation Genetics at the Kyoto University in Japan (Matsumura *et al.* 1996) studied 32 cases of basal cell carcinomas among Japanese patients – 16 of which were developed in sun-exposed areas and 16 developed in less-exposed areas. In both groups (consistent many other studies) the p53 gene was seen as the primary site of mutation.

Furthermore, 75% of the non-exposed group showed transversions – the exchange of nucleotides between purines and pyrimidines. This exchange of bases at the genetic level relates to the bonds making up the DNA molecule – creating a switching out between two different sequence types. Once again, the study's authors noted these results indicate a more complex mechanism other than simply sun exposure for skin cancer.

Transversions have been observed *in vitro* primarily within two mechanisms: From the impact of toxic molecules – including free oxygen species and various toxins like benzene – and from the impact of ionizing radiation. Ionizing radiation occurs from various electromagnetic sources such as microwaves and various electronic appliances.

While the sun might be considered a potential source of ionizing radiation, a molecular environment capable of creating ions at an intensity of radiation causing that ionizing must exist within the mechanism. More importantly, an environment within the body must exist where those ions – or reactive species – remain un-neutralized.

While a popular myth has spread that all free radicals are damaging at any level, research is revealing that exposure to reasonable amounts of free radicals, or oxidative species, is necessary for sustained health. In a study performed at the University of Jena in Germany (Schultz *et al*. 2007), free radicals formed in the cell through glucose inhibition significantly extended lifespan.

The effect was apparently because the immune system developed a resistance to the oxidative stress caused by the reactive oxidative species. Consistent with other observations of immune strengthening due to increased resistance, it appears that some free radical exposure is required by the body and its cells.

Yet we also know that an overexposure to free radicals is unhealthy and even carcinogenic. The question is where is the line between a healthy amount of free radicals and overexposure? As the above study illustrates, nature has a design for maintaining a healthy balance between antioxidants and free radicals.

This assumption also provides the basis for understanding why skin cancers (and so many other cancers and autoimmune disorders) are largely diseases of the modern industrialized societies, where sunlight and other natural inputs have been replaced by synthetic and often toxic versions.

We might closely consider the mutagenic effects that ultraviolet-B radiation has upon plants. (Yes, plant genes can also damaged by ultraviolet-B radiation, causing lesions.) Healthy plants have natural protective and neutralizing mechanisms and phytochemicals that mitigate this genetic damage. This becomes evident when we see some plants remaining green and healthy even as they sit in the intense sun all day long.

Other plants – even of the same species – that are poorly watered and/or poorly fertilized, will turn brown in the mid-day sun. On the cellular level, this browning effect would be comparable to the sun's exposure among poorly nourished human skin cells (Zaets *et al*. 2006).

This reality can be hard to swallow given the linear aspect of the sun-skin cancer link. In a review of numerous skin cancer studies by researchers from the University of Southern California's Keck School of Medicine, the researchers admitted, *"...controversy exists, especially in the use of sunscreens."* (Ivry *et al*. 2006)

A good case study in reduced sunshine and cancer is pancreatic cancer.

Research shows that less sunshine is linked to a greater prevalence of pancreatic cancer.

A study from the University of California at San Diego (Garland *et al*. 2015) found that pancreatic cancer risk is reduced in those regions that have greater ultraviolet-B radiation.

The study analyzed cancer data from 172 countries around the world. The countries with significantly less ultraviolet-B radiation had about 600 percent – or six times – more incidence of cancer compared to those countries with greater UV-B radiation – and thus less cloud cover.

This relationship remained when other risk factors known for pancreatic cancer were considered.

These regions with the highest rates of pancreatic cancer around the world include North America and Northern Europe, while those regions with the lowest rates include Asia and Africa.

On the other hand, those areas that have greater cloud cover and reduced ultraviolet-B radiation from the sun have the greatest incidence of pancreatic cancer.

The study was led by Dr. Cedric Garland, and Dr. Edward Gorham, both professors in the Department of Family Medicine and Public Health at UC San Diego. Dr. Garland is also a member of the UCSD Moores Cancer Center. Dr. Garland commented on the study:

"People who live in sunny countries near the equator have only one-sixth of the age-adjusted incidence rate of pancreatic cancer as those who live far from it. The importance of sunlight deficiency strongly suggests – but does not prove – that vitamin D deficiency may contribute to risk of pancreatic cancer."

According to the World Cancer Research Fund, pancreatic cancer is a leading cause of cancer, with some 338,000 new cases reported every year. It is also the fourth leading cause of cancer death.

Note that earlier research discussed in my book has found that the type of vitamin D produced from smart sun exposure is different than the vitamin D found in most vitamin supplements. We've also discussed that healthy sun exposure is linked to cognitive health.

Alcohol

A large study on breast cancer was conducted by researchers from the University of Southern Denmark and the University of Copenhagen (Dam *et al.* 2016). Here the researchers followed 21,523 women for 11 years. The researchers investigated the alcohol intake of the women and compared that with their incidences of breast cancer.

The researchers found that those who drank an average of four drinks a day had a 45 percent increased risk of breast cancer. Those who drank an average of three drinks a day had an 18 percent increased risk of breast cancer. Those who drank an average of two drinks a day had a 14 percent increase risk of breast cancer, and one drink a day on average increased the risk by 8 percent.

The researchers measured one drink as equivalent to 12 grams of ethanol. This is actually less than what most Westerners consider a single drink. For example, a 12-ounce bottle of beer (at 5% alcohol by volume) or a five-ounce glass of wine (at 12% ABV) will have about 14 grams of ethanol. For liquors, a 1.5 ounce shot of 80 proof (40% ABV) will have 14 grams of ethanol.

Furthermore, many beers have greater than 5% ABV and many wines have more than 12% ABV.

So let's convert this to realistic terms:

45 percent increased risk = 28 drinks/week x 12 grams = 336 grams divided by 14 = 24 drinks a week = 3.4 (conservative) drinks a day

18 percent increased risk = 21 drinks/week x 12 grams = 252 grams divided by 14 = 18 drinks a week = 2.57 (conservative) drinks a day

14 percent increased risk = 14 drinks/week x 12 grams = 168 divided by 14 = 12 drinks a week = 1.7 (conservative) drinks a day

The bottom line: Drinking significantly increases a woman's risk of breast cancer. And this risk, according to the research, goes right up into the five years before breast cancer diagnoses. Those who increased their consumption of alcohol in the five years before the diagnosis had a 30 percent increase in their breast cancer incidence.

And those who decreased their intake of alcohol over the five years had no increased incidence of breast cancer.

Research from Harvard University established that women who drink from 3-6 glasses of wine per week have a 15% increased likelihood of breast cancer, while those who drink more increase their risk by more than 50%. Furthermore, it was estimated that up to 20% of breast cancers result from excessive drinking.

The study, published in the *Journal of the American Medical Association* (Chen *et al.* 2011) followed 106,000 nurses from 1980 to 2008. The results were unmistakable: Drinking increases breast cancer incidence and 'binge drinking' - drinking more some nights than others - increased breast cancer incidence even further. The research was led by Dr. Wendy Chen of Harvard and the Brigham and Women's Hospital.

"Our results highlight the importance of considering lifetime exposure when evaluating the effect of alcohol, and probably other dietary factors, on the carcinogenesis process," she commented.

Dr. Steven Narod, a researcher from the Women's College Research Institute of Toronto, also commented about the study:

"For some women the increase in risk of breast cancer may be considered substantial enough that cessation would seem prudent."

Other research has confirmed this finding:

"The fact that small amounts of alcohol can increase women's risk of breast cancer has been known for at least a decade. This finding confirms what we already know," said Professor *Valerie Beral of University of Oxford.*

Another study, published in the *American Journal of Epidemiology* (Breslow *et al.* 2011) found that drinking increases other types of cancer. The study, done by researchers from the U.S. National Institute on Alcohol Abuse and Alcoholism, followed 323,354 participants.

The researchers found that both higher quantity drinking - drinking three or more drinks on drinking days - and higher frequency drinking - more drinking days increased cancer incidence. For example, higher quantity drinking increased deaths from all cancers among men by 24%; and higher frequency drinking increased deaths from all cancers among women by 32%.

Breast cancer deaths went up by 44% for higher frequency drinkers, and prostate cancer in men went up by 55% for higher frequency drinkers. Deaths from colon cancer nearly doubled among women who drank more.

While researchers wrestle with the conflicting evidence between the cardiovascular benefits of the antioxidant resveratrol, it is clear from other research that alcohol - ethanol - is clearly carcinogenic and toxic to the body.

This is why drinking damages the liver and why alcohol is responsible for an estimated 90% of all liver cirrhosis cases.

Ethanol is not the only toxin involved in alcohol. Alcohol consumption produces a compound in the body called acetaldehyde. This is also sometimes referred to as ethanal. The International Agency for Research on Cancer (IARC) has classified acetaldehyde as a Group 1 carcinogen.

Many other chemicals and toxins have also been associated with cancer. Illustrating the connection between smoking toxins and breast cancer, in March of 2011, researchers from the University of West Virginia (Luo *et al.* 2011) found, in an analysis of 79,900 women involved in the Women's Health Initiative, that active smoking was significantly linked to breast cancer incidence. The increase in incidence ranged from 9% for former smokers to 50% for long-time smokers.

Another study – this from Sweden's Karolinska Institute (Cottet *et al.* 2009) – followed 51,847 women for more than eight years. This study found that those women who drank more than 10 grams of alcohol per day had a 35% greater incidence of ER+/PR+ breast cancers. This was increased among women who were taking hormones.

The researchers noted that the ER+ relationship was important, as they stated in their conclusion:

"The observed association between risk of developing postmenopausal ER+ breast cancer and alcohol drinking, especially among those women who use postmenopausal hormones, may be important, because the majority of breast tumors among postmenopausal women overexpress ER."

What about Resveratrol?

We'll discuss resveratrol in more detail later. But as it relates to alcohol:

Certainly, resveratrol - a component heralded in wine - is a potent antioxidant. Resveratrol also fights cancer according to studies. But wine is not its exclusive source or even a significant source. Resveratrol is a component of grape skins, as well as many other foods.

Therefore, fresh red or purple grapes, or even juice, or many other fruits such as pomegranate, raspberries and others will typically have significantly more resveratrol content compared to wine. In fact, a glass of red wine will typically have no more than about 1 milligram of resveratrol content.

This means it would take a barrel of wine to render a significant amount of beneficial resveratrol.

Synthetic vitamin E

Medical researchers are surprised with study results that indicate taking a synthesized form of vitamin E in high doses significantly increased the risk of prostate cancer.

The study (Klein *et al.* 2011) was published in the *Journal of the American Medical Association*. The researchers gave rac-α-tocopheryl acetate, a synthesized molecule referred to (incorrectly) as vitamin E, or selenium, or both (or placebo) to 34,887 men in the U.S., Canada and Puerto Rico.

The study found that by 2011, those who had taken the synthesized vitamin E form during the trial period had a 17% higher incidence of prostrate cancer than the group that took a placebo during the trial period.

The trial dosing was discontinued in 2008, when the researchers found a 13% increased incidence of prostate cancer among the synthesized vitamin E (rac-α-tocopheryl acetate) group. The result surprised researchers because other vitamin E studies, including those on rats, have found that vitamin E prevents cancers of various types.

The dose of the synthetic rac-α-tocopheryl acetate vitamin E form was 400 IU (international units) - equal to 363 milligrams, which is 27 times higher than the 15 IU per day U.S. DV (daily value) for men over 50 years old for vitamin E.

Types of natural vitamin E

Natural vitamin E actually has eight different forms:

- ➢ alpha-tocopherol
- ➢ beta-tocopherol
- ➢ gamma-tocopherol
- ➢ delta-tocopherol
- ➢ alpha-tocotrienol
- ➢ beta-tocotrienol
- ➢ gamma-tocotrienol
- ➢ delta-tocotrienol

These different vitamin E forms work in a synergistic way within the body. The tocopherols are known antioxidants. But the tocotrienols have also been shown to have significant, if not sometimes greater antioxidant potency. Research has found that the tocotrienols have greater cancer prevention potential compared to the tocopherols.

While most consider vitamin E a single nutrient, there are at least eight forms of vitamin E. Four of them are tocopherols, which include alpha-tocopherol, beta-tocopherol, gamma-tocopherol, and delta-tocopherol. There are also four tocotrienol forms of vitamin E. This includes alpha-tocotrienol, beta-tocotrienol, gamma-tocotrienol, and delta-tocotrienol. The primary vitamin E form in most supplements is alpha-tocopherol. Most of the research on vitamin E has utilized only alpha-tocopherols.

Multiple studies (Ramadan *et al.* 2013) included a mix of tocotrienols have found that they support cardiovascular health. Diets can vary in terms of their vitamin E forms. Western diets are typically restricted to alpha-tocopherols and gamma-tocopherols. However, a mixed plant-based diet that includes coconut and palm foods, whole grain rice and other whole grains will render a mix of the tocotrienol forms.

Synthetic vitamin E (alpha-tocopherol in the form of rac-α-tocopheryl acetate) as offered by most commercial supplement producers, is a different molecule altogether than these forms of natural vitamin E. Illustrating this, research has shown that this synthesized version of isolated vitamin E, rac-α-tocopheryl acetate, has been shown to produce a foreign metabolite called alpha-CEHC (2,5,7,8-tetramethyl-2(2'-carboxyethyl)-6-hydroxychroman).

This metabolite is believed to be produced in the liver. α-CEHC analysis shows the molecule contains a truncated phytyl tail. In 1998, researchers from Germany's Institute for Human Nutrition (Traber *et al.* 1998) gave six humans 150 milligrams each of either the natural form of alpha-tocopherol vitamin E, d3RRR-α-tocopherol, or the synthesized version, rac-α-tocopheryl acetate.

The researchers tested plasma immediately, at six hours, twelve hours and 24 hours after the dosages. Urine was tested every day for the first five days, and then on day 8. The researchers found that while most of the natural form of alpha-tocopherol remained in the bloodstream, much of the synthesized vitamin E isolate *"preferentially metabolized"* to α-CEHC, which was excreted through the urine.

In general, the excretion of the synthetic vitamin E was two-to-three times the excretion of the natural form as measured over several days. After a thorough review of the results, the researchers concluded that the difference in the metabolite secretion wasn't simply the speed of metabolite production in the liver:

"The lower biological activity of synthetic vitamin E cannot be quantitatively attributed to its higher rate of metabolism."

Although nearly 3 times as much metabolite was made from synthetic compared with natural vitamin E, the amounts of the metabolite produced and excreted in the urine account for only a few percent of the deuterated vitamin E consumed. In other words, something else is going on with synthetic vitamin E metabolism.

Medical researchers from Rutgers School of Pharmacy (Wada *et al.* 2010) published results of various vitamin E trials, including a careful review of the research on vitamin E to date. They studied the various effects of vitamin E and the contrary results of several cancer studies.

Their research determined that the multiple forms of natural vitamin E acted synergistically within the body. For example, larger doses of alpha-tocopherol actually decrease levels of delta-tocopherol in the bloodstream and tissues.

They also found that gamma-tocopherol significantly decreased prostate tumor growth, as well as colon, breast and lung cancer. This research and others found that the different vitamin E forms had cross-signaling capability, and were not redundant in their effects. In other words, the different forms are interactive rather than duplicating. This issue also appears in some multi-vitamin use as well.

Unfortunately, medical researchers have not thoroughly investigated this. Another study, done by researchers from Ohio State University's Medical School, determined that less than 1% of the research on vitamin E even considered or tested the tocotrienol forms of vitamin E. They commented that:

"Tocotrienols possess powerful neuroprotective, anti-cancer and cholesterol lowering properties that are often not exhibited by tocopherols."

The researchers also warned of hasty conclusions about vitamin E using only one form - not to speak of that form being synthetic rather than the natural form:

"For example, evidence for toxicity of a specific form of tocopherol in excess may not be used to conclude that high-dosage "vitamin E" supplementation may increase all-cause mortality. Such conclusion incorrectly implies that tocotrienols are toxic as well under conditions where tocotrienols were not even considered."

The bottom line is that nature provides nutrients that are cancer-preventative, and nature's forms of vitamin E have been shown to be significantly antioxidant and anticarcinogenic.

However, problems arise when we make hasty assumptions and ignore nature's interactive and synergistic effects, and we try to reproduce these effects by synthesizing nutrients.

Occupational Cancer Risk

Carcinogens pervade our workplaces. Many occupations are exposed to cancer-causing agents, because most of the consumer exposures begin from manufacturing those products. Then there are other environmental agents.

Scientists from the University of Texas School of Public Health (McHugh *et al.* 2010) analyzed the data from the National Health and Nutrition Examination Survey to determine the relative risks of toxicity in different occupations.

They found that miners, health-care workers, and teachers have significantly higher rates of respiratory disorders than other occupations, including construction workers. Miners, for example had over four times the respiratory disorders incidence than construction workers. This of course relates to their exposure to indoor air pollutants at work.

Researchers from the National Institute for Occupational Safety and Health and the Centers for Disease Control (Greskevitch *et al.* 2007) investigated occupational conditions among agricultural workers using the 1988-1998 National Centers for Health Statistics' Multiple Cause of Death Data and the 1988-1994 Third National Health and Nutrition Examination Survey data (NHANES III).

They studied mortality ratios for eleven respiratory illnesses in crop farm workers, livestock workers, farm managers, landscapers, horticultural workers, forestry workers, and fishery workers.

Among the different occupations, the crop farm workers and livestock farm workers suffered significantly more deaths from cancer.

It is notable that these occupations each present particular toxins. In the case of miners, they are exposed to coal dust and soot, together with exhaust, with minimal ventilation. In the case of agricultural workers, landscapers and horticulture workers, they are exposed to chemical pesticides and herbicides. In the cases of teachers and healthcare workers, they are exposed to the contaminants that occupy their respective buildings and ventilation systems.

Exposure to cancer-causing toxins requires extensive ventilation and filtration systems. Whether these come in the form of protective breathing gear or building HVAC systems, the toxin exposures within a workplace must be minimized. Reducing exposure is, in fact, one of the driving purposes of the U.S. Occupational Safety and Health Administration (OSHA). Toxin exposure at the workplace has reached such significant levels that OSHA has put in place many regulations, such as Material Safety Data Sheets (MSDS), in efforts to protect workers from the effects of workplace toxins.

Why such an effort to protect workers from cancer-causing toxins? Today there are in the neighborhood of 100,000 different synthetic chemicals available in the marketplace.

The chemical industry has produced many workplace chemicals for industrial uses over the past century, and many of these chemicals have been subsequently found to be carcinogenic or otherwise toxic. Keeping track of the effects and safeguards of each of these chemical toxins is a dizzying affair. Yet it is theoretically the responsibility of any business to make efforts to protect its workers from these toxins.

Here is a small list of occupations and their carcinogenic toxins:

Occupation	Carcinogenic Exposures
Agricultural workers	Pesticides, herbicides
Plastics manufacturers	Plasticizers, VOCs, polymers
Painters	Paints/thinners (VOCs)
Drivers	Carbon, soot, formaldehyde, micro
Metal workers	Metallic dusts, heavy metals

Saw millers	Exhaust, preservatives
Janitorial and housekeepers	VOCs, cleaning chemicals
Home builders	VOCs, formaldehyde, asbestos
Health workers	SBS, viruses, chemicals

Chapter Three

Diet and Cancer

In this chapter we will discuss some of the research linking diet and cancer. We will discuss diets that increase the risk of cancer as well as diets that reduce the risk of cancer. Excuse any confusion as we go back and forth on some topics.

The Western Diet

The association between colon cancer and diets heavy in red meat has been shown conclusively in a multiple studies over the years. For example, an American Cancer Society cohort study (Chao *et al.* 2005) examined 148,610 adults between the ages of 50 and 74 living in 21 states of the U.S. They found that higher intakes of red and processed meats were associated with higher levels of rectal and colon cancer after other cancer variables were eliminated.

According to the World Cancer Research Fund and the American Institute for Cancer Research, in a report *Food, Nutrition and the Prevention of Cancer: A Global Perspective* (1997), 25-50% of all cases of cancer can be prevented by a vegetarian diet.

In the twelve year mortality study of 6,115 vegetarians and 5,015 meat-eaters mentioned earlier, vegetarians had a 40% lower risk of mortality from all cancers (Thorogood *et al.* 1994; West 1994).

Researchers from Uruguay's University of the Republic School of Medicine (De Stafani *et al.* 2012) found, in a study of 6,060 people that the risk of cancer of the kidneys, oral cavity, pharynx, esophagus, stomach, colon, rectum, larynx, lung, female breast, prostate and urinary bladder were significantly increased with higher consumption of processed meats. They found eating mortadella (large sausage), salami, hot dogs, ham, and salted meats even more associated with these cancers.

In a study (Kwan *et al.* 2009) of breast cancer survivors from the Life After Cancer Epidemiology Study, 1,901 patients diagnosed with early stage breast cancer were followed. Two eating patterns were found among the patients: One had greater consumption of fruits, vegetables, whole grains, and poultry (called the "Prudent pattern"). The other, called the "Western pattern" – had greater consumption of red and processed meats with refined grains.

The researchers found that those who adhered the closest with the "Prudent pattern" had lower rates of death from breast cancer or any other cause. Meanwhile those in the "Western pattern" suffered higher incidence of recurrent breast cancers, greater incidence of death from their breast cancer, and increased risk of death from any cause.

French researchers (Couto *et al.* 2011) have found that greater adherence to the Mediterranean diet reduces overall cancer risk. Researchers from the International Agency for Research on Cancer in Lyons, France, analyzed

142,605 men and 335,873 women from around Europe. They monitored cancer incidence and graded adherence to the Med diet using a 0-9 score. Among the study population, 9,669 men and 21,062 women contracted cancer.

The researchers found that for every two points increase in the Med diet score, there was a 4% reduction in cancer, and nearly 5% among men. The results did not include cancers related to smoking.

This study was the first to study the association between the Med diet and cancer risk overall.

Fiber content in diet critical in preventing cancer. This was illustrated in a study from University of Alberta researchers (Sharma *et al.* 2013) who followed 146,389 people. They found that Japanese men who had consumed more grain were only half as likely to die from cancer.

While some of these above studies did focus on cancer in aggregate, other research has focused on diet's relationship with individual cancers. Most of these have similar findings:

Cancer of the pancreas has one of the worst survival rates of any other cancer. Pancreatic cancer survival rates are about 25% for one year, and 6% for five years. In the U.S. 38,000 people were diagnosed with pancreatic cancer in 2011, and about 34,000 died of pancreatic cancer. It is the fourth highest cause of cancer deaths.

Swedish researchers have found that eating red meat significantly increases a man's risk of pancreatic cancer, and eating processed meats increases both men's and women's risk of contracting pancreatic cancer.

The research, from Sweden's National Institute of Environmental Medicine in Stockholm (Larsson *et al.* 2012), analyzed eleven clinical studies that followed 6,643 pancreatic cancer patients. The study found that eating more red meat increased a man's risk of pancreatic cancer by almost 30%.

The study, published in the *British Journal of Cancer,* determined that both men and women have an increased risk of pancreatic cancer – by almost 20% – from eating more processed meats.

The study gauged red meat consumption by categorizing those who ate 120 grams more red meat a day for the red meat analysis, and those who ate 50 grams more processed meat for the processed meat analysis.

This finding was confirmed by another study (Bosetti *et al.* 2013) from Italy, of 326 pancreatic cancer patients matched with 652 healthy control subjects (people who didn't have pancreatic cancer).

The researchers found that those who at higher intakes of animal products had double the risk of pancreatic cancer, while those whose diets had more plant-based foods ("vitamins and fiber" pattern) had a 69% reduced risk of pancreatic cancer.

A review of research by cancer scientists from Poland found 11 case-controlled studies comparing red meat consumption with pancreatic cancer risk. Their meta-analysis of these studies found that red meat consumption increases the risk of pancreatic cancer by 48%. They also found that eating more vegetables and fruit decreases pancreatic risk by 38% and 29% respectively.

Researchers from Spain's Programme of Epidemilogical Cancer Research in Barcelona (Gonzalez and Riboli 2010) conducted an analysis of 519,978 human participants from 23 centers among 10 European countries in Denmark, France, Germany, Greece, Italy, the Netherlands, Norway, Spain, Sweden and the United Kingdom. They found that gastric cancer was associated with higher consumption of red and processed meats, and lower risk was evident among those with higher phytonutrient (plant nutrients) plasma levels.

They also found that lung cancer was lower among those who ate more fruits and vegetables, even among smokers. And they found that higher breast cancer incidence was related to higher saturated fat consumption.

Researchers from the American Cancer Society (McCullough *et al.* 2013) studied 2,315 patients who had been previously diagnosed with colorectal cancer (colon and/or rectum cancer). Those who consistently ate higher intakes of red and processed meat before and after diagnosis had 79% higher risk of dying from colon cancer. Those who ate more meat also had a 63% higher risk of dying from cardiovascular disease compared to those with a reduced consumption of meat.

Researchers from the Harvard School of Public Health (Nimptsch *et al.* 2013) followed 19,771 women for nine years (between 1998 and 2007) and tracked their diets together with the incidence of colon cancer among them.

The researchers found that replacing a serving per day of red meat with poultry or fish reduced their risk of colon cancer by 35% and 41% respectively.

Multiple studies by cancer researchers have determined that a plant-based diet and less alcohol consumption significantly reduce the risk of breast cancer.

Scientists from Columbia University, Stanford University and UCLA (Link *et al.* 2013) followed 91,779 women for 14 years as part of the California Teachers study. The women were followed between 1995 and 2009.

The researchers tracked the number of breast cancers and tumors among the women during the women and matched these results with the respective diet patterns of the women. The researchers grouped the women into five basic diet patterns:

1) plant-based diet – high in fruits and vegetables

2) high-protein, high-fat diet – high in meats, eggs, fried foods, and fats

3) diet high in carbohydrates, processed and convenient foods, pasta, and bread products

4) ethnic diet – high in legumes, soy foods, rice, and dark-green leafy vegetables

5) salad and wine diet – high in lettuce, fish, wine, low-fat salad dressing, coffee and tea

Of these patterns, those who ate the most (highest quartile) plant-based diet pattern (1) had 15% less incidence of breast cancer and 34% less incidence of tumors that were estrogen receptor – negative and progesterone receptor – negative (ER-/PR-).

While the non-plant-based diets scored the lowest, the researchers also found that the "salad and wine diet" pattern produced a 29% higher incidence of estrogen receptor – positive progesterone receptor – positive (ER+/PR+) tumors.

With regard to the alcohol consumption, the researchers noted that alcohol was a contributing factor, but not the only contributing factor.

The researchers concluded that:

"The finding that greater consumption of a plant-based dietary pattern is associated with a reduced breast cancer risk, particularly for ER-/PR- tumors, offers a potential avenue for prevention."

Other studies have shown that a plant-based diet reduces the risk of breast cancer.

A study from France's INSERM scientists conducted a large study that followed 65,374 women for nearly 10 years (9.7 to be exact). The researchers divided the women into two primary eating patterns:

1) The Western diet – high in meat products, fried foods, cakes, mayonnaise, butter/cream and alcohol

2) The Mediterranean diet – high in vegetables, fruits, olive oil, sunflower oil and seafood

The Western diet plan resulted in a 20% greater incidence of breast cancer among those eating the most (highest quartile) of this diet, and 33% greater risk for ER+/PR+ tumors. Meanwhile, those eating the Mediterranean diet plan had 15% incidence of all breast cancers.

In fact, the evidence on fiber's ability to help prevent multiple cancers is pervasive. Studies have found links between lower dietary fiber intake and colon cancer, prostate cancer and others.

A large study connecting fiber and breast cancer from researchers at the Harvard School of Public Health (Maryam *et al.* 2016) utilized participants that took part in the Nurses' Health Study II. This included more than 90,000 women available for fiber consumption research.

At the end of the day, 44,263 women participated in the beginning through the end of the study, which followed the women from 1991, and analyzed their dietary habits from their high school years.

The dietary analysis of the women started with their high school years between 1960 and 1980 depending on the age of each woman. Then following the 1991 food frequency report, each woman updated their current diet every four years until 2007.

The women also were monitored for breast cancer incidence. Every other year the women reported breast cancer diagnoses or the lack thereof. The researchers found this reporting accuracy to be quite high as they sampled medical records.

The study also eliminated other variables known to influence breast cancer, such as smoking, weight, hysterectomy and other factors.

The researchers divided the fiber intake of the women into five levels – called quintiles. The lowest total fiber intake level (the lowest quintile) during early adult years averaged 12 grams of fiber per day. The next level was 15.3, and the highest fiber levels were a little over 26 grams of total fiber per day.

During their teenage years, this ranged from a low average of 16 grams per day to a high average fiber intake per day of 21.5 grams per day in the highest quintile.

The study found that diets higher in fiber during teenage years led to a reduced risk of breast cancer by between 16 and 20 percent.

And for every 10 grams of fiber increase there was a decrease in breast cancer incidence by 14 percent. This, according to lead researcher Dr. Maryam Farvid of Harvard, converts to a 30 percent reduction in breast cancer risk for someone who eats between 25 to 30 grams of total fiber per day.

For those women in their 20s, it's not too late to experience the anti-cancer benefits of fiber consumption. The Harvard study found that for every 10 grams of increased fiber per day there is a 13 percent reduction in breast cancer risk later on. This means that increasing fiber intake from 10 grams of fiber per day to 30 grams per day would decrease the risk of breast cancer later on by more than 25 percent.

This actually wouldn't be too hard to do. The average American consumes between 10 and 15 grams of total fiber per day according to the National Library of Medicine. Adding some additional grains, fruit and vegetables to ones diet can easily add up to 20 grams of fiber.

Dietary fibers include fiber that is fermentable by probiotics and non-fermentable fiber –also referred to as insoluble fiber.

Fiber is typically divided into soluble and insoluble fiber categories. This is defined by the fiber's ability to dissolve in water. Those fibers that dissolve in water also happen to be fermentable and thus provide food (prebiotics) for our gut's bacteria.

Foods high in insoluble fiber include grains, seeds and the skins of fruits. These balance bowel movements and our intestinal motility. These plant parts include cellulose, hemicellulose, and lignins. Other insoluble fibers include resistant starch and resistant dextrins.

Foods high in soluble fiber include oats, barley, nuts, fruits, beans and legumes. They contain mucilages, oligosaccharides and polysaccharides among others.

Soluble fibers have been found to absorb and remove cholesterol lipids that are not healthy in the bloodstream. They also feed our gut's microorganisms. Apparently, this synergistic decrease in bad cholesterol lipids and healthier probiotics decrease circulating estrogen levels. It is believed that this is because increased cholesterol levels increase estrogen levels.

This 25 to 30 grams of total fiber per day is the middle range of the recommended intake of fiber per day, according to the National Library of Medicine. That recommendation is for between 20 and 35 grams of total fiber per day. Natural medicine proponents often hike this to 35 to 45 grams of total fiber – though getting to that point is recommended gradually.

Dr. Farvid provides some practical advice:

"We recommend that parents of young daughters provide plenty of high-fiber foods at home and make sure their children eat enough fruits and vegetables, whole-grain pasta, dark bread or brown rice, legumes and nuts in their diet."

Other studies have shown that fiber and other foods eaten during a woman's teenage and early adult years can affect the risk of breast cancer. Another study from Harvard Medical School (Su *et al.* 2010) followed 29,480 women for ten years that included food questionnaires.

The study found those women who ate the highest levels of fiber during high school had 25 percent lower incidence of the breast cancer marker, proliferative BBD.

Furthermore, women who ate two or more servings of nuts per week during high school a phenomenal 36 percent reduced incidence of the breast cancer marker.

Another study from Harvard Medical School (Frazier *et al.* 2013) also studied early diets and breast cancer incidence. This study found that those who ate more fiber, vegetable oils, nuts and vitamin E foods had significantly lower risk of breast cancer later on.

This study also found that a greater consumption of animal fats, red meat and alcohol was associated with a greater risk of breast cancer later on.

The relationship between diet and breast cancer becomes more evident as we examine a study (Suzuki *et al.* 2008) of 51,823 Swedish women who were followed for more than eight years. Here the researchers found that those women who had the highest quartile of total fiber intake had a 34% decreased incidence of breast cancer and a 38% reduced incidence of ER+/PR+ tumors.

This study also found that among those taking hormones, the reduction of breast cancer incidence was a whopping 50%.

The researchers also found that those eating more cereal-based fiber (grains) had an even greater reduction in breast cancer incidence. A plant-based diet is naturally higher in fiber because whole fruits, vegetables and grains contain various plant fibers.

So it seems that fiber is a critical issue, and plant-based foods maintain higher fiber content, while the Western diet maintains lower fiber content.

Certainly this is compounded by the increased content of numerous anti-cancer phytochemicals in nuts, roots, grains, fruits and vegetables.

Animal Foods

After significant investigation of more than 40 years of research, the World Health Organization's research team has classified meat as carcinogenic. This includes both red meat and processed meat, though processed meat was classified as a more certain risk. The research was published in the British Medical Association's journal, *Lancet*.

The WHO's International Agency for Research on Cancer (IARC) investigated volumes of research on both processed meats and red meats. The IARC announced they found the prevailing research was strong enough to classify processed meat as a Group 1 carcinogen – the most certain classification. This means that the research was strong enough to identify processed meats as "carcinogenic to humans."

This puts processed meat in the same category given to tobacco and asbestos.

According to the WHO, this classification comes as a result of a series of studies that show that processed meats cause cancer. These studies include large-scale human population studies as well as clinical studies.

The IRAC's research (Simon *et al.* 2015) consisted of a meta-analysis that included more than 700 human epidemiological studies that reported on red meat, and more than 400 human epidemiological studies on processed meats. Because some of these studies investigated red meat and processed meat, the total study count included in the meta-analysis was 800. According to the WHO's press release:

"The IARC Working Group considered more than 800 studies that investigated associations of more than a dozen types of cancer with the consumption of red meat or processed meat in many countries and populations with diverse diets. The most influential evidence came from large prospective cohort studies conducted over the past 20 years."

The meta-analysis was conducted by 22 scientists (Bouvard *et al.* 2015) from 10 different countries. After each had performed their respective analytical calculations, they convened to come to a consensus on the research. This is the largest review of research done on meat and cancer so far.

Types of cancer clearly associated with processed meats include colorectal cancer, pancreatic cancer and pancreatic cancer. These are leading cancers throughout the world, especially among countries that consume the most meat.

The WHO reported that about on a global basis, some 34,000 cancer deaths per year worldwide are caused by processed meat diets. The estimate was calculated by a scientific research organization called the Global Burden of Disease Project.

The WHO's calculation of the cancer risk found a relationship between processed meat and cancer:

"In those studies, the risk generally increased with the amount of meat consumed. An analysis of data from 10 studies estimated that every 50 gram portion of processed meat eaten daily increases the risk of colorectal cancer by about 18%."

This means that for every 50 grams of processed meat eaten per day, ones cancer risk is increased by 18%. How much is 50 grams, you ask?

two slices of ham is about 50 grams

two slices of Canadian bacon is about 50 grams

one hot dog is about 50 grams

six slices of typical bacon is about 50 grams

five slices of salami is about 50 grams

The average American at 71 pounds of beef, lamb, veal and pork in 2013. If you divide 71 by 365 days in a year, we find that the average American ate 88 grams of meat every day.

About 60 percent of America's meat consumption is red meat, and only 22 percent is considered processed. But the average consumption per person also includes those who don't eat meat or only eat a little meat.

What meats are classified as processed?

A significant percentage of the total meat consumed in Western countries is processed. Processed meats include:

- Salami
- Corned beef
- Pepperoni
- Chicken nuggets
- Canned meats
- Sausages
- Hot Dogs
- Bologna
- Charcuterie
- Bacon
- Ham
- Beef jerky
- Meat sauces

Basically, a processed meat is any type of meat that has been:

- Cured
- Smoked
- Dried
- Salted
- Canned

The cancer risk doesn't end at red meat. The IARC also classified red meat as a carcinogen – giving it the classification of a Group 2A carcinogen. This classification is described as "probably carcinogenic to humans."

The reason for the difference in classification is the extent of the evidence. The evidence for processed meats is so strong that its classification is higher. There are very clear studies linking red meat with cancer, but just not as strong as that for processed meats.

Red meat, according to the WHO research, includes beef, veal, pork, lamb, mutton, horse, and goat.

The IRAC's research paper estimated that another 50,000 cancer deaths worldwide are likely to be caused by eating red meat.

Many of the studies have referenced processed meats. For example, Swedish researchers (Larsson *et al.* 2012) found that eating red meat significantly increases a man's risk of pancreatic cancer, and eating processed meats increases both men's and women's risk of contracting pancreatic cancer – considered one of the deadliest cancers.

The research, from Sweden's National Institute of Environmental Medicine in Stockholm, analyzed eleven clinical (human) studies that followed 6,643 pancreatic cancer patients. The study found that eating more red meat increased a man's risk of pancreatic cancer by almost 30%, but not in women.

However, both men and women have an increased risk of pancreatic cancer – by almost 20% – from eating more processed meats.

The study was published in the *British Journal of Cancer*.

Pancreatic cancer has one of the worst survival rates of any other cancer. Pancreatic cancer survival rates are about 25% for one year, and 6% for five years. In the U.S. 38,000 people were diagnosed with pancreatic cancer in 2011, and about 34,000 died of pancreatic cancer. It is the fourth highest cause of cancer deaths.

The study gauged red meat consumption by categorizing those who ate 120 grams more red meat a day for the red meat analysis, and those who ate 50 grams more processed meat for the processed meat analysis.

This is not the first study that has associated eating red meat and processed meats with cancer. Multiple studies have found that colorectal cancer, stomach cancer, liver cancer, throat cancer, lung cancer and other forms of cancer have also been associated with eating red and processed meats.

When meats are cooked, they become high in a number of compounds. Let's discuss a few:

Heterocyclic amines (HCA). HCAs are produced when meat is cooked at high temperatures. This includes frying, grilling and roasting. HCAs have been linked to cancer in a number of studies.

Polycyclic aromatic hydrocarbons (PAH). PAHs are also produced by cooking meats at high temperatures – again, frying, grilling and roasting.

Nitrites and nitrates. These are salts that are added to meat to preserve them. Nitrates have been shown to cause DNA damage.

Heme iron. This compound is found in red meat. These catalyze to form N-nitroso compounds, which have been suspected as cancer-causing.

To this, we can add significant research (Cogliano *et al.* 2011) illustrating that red meat stimulates the growth of certain pathogenic bacteria colonies.

These bacteria have been shown in other research to produce enzymes that have been linked with colon cancer and other cancers.

These pathogenic bacteria also produce an array of other byproducts, sometimes referred to as endotoxins. One type of these endotoxins – linked with cancer and an array of other conditions – are called lipopolysaccharides. We've also discussed some of the other conditions caused by lipopolysaccharides.

Dr. Christopher Wild, the director at the IARC, commented about the WHO research:

"These findings further support current public health recommendations to limit intake of meat."

A review of the WHO research by the American Cancer Society states:

"The American Cancer Society has long recommended a diet that limits processed meat and red meat, and that is high in vegetables, fruits, and whole grains."

Research from Harvard University and other institutions over the last decade has increasingly shown that cancer is positively linked to greater consumption of red meat. The link has been profound in colon cancer, prostate cancer and other forms of cancer.

And new studies keep coming in linking cancer to meat consumption. For example, one study (Guo *et al.* 2015) found that red meat intake increased the incidence of squamous cell carcinoma of the lung by 81 percent, and beef consumption more than doubled (222 percent) the incidence of this dangerous form of cancer. Squamous cell carcinoma of the lung has only a 15 percent five-year survival rate.

But the link between breast cancer and red meat consumption has been less obvious.

This doesn't mean that there isn't some clear evidence. A review of research provides some clarity. This study analyzed 26 studies through October of 2014, including 14 studies on red meat and 12 studies on processed meat. The researchers calculated relative risks for different intakes of red meat among the various studies.

Their research found that for every increase of 120 grams of red meat per day, breast cancer incidence increased by 11 percent. And for every increase of 50 grams of processed meat per day, breast cancer incidence increased by 9 percent.

That said, some of the studies showed even higher associations. This included up to 16 percent increased breast cancer incidence for every 120 grams of red meat consumption, and 16 percent for every 50 grams of processed meat consumption.

Some have hypothesized that the reason for the difference in studies relates not just to the type of meat, but the amount of iron in the meat. Others have pointed to the levels of potential nitrites in the meat. Processed meat is typically higher in nitrites.

This review has prompted cancer researchers to investigate the link between breast cancer and meat intake more definitively.

One group of cancer researchers has significant clout and resources at its disposal to investigate this more definitely: Scientists at the National Cancer Institute of the National Institutes of Health, to be specific.

The NIH's National Cancer Institute has 69 cancer centers throughout the U.S., where doctors conduct research and provide treatment for patients. The combined budget for the National Cancer Institute in 2013 was $4.789 billion.

One thing the NIH is good at is population research. In this topic in particular, the research clout and funding provides some significant clarity in the case of breast cancer and meat consumption.

The NIH researchers (Inoue-Choi *et al.* 2015) followed 193,742 postmenopausal women for 11 years – between 1995 and 2006. The researchers conducted food frequency questionnaires to determine meat intake, along with nitrite intake and heme iron.

The researchers categorized the different women into groups rated by their intakes. These were divided into quintiles. This means the women were divided into five groups for each of the intakes. This allowed the researchers to compare the number of cancers among the different diets among the women.

The research found that those in the highest quintile red meat consumption group had 25 percent higher incidence of localized breast cancer compared to the lowest quintile of red meat consumption.

The processed meat consumption was a little higher. Those in the highest group had 27 percent increased incidence of localized breast cancer compared to the lowest quintile of processed meat consumption.

Nitrite consumption also increased the incidence of breast cancer. Those in the highest group of nitrite consumption had 23 percent greater incidence of breast cancer compared to the lowest group. Heme iron consumption also increased the incidence.

The researchers concluded that the heme iron and nitrites may increase the cancer risk notably because meat contains heme iron and nitrites. But they were clear that meat consumption provided significant risk:

"Our findings suggest that high consumption of red meat and processed meat may increase risk of postmenopausal breast cancer."

It should be noted that this study only compared those who ate the most meat to those who ate the least, in five increments. It did not compare those who ate meat with those who did not eat meat. Logically, this should equate to a significantly higher difference.

Greater breast cancer risk has been found in studies on processed meats. For example, one study (Mourouti *et al.* 2015) of 500 women – including 250 women with breast cancer – found that processed meats eaten once or twice a week increased the risk of breast cancer among the women by 265 percent – that is, nearly 2.7-fold risk.

Why Does Meat Increase Cancer Incidence?

There are a number of reasons, according to the research. These relate to our gut bacteria, to toxin intake and many others. One proposal has been gaining evidence: The notion that the heterocyclic amines that are formed when meat is cooked increases free radicals within the body.

This theory was tested by scientists from Brazil's University of Sao Paulo (Carvalho *et al.* 2015). The researchers tested 561 adults. The researchers conducted a 24-hour dietary recall with each of the subjects. They also tested each of the human subjects' levels of oxidative stress. The researchers used malondialdehyde concentration testing to find that heterocyclic amine consumption linked to greater oxidative stress.

But heterocyclic amines intake is not the only toxin to be concerned about. A study from Germany's German Cancer Research Center (Rohrmann *et al.* 2009) studied the breast DNA adducts of 44 women who underwent breast reduction.

A DNA adduct is a portion of DNA that has bonded with a chemical linked with cancer.

The researchers found that DNA adducts were linked with higher intakes of fried meat, beef and total heterocyclic amine intake. Because the DNA adducts were not all specific to heterocyclic amines: They concluded that there were other potential cancer-causing agents in the meat, including polycyclic aromatic hydrocarbons.

Low-Carb Diets

Low-carb diets have become extremely popular over the past decade, with the advent of the Adkins diet, the Paleo diet and the Keto diet. But are low-carbohydrate diets safe?

Research from the Harvard School of Public Health (Clifton *et al.* 2011) has found that low-carbohydrate, high-animal-protein diets significantly increase the risk of early death. The researchers followed 85,168 women between 34 and 59 years old for 26 years, and 44,548 men between 40 and 75 years old for 20 years. At the beginning of the study, none had cancer, heart disease, or diabetes.

During the study there were 12,555 deaths. Of these, 2,458 were heart disease, and 5,780 were cancer among the women, and 2,746 were heart disease and 2,960 were cancer among the men. Those eating low-carbohydrate, high-animal protein diets were 23% more likely to die from any cause, and 28% more likely to die from cancer. The Low-carb animal protein dieters were also 14% more likely to die from heart disease.

However, those eating a diet high in vegetable-protein and low in carbohydrates had a 20% lower risk of early death. But because so many low-carbohydrate eaters utilize animal proteins, the overall total low-carbohydrate dieters - including those using animal protein and vegetable protein - had an increased mortality rate of 12% over those not using the low-carb diet. This of course means that the low-carb animal protein dieters had an even more significant risk of early death.

"A low-carbohydrate diet based on animal sources was associated with higher all-cause mortality in both men and women, whereas a vegetable-based low-carbohydrate diet was associated with lower all-cause and cardiovascular disease mortality rates," concluded the Harvard researchers.

A study at the Ontario Cancer Institute (Martin *et al.* 2011) has found that lower intakes of carbohydrates increases the risk of breast cancer among women. The study followed 4,690 women for an average of ten years who had extensive mammogram density. They were randomized and split into two groups.

One group reduced fat intake and increased carbohydrate levels. The other group had higher levels of fat intake. Both groups were monitored closely and their diets were measured periodically. During the study period, 210 women had suffered from invasive breast cancer.

The researchers found those women with higher levels of carbohydrates in their diet had lower incidence of breast cancer. They also found that higher weight levels were associated with greater incidence of breast cancer. The research found no relationship between fat intake and breast cancer.

What about Low-Carb Diets for Cancer Patients?

As we'll discuss later, refined sugar increases the risk of cancer. And cancer cells tend to grow faster in the presence of greater levels of sugar and glucose. Does this mean a low-carb diet is better for a cancer patient?

A 2011 study (Schmidt *et al.*) from Germany's University Hospital of Wuerzburg tested 16 patients with advanced metastatic tumors with no conventional treatment options. They were instructed to follow a Keto diet with less than 70 g of carbs a day.

Out of sixteen patients, only 6 could tolerate the diet for more than 8 weeks. Most could not tolerate the diet. Five had significant progression of the cancer, and 2 died early. Those who could tolerate the diet reported "no severe side effects."

So was the diet successful? A little more than a third of those tested could tolerate the diet or didn't die while doing the diet. Five of the patients who tolerated the diet reported some improvement in emotional functioning and some insomnia improvement.

Reducing carbohydrates in itself is not bad. Reducing glucose supply for hungry cancer cells isn't bad either.

But most low-carbohydrate diets typically focus on red meat and even processed meats and dairy, all of which has been linked to a greater risk of cancer.

Meat-based foods also have increased levels of saturated fats, synthetic hormones and antibiotics used to fatten up commercial livestock. The livestock bioaccumulates these toxins within their fat cells. Then these are passed on to those who consume meat foods.

Does this mean that grass-fed beef is the answer? Beef will still bioaccumulate toxins in their fat cells - whatever toxins are in the air and in the ground. These toxins then accumulate in our bodies as a result.

A plant-based low-carb diet may have an altogether better result. Reducing refined carbohydrates and focusing on raw or minimally processed plant-based foods.

The reality is that fiber-rich carbohydrates are necessary for the human body to maintain health. Our digestive tracts were designed for fermenting (with probiotics) fiber-rich whole carbohydrates. If we were meant to eat only meat we would have basically straight tubes for intestines. Instead, our digestive tracts are windy and meant to ferment and digest fiber.

This is why our salivary glands and gastric cells produce amylase and other enzymes that break down start. Its also why our digestive tracts mirror those of other plant-eaters in the animal kingdom. Our bodies were designed to eat plant-based fibers.

Many low-carb dieters do not realize that vegetable-source proteins are a viable alternative. According to a Harvard School of Public Health review of the research:

"Vegetable sources of protein, such as beans, nuts, and whole grains, are excellent choices, and they offer healthy fiber, vitamins, and minerals. Nuts are also a great source of healthy fat."

Many of the food mentioned in this quote do reduce the risk of cancer. We'll discuss that research later on.

Good Carbs versus Bad Carbs

Typically, low-carb diets are focused on reducing refined and overly-processed carbohydrates. These include donuts, cookies, breads and other baked goods made with refined sugar, refined flours, preservatives and other false food ingredients. They also include candy bars, white rice, and many other false foods.

Removing those kind of carbs from our diet is a good thing. But this doesn't mean we have to throw out the baby with the bath water – so to speak. In other words, there are good carbs and bad carbs.

Good carbohydrates are found in plant-derived foods. Plant-based carbohydrates contain a host of nutrients and natural fibers. They will typically contain polysaccharides and oligosaccharides, often referred to as starches. Prior to refining, these starches offer us significant fiber, which reduces our risk of gastric cancer, colon cancer, rectal cancer and prostate cancer.

Greater levels of fiber in the diet have been associated with reducing the risk of other types of cancer as well.

Greater fiber levels have also been associated with lower levels of LDL cholesterol in the blood. This is because fiber attaches to LDL cholesterol in the gut, inhibiting LDL release into the bloodstream. In other articles, we've discussed how plant-based low-carb diets are different than meat-based low-carb diets. That research shows that plant-based low-carb diets reduce the risk of diabetes and reduce bad cholesterol.

Diets high in plant-based proteins also provide an array of plant nutrients, which include a myriad of vitamins, minerals and plant polyphenols. Plant-based diets also reduce heart disease and cancer risk according to other research.

Low carbohydrate diets with high intakes of red meat have become popular over the past few years. But questions surrounding their safety have continued to plaque these diets. We've discussed other research showing the low-carb high-meat diets increase the risk of early death and heart disease. Now we find that these types of low-carb diets also increase the risk of breast cancer.

The Mediterranean Diet

The connection between cancer and red meats has also been made among European research studying the Mediterranean diet. The Med diet is known for its reduced intake of red meats, and increased intakes of fruits, vegetables, monounsaturated fats and low levels of saturated fats.

Fruits and vegetables are the mainstay of the anti-cancer Mediterranean diet. If you wanted the most effective way to reduce your cancer risk, you might consider the Mediterranean Diet. This is the conclusion of multiple studies that have been done on large populations of people.

Researchers from the International Agency for Research on Cancer in Lyon, France (Couto *et al.* 2011) have found that the Mediterranean diet reduces cancer risk. The researchers studied 142,605 men and 335,873 women. They graded adherence to the Mediterranean diet with a 0-9 score. Among the whole population, 9,669 men contracted cancer and 21,062 women contracted cancer.

They found that a two point better Med diet score resulted in a 4% reduction in cancer. The results cancelled out cancers relating to smoking. The Med diet is known for its reduced intake of red meats, and increased intakes of fruits, vegetables, monounsaturated fats and low levels of saturated fats. This study was the first to analyze the association between the Med diet and cancer risk overall.

Other studies have found that the Med diet reduces risk in particular cancers. For example, a study by researchers from Spain's Programme of Epidemilogical Cancer Research in Barcelona (Gonzalez *et al.* 2010) tested 519,978 human participants from 23 centers among 10 European countries - Denmark, France, Germany, Greece, Italy, the Netherlands, Norway, Spain, Sweden and the United Kingdom.

This study found that gastric cancer was associated with red and processed meats, and lower risk was evident among those with higher plasma levels of phytonutrients (plant nutrients). The research found that lung cancer was lower among those who ate more fruits and vegetables, even among smokers. They also found in this study that higher breast cancer incidence was related to higher saturated fat consumption.

They found that higher consumption of dairy protein and calcium from dairy products, along with high serum concentration IGF-I (found higher among dairy and cattle given growth hormones) were all associated with increased incidence of prostate cancer. The Med Diet also decreases heart disease risk according to studies. It also helps prevent metabolic disease.

Fats that Fuel Cancer

Our bodies produce cancer cells every day. The immune system is constantly scanning our body for these mutations. And will trigger a killswitch within such a cell when it finds one. The killswitch initiates the destruction of the cancerous cell before it has a chance to replicate. The immune system follows by breaking down the cell and sweeping it from the body.

Occasionally, however, such a mutated cell will replicate faster than the immune system can kill them. What makes a cancerous cell grow and expand so quickly? Scientists have been asking this question for decades. A breakthrough discovery has found the answer. And it ties right into other research linking certain diets with cancer.

Research on cancer has revealed that a saturated fat prominent in Western diets makes cancer cells grow faster. The fatty acid is palmitic acid.

This fatty acid is a central fat contained within animal-based foods.

Over the past two decades, research from around the world has consistently found a correlation between diets rich in animal fats and higher cancer rates. We're talking all types of cancer here – from breast cancer to colorectal cancer.

In research funded by the Worldwide Cancer Research at the Institute for Research in Barcelona (Pascual *et al.* 2016) found a type of protein – called CD36 – on the cell membranes of cancer cells. This protein signals cancer cells to metastasize. (To metastasize means to spread).

The CD36 protein is stimulated by a certain type of saturated fatty acid – palmitic acid.

Professor Salvador Aznar Benitah at the Institute for Research headed up the research. It was published in the prestigious journal, Nature.

Dr. Benitah's team consistently found the CD36 proteins on metastatic cancer cells from a host of patients with a variety of different cancers. These included oral cancer, skin cancer, ovarian cancer, lung cancer and breast cancer.

Dr. Benitah's team confirmed the CD36's role in cancer by applying CD36 to non-metastatic cancer cells. The application led these cells to become metastatic.

Dr. Benitah stated:

"Although we have not yet tested this in all tumor types, we can state that CD36 is a general marker of metastatic cells, the first I know of that is generally specific to metastasis."

The researchers then tested cancer cells against different types of diets, and found that high-fat diets stimulated the CD36 protein. This in turn produced greater cancer cell metastasis.

Then the researchers focused upon which fatty acids in high-fat diets initiated more cell growth. They ended up finding that palmitic acid specifically sparked metastatic cancer growth.

"Fat is necessary for the function of the body, but uncontrolled intake can have an effect on health, as already shown for some tumors such as colon cancer, and in metastasis, as we demonstrate here."

Other research has revealed the mechanisms involved in palmitic acid's role in cancer growth. But other studies have also implicated palmitic acid's role in cancer. Multiple studies have indicated this.

In one study, palmitic acid fueled the growth of liver cancer cells in the laboratory (Tu *et al.* 2014). In another, palmitic acid was shown to fuel the cascaded growth of liver cells (Wang *et al.* 2011).

In yet another (Lou *et al.* 2014), palmitic acid-fueled liver cancer was found to involve an uncoupling protein (uncoupling protein-2). The researchers stated:

"Results demonstrated that uncoupling protein-2 was associated with autophagy during palmitic acid-induced hepatic carcinoma cells injury."

Other studies have shown how palmitic acid is related to metabolic abnormalities. A study that involved researchers from University of Hawaii at Manoa (Zhao *et al.* 2016) studied 312 people for ten years in China. They found that those whose diets had lower levels of palmitic acid and stearic acid also had lower rates of metabolic abnormalities.

Research from Germany's Friedrich Schiller University (Knoll *et al.* 2006) found that one of the byproducts of palmitic acid consumption is 2-Dodecylcyclobutanone. And 2-Dodecylcyclobutanone appears to produce mutations among human colon cells. These are linked with colon cancer.

Researchers from Hong Kong Baptist University found that melanoma cell cultures and tissue cultures where melanoma was growing had higher concentrations of palmitic acid. They also found that cancer cells pretreated with palmitic acid grew into significant tumors. The researchers stated:

"Recently, an isotopic fatty acid tracing-based metabolomics study revealed that cancer cells including melanoma incorporated exogenous palmitic acid into structural and signaling lipids, suggesting that exogenous fatty acids, such as palmitic acid, also play an important role in melanoma pathogenesis."

Researchers from Poland's Lodz University of Technology identified several Raman diagnostic markers for early identification of breast cancer. One of these markers is significant to our discussion: Palmitic acid.

Why? Because Raman imaging found high levels of palmitic acid within ducts during cancer growth.

Note that Dr. Benitah referred to uncontrolled fat intake. This is a key component of the Western diet – where palmitic acid consumption is prevalent to the extreme.

More specifically, palmitic acid is most prevalent in animal foods – meat and dairy. This includes red meat, poultry, eggs, fish and game meat.

Full fat dairy will also contain a considerable amount of palmitic acid. The butterfat content of whole milk can contain 29 to 31 percent palmitic acid. Whole milk will typically contain 3.25 percent butterfat. Low-fat milk will contain 1 percent butterfat, while a skim milk or nonfat milk can contain virtually no butterfat, and thus none or little palmitic acid.

Palm oil can contain, as a percentage of total fat, 44 percent palmitic acid.

Coconut oil and vegetable oils also contain a small amount of palmitic acid – 9 or 10 percent of total fat content or so. These are a fraction of the levels compared to animal foods due to the smaller addition of vegetable oils in foods. Vegetable fats also contain significantly higher levels of monounsaturated and polyunsaturated fatty acids, which significantly overtake their fractional saturated fat content.

These fat content percentages are deceiving when comparing plant-based diets to the Western diet. This is because plant-based foods have a very low fat content in general compared to animal-based foods. Plant-based foods contain significantly lower fat content by weight. And a significantly lower fat content per calorie.

This research is significant, first, for those who have been diagnosed with some form of cancer. Decreasing consumption of saturated fats and specifically, palmitic acid, should help reduce the metastasis of their cancer.

Plant-based Diets

Scientific research has confirmed that fiber-rich whole plant-based foods decrease the risk of most cancers and extend longevity in general.

There is an incredible supply of clear evidence proving this.

For example, phytosterols, which come from fiber-rich whole carbohydrates from plant sources, have been shown to decrease the risk of many types of cancers.

In a review of the research, University of Manitoba (Kunzmann *et al.* 2015) scientists concluded:

"Phytosterols have been reported to alleviate cancers of breast, prostate, lung, liver, stomach and ovary."

The "phyto" in phytosterols means these come from plants.

Fiber-rich plant-based grains and cereals have also been proven in many studies to reduce the risk of other cancers, such as colorectal and prostate.

For example, a study from the Queen's University in Belfast (Johnsen *et al.* 2015) followed over 57,000 people for three and five years. They found those who ate the highest amount of dietary fiber had a 24 percent decreased risk of distal colorectal cancer, and a 38 percent decreased risk of distal colon cancer.

In another study, scientists from the Danish Cancer Society Research Center (Kyrø *et al.* 2013) followed 108,000 people for 11 years. They found those who ate the highest amounts of whole grains had a 34 percent lower risk of colorectal cancer compared to those who ate the lowest amounts of whole grains. These included whole-wheat bread and cereals.

They also found that the risk of colorectal cancer fell by six percent for every 50 grams of additional whole grain eaten a day.

Even whole-wheat bread and high-fiber cereals have been shown to reduce the occurrence of cancer, and a longer life in general.

Illustrating this, Danish and Swedish medical researchers (Kyrø *et al.* 2015) followed more than 120,000 people. They tracked their diets between 1992 and 2009. The researchers found that those who ate more fiber-rich breakfast cereal and non-white bread (basically, whole wheat breads) had a 32 percent reduced risk of death from all causes during the period.

This translates to those who eat whole grains living longer – nearly a third longer.

Italy's University of Florence conducted a meta-analysis of studies that compared veggie diets to omnivore diets and found no less than 96 studies.

Yes, that is a lot of studies. The sheer volume of research allows medical researchers to come to clear conclusions.

The research found that plant-based diets – vegan or vegetarian – resulted in reduced body mass index levels, reduced total cholesterol, reduced LDL-cholesterol, and reduced glucose intolerance as compared to omnivore diets.

But the bigger result this meta-analysis found is that deaths of any cancer are reduced by 15 percent for vegans compared to omnivore diets, and 8 percent for eating any other type of primarily plant-based diet.

That does mean that those eating a plant-based diet won't get cancer. But the risk is reduced.

There are many causes for cancer and heart disease outside of diet as we've been discussing. But a vegetarian or vegan diet alone could save between 47,000 and 71,000 Americans every year from cancer, relatively.

Fruit and Cancer

Researchers from Harvard University's School of Public Health, along with the Dana-Farber Cancer Institute (Farvid *et al.* 2016) followed over 130,000 women. Over 90,000 women between 27 and 44 years old were followed from 1991 to 2013. And over 44,000 women were followed between 1998 and 2013.

The women completed questionnaires on diet, and their instances of breast cancer were compared with their diets. Every four years, the women answered another diet questionnaire to test their diets at the time.

The research found that those who ate the most fruit during their teenage years had an average of 25 percent less incidence of breast cancer. This was even higher – between 26 and 31 percent less incidence – for postmenopausal breast cancers.

Prominent fruits during teenage years among those with reduced incidence included bananas, grapes and apples.

Breast cancer incidence also went down for those with higher intake of vegetables during their teenage years. The decreased risk ranged from 25 percent to 16 percent among the different groups.

Higher intake of both fruits and vegetables during younger adult years also reduced the risk of breast cancer, but not as much as produced during the teenage years according to the research. Young women who ate higher amounts of fruits and vegetables rich in carotene – especially alpha-carotene found in yellow or orange vegetables – had as high as 15 percent less incidence of breast cancer.

Oranges and kale were prominent among diets of young adult women who avoided cancer.

Those women who ate more vegetables during their teenage years and early adult years had a 26 percent reduced incidence of premenopausal breast cancers.

The researchers concluded:

"There is an association between higher fruit intake and lower risk of breast cancer. Food choices during adolescence might be particularly important."

What about fruit juices?

Sorry, but no. The research found that drinking more fruit juice – through to the menopausal years – actually increased the risk of premenopausal breast cancer by 18 percent. Otherwise, fruit juice did not decrease other types of breast cancer risk.

But why, you ask? First, fruit juices typically have little or much less fiber from the fruit. These fruit fibers are critical because they contain many nutrients.

In addition, many of the phytonutrients within fruit are heat sensitive. So they are lost during the pasteurization process.

It is also important to note that adding back some ascorbic acid to lift the juice's level of vitamin C does not replace the pure vitamin C in the raw fruit. As discussed in other articles, vitamin C is more than ascorbic acid. It contains bioflavonoids, rutins, and other complexes that together make it vitamin

C. This is why, for example, ascorbic acid will not cure scurvy – while most vitamin C-rich raw fruits will.

Refined Sugar

Positron emission tomography scans have determined that cancer cells multiply faster than normal human cells. And they consume 10 to 12 times more sugar than healthy cells.

Indeed, laboratory studies have found that glucose increases the proliferation of cancer cells (Shimoda *et al.* 2017).

In 2020, researchers from the French National Institute of Health and Medical Research (INSERM), the Nutritional Epidemiology Research Team (EREN) and the Epidemiology and Statistics Research Center at the University of Paris (Debras *et al.* 2020) completed a large study to understand the relationship between sugar and cancer.

The researchers followed 101,279 people for ten years. They had an average age of 41 years old. Their sugar consumption was compared to their incidence of cancer after adjusting for other known risk factors for cancer.

The researchers found that those who consumed more sugar had a 51 percent higher incidence of breast cancer. And those who consumed more sugar had a 17 percent higher incidence of all cancers.

Junk foods cover the aisles of most markets. Yet research from the University of Texas MD Anderson Cancer Center in Houston (Melkonian *et al.* 2016) linked diets rich in junk foods to lung cancer.

The research assessed the diets of 1,905 people who were recently diagnosed with lung cancer, and compared these to the diets of 2,413 healthy people. In particular, they assessed their glycemic consumption, according to the glycemic index.

The researchers found those with diets with more foods high on the glycemic index had a 48 to 49 percent increased risk of lung cancer.

High glycemic foods are basically generalized as carbohydrate-based foods that have been refined in some form. In the case of grain-based foods, these are foods that have had the fiber removed.

There are other types of refined foods that have high glycemic index levels. These include fruits where the pulp (fiber) has been removed. Or grains that have been stripped of their fiber, leaving a white flour. Or sugar cane where all the plant fibers are removed, leaving a refined sugar. Or corn where all the corn fiber and nutrients have been removed, yielding corn syrup.

These types of foods are highly glycemic because they are devoid of the natural plant fibers and micronutrients that naturally slow down the absorption of the glucose contained within the food. These refined foods surge glucose into the blood – and thus increase what is called our glycemic load.

Yes, our bodies do need glucose for our cells to operate efficiently. But too much too fast is not healthy.

In such a refined state, these high glycemic foods dramatically increase the amount of sugar (glucose) in the blood. Such a condition puts pressure on all of the body's sugar-handling systems. These include the pancreas that produces insulin, the cells that receive the insulin and sugars, and the entire cardiovascular system that must fend off from the over-supply of sugar in the bloodstream.

For some clarity on the index itself, here is a searchable glycemic index based upon the USDA list of foods.

Free Glucose and Free Radicals

Free glucose blood sugars can oxidize if they are not immediately utilized by cells. This over-supply of sugar in the bloodstream produces an influx of oxidized free radicals. These free radicals damage everything from blood vessels to any organ that is fed by the blood.

Such a condition also produces type-two diabetes, as the body reacts with an inflammatory response to this dramatic influx of free glucose. Involved with type two-diabetes is insulin and glucose resistance within the cells. This produces a vicious cycle of increase free glucose in the blood.

The damage to the body, as a result, includes the lungs. The lungs are also made of cells and these must also have a good supply of well-timed energy. Lung cells must also be protected against free radicals. Free radicals on the loose within the bloodstream do more than produce atherosclerosis and dementia. They also are implicated in lung conditions such as asthma and COPD.

But these free radicals produced by free glucose can also damage the DNA of cells. When this happens, the risk of any type of cancer is increased. The researchers of this study confirmed this as they stated:

"Postprandial glucose and insulin responses play a role in carcinogenesis."

The term "postprandial glucose" refers to high glucose levels that result from eating a meal of refined foods – outside of the body's normal healthy insulin response when whole foods are eaten.

Refined carbohydrates are basically junk foods. Junk foods such as white bread, cakes, cookies, candies, soda pop and so many others are the foods with the highest glycemic levels.

Some of these junk foods have become staples in the Western diet. Such is the case for white bread, cake, donuts and so on.

Some of these foods might even be labeled as "natural" or "organic." But we must look for their tell-tale signs – their processed, refined ingredients. These will reveal that what might have originally been a healthy fiber-rich plant food, is not a high glycemic index junk food.

Some fruits have high glycemic load numbers. However, fresh whole fruits also contain pulp and numerous anticancer micronutrients, as we'll discuss below. These balance and neutralize free radicals.

Dairy

The China Study by Dr. T. Colin Campbell (2006) of Cornell University documented a 20-year study on the Chinese population as it evolved from a predominantly fish and plant-based diet to a Western Diet.

The primary study documented in this book was the China–Cornell–Oxford Project, was a 20-year-long study that followed 6,500 people from 65 counties in rural China. Their diets were tracked along with their history of cancers in others across the country as well as Western countries.

Dr. Campbell's research concluded that cancer levels were significantly higher among those that ate more animal-based foods.

This contrasted with those with diets containing more plant-based foods. They had dramatically lower rates of cancers and early mortality.

According to Dr. Campbell, dairy stood out as one of the significant risk factors for cancer in the research.

Research has linked growth hormone use for producing milk with cancer. So it is important that we know which milk brands don't come from cows that are receiving growth hormone injections or growth hormones in their feed.

After a significant review of the available research on growth hormones and cancer, the American Public Health Association - an association of physicians and public health officials - included the following statement in a 2009 Policy Release regarding the use of growth hormones in dairy cows, after a review of the evidence: *"elevated IGF-1 levels in human blood are associated with higher rates of colon, breast, and prostate cancers."*

There is also concern that hormone-treated milk is responsible for girls reaching puberty earlier. Indeed, researchers from the University of Cincinnati's College of Medicine (Biro *et al.* 2010) studied 1,239 girls from 6-8 years old. They found that girls in this age group are reaching puberty at double the rate they did just ten years ago. The question is whether this is all related to dairy from supplemented-hormone cows.

A 2007 study from the International Agency for Research on Cancer in France (Norat *et al.* 2007) studied the possible dietary sources for increased IGF-1 levels in the blood. They studied 2,109 women who were questioned on diet and tested for circulating IGF-1 levels.

This research indeed confirmed that circulating IGF-1 levels were "modestly related" with the consumption of dairy products. However, they were also related to the intake of protein, minerals such as calcium, magnesium and phosphorus, and vitamins B6 and B2. This study also found that IGF-1 levels were reduced with greater consumption of vegetables. The study did not test the effects of plasticizers such as BPA on IGF-1 levels.

For these reasons, it is important that consumers know which milks don't come from cows injected or fed growth hormones. In 2011, a Sixth Circuit Court of Appeals found that the State of Ohio restricted free speech when it ruled that organic milk farmers and bottlers. They were mandated by the state they could not list on their labels that their dairy products were made without synthetic hormones, pesticides, herbicides and antibiotics.

The state of Ohio responded by agreeing to allow such statements on dairy labels. This ended the legal battle between the State of Ohio and the Organic Trade Association, the International Dairy Food Association (IDFA), and organic milk producers.

The finding by the Sixth Circuit Court of Appeals determined that Ohio State's rule was unconstitutional because it restricted speech. The label claims that had been banned included "rbGH Free," "Hormone Free," "rbST Free," and "No Artificial Hormones." "Ohio's abandonment of this misguided rule is a victory for consumers, farmers and manufacturers alike.

Consumers have the right to make informed choices about the foods they eat, and farmers and manufacturers can continue to communicate truthfully with consumers," said the executive director of the Organic Trade Association, Christine Bushway, in an interview with NewHope360 (Baginski *et al.* 2011).

The lawsuit was filed in 2008 after Ted Strickland, Governor of Ohio, announced Executive Order 2008-03s, "Immediate Adoption of Rule to Define What Constitutes False and Misleading Labels on Milk and Milk Products." This rule stated that *"there is no significant difference between milk produced for cows supplemented with rbST and milk produced from cows not supplemented with rbST."* It also stated that *"Ohio's citizens are best served when they have complete and accurate information with which to make choices about the products they buy."*

This statement in the order apparently helped the case for consumers knowing whether the cows were supplemented with hormones. The critical issue many have with milk produced from cows supplemented with synthetic hormones is the possibility of elevated circulating levels of IGF-1 resulting from consuming those dairy products.

Organic Foods

Consuming organic foods can significantly reduce our risk of contracting cancer according to medical scientists.

Organic foods have been found to taste better according to some research. And they have been found to contain more vitamins and minerals according to others. Still other studies have shown that organic foods provide a significant increase in antioxidants and other medicinal elements in plants.

Are all of these connected? Quite possibly. Let's review that after taking a look at a study on organics and cancer.

The study was published in the *Journal of the American Medical Association.* The researchers (Baudry *et al.* 2018) were from France's government research institution INSERM (French National Institute of Health and Medical Research) and the University of Paris.

The researchers conducted a population study of 68,946 middle-aged adults from France. The participants reported on how much organic food they consumed, of 16 typical food groups. The researchers also conducted intake records that tested their daily food consumption.

Then the researchers followed the population for seven years, from mid-2009 through late 2016.

The researchers measured the number of cancer diagnoses through this period and compared this with the amount of organic food that was consumed by each person.

The most prevalent cancers among the population were breast cancer, then prostate cancer, then skin cancers, colorectal cancers, and lymphomas.

The researchers found that a greater frequency of organic food consumption reduced the incidence of cancer by an average of 25 percent. Moderate organic consumers also had a lower cancer incidence.

However, organic food consumers also had 76 percent lower incidence of lymphomas, and 86 percent lower incidence of non-Hodgkin's lymphomas.

Organic food consumers also saw their incidence of breast cancer reduced by 34 percent.

The researchers eliminated risks related to alcohol use, smoking, family cancer history, weight and relative exercise rates.

As mentioned above, other research has shown that organic foods tend to have more vitamins and minerals and more phytochemicals. Phytochemicals are compounds in plant foods that stimulate the immune system and also help the body detoxify.

Some plant chemicals also reduce the ability of cancer cells to metastasize.

These are certainly enough, but they aren't the only reasons organic foods can reduce the risk of cancer.

A number of chemical pesticides and herbicides have been linked to cancer incidence. Because organic foods will contain fewer chemical pesticides and herbicides, consumers can see their cancer risk going down.

A study from Stanford University researchers (Smith-Spangler *et al.* 2012) analyzed 240 studies on organic foods and found that studies showed reduced urinary pesticide levels, including two among children. The researchers found that pesticide residues were significantly lower among those who ate organic foods.

Besides that, as also reported, organic foods tend to taste better.

The only downside is cost. Yes, the prices for organics can be significantly higher than conventional foods. But the more we each purchase organic, the more prices can come down as more farmers will switch to organic production. This has become evident over the past few years as organic food consumption has increased.

The Alkaline Diet

This discussion of an anticancer diet should also include the reflective effects of an alkaline diet: The proper acid-alkaline balance among the blood, urine and intercellular tissue regions.

The reference to acidic or alkaline body fluids and tissues has been made by numerous natural health experts over the years. Is there any scientific validity to this?

Many nutritionists condemn an acidic metabolism and loosely call appropriate metabolism as a *state of alkalinity.* Strictly speaking, however, an alkaline environment is not healthy. The blood, interstitial fluids, lymph and urine should be *slightly acidic* to maintain the appropriate mineral ion balance. Let's dig into the science.

Acidity or alkalinity is measured using a logarithmic scale called pH. The term pH is derived from the French word *pouvoir hydrogene,* which means 'hydrogen power' or 'hydrogen potential.' pH is quantified by an inverse log base-10 scale. It measures the proton-donor level of a solution by comparing it to a theoretical quantity of hydrogen ions (H+) or H_3O+.

The scale is pH 1 to pH 14, which converts to a range of 10^{-1} (1) to 10^{-14} (.00000000000001) moles of hydrogen ions. This means that a pH of 14 maintains fewer hydrogen ions. It is thus *less acidic* and *more alkaline* (or basic).

The pH scale has been set up around the fact that water's pH is log-7 or simply pH 7—due to water's natural mineral content. Because pure water forms the basis for so many of life's activities, and because water neutralizes and dilutes so many reactions, water was established as the standard reference point or neutral point between what is considered an acid or a base solution. In other words, a substance having greater hydrogen ion potential (but lower pH) than water will be considered acidic, while a substance with less H+ potential (higher pH) than water is considered a base (alkaline).

Now the solution with a certain pH may not specifically maintain that many hydrogen ions. But it has the same *potential* as if it contained those hydrogen ions. That is why pH is hydrogen power or hydrogen potential.

In human blood, a pH level in the range of about 6.4 is considered healthy because this state is slightly more acidic than water, enabling the bodily fluids to maintain and transport minerals. It enables the *potential* for minerals to be carried by the blood, in other words. Minerals are critical to every cell, every organ, every tissue and every enzyme process occurring within the body. Better put, a 6.4 pH offers the appropriate *currency* of the body's fluids: This discourages acidosis and toxemia, maintaining a slight mineralized status.

Acidosis is produced with greater levels of carbonic acids, lactic acids, and/or uric acids among the joints and tissues. These acids are readily oxidizing, which produces free radicals. And as we've discussed, an overload of oxidative free radicals is one of the hallmarks of cancer cell development and proliferation.

However, an overly alkaline state can precipitate waste products from cells, which can also flood the system with radicals. For this reason, *toxemia* results from either an overly acidic blood-tissue content or an overly alkaline blood-tissue content. In other words, pH *balance* is the key.

Therefore, balance should also be concurrent with an anticancer diet.

A study from the National Cancer Institute of the NIH (Wright *et al.* 2005) followed 27,096 male smokers between 50 and 69 years old. The research found having a higher acidic diet had a 15 percent greater risk of bladder cancer.

Among those who smoked for more than 45 years, the incidence of bladder cancer was 72 percent higher for those with a higher acidic diet.

This correlates with the understanding that those who have smoked for a longer period will typically have a greater level of free radicals and a greater cancer risk. In these cases, an alkaline diet will have a greater effect.

A study from Japan's Karasuma Wada Clinic and the Cleveland Clinic (Hamaguchi *et al.* 2017) studied 11 patients with non-small cell lung cancer. The researchers found an alkaline diet increased the effectiveness of their treatment, using epidermal growth factor receptor.

Ions from minerals like potassium, calcium, magnesium and others are usually positively oriented—with alkaline potential. But to be carried through a solution, the solution must have the pH potential to carry them.

Besides being critical to enzymatic reactions, these minerals bond with lipids and proteins to form the structures of our cells, organs and tissues—including our airways, nerves and mucosal membranes.

Natural health experts over the past century have observed among their patients and in clinical research that an overly acidic environment within the body is created by a diet abundant in refined sugars, processed foods, chemical toxins and amino acid-heavy animal foods.

The evidence has connected this acidic state to toxemia. The toxemia state is a state of free radical proliferation, which damages cells and tissues. It is also a state that produces systemic inflammation, because the immune system is over-worked as it tries to remove the cell and tissue damage.

As mentioned earlier, animals accumulate toxins within their fat tissues. They are bioaccumulators. Thus, animals exposed to the typical environmental toxins of smog and chemical pollutants in their waters and air—along with pesticides and herbicides from their foods—will accumulate those toxins within their fat cells and livers. And those who eat those animals will inherit (and further accumulate) these accumulated toxins. In addition, animals secrete significant waste matter as they are being slaughtered.

Plants are not bioaccumulators. While they can accumulate some pesticides and herbicide chemicals within their leaves and roots, they do not readily absorb or hold these for long periods within their cells. This is because many environmental toxins are, as mentioned, fat soluble. Because plants have little or no fat, they can more easily systemically rid their tissues of many of these toxins over time.

Further, as the research has shown, a diet heavy in complex proteins—which contain far more amino acids than our bodies require—increases the risk and severity of inflammation. Amino acids are the building blocks of protein. A complex protein can have tens of thousands of amino acids. While proteins and aminos are healthy, a diet too rich in them will produce deposits in our joints and tissues, burdening our immune system.

Diets rich in red meats also produce byproducts such as phytanic acid and beta-glucuronidase that can damage our intestinal cells and produce a greater risk of colorectal cancers.

The complexities of digesting complex proteins produce increased levels of beta-glucuronidase, nitroreductase, azoreductase, steroid 7-alpha-dehydroxylase, ammonia, urease, cholylglycine hydrolase, phytanic acid and others. These toxic enzymes deter our probiotics and produce systemic inflammation. Not surprisingly, they've all been linked to colon cancer.

By contrast, plant-based foods contain many antioxidants, anti-carcinogens and other nutrients that strengthen the immune system and balance the body's pH. Plant-based foods also discourage inflammatory responses. Plant-based foods feed our probiotics with complex polysaccharides called prebiotics. They are also a source of fiber (there is little fiber in red meat)—critical for helping prevent colon cancer.

Nutrition for Cancer Patients

Diet is critical to cancer care. Diet and nutrition has maintained an untouchable status among cancer treatment, new research is finding that a cancer patient's choice of diet is critical to their chances of survival.

Researchers from Philadelphia's Thomas Jefferson University (Anthony *et al.* 2013) confirmed that diet and nutrition choices are critical in cancer treatment.

The researchers investigated the use of nutrition and diet during cancer treatment – not as a primary treatment, but as supportive treatment – also called palliative cancer care.

Utilizing decades of research that have shown that particular types of diets and foods help prevent cancer, the researchers determined that there are several topics of concern when considering diet during cancer treatment:

Ensuring enough calories yet preventing problems with glucose control – which encourages metastasis – comes with new research that glucose control is related specifically to whether the carbohydrates in the diet come in the form of whole foods or refined, processed carbohydrates, according to the researchers:

"… and such an approach may not only satisfy caloric requirements but also positively impact secondary problems related to sugar consumption, insulin resistance, inflammation, and others …"

152

This has been summarized from the American Cancer Society's guidelines regarding diet:

"choosing whole grains instead of refined grain products"

The researchers also investigated the role of red meat and processed meats in cancer care. They reviewed the research which has linked these foods with cancer, and found that prevailing cancer care advice has advised patients to lower red meat and processed meat intake, as recommended by the American Cancer Society:

"limiting the amount of processed and red meat eaten"

The researchers also acknowledged the research associated with reduced cancer and remission risk with greater consumption of fruits and vegetables, and again this has been recommended by the ACS:

"eating at least two and a half cups of vegetables and fruits each day"

The researchers also found that increased consumption of refined carbohydrates, and refined fructose (such as high-fructose corn syrup). The research suggests that refined carbs *"has been associated with cancer in general"* and refined fructose has been linked with greater obesity – which they and most other clinicians discourage in cancer care.

The issue of weight control is important in cancer care, because, as stated by the researchers:

"However, many patients are overweight at the time of diagnosis or become so after treatment."

They also acknowledged that:

"Women diagnosed with early-stage breast cancer might improve overall prognosis and survival by adopting more healthful dietary patterns."

With regard to certain diets, the researchers stated that:

"Red and processed meat consumption has consistently gained a reputation as a contributor to disease, including cancer. Data is emerging that red and processed meats may influence disease recurrence and mortality as well, for example, for colorectal cancer survivors. Evidence shows that consumption of red meat can activate cancer genes in the colon such as the MDM2 and ubiquitin genes as well as the WNT gene signaling pathway which is involved in epithelial proliferation and differentiation. Such genetic modulation can facilitate cellular progression to colon cancer."

The research has also supported the implementation of healthy lifestyles:

"Prospective observational studies have shown that increased exercise after diagnosis and avoidance of a Western pattern diet (high intake of red and processed meats and refined grains) are associated with a reduced risk of cancer recurrence and improved overall survival in early-stage colorectal cancer after standard therapy."

The researchers also clarified that red meat stimulates inflammation and cancer. Here is their statement:

"The data also suggests that red meat, in particular, is pro-inflammatory and procarcinogenic. For example, the European Prospective Investigation into Cancer and Nutrition-Potsdam study of 2,198 men and women found that the consumption of red meat was significantly associated with higher levels of the inflammatory markers GGT and hs-CRP

when adjusted for potential confounding factors related to lifestyle and diet. Another study showed that when people were given a 7-day dietary red meat intervention, fecal water genotoxicity significantly increased in response to the red meat intake. These effects included modifications in DNA damage repair, the cell cycle, and apoptosis pathways."

Noting the data, the researchers made a direct recommendation:

"*Thus, red meat should be minimized or eliminated from the diet of palliative care patients.*"

The researchers also linked red meat intake with bladder cancer and bladder cancer survivorship.

The researchers recommendations were confirmed by a study of breast cancer survivors from the Life After Cancer Epidemiology Study (Kwan *et al.* 2012). Here 1,901 patients who were diagnosed with early stage breast cancer were followed. Two eating patterns were found among the patients: One had increased consumption of fruits, vegetables, whole grains, and poultry (called the "Prudent pattern"). The other, called the "Western pattern – increased consumption of red and processed meats with refined grains.

The researchers found that those who adhered the closest with the "Prudent pattern" had lower rates of death from breast cancer or any other cause. Meanwhile those in the "Western pattern" suffered higher incidence of recurrent breast cancers, greater incidence of death from their breast cancer, and increased risk of death from any cause.

The researchers summarized their findings:

"*Overall, the cumulative data suggests that refined carbohydrate and red meat consumption should be avoided or significantly reduced in the diet of patients with cancer as there are many other healthier sources of caloric intake. Achievement and maintenance of a healthy body composition via a plant-based diet high in fruits, vegetables, and whole grains and low in saturated fats and red or processed meats should be the guidelines imparted to patients from their health care providers.*"

Diets that reduce inflammation and oxidative stress

The researchers also investigated dietary choices that reduced inflammation in the body, and minimized free radicals – referred to as oxidative stress – stating:

"*The literature indeed shows more studies exploring the link between cancer and inflammation. Inflammation itself is associated with high levels of oxidative stress that can damage most of the body's tissues and genetic material which ultimately can lead to cancer formation.*"

The researchers then investigated different diets found in the research to be anti-inflammatory, particular Ayurvedic diet:

"*Ancient cultures also developed and used anti-inflammatory diets, such as in Ayurvedic (a system of traditional medicine native to the Indian subcontinent that stresses plant based treatment), which are now investigated using modern criteria.*"

Another study (Venil *et al.* 2012) investigated the use of the Ayurvedic diet in cancer therapy. The research, from the Indian Institute of Technology of Madras, found that Ayurvedic diets offered several avenues for reducing inflammation and halting the "Shared Pathology" between cancer and pro-inflammatory diets.

Anti-inflammatory components of the Ayurvedic diet highlighted included triterpenes, which included betulinic acid, boswellic acid, diosgenin, madecassic acid, maslinic acid, momordin, saikosaponins, ursolic acid, and withanolide. These of course are derived from some of the herbs and spices found among Ayurvedic diets, including turmeric, Ginger, boswellia and ginseng.

Other areas of interest in palliative cancer treatment that were highlighted by the researchers included vitamin D, probiotics and prebiotics, multivitamins and antioxidants including polyphenols and others.

Chapter Four

Anticancer Superfoods

There are foods and then there are superfoods. For the purposes of this book, we will classify any food that has been shown to be anticancer as a superfood.

This doesn't meant other natural foods don't also reduce the risk of cancer. As the previous chapter showed, certain diets – and the foods they contain – can help prevent cancer incidence.

Citrus

Citrus fruits are tangy and tasty, yet they also combat ulcers and help prevent stomach cancer. One might think the acidic nature of fresh citrus would exacerbate an ulcer, but the opposite is true.

These conclusions have been borne out of multiple studies over the years. These have included large population studies, clinical tests and laboratory studies. These have looked at the myriad of compounds in fresh citrus fruits.

And because ulcers have also been linked with stomach cancer, the notion that fresh citrus fruits can ease ulcers as well as reduce stomach cancers is a natural conclusion.

A study from South Korea's Jeju National University School of Medicine (Bae *et al.* 2016) analyzed five large population studies that tracked stomach cancer. The studies were from the U.S., the Netherlands, Europe, China and Japan. These five studies followed 490,802 people, 4,035 people, 477,312 people, 132,311 people and 42,470 people, respectively.

Yes, these were large population studies conducted by researchers from those respective countries.

Using the combined data from these studies, the researchers determined that eating fresh citrus fruits significantly decrease the incidence of stomach cancer.

They found that eating just 100 grams of citrus per day reduces the incidence of cardia gastric cancer by 40 percent. And the risk of any type of stomach cancer was reduced by 13 percent by citrus consumption.

The researchers also found a dose dependency in the relationship between citrus fruits and cardia stomach cancer. Eating 100 grams a day resulted in a 40 percent reduction in the cancer incidence. But eating 50 grams a day cut the risk by 23 percent.

According to the USDA, an average orange weighs 131 grams. This means that by eating just one orange a day, we can exceed the 100 grams a day.

Eat two oranges a day? Even better. We can assume from the dose-dependency relationship that this will reduce our risk of gastric cancer even further.

Helicobacter pylori is a bacteria species that often infects the stomach wall. It is often associated with many cases of ulcers.

In addition to being linked to ulcers, H. pylori infections have also been linked to approximately 74 percent of gastric cancer cases.

A majority of people have H. pylori in the gut. However, research has established a more destructive form of H. pylori can infect the gut. This is called CagA-positive H. pylori. The CagA stands for cytotoxin-associated gene.

This particular type of H. pylori is highly resistant to most antibiotics. We discussed how this strain of H. pylori differs from most strains that naturally inhabit many guts.

Our point here is that eating fresh citrus fruits has been shown to reduce H. pylori infections.

Researchers from Italy's University of Messina (Giuseppina Mandalari *et al.* 2017) studied the relationship between citrus and ulcers and H. pylori infections. These included laboratory studies to test citrus against H. pylori.

Types of citrus shown to fight H. pylori among multiple studies (Zhang *et al.* 2015; Dong *et al.* 2014; *et al.*)

- Mandarins (*Citrus reticulata*)
- Oranges (*Citrus sinensis*)
- Grapefruits (*Citrus paradise*)
- Lemons (*Citrus lemon*)
- Satsuma Mandarins (*Citrus unshiu*)

These are just the types of citrus tested against H. pylori. Other citrus fruits will share many of the compounds of these above.

The research determined that citrus has two effects upon the microbial nature of the gut. The first is that it decreases H. pylori content. This is achieved by citrus' antibacterial qualities.

Components in citrus that have been shown to inhibit H. pylori include neohesperidin, hesperetin, neoeriocitrin, naringin, eriodictyol, naringenin, hesperetin, geranyloxyferulic acid, boropinic acid, sudachitin and demethoxy-sudachitin.

Besides inhibiting *H. pylori*, the research has found that citrus inhibits other bacteria, including *E. coli*, Pseudomonas and Salmonella species. We have discussed how citrus can rival antibiotics against resistant bacteria.

The research found these components of citrus work synergistically to inhibit the growth of *H. pylori*. Some of the research also indicated that citrus reduces the effectiveness of urease enzymes produced by *H. pylori*. By blocking the urease enzymes, citrus helps block the growth of the bacterium.

The other component discovered by the researchers was citrus' ability to feed the gut's probiotic populations. This makes citrus an effective prebiotic.

The researchers found that pectin oligosaccharides present in the inner peels of citrus provide prebiotic properties. The research showed that these oligosaccharides increased populations of bifidobacteria and lactobacilli probiotics within the gut.

We have discussed how probiotics reduce cancer and pathobiotics cause cancer. We'll dig into that more later.

This prebiotic property of citrus increases populations of these healthy bacteria. The researchers stated:

"The results obtained demonstrated that bergamot oligosaccharides resulted in a high increase in the number of beneficial bacteria, such as bifidobacteria and lactobacilli, whereas the clostridial population decreased."

Connecting all these realities and studies together creates a grander image of how fresh citrus fruits fight ulcers and stomach cancers.

The various plant compounds in fresh citrus provide a myriad of benefits. These include stimulating healthy stomach lining, inhibiting H. pylori outbreaks, and preventing cancer cells from growing.

We should note that pasteurized citrus juices won't necessarily maintain the same properties as fresh citrus fruits. That's because the pasteurization process removes many of the flavonoids and other critical compounds. This is because many of these are heat sensitive.

Pasteurization also tends to increase the acidic content of the juice at the same time. These acids may actually exacerbate an ulcerative condition.

In addition, many of these compounds are contained within the pulp and the rind of the citrus. Juices are often stripped of these essential parts of the citrus fruit during processing. Yet these are the very elements that really help the stomach.

Should we expect less from such a tangy and tasty fruit?

Citrus Peels

Citrus peels contain several polymethoxylated flavonoids (PMFs). Nobiletin is a O-methylated flavone. It renders a hydroxyl group that mediates a reaction called O-methylation. Methylation allows for the donation of methyl groups, which provide radical-neutralizing effects, as well as the inhibition of lipid peroxide-friendly LDL cholesterol apoprotein B.

Other O-methylated flavones include tangeritin (first found in tangerine oil), wogonin (found in the herb baikal scullcap), and sinensetin, found in the Java tea herb *Orthosiphon stamineus.*

Citrus peels can contain as much as 70% oil. The oil contains a number of other healthful components including limonene and linalool. Limonene is monoterpene known for its antimicrobial and radical-scavenging abilities. Most applications of citrus remove the peel and toss it out. In a good year, over 700,000 tons of peel solids will be discarded or sold for feed.

Citrus peel is typically a quarter inch or more thick. It begins at the outer layer where the pigment is located, ending at the citrus segments. Even when we peel a citrus fruit by hand there is a thin layer of peel remaining over the segments of the fruit.

Certainly, eating more citrus peel is a good idea. We have discussed some of the health benefits of citrus peel in previous articles.

A useful strategy might be to toss the whole unpeeled citrus fruit into a blender together with other fruit. This can make a wonderful and tangy fruit smoothie. If the outer rind of the fruit seems a bit damaged, we can cut the outer rind off, still leaving much of the peel intact.

Eating the rind and the citrus fruit like an apple is obviously one strategy. Another strategy would be to just peel or slice off the very outer rind and leave as much of the inner peel as possible. The bitterness of the peel may take a bit to get used to, but after awhile it will take on a taste of its own and complement the sweeter inner fruit.

Another anticancer agent in citrus peels is nobiletin. Nobiletin is what is called a polymethoxylated flavone. A flavone is a type of flavonoid – which are often found among citrus plants and a number of herbal medicines. Flavones have a number of medicinal effects upon the human body. They are antioxidants, but also tend to be antimicrobial and anticancer as well.

In particular, this nobiletin flavone is found most often among citrus peels. These include oranges, mandarins, tangerines and other citrus. Other polymethoxy flavones in citrus include tangeretin, hesperidin and hesperetin, and other important citrus flavonoids include naringenin, and naringin.

But nobiletin has gained significant traction in medical research due to its outstanding benefits to our health. As a result, over the past decade, nobiletin has been studied extensively by medical researchers from around the world.

Researchers from Japan's NARO Western Region Agricultural Research Center (Saito *et al.* 2015) found that nobiletin inhibits the growth of leukemia by modulating the natural killer cell function. This was accomplished through the biochemical modulating the genetic processes of these natural killer cells.

Another study (Uesato *et al.* 2014) found that nobiletin inhibits the growth of lung cancer cells through a process called notch signaling.

Researchers from West Virginia's Alderson Broaddus University (Chen *et al.* 2014) found that nobiletin isolated from citrus peels inhibited the growth of two types of prostate cancers. This was accomplished through another complex genetic modulation, including the blocking of VEGF.

Researchers from Taiwan's Chung Shan Medical University (Hsiao *et al.* 2014) also studied the effects of nobiletin on leukemia cells. In this study they found that nobiletin blocked the proliferation of the leukemia cells. This means that the citrus peel extract blocked the growth of leukemia.

Researchers from Japan's Nakamura Gakuen University (Chen *et al.* 2014) found that nobiletin blocked the growth of three different types of breast cancers. Once again the mechanisms were complex, but in general, they suppressed the growth of the cancer cells through genetic switching.

Research from Japan's Kansai University and Mukogawa Women's University tested nobiletin on non-small-cell lung cancer cells. Once again, they found the citrus peel extract inhibited the growth of the cancer cells in laboratory tests.

Research from Japan's Nakamura Gakuen University, studied several human lines of breast cancer cells. These included the cell lines MCF-7, HER2-positive SK-BR-3, and triple-negative MDA-MB-468. These represent a significant swath of potential breast cancers that occur among women.

The researchers found the citrus peel extract nobiletin inhibited the growth of all three breast cancer lines, with the most being the MDA-MB-468 cell line. This was extracted from a 51-year old African American woman with adenocarcinoma – breast cancer.

The significant point about this study is that the citrus peel extract blocked tumor growth on a dose-dependent manner. This means the effect was definite – the more dose, the greater the inhibition.

The inhibition was also time-dependent. This means the effect continued over the duration of the treatment.

This research is confirmed by another study on non-small cell lung cancer and nobiletin from the Xinjiang Medical University (Da et al. 2016).

It doesn't stop there. Sichuan University researchers (Meiyanto et al. 2012) studied human liver cancer cell lines with nobiletin and found the extract halted the growth of SMMC-7721 tumor cells.

In this study also, the tumor inhibition effect was found to be dose-dependent. The greater the nobiletin dose, the more tumor cells died.

Researchers from Korea's Jeju National University (Moon et al. 2013) tested nobiletin against human stomach cancer cells. Again they used a human gastric cancer cell line, the SNU-16 cell line.

Again they found that the citrus peel extract halted the growth of the cancer cells, against in a dose-dependent manner. When the researchers tested the nobiletin together with the chemotherapy drug 5-fluorouracil, the cancer-killing effect was increased as compared with the chemotherapy drug alone.

This strategy of combining nobiletin with chemotherapy drugs has been tested in other studies. For example, nobiletin research from Japan's Osaka University of Pharmaceutical Sciences found that the citrus extract nobiletin inhibits the growth of non-small-cell lung cancer in human cells.

Non-small-cell lung cancer often escapes chemotherapy solutions. The researchers tested two human non-small-cell lung cancer cell lines A549 and H460. They tested paclitaxel and carboplatin with the cancer cells and then added nobiletin in combination and found that the nobiletin killed the non-small lung cancer cells the chemotherapy missed.

Other cancers, such as leukemia, have also been found to be potentially treated with nobiletin.

In many of these studies, the mechanisms involved in the citrus peel extract's ability to halt the cancer growth was the stimulating or modulating a genetic change that helps the body kill tumor cells.

In other words, the citrus peel extract actually stimulates the body's own mechanisms for killing cancer cells.

Even the healthiest of us must deal with cancer cells all the time. A cancerous cell growth will occur quite often. But a healthy body will initiate what is called apoptosis – the killing of the cancer cell. This is initiated through the Bcl-2 protein and others – typically driven by the immune system.

But when our body and its immune system is overburdened, the cancer growth can get out of hand.

Remember that a strong liver will reduce cancer risk. We can now add liver health to the above benefits of nobiletin. Researchers from Japan's College of Life Sciences in Kusatsu (Yoshigai *et al.* 2013) produced a nobiletin extract from the peels of the chinpi fruit – *Citrus unshiu.*

They then tested liver cells in a laboratory and found using chromatography that the nobiletin stimulated a healing process among the cells by limiting the produced nitric oxide and stimulated a genetic change (blocking iNOS) that produced a healing effect.

The researchers concluded from this finding that nobiletin has a healing effect upon the liver:

"The suppression of iNOS induction by nobiletin suggests that nobiletin may be responsible for the anti-inflammatory effects of citrus peels and have a therapeutic potential for liver diseases."

Another compound found in citrus peels is modified citrus pectin. Other research finds MCP helps the body detoxify and boosts immune function. Citrus peels also inhibit bacteria according to other research.

Modified Citrus Pectin

Modified citrus pectin (MCP) has been shown to boost immunity, increase detoxification, lengthen lifespan, reduce heart disease and fight cancer.

A study led by anti-aging expert, Dr. Isaac Eliaz (Eliaz *et al.* 2019) has found that modified citrus pectin reduces disease by blocking the destructive Galectin-3.

Dr. Eliaz presented to the 19th Annual World Congress on Anti-Aging Medicine and Regenerative Biomedical Technologies new findings that show citrus pectin blocks the biomarker Galectin-3 – found to increase life-threatening disease incidence and early death.

"MCP offers unprecedented health benefits by binding and blocking excess Galectin-3 molecules throughout the body. With the latest research linking Galectin-3 to the progression of numerous diseases, this presentation felt like a breakthrough moment where a new tool in medicine is being introduced to a whole medical community for the first time," said Dr. Eliaz.

The anti-aging conference was attended by more than 1,000 physicians, health practitioners, and scientists.

Dr. Eliaz' research data revealed that the modified citrus pectin, derived from the pith of citrus fruit peels, blocked unhealthy levels of Galectin-3 molecules circulating within the body. Elevated levels of Galectin-3 has been shown to be associated with heart disease, tissue fibrosis, cancer, and diseases of other organs. So far, MCP has been found to be the only natural Galectin-3 blocker available today. MCP binds to excess Galectin-3 molecules, preventing them from damaging tissues.

MCP reduces the risk of tumor growth and helps prevent tumors from forming. For example, one study (Fang *et al.* 2018) found that MCP significantly inhibited the growth and survival of bladder cancer cells.

Another study (Hossein *et al.* 2019) found that MCP prevents ovarian cancer cells from migrating and further invasion.

Another study (do Prado *et al.* 2019) found that MCP inhibits migration of cancer cells, halts proliferation and aggregation of cancer cells.

Another study (Conti *et al.* 2018) found that modified citrus pectin reduces migration of prostate cancer cells.

Yet another study (Guess *et al.* 2003) tested 10 men with recurring prostate cancer. After one year of taking MCP, 70 percent of the men had significantly reduced growth rates of the prostate cancer cells.

Circulating levels of Galectin-3 are now measurable with a blood test, and the test has been approved by the FDA to help determine higher risks of heart disease and damage to other organs.

Dr. Eliaz' research has also shown that modified citrus pectin enhances immunity. One of his studies showed that MCP activated B-cells and activated T-cells and natural killer cells. The NK-cells' stimulated activity was found to kill leukemia cancer cells, as published in the journal BMC Complementary and Alternative Medicine.

MCP has also been shown to stimulate detoxification. Dr. Eliaz found that MCP reduces heavy metal levels within the body.

"When the toxic burden is high, I recommend a gentle yet highly effective heavy metal detoxification program using Modified Citrus Pectin. MCP is clinically proven to significantly reduce dangerous heavy metals, including lead, mercury, arsenic, and cadmium, without lowering levels of essential minerals," added Dr. Eliaz.

A number of studies have also found MCP to be a natural detox agent. In a 2019 study, a team of doctors studied six people in the Phoenix Arizona area, who had uranium exposure.

The doctors tested their blood, urine and fecal matter beforehand, and gave them three 750 milligram capsules of MCP twice a day for six weeks. They tested the patients after six days and six weeks, and then again six weeks after halting the supplementation.

The researchers found all the subjects had increased levels of uranium in their feces. The supplementation increased their uranium counts in their feces with supplementation. And six weeks after stopping, five of the six patients then showed significantly decreased levels of uranium.

One study (Glinsky *et al.* 2008) tested hospitalized children with toxic lead poisoning (levels over 20 micrograms per deciliter). The researchers gave some of the children MCP in three doses per day. The researchers found the children had dramatically decreased levels of lead in their blood and urine samples.

Blood levels of lead went down by an average of 161 percent and urine levels of lead went down by 132 percent on average. The doctors reported:

"The need for a gentle, safe heavy metal-chelating agent, especially for children with high environmental chronic exposure, is great. The dramatic results and no observed adverse effects in this pilot study along with previous reports of the safe and effective use of MCP in adults indicate that MCP could be such an agent."

A number of studies have also found MCP to be a significant antioxidant. In one study (Ramachandran *et al.* 2017) scientists found that MCP had a significant antioxidant effect, helping to inhibit TNF-alpha levels, nuclear factor-kappa B activity and lipid peroxidation levels.

The researchers also found MCP reduced inflammation and was a potent antioxidant.

Another citrus peel compound is nobiletin. Research has found that nobiletin helps the heart and the liver, and fights cancer. Citrus peels also fight bacteria according to other research.

The bottom line? Don't be so hasty about cutting away all the peel from your citrus fruits.

Cruciferous Vegetables

Cruciferous vegetables such as broccoli, cabbage, cauliflower and watercress contain several compounds that inhibit cancer growth

Increasing evidence is finding that isothiocyanates and sulforaphane from cruciferous vegetables inhibit the development of cancer in the body. As the research has matured, active anticancer compounds in cruciferous vegetables are getting more attention among researchers.

Researchers from the University of Minnesota (Yuan *et al.* 2016) tested 82 smokers for what is called NNK activation. NNK is a carcinogen – long form is also known as 4-(methylnitrosamino)-1-(3-pyridyl)-1-butanone. It is a leading cause of cancer from smoking. The smokers were given either the active compound in watercress – phenethyl isothiocyanate – or a placebo for a week. Previous research has established that phenethyl isothiocyanate or PEITC is significantly anticancer.

The researchers gave the smokers special cigarettes so they could measure NNK metabolism. They found that in just one week, NNK activation was reduced by 7.7 percent. That's not bad for chain-smokers!

The researchers concluded:

"The results of this trial, while modest in effect size, provide a basis for further investigation of PEITC as an inhibitor of lung carcinogenesis by NNK in smokers."

As hinted at above, this is not the first study showing cruciferous vegetables' anticancer ability.

A study from the Czech Republic's Faculty of Medicine and Dentistry, Palacky University Olomouc (Vanduchova *et al.* 2019) studied isothiocyanate and sulforaphane. They found that both inhibited cancer cells and tumor growth in laboratory studies.

A study from University of Pittsburgh School of Medicine (Singh *et al.* 2019) showed similar findings. They found that sulforaphane halted the progression of prostate cancer in laboratory studies.

They also found that cancer markers showed improvements among prostate cancer patients. They stated:

"Examination of plasma lactate levels in prostate cancer patients following administration of an SFN-rich broccoli sprout extract failed to show declines in its levels."

A study from Britain's Edinburgh Napier University (Fogarty *et al.* 2012) found that watercress reduces DNA damage and oxidative stress – two main components of cancer development.

The researchers studied ten healthy young men (average age 23) for four months. The men were tested before and after the study, and on a daily basis, before and after exhausting aerobic exercise. During one eight-week period, the subjects took 85 grams of watercress supplements daily. They took the supplements two hours before exercise. During the other eight-week period, they worked out without the supplements.

When given the watercress supplement, the men showed a significant reduction in reactive oxygen species levels, and reduced DNA damage. Blood samples also revealed that levels of lipid peroxidation – the major cause of artery disease – were also significantly lower when taking the watercress.

Strenuous exercise typically produces DNA damage, which the body will hopefully repair. The ability of watercress to reduce DNA damage confirms earlier research showing that watercress reduces mutation and cancer growth.

The researchers commented on this aspect of the study:

"The study demonstrates that exhaustive aerobic exercise may cause DNA damage and lipid peroxidation; however, these perturbations are attenuated by either short- or long-term watercress supplementation, possibly due to the higher concentration lipid-soluble antioxidants following watercress ingestion."

A study from China's First Affiliated Hospital of Guiyang Medical College (Wang *et al.* 2014) found that Phenethyl isothiocyanate halted the growth of leukemia cancer cells.

Another study, from the University of Pittsburgh (Sakao *et al.* 2015) found that isothiocyanate and sulforaphane – also present in watercress as well as broccoli and other cruciferous vegetables – can halt the growth of prostate cancer.

Georgetown University researchers (Wang *et al.* 2011) established that isothiocyanate inhibited the growth of cervical cancer and breast cancer cells.

Cancer researchers love to hone in on one special anticancer agent. They are looking for single bullets. But nature doesn't work like that. Nature's anticancer foods like watercress will contain other anticancer agents to fight cancer. Yes, nature fights cancer.

Besides isothiocyanate and sulphorophane, watercress contains a host of antioxidant nutrients, including xanthophyll, beta-carotene, alpha-tocopherol and gamma-tocopherol (two forms of vitamin E), each of which have been shown to slow free radical formation in the body. As other studies have shown, this in turn can reduce the rate of DNA damage and cancer formation in the body.

Avocados

Avocados fight cancer. Science is now confirming that avocado fights cancer and the free radicals that cause it. Avocados are serious antioxidants. This in addition to the incredible array of health properties of the humble avocado.

Researchers from the School of Medicine of Mexico's Monterey College of Technology (Rodríguez-Sánchez *et al.* 2013) studied the L-ORAC of the avocado (*Persea americana*).

The ORAC (oxygen radical absorbance capacity) test measures the antioxidant capacity of a food. This is done using by using chromatography after a food has been fractioned.

In this case, the researchers used a lipid fraction to conduct the ORAC test – measuring the lipophilic elements of the avocado's pulp. Lipophilic roughly means "fat-loving" – the ability of a certain compound to dissolve in or have affinity with fats, also called lipids.

The avocado's lipophilic phytonutrients, which include tocopherols, sterols, monusaturates, carotenes and acetogenins, provide the bulk of these antioxidant benefits.

The acetogenins in avocados have been found to provide more than just antioxidant benefits. Researchers from Ohio State University (D'Ambrosio *et al.* 2011) found that two of avocados' acetogenins – dihydroxyheptadecenyl acetate and dihydroxyheptadecynyl acetate – inhibited the growth of cancer cells.

The researchers found that these two acetogenins blocked the phosphorylation process of oral cancer cells. This effectively stops their ability to expand and metastasize.

So far, five acetogenins have been found in avocado. The Monterey researchers found two addition acetogenins in their research.

Avocados reduce LDL-c and Triglycerides

Other research has found that avocados reduce low-density lipoprotein – a carrier for cholesterol in the body that is subject to peroxidation – which damages the blood vessel walls.

For example, 15 women were studied at the Wesley Hospital in Brisbane, Australia. Those who ate a diet rich in avocados for three weeks found their total cholesterol reduced by over 8%, and LDL-c levels also went down significantly.

Another study of 12 diabetic women found that a four-week diet rich in avocados reduced triglycerides by 20%. The study also found that the avocado diet increased their glycemic control as well.

Another study tested 67 volunteers – a third of which had high cholesterol – with either an avocado-enriched diet or a control diet. After only seven days, those on the avo-rich diet showed a reduction of total cholesterol by 16%-17%, an LDL-c reduction of 22%, and a 22% reduction in triglycerides. Those on the avocado-rich diet also had an average increase of 11% in HDL-c – the "good" lipoprotein.

Avocado contains a fatty alcohol or triol, called avocadene. Avocadene has a molecular structure of 16-heptadecene-1,2,4-triol. Avocadene has been shown to be antibacterial as well as anti-inflammatory.

Avocados also contain numerous other nutrients, and one of the best sources of B vitamins. Avocados contain 28% RDA (recommended daily amount) of vitamin B5, 20% RDA for vitamin B6. 20% RDA for folate (B9), 12% RDA for niacin and 9% RDA for vitamin B2.

Avocados also contain significant amounts of vitamin A, vitamin E, potassium, magnesium, copper, iron and zinc.

Avocados also contain good fiber – about five grams for a medium avocado, equating to about a gram of fiber per ounce.

Most of avocado's calories are derived from monounsaturated fat. Monounsaturated fats like oleic oil have been found to reduce heart disease, reduce dementia risk and lower cholesterol levels.

Most people think that avocados are fatty foods that increase weight. Not true. In a study of sixty-one persons, with a control group on a calorie-restricted diet, those who ate avocado oil to replace their other oil sources had comparable weight loss with the other participants on diet.

The research was conducted by researchers from South Africa's Potchefstroom University for Christian Higher Education (Pieterse *et al.* 2005). Their stated purpose was to *"dispel the myth that avocados are fattening."*

They gave part of a group of sixty-one obese persons on a weight loss regimen avocado oil to replace their other fat and oil sources. At the end of six weeks, the avocado oil subjects had similar weight loss results as with the other weight loss subjects.

The research included 13 men and 48 women, with BMIs (body mass index) of 32 +/- 3.9. They were paired and assigned to either a group who consumed 200 grams per day of avocados, each containing over 30 grams of fat on average. This served as a substitute for 30 grams of other dietary fats in their diets. The other group excluded avocado from their diets, while on a reduced-calorie diet for 6 weeks.

Parsley

Parsley (*Petroselinum crispum*) fights cancer and reduces inflammation.

Parsley may be a great garnish. And it can seriously freshen the breath. But research proves that parsley also boosts the immune system, reduces inflammation and fights off cancer.

Multiple studies show that parsley contains significant anti-inflammatory properties, boosts liver health, is antioxidant and even anti-carcinogenic. It also supplies numerous nutrients and relaxes smooth muscles.

A study from Germany's University of Rostock (Schröder *et al.* 2017) studied parsley root extract. They tested the extract against malignant and benign breast cancer cells.

The researchers found the parsley extract killed the breast cancer cell lines at a rates ranging from 70 percent to 80 percent.

This and other research has connected parsley's apigenin to cancer inhibition. Apigenin is a flavone. A 2016 study from Texas A&M University found that apigenin from parsley inhibited the growth of uterine cancer cells.

Research from China's Jiangsu Polytechnic College of Agriculture and Forestry (Liu *et al.* 2011) found that apigenin also blocked the action of MEK kinase 1, which in turn prevented bladder cancer cells from migrating and thus inhibited tumor growth.

In this case, the apigenin compound was found with the ability to stop tumor growth by blocking tumors from creating blood vessels.

Hungarian researchers (Pápay *et al.* 2012) confirmed that parsley boosted the body's ability to fight inflammation.

The research found that parsley contained numerous nutrients and bioactive constituents, including several flavonoids and cumarins. They found that in addition to its anti-cancer properties, Parsley slows inflammation and neutralizes oxidative radicals (free radicals).

Parsley's ability to encourage healing has also been shown in other studies. For example, a study from Turkey's Hacettepe University Faculty of Medicine (Tavil *et al.* 2012) found that increased parsley consumption was associated with fewer complications after hematopoietic (bone marrow) stem cell transplantation in children.

In this study, the diets of 41 children who underwent the stem cell transplantation were analyzed. Improved outcomes were seen among those eating more Parsley, as well as those children who ate onions, bulgur, yogurt and bazlama (a Turkish yeast bread).

Furthermore, Denmark's Institute of Food Safety and Toxicology (Nielsen *et al.* 1999) conducted a study on 14 people using parsley. In two study periods, the subjects included about four milligrams of parsley every day for one of two weeks.

The researchers found that taking Parsley boosted levels of erythrocyte glutathione reductase and superoxide dismutase in the subjects. These two enzymes increase detoxification efforts of the body, as they help remove oxidization agents that can harm tissues and blood vessels.

Parsley is also rich in numerous antioxidant nutrients, including vitamin A, vitamin C, vitamin E, beta carotene, lutein, cryptoxanthin, zeaxanthin, folate and is one of the greatest sources of vitamin K, with 1640 micrograms per gram – over 12 times the U.S. DRI (dietary reference intake) of 90-120 micrograms per day. One hundred grams of Parsley also contains more than double the RDA for vitamin C and almost triple the RDA of vitamin A.

The ability of Parsley to relax smooth muscles appears to come from its blocking of the polymerization of actin. This has significant importance to asthmatics, as a severe asthmatic attack will accompany the over-contraction of the smooth muscles around the lungs. Relaxing those smooth muscles is one key component of urgent care in asthmatic attacks.

Other bioactive constituents in Parsley include eugenol, crisoeriol, luteo-lin and apiin. Eugenol has been used by traditional doctors as an antiseptic and pain-reliever in cases of gingivitis and periodontal disease, and has been shown to reduce blood sugar levels in diabetics.

Cumarins are natural blood thinning agents, as they provide anti-coagulating properties. This can aid circulation, especially in cases of edema (swelling). However, the cumarin content in Parsley is minor, and balanced by its many other nutrients. So it does not come with the side effects known for wayfarin and other isolated anti-coagulants.

The antioxidant nutrients in parsley have been shown in other research to reduce the oxidation of lipids, relating directly to vision disorders, heart disease, dementia and other inflammation-related conditions.

Nuts

A number of large and small studies have shown that nuts decrease our risk of cancer.

Harvard Medical School researchers (Bao *et al.* 2013) followed 75,680 women in the Nurses' Health Study – started in 1976 and expanded in 1989. The researchers measured nut consumption among the subjects and updated it every two to four years.

Those who ate at least one ounce of nuts twice a week had a 35% lower incidence of pancreatic cancer and a 32% lower incidence of diabetes.

This effect remained after canceling out other known causes of pancreatic cancer. Those included higher BMI, less physical activity, greater consumption of red meat and less consumption of fruits and vegetables.

Tree Nuts

Tree nuts are distinguished from nuts such as peanuts, which are technically legumes. We have discussed how tree nuts have cardiovascular benefits. Popular tree nuts include:

> ➢ Almonds

- Brazil nuts
- Chestnuts
- Cashews
- Hazelnuts
- Macadamia nuts
- Pecans
- Pine nuts
- Pistachios
- Walnuts

Researchers from the Dana Farber Cancer Institute (Fadelu *et al.* 2017) conducted a study on stage III colon cancer patients. They utilized a questionnaires and cancer history for 826 patients. The study began in 1999 and continued through the years.

Each patient completed a dietary questionnaire after they finished their chemotherapy treatment. This covered their various diet habits. The questionnaire included nut intake because of other research linking nuts to metabolic disease and obesity.

The researchers found those patients who consumed two or more ounces a week of any type of nut experienced a 42 less incidence in their colon cancer recurring.

Those who ate two or more ounces a week of tree nuts in particular experienced a 46 percent reduced incidence of cancer recurring.

This effect was found regardless of other factors, which included age, gender, tumor type and body mass index.

Only 19 percent of the patients ate two or more ounces of nuts a week.

The researchers also found that those patients who ate two ounces of nuts per week had a 57 percent reduced chance of dying during the period of follow-up.

Depending upon the type and when it is diagnosed, colon cancer five-year survival rates range between 70 and 90 percent.

Tree nut consumption alone reduced the risk of dying during the follow-up period by 53 percent.

The researchers also analyzed peanut and peanut butter consumption and determined that most of the benefit came from the consumption of tree nuts.

Daniel F. Hayes, MD, one of the study authors, commented on the benefit:

"It should be emphasized that the authors are not suggesting that eating nuts should be considered a substitute for standard chemotherapy and other treatments for colon cancer, which have dramatically improved survival. Rather, patients with colon cancer should be optimistic, and they should eat a healthy diet, including tree nuts, which may not only keep them healthier, but may also further decrease the chances of the cancer coming back."

A study from Spain's University of Castille-La Mancha (Tárraga López *et al.* 2014) analyzed data from 145 clinical studies with tens of thousands of people. These included research on the effect of different foods on colorectal cancers.

The data researchers found that frequent consumption of nuts reduced the incidence of cancer among population studies – along with vegetables, brown rice and reduced meat intake.

The hypothesis that walnuts suppress breast cancer doesn't come without cause. A 2015 study from Mexico's University of Colima investigated 97 patients with breast cancer, along with 104 healthy people (Soriano-Hernandez *et al.* 2015).

The researchers conducted a review of the subjects' diets. They found that those who ate more walnuts, peanuts and/or almonds had a decrease in their risk of breast cancer by two to three times. Those who ate only small amounts of these nuts had negligible effects.

A study from the World Health Organization's International Agency for Research on Cancer (Jenab *et al.* 2014) followed 478,040 people from Europe. They found women who ate the highest amounts of nuts had a 31 percent reduced risk of colorectal cancer.

A study from Spain's Catalan Institute of Oncology found nuts exert a "protective effect" against cancer.

Other laboratory studies have made similar conclusions.

Walnuts

Walnuts in particular have a number of phenolic acids that apparently deter cancer cells. Research from Portugal's University Fernando Pessoa (Carvalho *et al.* 2009) studied human cancer cells.

They found that walnuts in particular inhibited human kidney cancer cells, human rectal cancer cells and human colon cancer cells. And they found the phenols seemed to have a serious cancer inhibitory effect.

Intensive research is indicating that walnuts (*Juglans regia*) can suppress breast cancer tumors and help prevent breast cancer. This is the conclusion derived from laboratory research, research on animals and human clinical research.

Research is indicating that walnuts can inhibit breast cancer tumors and reduce the risk of breast cancer.

Breast cancer is by far the most common form of cancer affecting woman around the world. In 2018 there were more than two million new cases of breast cancer. Western countries by far had the most cases, with countries such as France, Australia, UK, Italy, New Zealand, Germany, the U.S. and Canada all rounding out the top 25 countries in the world in terms of breast cancer incidence. (Western diet anyone?)

Approximately 12 percent of U.S. woman will develop invasive breast cancer during their lifetimes according to the newest research. This equates to one in eight U.S. women. Over 40,000 women will die from breast cancer in 2019 in the U.S.

Note that men also contract breast cancer. A man's risk of breast cancer is much lower than a woman's, at about 1 in 883.

After studying walnuts for breast cancer in laboratory research, doctors at Marshall University investigated breast cancer in 10 women whose biopsies indicated they had breast cancer tumors (Hardman *et al.* 2019).

After their biopsies, the researchers had half of the women consume two ounces of walnuts per day for about two weeks. This occurred in between their biopsies and their surgeries to remove the tumors.

The doctors took another biopsy after two weeks – prior to their surgery. The researchers found the walnut group's tumors had radically changed genetically. They found that in the walnut group that gene expression had changed in 456 different genes. These included gene expressions that suppress tumor growth. This finding is significant, because it shows the extent of the effects of walnuts upon the tumors.

Dr. Elaine Hardman, who led the study, stated,

"These results support the hypothesis that, in humans, walnut consumption could suppress growth and survival of breast cancers."

Another study tested walnuts on human breast cancer cells and colon cancer cells (Liao *et al.* 2016). The researchers found that walnut proteins inhibited breast cancer cells by about 63 percent. Walnuts also inhibited the colon cancer cells by 51 percent.

Another 2016 study tested walnut against MCF-7 human breast cancer cells (Jahanbani *et al.* 2016). These researchers found that exposure to small amounts or walnut proteins halted cancer proliferation and killed cancer cells at a rate of about 80 percent.

Other breast cancer cell research has showed similar findings.

Walnuts contain a chemical called juglanin. Juglanin was investigated in a 2017 study from China's Henan University (Sun *et al.* 2017). The researchers tested juglanin on human breast cancer cells in the laboratory.

The scientists found that the juglanin killed breast cancer cells. It also acted as a free radical scavenger to help prevent further breast cell damage.

Green walnuts tend to contain more Juglanin.

The scientists also found that juglanin stopped tumor growth in mice with breast cancer.

Another study from Marshall University also studied breast cancer in mice (Hardman *et al.* 2014) and found that whole walnut added to the diet reduced mammary gland tumors. They found that multiple compounds in walnuts (including juglanin) had a synergistic anticancer effect.

A number of studies on mice have shown that walnuts inhibit colon and rectal cancers. Other studies have shown that walnuts inhibit breast cancers (Hardman *et al.* 2009).

Here are the primary phenolic acids in walnuts:
- Coumaric acid
- Ferulic acid

- ➤ Juglone
- ➤ Myricetin
- ➤ Syringic acid
- ➤ Vanillic acid

Peanuts

We're including peanuts in the "nuts" category because most people do. Peanuts are powerhouses for healing and preventing disease. The proof might have been in the PB for a long time now. But now we have the whole nut, so to speak.

Research finds that peanuts reduce the risk of early death from heart disease, cancer and a host of other conditions. Peanuts even drop the risk of early death from any cause.

I have been a fan of peanuts for many years. Peanuts and unsweetened peanut butter have continued to offer me and millions of other 'peanut heads' antioxidant healing benefits packaged within a convenient complete protein snack or meal.

Peanuts also provide many other nutrients. It is for this reason that peanut butter is a primary ingredient food used to save children with Severe Acute Malnutrition – or SAM.

Yes, Doctors Without Borders, UNICEF and other agencies have brought millions of starving children back from the brink using a combination of peanut butter and powdered milk. They found that many other foods don't work so fast – but peanut butter does for some reason. Many have dubbed peanut butter a "miracle food" as a result.

Peanuts are only one essential amino acid short of being a complete protein. A complete protein means the food contains all nine essential amino acids. Peanuts contain all but one – methionine.

However, when peanuts or peanut butter are combined with a grain – such as whole wheat bread or oats – the combination provides us with a complete protein meal or snack.

After all, who eats peanut butter alone?

Peanuts are packed with protein. Just two tablespoons of peanut butter will provide a solid 8 grams of protein. A considerable amount of your day's protein needs.

Peanuts are packed with more than 30 other nutrients. These include healthy doses of minerals, including magnesium (346 milligrams per cup of peanut butter), calcium (111 mg), potassium (1674 mg), zinc (7.5 mg), copper (1.2 mg), selenium (14 mcg), iron (4.8 mg) and phosphorus (924 mg).

Peanuts also contain decent levels of vitamin E, vitamin K, thiamine, riboflavin, niacin, B6, folate, pantothenic acid, choline and betaine.

Peanuts also contain considerable omega-3 fatty acids, at 196 milligrams, and over 61 grams of monounsaturated fats. Furthermore, peanuts also contain sterols – an incredibly healthy type of fat that helps reduce low-density lipoprotein levels (LDL-c). Sterols also produce antioxidant effects among the fat portions of our metabolism.

Researchers from a consortium of universities, including Harvard University, Oslo University, Imperial College of London, Mount Sinai School of Medicine, University of Leeds and others (Agune *et al.* 2016) investigated the effects of eating peanuts and tree nuts.

The researchers conducted a meta-analysis study that analyzed 20 different studies and 819,448 human participants. These included studies that tested nut consumption on rates of cancer, cardiovascular disease, coronary heart disease and respiratory diseases. And yes, deaths from any cause.

The researchers found that increasing peanut or other nut consumption by 28 grams per day reduced the incidence of cancer by 15 percent.

As mentioned, this was a meta-analysis of multiple studies. Some of these were quite large.

An example of one of these is a 2015 study from The Netherlands' Maastricht University (van den Brandt *et al.*). In this study, 120,852 Danish men and women aged between 55 and 69 years old were followed since 1986.

The research found similar results as quoted in the meta-analysis, including cancer, diabetes, cardiovascular disease, respiratory disease and neurogenerative diseases. They also found peanut consumption decreased all-cause mortality.

Peanut butter didn't decrease mortality in this study. Why? We might offer that most peanut butters include sugar. This has the opposite effect of peanuts, as we discussed in a previous chapter.

Peanuts and unsweetened peanut butter incurs a reduced glycemic response as well. This is good for helping to prevent cancer as we've discussed.

For example, a study from Brazil's Federal University of Viçosa tested 15 obese women. They compared their blood sugar levels after eating breakfast meals with and without peanut butter.

They found that including peanut butter with breakfast reduced their blood sugar and steadied their glycemic response for the day. It also helped reduce their appetites throughout the day. The researchers concluded:

"Inclusion of peanut butter, and probably whole peanuts, to breakfast may help to moderate glucose concentrations and appetite in obese women."

Other studies have found similar effects of peanuts. Some studies have also found that peanuts reduce body fat.

These results indicate that peanuts fall into the category of plant medicines. This includes such medicinal roots like turmeric, ginseng and carrots. Now it's not that peanuts maintain the same healing properties and the same medicinal compounds as these. But peanuts do promote similarly incredible effects upon our health.

I say this also because I am sure that more medicinal effects of peanuts will soon be exposed by research. The ability to reduce rates of heart disease and cancer and other conditions doesn't happen in a vacuum. Currently, most research on peanuts – outside of the studies discussed here – have focused upon either peanut allergies or peanuts' improved glycemic response.

What about peanut allergies?

Yes, a small fraction of people have peanut allergies. Only about 0.6 percent of Americans. But as I discuss in my book on the topic, there are some scientifically-backed ways to reverse food allergies.

Nuts are Serious Prebiotics

One of the central reasons for nuts' ability to inhibit cancer is that they feed and promote healthy gut probiotics. This means that nuts are serious prebiotics.

A study from Friedrich Schiller University Jena (Schlörmann *et al.* 2017) investigated fermented nuts and colon cancer. The reason for this is because nuts become fermented by gut bacteria as they are digested in the gut.

The researchers found the chemicals produced by the nut fermentation significantly inhibited colon cancer cells. Their ability to stop DNA mutations and free radical formation ranged up to four times than normal. These effects together stopped cancer cell growth and killed cancer cells. The researchers concluded:

"The differential modulation of genes involved in detoxification and cell cycle together with an inhibition of proliferation and induction of apoptosis in adenoma cells might contribute to chemopreventive effects of nuts regarding colon cancer."

Friedrich Schiller University (Lux *et al.* 2012) scientists also studied fermented nuts in the laboratory. Once the nuts were fermented by gut bacteria, the researchers found the nuts produced significant amounts of short chain fatty acids (SCFAs). SCFAs are good for the large colon because they help to provide a toxin-free environment to the colon.

The main SCFAs are acetic acid, butyric acid and propionic acid.

Short chain fatty acids are produced by healthy probiotics, but also encourage the growth of more healthy probiotics in the gut.

These healthy probiotics in turn produce healthy enzymes. SCFAs also discourage pathogenic bacteria, which produce enzymes found to cause colon cancer. These relative levels of bacteria determine levels of propionates and butyrates in the gut.

We can safely conclude that simply munching on nuts every day has an incredible effect upon our colon health. It's simply nuts.

Legumes

The evidence is mounting that legumes, which include beans, peas and lentils, fight cancer in a serious way. This also includes bean sprouts. Research has confirmed that legumes reduce a myriad of cancer types with several mechanisms.

Let's survey some of the latest research evidence.

A study from Spain's Centro de Investigación Biomédica en Red Fisiopatologia de la Obesidad y la Nutrición (CIBEROBN) (Papandreou *et al.* 2018) followed 7,216 people for an average of six years. The researchers analyzed their diets, and in particular, their consumption of legumes – including dry beans, chickpeas, lentils and fresh peas.

The researchers found that those who ate more legumes had a half the number of cancer deaths compared to those who ate fewer legumes. Yes, they found a 49 percent lower incidence of death from cancer by eating more legumes.

Legume foods are not only nutritious: Research is uncovering their ability to significantly reduce the risk of cancer.

A legume is typically considered a type of bean or seed derived from a pod. This limited definition, however, causes some confusion for some because there are seeds and nuts that are not really legumes. The more blunt definition is that legumes come from plant species in the Leguminosae family – also called Fabaceae.

This is a gigantic family of plants – and over eighteen thousand species of plants belong in this family. Further complicating the definition is that many plants in the Leguminosae family are not typically eaten as a nut, bean or seed. Some, such as those in the Astragulus genus, are medicinal herbs. Some legume species are ornamental plants.

Yet within this large family of plants we find some of the most nutritious foods. These include lentils (of different colors), black-eyed peas, green peas, snow peas, dwarf peas, pinto beans, navy beans, green beans, adasazi beans, black beans, garbanzo beans, pinto beans, soybeans, wax beans, adzuki beans, mung beans and some other beans. Surprising to most, legumes also include peanuts, alfalfa, clover and lespedeza – also called bush clover.

More specifically, research confirms that legumes reduce the risk of colorectal cancer. Legumes along with the consumption of whole cereal grains and cereal grains – many of which share compounds with legumes – has also been found to significantly reduce the risk of colorectal cancer.

Colorectal cancer is a leading form of cancer. Among both men and women in the U.S., colorectal cancer is the third most common form of cancer. Worldwide, one in ten cancer cases is colorectal cancer.

A study that underscores the ability of legumes to reduce the risk of colorectal cancer came from the Republic of Korea's National Cancer Center and the Seoul National University College of Medicine and Hospital (Shin *et al.* 2015).

The researchers studied the diets of 901 colorectal cancer patients along with 2,669 control subjects. The number of control participants was based upon a multiple of three controls for every cancer patient.

The diets of the 3,740 people were analyzed for 106 different foods and graded for frequency. The researchers utilized a ten-year frequency basis. The analysis closely investigated the intake of foods that contain isoflavones. This is because several studies have shown that the intake of isoflavones decreases the risk of cancer.

The research results indeed confirmed this. Those who ate the most isoflavone-containing foods had a significantly less incidence of colorectal cancer.

The isoflavone-containing foods that decreased cancer risk included soybeans. Women who consumed the highest quartile of soy foods saw their risk of colorectal cancer reduced by between 38 and 46 percent. Men in the highest quartile of soy foods had between 33 and 44 percent reduction of colorectal cancer. But those who consumed the middle ranges of soy foods had increased risk ranging from 28 percent to 34 percent.

But it was the legumes that provided the biggest and most consistent reduction in colorectal cancer risk. Those who ate the most legumes (highest quarter) saw their incidence of colorectal cancer drop by over 50 percent – with women as high as 56 percent lower incidence.

Furthermore, this reduced incidence also occurred with the other quartiles of legume consumption. As legume consumption increased, the incidence of colorectal cancer was reduced.

Similar results were found by researchers from Moores Cancer Center at the University of California at San Diego along with researchers from Jordan's King Hussein Cancer Center and Hashemite University in Jordan(Tayyem *et al.* 2015).

The researchers studied 501 people, including 220 colorectal cancer patients. Once again, the diets of all the participants were reviewed and analyzed. This analysis found that those people who ate the most refined wheat bread (AKA white bread) had over three times the incidence of colorectal cancer compared to those who ate the least amount of white bread. And those who ate the most white rice also had triple the risk of colorectal cancer.

But those who ate more legumes and whole cereal grains had a significantly reduced incidence of colorectal cancer. For example, those who ate the highest amounts of whole wheat bread had a 56 percent reduction in colorectal cancer incidence.

Yes, we can conclude that these foods – legumes and whole grains – help prevent colorectal cancer. But what about other cancers?

Research has also found that legumes and whole grains reduce the risk of prostate cancer as well. A study from Harvard Medical School (Yang *et al.* 2015) found that those who ate the most legumes and whole grains – along with more fruits, vegetables and fish – had a 46 percent reduction in prostate incidence. This study followed 926 men that participated in the Physicians' Health Study.

Aren't legumes and whole grains just good roughage? Why do they help protect against cancer? Is it just because they have good fiber?

No, it is not just the fiber content of these foods. Yes, they do contain good fibers – both soluble and insoluble fiber. Fiber-rich foods have the effect of keeping the intestinal tract regular, but they do much, much more.

Legumes and many whole grains contain compounds called isoflavones. As mentioned briefly above, these compounds have been found in studies to reduce the risk of cancer – particularly colorectal, breast and prostate cancers.

One of the mechanisms found for this is that isoflavones seem to increase anticancer cytokines (such as natural killer (NK) cells) and decrease cytokines that allow cancer cells to operate.

Another element of isoflavone-containing legumes and grains is that diadzen will stimulate the release of S-equol by gut bacteria. S-equol had been shown in a number of studies to reduce several cancers, including breast and prostate cancer.

Legumes and whole grains also provide a potent source of antioxidants in the form of polyphenols and anthocyanins. These help prevent free radicals from forming, whether in the gut or bloodstream. Free radicals can damage DNA, causing mutations that can form cancerous cells.

Legume foods and many whole grains also provide phytosterols that help reduce the release of low-density lipoproteins – also referred to as LDL. LDL particles are easily oxidized in the bloodstream. These oxidized particles damage the walls of our blood vessels, causing atherosclerosis and other cardiovascular problems.

But one of the greatest benefits of legumes and whole grains is that they provide potent prebiotics to our gut bacteria. These prebiotics feed those lactobacilli and bifidobacteria and thus increase their colonies. When probiotic colonies are increased, colorectal cancer risk is lessened.

Bad bacteria in our gut increases the risk of colorectal cancer. This is because these bad bacteria produce enzymes that damage the cells of our intestines. They effectively cause genetic mutation, which produces cancer.

Legumes are best eaten after being soaked and cooked. Soaking and cooking will effectively reduce phytates, allowing for better mineral absorption.

A study from the University of Colorado School of Medicine (Borresen *et al.* 2016) tested 37 patients who survived colorectal cancer. For four weeks, they gave the patients a regimen of 35 grams of navy beans or 30 grams of rice bran, along with a control group that ate neither.

The researchers found those who consumed the navy beans had longer telomere lengths and significantly lower levels of inflammation. They concluded these patients had a greater survival potential as a result of their navy bean consumption.

A 2014 study from Mexico's Universidad Autónoma de Querétaro (Luna *et al.*) found that bean proteins inhibited human colorectal cancer cells.

We've also shown research proving that nuts also fight colorectal cancers.

Multiple studies have investigated lectins in beans that have specific anti-cancer effects. For example, researchers from Japan's Kibi International University (Une *et al.* 2018) tested Japanese red sword beans (*Canavalia gladiata*) for anti-cancer properties. They found the beans contain a particular lectin that significantly boosts the immune system's ability to fight cancer.

They found the RSB lectin boosted interleukin-2 and inhibited melanoma cancer cells from growing.

A study from the University of Hong Kong (Chan *et al.* 2016) tested another bean lectin, from the white kidney bean (*Phaseolus vulgaris*). The researchers found that the white kidney bean lectin inhibited breast cancer and sinus cancer cells.

A study from Babol University of Medical Sciences (Joghatai *et al.* 2018) found that mung bean proteins inhibited human breast cancer cells, cervical cancer cells, and skin cancer cells.

They also found that the mung bean proteins help prevented radiation damage to skin cells. This means they help guard against sunburn-related skin cancers.

A study from the All India Institute of Medical Sciences (Kumar *et al.* 2017) found that black turtle beans (or black beans) have anti-cancer properties. The researchers tested the bean extracts against two types of human breast cancer cells. They found the extracts inhibited the growth of breast cancer cells. They also found the bean extracts killed many cancer cells (apoptosis) outright.

This ability to kill cancer cells occurred by the bean extracts damaging the mitochondria and producing DNA fragmentation in the cancer cells.

A study from Italy's CREA institute (Ombra *et al.* 2016) analyzed twelve different varieties of common beans (Phaseolus vulgaris). They found a number of known anti-cancer compounds, including gallic acid, chlorogenic acid, epicatechin, myricetin, formononetin, caffeic acid, and kaempferol.

They also found the bean extracts inhibited the growth of human colorectal cancer and human breast cancer cells.

In a study from the Complutense University of Madrid (Guajardo-Flores *et al.* 2013) raw, cooked and germinated black beans (Phaseolus vulgaris) all had anti-tumor effects, particularly with colorectal and breast cancer as well as melanoma cancer cells. The raw beans had the most anti-tumor effects in this research.

This doesn't mean that sprouted beans don't also inhibit cancer. In fact, they may well have a greater effect due to their increased assimilation.

In a 2013 study, researchers from Mexico's Monterrey Institute of Technology (López *et al.*) determined that black bean sprouts are anticarcinogenic against breast cancer, liver cancer and colon cancer cells.

The researchers sprouted black beans (Phaseolus vulgaris) and then tested them and their constituents against cancer cell lines of various types of cancers. The researchers found that after three days and five days of germination, the phytonutrient extracts isolated from the sprouts were able to inhibit the growth of all the cancer cells tested.

They also tested the same sprout isolates against non-cancerous (healthy) cells as controls and found no negative impact upon healthy cells. (Many of the above studies also did this as well.)

The researchers then isolated some of the constituents of the sprouted beans and found that the saponins and flavonoids had the greatest inhibition against liver and colon cancer cells. Meanwhile, the genistein content of the sprouts was found to inhibit the breast cancer cells.

The researchers also found the black bean sprouts to be particularly high in antioxidants.

What about Phytates?

Early sprout research as documented by Hofsten (1979) and others determined that sprout germination increases many nutrients and others are made more available for assimilation.

Other research (Chen and Pan 1977) found that germination decreased phytic acid in soybeans by 22% while the enzyme phytase increased 227% after five days of soybean germination.

Cooking beans also decreases their phytic acid content and increases their phytase content.

Because phytic acid/phytate can bind some minerals, eating raw beans is not advised. Nutrients like calcium and zinc are more assimilable from sprouted or cooked beans.

Also, the oligosaccharides that produce flatulence are hydrolyzed during sprout germination and to a lesser degree by cooking, making bean sprouts and well-cooked beans easier to digest.

Beans are particularly high in a number of phytonutrients, including flavonols like quercetin and kaempferol, and anthocyanins. They are also high in polyphenols like ferulic acid and chlorogenic acid. All of these are potent antioxidants shown to stimulate the immune system.

Grapes

A study from the University of Barcelona (Matito *et al.* 2011) found that procyanidins from grapes protect against the damaging effects of UVA rays from the sun, including cancer and cell death.

The study, performed in the Department of Biochemistry and Molecular Biology at the university, found that the antioxidant polyphenols in grapes protect the cells of the skin - keratinocytes - against damage from reactive oxygen species (ROS). Reactive oxygen species, also called free radicals, damage skin cells by producing lipid peroxidation.

We've discussed how this has been shown to damage cell membranes, produce DNA mutation, turning a healthy cell into a cancerous cell.

Lead researcher Dr. Marta Cascante, a Professor of Biochemistry explained this process:

"These polyphenolic fractions inhibit the generation of the ROSs [reactive oxygen species] and, as a result, the subsequent activation of the JNK and p38 enzymes, meaning they have a protective effect against ultraviolet radiation emitted by the sun."

The p38 and JNK1/2 enzymes are stimulated by both ultraviolet-A and ultraviolet-B radiation from the sun. In the experiment, they were inhibited by the grape extracts. These two enzymes are implicated in the production of the free radicals that harm the cells.

The phytochemicals in the grapes are procyanidin oligomers and gallate esters. Procyanidins have been found in a number of other plant foods, as has gallic acid. This study confirms others that have found that certain plant antioxidants protect against sun damage. These same antioxidants also help plants protect themselves against sun damage.

Papaya Leaf

Research has found that extracts from papaya leaf inhibit cancer cells and the growth of cancer. A study from University of Tokyo's Institute of Medical Science (Otsuki *et al.* 2010) studied leaf extracts from the plant *Carica papaya* Linn - the common papaya tree.

The researchers tested extracts of different strengths against several human tumor cell lines and human peripheral blood mononuclear cells (PBMC). They found that the extract inhibited the growth of tumor cells, and increased the production of cytokines such as IL-2 and IL-4 among the PBMC cells. The cytokines were then analyzed *in vitro* by ELISA, microarray and real-time RT-PCR testing.

Leading the research study was Nam Dang, M.D., Ph.D., a professor of medicine at University of Florida. Dr. Dang is a Harvard Medical School graduate and leading cancer researcher. The research also documented anecdotal experiences with patients with advanced cancers who achieved remission after drinking teas or tea extracts made from papaya leaves.

The paper, published in the *Journal of Ethnopharmacology,* explains that papaya leaf boosts activity and production of the signaling molecules called Th1-type cytokines. These regulate the immune system, meaning that papaya leaves could have many other immunotherapeutic benefits.

"Since Carica papaya leaf extract can mediate a Th1 type shift in human immune system, our results suggest that the CP leaf extract may potentially provide the means for the treatment and prevention of selected human diseases such as cancer, various allergic disorders, and may also serve as immunoadjuvant for vaccine therapy."

Papaya fruits also contain many of the constituents, such as papain, that are also present in the leaves. Papayas, and more specifically green papayas, have also been used in traditional Polynesian medicine for many centuries to heal various disorders.

Papaya fruit contains linalool, benzylisothiaocyanates, chitinase and alkaloids such as carpaine and benzyl-glucosides.

The leaves contain carpain, pseudocarpain, choline, carposide, choline, and dehydrocarpaine among others. Chitinase from papayas has been found to have antibacterial activity, and carpaine and carpasemine (a benzylisothiocyanate) have been shown to have antihelmintic (inhibits parasites) properties.

The fruits have long been used in traditional medicine for digestive ailments, ringworm, skin issues and urinary tract issues. Other research shows that fermented papaya stimulates the immune system.

Garlic and Onions

Eating garlic and onions have proven to reduce the risk of breast cancer.

More women die from breast cancer than any other form of cancer. The World Health Organization has estimated that 627,000 women died from breast cancer in 2018. In 2019, over 40,000 women are expected to die from breast cancer just in the U.S., with over 265,000 new cases expected. About 1 in 8 U.S. women will develop breast cancer during their lifetimes in the U.S.

It is notable that breast cancer rates are highest among more developed countries according to the World Health Organization.

Garlic (*Allium sativum*) and onions (*Allium cepa* L.) belong to the Allium plant family. This group also includes over 500 plants, including shallots (Allium ascalonium), scallions (*Allium fistulosum*), leeks (*Allium ampeloprasum* var. porrum) and chives (*Allium schoenoprasum*). These medicinal foods have been used in traditional medicines around the world for thousands of years. Their medicinal abilities stem from a number of compounds that are common in onions and garlic. These include organosulfur compounds such as:

> ➤ aliin (S-allyl cysteine sulfoxide)
> ➤ allicin (diallyl thiosulphate)
> ➤ ajoene (trithiadodeca trieneoxide)
> ➤ allylpropyl disulfide
> ➤ diallyl disulfide
> ➤ diallyl trisulfide
> ➤ sallylcysteine
> ➤ vinyldithiines
> ➤ S-allylmercaptocysteindiallyl sulfide
> ➤ S-allylcysteine
> ➤ isothiocyanate sulforaphane

These organosulfur compounds have been found to stimulate the liver's production of glutathione products such as glutathione transferase, glutathione peroxidase and glutathione dismutase.

These collectively aid the body in reducing oxidative stress and toxicity throughout the body. Indeed, garlic and its cousins also contain enzymes, including allinase, myrosinase and perosidases.

For this reason and more, allium foods have been found to stimulate immunity and help the body fight onslaughts, including cancer.

Garlic, onions and other allium foods also contain tremendous phenols and flavonoids. These include quercetins and caffeic acid. These stimulate the immune system and discourage the growth of cancers. Quercetin in specific has been shown to depress the body's expression of p52 proteins among breast cancer cells. This helps knock down those cells to help the body's immunity conquer them.

Researchers from the University at Buffalo and the University of Puerto Rico (Desai *et al.* 2019) studied 670 women between 30 and 70 years old, including 314 that had been diagnosed with breast cancer. The researchers studied their diets in particular, along with their age, education, BMI, family history, smoking and so on.

After every other association was examined, the researchers found those who regularly consumed more garlic and onions had a 49 percent reduced risk of developing breast cancer compared to those who consumed less garlic and onions.

Those women who regularly ate a moderate amount of garlic and onions also had reduced risk, to the tune of 41 percent less incidence of breast cancer.

Moreover, the scientists also found that those who ate a sofrito dish more than once a day saw their incidence of breast cancer go down by a whopping 67 percent. Sofrito is a Puerto Rico traditional dish that contains both fresh garlic and onions.

This is not the first study to find that eating garlic and onions or other allium foods reduces the risk of breast cancer.

A 2016 study published in the Journal of Breast cancer (Pourzand *et al.* 2016) tested 285 women between 25 and 65 years old. They found that those who consumed higher quantities of raw onion had a 37 percent reduced risk of breast cancer.

A 2012 study of over 6,900 women in China (Bao *et al.* 2012) found that those women who ate the most allium vegetables had the lowest risk of breast cancer. They were graded for various other foods and allium vegetables had the most anti-cancer effect.

The reduced risk was smaller due to the fact that they compared eating more than 14.75 grams per day versus a moderate intake of 3 grams per day. As the study above showed, moderate consumption of garlic and onions also significantly decreases cancer risk for women.

garlic and onions and breast cancer risk

Even moderate consumption of fresh onions and garlic significantly decreases the risk of breast cancer.

A study from Mexico (Torres-Sánchez *et al.* 2000) studied the diets of 198 women between 21 and 79. They found that eating a slice of onion or more per day resulted in a 70 percent decrease in breast cancer.

A 1998 study from France (Challier *et al.* 1998) tested 690 women, of whom half had been diagnosed with breast cancer. They found that those women who ate more garlic and onions also had a 70 percent decreased risk of developing breast cancer.

These studies are also supported by laboratory studies showing garlic and onions' ability to deter cancer cells.

Because many of the compounds in onions and garlic are particularly heat-sensitive, cooking may not yield the same effects. As expected, research on garlic supplements and cooked allium foods, for example, has been less encouraging when it comes to reducing breast cancer risk.

For example, a study from the Netherlands (Dorant *et al.* 1995) found that garlic supplements and [cooked] leaks and onions were not associated with reduced breast cancer risk reduction. In one of the studies discussed above, (Pourzand *et al.* 2018) for example, found increased breast cancer risk among those who ate more cooked onions. This may be because cooked onions are often served with meat dishes, which have been linked with greater breast cancer risk.

Note that sofritos utilize fresh onions and garlic.

In a 2016 study from The State University of New York (Myneni *et al.*), researchers collected population data from Taiyuan China. Data came from 399 lung cancer patients and 466 healthy people. They found that those who ate raw garlic twice a week or more had a 50 percent reduced risk of contracting lung cancer.

Researchers from the Peking University Cancer Hospital and Institute (Li *et al.* 2016) followed over 6,500 people for 22 years. Many of them had been diagnosed with H. pylori. The researchers found that garlic supplementation for seven years reduced gastric cancer risk by 44 percent.

Some research has found that aged garlic extract can be significantly more anticancer than fresh garlic. This is based upon laboratory studies to date (Lv *et al.* 2019).

Other research (Nicastro *et al.* 2015) has found that both garlic and onions can help prevent cancer. Most agree that that the organosulfur compounds in these foods give them much of their anticancer properties.

The bottom line is that eating fresh garlic and onions is a proven way to reduce breast cancer risk. But cooking them may not yield the same benefits.

Carrots

Several studies have illustrated and confirmed that carrots provide anti-cancer benefits, at least in the cases of gastric and prostate cancers.

Five international studies – which studied more than 200,000 people in different countries – have proven the case for carrots' ability to help prevent stomach cancer. The studies were done in Japan, Sweden, the Netherlands and Lithuania.

When the results of these studies were combined and reduced, researchers found that increased carrot consumption reduces the risk of gastric cancer by 26 percent. The research was published in the *Journal of Gastric Cancer* (Fallahzadeh *et al.* 2015)

Carrots reduced the risk of another cancer - gastric cardia cancer – by even more. The combined research calculated that gastric cardia cancer risk was reduced by 38 percent from carrot consumption. Gastric cardia cancer is when cancer attacks the topmost portion of the stomach – known as the cardia.

How many carrots did it take to get these results? The largest study, of 120,852 people (Steevens *et al.* 2011), used 25 grams per day of carrots. The next largest, from Japan, studied over 60,000 people using three or more carrots per week.

The Lithuania study that included 1,137 people used between 1 and 6 carrots per week. This resulted in a 47 percent reduction of gastric cancer.

So we're not talking a lot of carrots here. One serving of carrots according to the FDA will contain 128 grams. This is equivalent to one cup of chopped raw carrots.

One serving per day would thus equate to more than five times the carrot consumption that resulted in the 26 percent reduction of risk.

This would also mean that one serving per day of carrots should also result in an even greater reduction of cancer risk.

Stomach cancer isn't the only type of cancer that carrots will help prevent. In research published in the *European Journal of Nutrition* (Xu *et al.* 2014), researchers conducted a meta-analysis of available research correlating carrot consumption and prostate cancer prevalence.

The meta-analysis done by the researchers found that carrot consumption reduced the risk of prostate cancer by 18 percent.

The researchers also calculated the relationship on a dose-response. This found that for every 10 grams per day of carrot consumption, prostate cancer risk is decreased by 5 percent.

Remember that one serving of carrots – about a cup chopped – is 128 grams. This means that just one serving of carrot per day would equate to a 64 percent reduced risk of prostate cancer according to the dose analysis.

Carrots seem innocent enough in terms of vitamin content. Yes, a serving of fresh carrots can provide 21,383 IU of vitamin A (428% Daily Value). And nearly 17 micrograms of vitamin K (21% of Daily Value). And a serving of carrots provides over 24 micrograms of folate (6% of Daily Value).

Outside of the vitamin A content, there doesn't seem much else that special about carrots from the vitamin-mineral data. Yes, they do contain a fair amount of calcium, magnesium, phosphorus and potassium. But these are mostly in the single digit Daily Value levels. And its vitamin C levels – at 7.6 milligrams per serving – is only 13% of Daily Value.

But carrots provide a phytonutrient sneak attack in the form of special compounds. These include compounds called polyacetylenes. These are natural polymers of acetylenes that occur in certain herbal medicines – and notably in carrots. The most prevalent polyacetylenes in carrots include falcarinol and falcarindol.

Polyacetylenes are notable because they have been shown to increase the rate of DNA repair within cells. When DNA repair is slowed, cancer risk is raised.

A study from the *European Journal of Pharmacology* (Christensen *et al.* 2014) found that falcarinol polyacetylenes inhibited the breast cancer resistance protein.

Another secret weapon carrots have is their beta-carotene and alpha-carotene content – and to a lesser degree, gamma-carotene. These carotenoids help stop free radical formation with their antioxidant properties. Many free radicals get that way from oxidation. With greater carrot consumption, our cells are exposed to fewer attacks from free radicals.

Carrots have greater levels of the E-beta-carotene isomer. This is a stronger isomer than the Z-isomer (cis). This E-beta-carotene molecule is also more durable in storage.

Carrots also contain the phytocompounds zeaxanthin and lutein. This is a particularly important nutrient to the health of the eyes – but also provides antioxidant benefit in other parts of our physiology.

Carrots also contain phenolic hydroxycinnamic acid compounds such as caffeic acid, ferulic acid and coumaric acid. These, together with anthocyanidins, provide unique antioxidant and healing benefits that will help reduce our risk of any cancer.

Carrots also contain a beneficial amount of fiber, at 2.8 grams. More than half of this is insoluble fiber, which is extremely beneficial for the digestive tract and its microbes.

There are a number of different varieties of carrots. They can be generally classified by their color pigments. The general carrot species is *Daucus carota* subspecies Sativus. But there are several cultivars, which include Chantenays and Nantes.

But there are also different pigment varieties. These include purple and yellow carrots. The typical orange carrots are high in the beta-carotene. But purple and red carrots are higher in anthocyanins. And yellow carrots are particularly high in lutein.

These different carrots can also taste a little different – but still most carrots are sweet.

Like to juice? Fresh carrot juice will also contain many of these compounds, but with less than a third of its fiber content.

Carrot consumption has also been linked with reduce cardiovascular disease as well.

Olives

Scientists have proven that olives are more than a bit healthy. Studies have found that a constituent of olives and olive oil inhibits the growth of cancer.

A study from the University of Texas (Peluso *et al.* 2017) has shown that olives stop an important pathway that cancer cells use to grow.

The signaling pathway uses mitogen-activated protein kinases or MAPKs to express certain genes. This signals the growth of the cancer cells, producing metastasis.

The researchers found that a compound in olive called squalene, helps block the MAPK signaling system. The researchers concluded that virgin olive oil could be used as an adjuvant to other cancer therapies, calling virgin olive oil a "natural delivery system."

Scientists at the King Saud University (Hassan *et al.* 2012) treated human breast cancer cells with another constituent of olives known as oleuropein. The testing found that Oleuropein produced genetic changes among breast cancer cells that serve to inhibit their ability to metastasize and grow throughout the body.

One of the two key genetic changes influenced by the oleuropein was the inhibition of the matrix metalloproteinase (MMP) enzymes. These MMPs – specifically MMP2 and MMP9 – usher the process of metastasizing. The MMP enzymes were blocked, effectively inhibiting the spread of the cancer.

The oleuropein extract also stimulated a genetic expression of the TIMP gene. When these genes are expressed, through a polymerase chain reaction, tumor growth is halted.

The researchers concluded that:

"Treatment of breast cancer cells with oleuropein could help in prevention of cancer metastasis by increasing the TIMPs and suppressing the MMPs gene expressions."

While olives contain a number of polyphenols, oleuropein and squalene are two of the best known. Other polyphenols within olives and olive oil can include hydroxytyrosol, tyrosol and verbascoside (Waterman *et al.* 2007).

Along with these benefits, oleuropein has been found to dilate the blood vessels, reducing blood pressure and increasing bloodflow. Olive's high level of antioxidants also gives it a tremendous anti-inflammatory capacity, especially among the cardiovascular system. Olive leaf has been found to be antiviral. It appears to inhibit virus' ability to replicate, preventing viral shedding and budding within the cells and cell membrane.

Olives are also rich in a host of other beneficial nutrients, including copper, vitamin E and iron.

The olive also contains a unique monounsaturated fatty acid called oleic acid. Olive oil also contains linoleic, palmitic, stearic and linolenic fatty acids. The combination of fats in olive helps balance pro-inflammatory fats such as saturated fats and arachidonic acids in other foods.

This blend of fatty acids, along with its antioxidants, gives olives and olive oil its proven ability to reduce the risk of cardiovascular disease and help prevent inflammatory diseases such as arthritis.

Olive oil comes with a variety of labels, including virgin or extra virgin. Virgin oil must maintain a standard of less than 1.5-2% acidity (depending upon the country or origin), while extra virgin must maintain less than 0.8% acidity. A misnomer is that extra virgin is supposed to be from the first pressing. Rather, oil manufacturers find that certain seasonal pressings of certain olive varietals will produce the desired lower acid levels.

Many also assume that extra virgin oil utilizes only a mechanical press, but virgin olive oil also must be mechanically pressed. This contrasts to using chemical solvents to extract the oil.

Most conventional vegetable oils are chemically extracted, while most olive oils are mechanically pressed. It should be noted that some mechanically pressed olive oils are blended with others to achieve the lower acidity – which is regulated by the Italian, Greece and government agencies.

In addition, high quality extra virgin olive oil is typically cold pressed, because it is mechanically pressed and utilizes less heat in the process. Most of the high quality extra virgin olive oils are cold pressed. Mechanical cold pressing helps preserve some of the heat-sensitive polyphenols and other nutrients contained within a fresh olive.

Pickling olives in a vinegar solution is one of the easiest and more delicious ways to preserve the polyphenol content of fresh olives.

Mango

A multitude of scientific studies have concluded that mango offer significant health benefits, including inhibiting cancer growth and reducing inflammation.

Much of the research has focused upon a compound found in mangoes called mangiferin. Mangiferin is a xanthonoid that contains a C-glucosyl molecular bond structure. It is this structure that appears to produce many of mango's anti-inflammatory, anti-cancer benefits.

One study (Deng *et al.* 2018) tested mangiferin against breast cancer cells. The researchers found that the mango compound mangiferin inhibited malignancy and the progression of breast cancer. The research also found mangiferin blocked the ability of the cells to signal each other in order to expand.

A study from University of Missouri (Al-Yasiri *et al.* 2017) studied mangiferin with prostate tumors. The researchers found that mangiferin reduced tumor size by five times after three weeks of treatment.

Mangoes also help prevent several types of cancer.

Another study, from Detroit's Karmanos Cancer Institute found that mangiferin blocks the inflammatory NF-$\varkappa$B signaling pathway, which in turn inhibits cancer cell formation and growth.

A metabolite of mangiferin called norathyriol was found by University of Minnesota researchers (Li *et al.* 2012) to inhibit the growth of skin cancer. Skin cancers were suppressed amidst UV radiation. These researchers also found the NF-𝜘B pathway was blocked.

Researchers from Cuba's Center for Pharmaceutical Chemistry (García-Rivera *et al.* 2011) found that mangiferin extracted from mango bark also contained these anti-tumor effects. In this study, they found the mango tree contained another anticancer compound called gallic acid, which seemed to work in conjunction with the mangiferin compound.

They called this particular extract Vimang. Vimang blocked the growth of a number of cancer cell types.

Mangoferin is also contained within mango leaves. Researchers from Taiwan and Japan found that mango leaves contain significant mangiferin content, and this mangiferin produced similar anti-cancer activity.

Other research has established that mangiferin may be useful in a number of inflammatory-related disorders, including diabetes and heart disease.

Scientists presented research at San Diego's Federation of American Societies for Experimental Biology (FASEB) that reported that people who eat mangos have a better diet and fewer health issues.

The research compared the diets of over 13,000 individuals participating in the National Health and Nutrition Examination Survey (NHANES) between 2001 and 2008 to the Healthy Eating Index (HEI). Those who ate mangos regularly scored higher on the HEI than those that did not.

Compared to non-mango consumers, mango consumers had increased intake of vitamin C, magnesium, potassium and dietary fibers, and had a lower average body weight.

Mango eaters also had significantly lower levels of the inflammatory marker C-reactive protein.

"We found that adults who ate mangos tended to have a lower body weight, higher intake of fiber and lower intake of fat, all of which are associated with better cardiovascular health," stated Dr. Victor Fulgoni, the lead researcher of this study.

Another exploratory study presented at FASEB conducted at Texas A&M University found that mangiferin is toxic to breast cancer cells.

"In summary, the anti-carcinogenic and anti-inflammatory activity of mango polyphenolics in breast cancer cells were at least in part due to targeting proteins that play an important role in the survival of breast cancer cells," noted one of the study's lead researchers, Dr. Susanne Talcott. "The ability for bioactive components in mangos to reduce cancer promoting cells may be the next big thing in the battle against breast cancer, but more research is needed at this time."

A study from Spain's University of Cadiz (Fernández-Ponce *et al.* 2017) tested mango leaf extracts against different degrees of invasive breast cancer. They found that the extracts provided protection against minimally invasive breast cancer as well as highly invasive breast cancers. The researchers found that compounds called gallotannins killed breast cancer cells.

Mangoes contain more than 20 vitamins, minerals and antioxidants. They also contain significant amounts of a special antioxidant called beta-carotene. Beta-carotene is known to help protect the eyes from macular degeneration. Carrots also contain significant beta-carotene. And carrots also help prevent some cancers.

Mango is one of the world's most popular fruits outside of the U.S. Mangos typically grow in warm, tropical climates. And mangoes have become more plentiful on the world market in recent years. Mango availability per capita has increased steadily over the past decade and can now often be found at different markets. The delicious and healthy fruit may very well be at your local market.

Pomegranate

A host of studies have found that Pomegranate can inhibit the growth of colon cancer cells, lung cancer cells, prostate cancer, breast cancer and skin cancer.

Researchers from the University of Alabama at Birmingham (Sharma *et al.* 2017) reviewed the research and found a variety of laboratory studies illustrated pomegranate's ability to inhibit cancer cell growth. They stated:

"The pomegranate (Punica granatum L.) fruit has been used for the prevention and treatment of a multitude of diseases and ailments for centuries in ancient cultures. Pomegranate exhibits strong antioxidant activity and is a rich source of anthocyanins, ellagitannins, and hydrolysable tannins. Studies have shown that the pomegranate fruit as well as its juice, extract, and oil exert anti-inflammatory, anti-proliferative, and anti-tumorigenic properties by modulating multiple signaling pathways, which suggest its use as a promising chemopreventive/chemotherapeutic agent."

Greenfoods

A greenfood is a category of foods that are considered nutritionally superior than the typical fruits and vegetables. Greenfoods include the wheat grasses, sprouts, algae, and sea vegetables.

Greenfoods provide practically every nutrient imaginable, including enzymes, minerals, trace elements, essential and non-essential amino acids, vitamins, antioxidants and various phytonutrients. Many will provide over 1,000 nutrients.

A big benefit of greenfoods is their alkalinity. This gives them the ability to neutralize radicals and lipid peroxides.

Much of this alkalinity comes from greenfoods' bioavailable mineral content. Many of these minerals are also are colloidal. They tend to be hydrophobic, and maintain a positive electrical charge—rendering them alkaline.

Cereal Grasses

Wheat grass is the young grass of the wheat species, *Triticum aestivum*. In addition to a plethora of vitamins, minerals, amino acids, phytonutrients, metabolic enzymes—including superoxide dismutase and cytochrome oxidase—wheat grass maintains up to 70% chlorophyll.

Early research by Dr. Charles Schnabel, Dr. George Kohler and Dr. A.I. Virtanen in the 1925-1950 era found that cereal grasses like wheatgrass achieved their highest nutrient content at around 18 days—right before the first jointing.

Researchers from the Singhad Dental College in India (Gore *et al.* 2017) studied wheatgrass extract against oral squamous cell carcinoma. The researchers applied the wheatgrass to human oral cancer cells and found that within 24 hours, the extract had inhibited the cells by 41 percent.

Wheat grass can increase blood hemoglobin levels. Wheat grass tablets decreased blood transfusion needs by 25% among 20 children requiring frequent blood transfusions in a study.

Barley grass maintains similar properties. Research has found that barley grass is a potent free radical scavenger; significantly reduces total cholesterol and LDL-cholesterol; and inhibits LDL oxidation. Barley grass juice powder can have 14 vitamins, 18 amino acids, 15 enzymes, 10 antioxidants, 18 minerals and 75 trace elements.

Another cereal grass is Kamut grass. The khorasan wheat has higher protein levels than most wheat varieties, and contains higher zinc, selenium and magnesium content. Selenium is known for stimulating glutathione activity as we've discussed.

Sprouts

Sprouts and their powders are nutritional powerhouses. They have exponential nutritional value, well above the nutrient content of their seeds or the fully-grown plants. This was confirmed in 1970s experiments by former Hippocrates

Health Institute Director of Research, Viktoras Kulvinskas, M.S. Kulvinskas, who found that ascorbic acid levels in soybean sprouts increased from zero to 103 milligrams per 100 grams by day six—about the ascorbic acid content found in lime juice. These levels fall off significantly within days.

Each plant has a different nutrient peak. Ascorbic acid content in broad bean sprouts—used to cure scurvy during World War I—peaks in three days, after which the levels fall off.

Many believe that sprouts produce this greater antioxidant content to defend themselves against threats from the soil.

This likely translates to cancer prevention. Especially in the case of broccoli sprouts. Researchers from Oregon State University (Beaver *et al.* 2017) found that broccoli sprouts fed to mice reduced their incidence and occurrence of prostate cancer significantly.

Great nutritional sprouts include wheat grass sprouts, barley, oats, beans, broccoli and cabbage. The latter two provide a class of nutrients called glucosinolates. These glucosinolates yield sulfur compounds and indole-3 carbinols. Both have shown to have significant anticarcinogenic and anti-inflammatory effects in the body.

Seed selection is critical. A good quality seed will germinate at least 50%. Heirloom seeds often germinate at much higher rates.

Spirulina

Spirulina use dates back to the Aztecs. A good source of carotenoids, vitamins (including vegan B12 according to independent laboratory tests) and minerals, spirulina contains all essential and most non-essential amino acids, with up to 65% protein by weight. It also contains antioxidant phytonutrients such as zeaxanthin, myxoxanthophyll and lutein. It also will contain antioxidant carotenoids, vitamins and minerals.

Spirulina also contains phycobiliprotein, a unique blue pigment anti-inflammatory and antioxidant. Research has showed that phycobiliproteins can protect the liver and kidney from toxins. They are also anti-viral, and stimulate the immune system.

A number of studies have shown that spirulina can inhibit cancer growth. For example, a study from Maria Curie-Skłodowska University in Poland (Czerwonda *et al.* 2018) found that spirulina inhibited the proliferation of human non-small-cell lung carcinoma cells. They also found that the spirulina inhibited skinc cancer cells by changing the way the cells expressed certain cytokines.

Researchers from the medical school at Greece's University of Crete (Stancioiu *et al.* 2019) treated 34 patients with benign thyroid nodules with a combination of spirulina, curcumin and Boswellia or a placebo. After 12 weeks of treatment in a cross-over method (where both groups take each), the researchers found that the spirulina combination significantly reduced the size of the thyroid nodules.

Spirulina also boosts blood health. In one study from the University of California-Davis, 12 weeks of 3000 milligrams of Hawaiian spirulina per day significantly increased hemoglobin concentration and mean corpuscular hemoglobin among 30 adults over the age of 50. IDO (indoleamine 2,3-dioxygenase) enzyme activity—a sign of increased immune function—was also higher among the subjects.

Chlorella

More than 800 published studies have verified the safety and efficacy of *Chlorella pyrenoidosa, Chlorella zofingiensis* and *Chlorella vulgaris*. Chlorella's reputation of drawing out heavy metals and other toxins make it a favorite among health practitioners.

Chlorella also fights cancer. Researchers from Peking University (Zhang *et al.* 2019) found that chlorella scavenged hydroxyl radicals significantly. It also inhibited the growth of human colon cancer cells.

Chlorella maintains considerable vitamins minerals, and phytonutrients—including chlorella growth factor (CGF), known to stimulate cell growth. It is also a complete protein, with about 60% protein by weight and every essential and non-essential amino acid. Clinical studies have shown that chlorella stimulates T-cell and B-cell activity and contributes to the improvement of fibromyalgia, ulcerative colitis and hypertension. Another study showed that chlorella increases IgA levels and lowers dioxin levels in breast milk.

Chlorella's tough cell wall must be broken down mechanically to allow these nutrients' bioavailability. Our digestive enzymes cannot digest these outer cell walls. For this reason, quality chlorella growers will pulverize this tough outer cell wall.

Haematococcus and Astaxanthin

Another greenfood algae is *Haematococcus pluvialis,* known for its high astaxanthin content. Astaxanthin is a strong carotenoid similar to beta-carotene. For this reason, astaxanthin is one of the most powerful natural antioxidants known. It also has anti-inflammatory effects, and has been used for eye health, joint healthy, muscle soreness, cardiovascular health, and skin health. It can also protect against damage from UV radiation.

Several studies have shown that astaxanthin inhibits cancer growth. Several laboratory studies have shown it prevents cancer cell proliferation (Kowshik *et al.* 2019).

Superfood Compounds

Superfoods contain thousands of compounds, some of which have been isolated, and others that have not been identified.

The number of plant compounds – phytonutrients – is gigantic. Categories include isoflavonoids, flavones, procyanidins, flavanols, flavonols, carotenoids and many others. I know this may be a little confusing. But let's take a look at the science for some of these found to inhibit cancer.

Flavanols

Flavanones are significant in citrus, while the flavones are in many vegetables and herbs. Anticancer parsley contains flavanols. Tree nuts – found to reduce colon cancer – are also high in flavanols. Legumes also contain flavanols. And several medicinal mushrooms contain anticancer flavanols. In addition, olives and olive oil contain anticancer flavanols.

In a study from Poland's Medical University of Lodz (Owczarek *et al.* 2017) researchers studied human colon cancer cells. In particular, they tested an extract of the Japanese Quince fruit (*Chaenomeles japonica*). The extract isolated a collection of compounds called flavanols. This flavanol extract contained polyphenols such as procyanidin monomers and oligomers. These are components of the fresh quince fruit as well as other foods, as we'll discuss below.

The researchers found that the flavanol extract significantly blocked the ability of the cancer cells to continue to expand. After 72 hours, they found the quince extract blocked the genetic expression of proteins by up to 77 percent. It also inhibited the MMP-9 levels in the cells. MMPs are linked to tumor progression. The quince extract also inhibited the production of key enzymes that allow the cancer cells to migrate and expand.

Okay, but do flavanols protect against colon cancer when people eat more foods containing them on a daily basis?

A review of research that included nearly 400,000 people from China's National Center of Colorectal Surgery (Jin *et al.* 2012) determined that certain phytonutrients, specifically flavonoids and flavanols, have the ability to significantly reduce the risk of colorectal cancer.

After an extensive review of the evidence, the researchers narrowed the research down to eight studies, which included 390,769 people. These included a range of protocols, including large population studies as well as controlled randomized studies.

The researchers utilized the Cochrane library and the Cochrane protocol for reviews. This process helps quantify the results – often creating more conservatism among the results due to strict result comparisons.

The research found that foods containing flavanols – more technically referred to as flavan-3-ols – resulted in a significant reduction in incidence in colorectal cancer. The greater the flavanol consumption, the greater the association. More specifically, they found that greater consumption of epicatechin – a flavanol – significantly decreases the risk of colorectal cancer.

Flavanols include the category of catechins, which includes epicatechin, gallocatechin and epigallocatechin. Depending upon the molecular classification, they can also include kaempferol. Collectively these and others are also referred to as polyphenols.

Plant polyphenols like catechins are found in many fruits and vegetables and vinegar. They are also found in herbal teas and green tea, as well as cocoa (from *Theobroma cacao*). Significant flavanol content has also been found in apples, onions and some beans.

The research also found that the consumption of procyanidins and phytoestrogens also reduced colorectal cancer incidence. The researchers characterized the association of these as "medium quality," meaning there was a definite association between the consumption and colon cancer, but not as strong as the polyphenol association.

Procyanidins and Phytoestrogens

The research also found that the consumption of procyanidins and phytoestrogens also reduced colorectal cancer incidence. The researchers characterized the association of these as "medium quality," meaning there was a definite association between the consumption and colon cancer, but not as strong as the polyphenol association.

Two other phytocompounds found to reduce colorectal cancer was genistein and formononetin. These are considered isoflavonoids but also phytoestrogens because they have the ability to bind to the body's estrogen receptors. This can be significant because as people age – especially women – estrogen availability slows and this can be pro-inflammatory. When phytoestrogens are in the diet, these can help dampen the effects of estrogen reduction as we age.

The phytoestrogens genistein and formononetin are significantly found in beans, soy, red clover and some whole grains.

Flavonoids

Flavonoids have a variety of health benefits. Most flavonoids are free radical scavengers – antioxidants. They reduce inflammation and many have been found to prevent cancers of different types.

Some of the more well known flavonoids include quercetin – a nutrient found in apples, onions, garlic and other foods; hesperidin and rutin from citrus products; epicatechins from vegetables, green tea, herbs and cocoa; kaempferol from cabbage, Brussels sprouts, kale, leeks, grapes and apples; and proanthocyanidins from oats, barley and flax. Other research has found that legumes and beans help prevent cancer. Olives and olive oil are also anticancer.

In a large study from ten European countries, Italian researchers have found that diets containing higher levels of flavonoids significantly reduce the incidence of gastric cancer.

In this subset of the European Prospective Investigation into Cancer and Nutrition study (Zamora-Ros *et al.* 2012) the researchers from the Catalan Institute of Oncology followed 477,312 people – the majority of whom were women. The subjects answered extensive diet and lifestyle surveys, and they were followed for ten years.

The compositions of their diets were compared to the USDA's database on food-composition along with the Phenol-Explorer database to determine their flavonoid content.

Those women who had diets with greater amounts of total flavonoid content had nearly 20% lower incidence of gastric cancers than those women with lower flavonoid diets. The inverse association was even greater among intestinal tumors. And specific flavonoid types also had greater association with cancer prevention – anthocyanidins, flavonols, flavones, and flavanols.

There are six major types of flavonoids. These include isoflavonoids, flavones, anthocyanidins, flavanones, flavanols and flavonols.

Some types of flavonoids – most specifically those in citrus – have been dubbed 'bioflavonoids' but the broader term flavonoid has a greater specificity among the various food groups.

Diets that contain significant quantities of these constituents are typically diets high in fresh foods – as many flavonoids are heat sensitive. Diets high in fresh foods also have many other benefits, because these foods are nutrient-dense and rich in fiber.

The researchers' study confirmed this. Their conclusion: *"Total dietary flavonoid intake is associated with a significant reduction in the risk of gastric cancer in women."*

According to the World Health Organization, gastric cancers cause some 800,000 deaths globally. Gastric cancers typically start in the walls of the stomach, but tumors often grow in the intestines and esophagus. From there, they can metastasize into the lymph nodes and spread elsewhere. Gastric cancer comes with only a 65% average six month survival rate.

One of the studies included in the review was from the U.S. National Cancer Institute (Bobe *et al.* 2008). The study followed 1,905 people and their diet with an average age of 61.

The researchers compared the consumption of 29 different flavonoids together with the incidence of the occurrence of adenomatous polyps – a frequent symptom of colorectal cancer. The research used colonoscopies to determine polyp incidence.

This study also showed that switching to a high-fiber diet also significantly reduced polyp incidence and subsequent colorectal cancer.

Furthermore, the study found that colorectal cancer prevention occurred most significantly among those who consumed the higher levels of flavonol foods. In other words, just adding a few veggies to the diet won't necessarily tip the scale.

Carotenoids

Carotenoids found in tomatoes, carrots and other foods help prevent cancer growth according to studies.

For example, breast cancer risk is significantly decreased by eating more foods with carotenoids according to several studies. Here is a survey of the scientific evidence and a listing of foods that are high in the carotenoids shown to reduce breast cancer incidence.

A study from Harvard University (Eliassen *et al.* 2018) tested 32,826 women for levels of carotenoid levels in their blood. Of these, 18,743 were tested again 12 years later. The women were then followed for the next ten years. So the women were followed for over 20 years for incidence of breast cancer.

The researchers found that those women with less carotenoids in their blood had a higher incidence of breast cancer. Higher levels of alpha-carotene, beta-carotene, lycopene and total carotenoids had up to 28 percent lower incidence of breast cancer according to the research.

In another study (Wang *et al.* 2014) scientists also found that women who eat more carotenoids have a significantly reduced risk of breast cancer.

The study, published in the British Journal of Nutrition, followed 561 women who had been diagnosed with breast cancer along with 561 healthy women who were matched for age and where they lived.

Each of the women were interviewed directly the researchers and given a food frequency questionnaire.

The researchers used a quartile system – meaning they compared those whose consumption of carotenoids were in the highest 25 percent with those who were in the lowest 25 percent of carotenoid consumption.

The researchers found the highest quartile of beta-carotene dietary consumption had a 46 percent reduced incidence of breast cancer. Those who consumed the highest quarter of alpha-carotene in their diets had a 39 percent reduced risk of breast cancer.

And those who consumed higher amounts of beta-cryptoxanthin within their diets had a 62 percent reduced risk of breast cancer. Furthermore, those who consumed more luteins and zeaxanthins resulted in 51 percent reduction in breast cancer risk.

This result confirms another study done several years ago (Huang *et al.* 2007) of 122 women with breast cancer along with 632 healthy women. This study found that greater lycopene consumption reduced breast cancer risk by 74 percent, beta-carotene reduced risk by 62 percent and greater beta-cryptoxanthin reduced breast cancer risk by 57 percent.

This study also found that total carotenoid consumption reduced breast cancer risk by 63 percent.

A study from researchers from the American Cancer Society (Wang *et al.* 2015) also tested a large population of women. This study found that higher alpha-carotene levels reduced the incidence of breast cancer by between 40 and 43 percent. Among women who also ate higher levels of fruits and vegetables, the higher alpha-carotene levels reduced breast cancer incidence by 50 percent.

Yes, breast cancer rates were double for those women who ate less carotenoids along with fruits and vegetables in general. This supports other diet and breast cancer research.

Lutein

In another study, doctors at the Paul L. Foster School of Medicine at Texas Tech University (Gong *et al.* 2018) studied several carotenoids against human breast cancer cells. The researchers tested beta-carotene, lutein and astaxanthin. The researchers found that lutein in particular inhibited the growth of breast cancer cells similar to chemotherapy drugs. These chemotherapy drugs include taxanes, paclitaxel and docetaxel.

That means that the carotenoid lutein works like these chemotherapy drugs. Carotenoids are the color pigments in vegetables and some fruits.

Foods high in carotenoids
  ➢ Carrots
  ➢ Pumpkins
  ➢ Sweet potatoes
  ➢ Collard greens

- ➤ Sources of alpha-carotene include:
- ➤ Pumpkin
- ➤ Squash
- ➤ Green beans
- ➤ Leafy greens
- ➤ Sources of beta-cryptoxanthin include:
- ➤ Peppers (hot or sweet)
- ➤ Squash
- ➤ Persimmons
- ➤ Apples
- ➤ Pumpkins
- ➤ Carrots
- ➤ Tangerines
- ➤ Oranges
- ➤ Papayas
- ➤ Some sources of lutein and zeaxanthins:
- ➤ Romaine
- ➤ Broccoli
- ➤ Corn
- ➤ Spinach
- ➤ Saffron
- ➤ Kale
- ➤ Yellow carrots
- ➤ Chard
- ➤ Turnip greens
- ➤ Peas
- ➤ Goji berries

While the protective capacity of these foods was across the board in terms of the above percentages, the researchers noted that even greater protection was provided by these foods to those women who were pre-menopausal.

This of course means it is better not to wait to long to start changing the diet.

Also, those women who were exposed to second hand smoke also had a greater amount of protection from breast cancer from the above carotinoid foods.

One of the main reasons for this reduction is the fact that these carotenoids are significant free radical neutralizers. The bind to free radicals before they can seriously damage our tissues, and thus prevent that damage.

Furthermore, these free radical scavengers each collect different types of free radicals – namely some of those involved in lipid peroxidation.

Significant research has established that free radicals play a critical role in tumor creation and production, along with cardiovascular disease.

It should be noted that men also get breast cancer.

Chlorophyll

If you are eating anything green, you are eating chlorophyll. And research is finding that chlorophyll helps prevent cancer from growing in the body.

A study from Oregon State University (McQuistan *et al.* 2011) has confirmed that chlorophyll protects against the formation and growth of tumors.

The research first analyzed a number of studies that have been done testing chlorophyll for cancer prevention, including those involving rainbow trout, mice and humans. In the human study, cellular uptake of the carcinogen aflatoxin was blocked by chlorophyll.

The researchers then focused on what is called the dose-response relationship between chlorophyll and the prevention of tumor-genesis – or cancer formation.

Chlorophyll is a primary constituent of green vegetables. It is the pigment that makes plants green. Plants use chlorophyll to help convert the sun's energy into nutrition in a process called photosynthesis.

The research utilized 12,360 rainbow trout, treated with chlorophyll after exposure to dibenzochrysene – a toxic carcinogen. Those trout given chlorophyll had from 29 to 64 percent fewer liver tumors, and 24 to 45 percent fewer stomach tumors. The mechanism involved again appears to be that chlorophyll blocks carcinogen absorption and use by the cells.

However, when carcinogen exposure was significantly increased, chlorophyll did little to reduce tumors, and even accompanied an increase in the number of tumors. However, the researchers characterized this level of toxin exposure as "unrealistic."

In other words, when considering the typical exposure to toxins, and the healthy inclusion of vegetables in the diet – within the parameters that resulted in chlorophyll's ability to reduce tumors – there is a clear cancer prevention benefit from eating dark green leafy vegetables and other chlorophyll sources.

The researchers concluded:

"These results show that chlorophyll concentrations encountered in chlorophyll-rich green vegetables can provide substantial cancer chemoprotection, and suggest that they do so by reducing carcinogen bioavailability."

Nutritionists and traditional doctors have long held that chlorophyll provides numerous health benefits. Besides the array of vitamins, minerals and other phytonutrients, this research provides yet another reason to eat our vegetables. Other research finds that eating more vegetables can extend life. For this same reason, the Mediterranean Diet helps cognitive health.

Another way to increase chlorophyll in the diet is to supplement with spirulina and/or chlorella. Both of these are algae that produce a tremendous amount of chlorophyll.

Plant Lectins

Lectins from a variety of plant foods inhibit cancer naturally.

Researchers from the University of Tokyo (Soga *et al.* 2013) discovered that a lectin naturally contained in Wisteria japonica seeds selectively binds to several types of cancer. And other plant lectins have been found to have this capability.

The researchers conducted laboratory tests using seeds from three different plants – *Wisteria floribunda* (Japanese wisteria), *Wisteria brachybotrys*, and *Wisteria japonica* (Japonica). The researchers extracted agglutinizing lectins from each of the seeds of these three plants.

Agglutinizing lectins often play a protective role in nature, where they protect their host from the intrusion of certain molecules or even bacteria or viruses. For this reason practically every plant will contain some lectins.

Agglutinizing lectins appear throughout nature within many different species. The word agglutinin comes from agglutinare, which means "to glue."

Agglutinizing lectins will thus bind with and sometimes "clump" different types of elements. They may bind to bacteria, or they might bind to red blood cells. Or they may simply bind to sugars, or even antibodies.

In the case of the lectins within the Japonica tree, and compared to the other three species of Wisteria, the researchers extracted and purified lectins that were found to bind to N-acetylgalactosamine. This is a galactose sugar combined with an amino acid—a component of living cells involved in intercellular communication and thus a part of most of most living cells.

But in this case, the researchers found these lectins were smart – and one was smarter than the other two. The researchers tested all three against a host of different cells, including human cancer cells that had been collected from cancer patients.

These included human squamous cell carcinoma, cancer cells from the kidney, liver cancer cells and lung cancer cells among others. The researchers also tested the Wisteria lectins against normal (healthy) cells.

The two Wisteria plants were found to bind with all of the cancer cells.

But the lectin from the Wisteria japonica was found to bind only with the skin cancer cells, the kidney cells and the lung cancer cells.

The researchers indicated this meant the Wisteria japonica lectin could be used as a diagnostic tool – and possibly even a treatment tool – against these forms of cancer.

The researchers noted:

"In addition, histochemical analysis of human squamous cell carcinoma tissue sections demonstrated that Wisteria japonica lectin specifically bound to differentiated cancer tissues but not normal tissue. This novel binding characteristic of Wisteria japonica lectin has the potential to become a powerful tool for clinical applications."

The fact that lectins will selectively bind to cancerous cells have been seen among other types of plant lectins, including wheat germ agglutinin (WGA) and others. In a university study from Argentina (Glavas-Dodov *et al.*

2013) WGA was found to selectively bind to polycystic ovary cells. Other studies have shown WGA will not only bind but inhibit growth of colon cancer cells in the gut.

In this research, the WGA and other lectins would selectively differentiate between the cancer cells and the healthy cells around them—leaving the healthy cells intact.

The general take-away relates to utilizing those elements in nature that can help protect us. Lectins within plants help protect the plant from foreign forces that endanger the plant's survival. Now we are finding that these same elements can help us protect our own bodies.

This is really not a new thing – though our realization might be. For decades researchers have known that the same antioxidants that help neutralize free radicals within our bodies are produced by plants to help protect themselves from the environment around them.

And surely we are slowly learning just how smart nature is. Hopefully we will all learn this sooner so we can halt the continuing decimation of so many smart plant species around the world.

Resveratrol

A flurry of research published over the past 30 days has found that resveratrol blocks a number of different cancers, including breast cancer, skin cancer and leukemia.

Resveratrol is a compound found in the skin and stems of many red fruits including red grapes, but is also found among other plant-based foods such as peanuts. The plant compound has been linked with longer lifespan and reductions in heart disease. Now we find that its ability to stop cancer is pervasive.

A study from South Korea's Kongju National University (Gweon *et al.* 2013) found that resveratrol stopped the progression of a connective tissue cancer called fibrosarcoma. The researchers tested human fibrosarcoma cell growth after treatment with resveratrol and found the potent polyphenol stopped the fibrosarcoma cells in their tracks. Several doses of resveratrol were applied in this study, and all doses resulted in the cancer cell inhibition.

The mechanism found by the researchers related to the ability of resveratrol to regulate cell enzymes called matrix metalloproteinases (MMPs). MMPs govern the process of cell breakdown and tissue expansion.

The researchers also found that resveratrol triggered the p38 and PI-3K pathways within the cancerous cells, stopping them from metastasizing.

Meanwhile, research from the Sackler School of Medicine at Israel's Tel-Aviv University (Bergman *et al.* 2012) found that resveratrol inhibited the growth of colon cancer cells. In this study, resveratrol slowed the production of certain inflammatory cytokines among human colon cancer cells including IL-6 and IL-10. At the same time, the resveratrol increased the TNF-alpha cytokine, which stimulates cell death among cancerous cells.

Researchers (Kostyuk *et al.* 2012) from Rome's Dermatological Institute of the Immaculate – a leading skin research college – found that resveratrol and related plant polyphenols inhibited skin cancer growth on cells that suffered from ultraviolet radiation. Some of this effect was seen to be an alteration of the cytokines, but also by stimulating cancer-cell beating cytokines such as NFkappaB.

Scientists from the Southern Illinois University School of Medicine (Pandey *et al.* 2012) have found that resveratrol inhibited the growth of breast cancer by stopping the stem-like cells that form into breast cancer tumors. This was accomplished by the resveratrol inhibiting DNA expression, preventing the cells' maturation into full blown tumor cells. The researchers concluded that the finding *"provides us with a strong rationale to use this agent for chemoprevention against ductal carcinoma in situ of breast cancer."*

Researchers from Spain's University of Murcia (Fernández-Pérez *et al.* 2012) also studied resveratrol's ability to stop breast cancer growth, along with human leukemia. Once again, the researchers found that resveratrol inhibited the growth of three different cancer cell lines by altering the genetic expression among these cells.

German researchers (Macke *et al.* 2012) found that resveratrol contains a chemical structure called a γ-lactam ring, which appears to be a critical factor that stops cancer cell growth by stimulating anti-cancer DNA expression.

Researchers from Turkey's Hacettepe University (Aydin *et al.* 2012) found that resveratrol stops human cancer growth of breast cancer, prostate cancer, colon cancer, pancreatic cancer, and thyroid cancer in lab studies. They found that resveratrol stops and may even reverse DNA damage among cells that are becoming cancerous.

Scientists from China's Tongji University School of Medicine (Wang *et al.* 2012) have found that resveratrol inhibits the growth of lung cancer cells. The researchers found that resveratrol stopped what is called the epithelial-to-mesenchymal transition – the ability of the cells to mature into tumor-like cells. They also found that resveratrol stopped the ability of the cancer cells to adhere to tissue systems.

Scientists from South Korea's Soonchunhyang Medical Research Institute at Soonchunhyang University (Lee *et al.* 2012) found that resveratrol stopped the growth and expansion of malignant mesothelioma cells – a type of lung cancer often caused by asbestos exposure. The research found, once again, that resveratrol altered DNA expression and halted the ability of these cancer cells to metastasize.

Research has so far found that over 100 different gene expression pathways are altered by resveratrol. These include not only those that inhibit various types of cancer cells, but also those that regulate artery health, liver health, brain cell health and other health factors.

While resveratrol has become popular because it is a component of wine, the resveratrol content in wine is actually quite small, and its effectiveness may well be eliminated by the wine's alcohol content.

The effective dose of resveratrol found in several studies has been established as between 1.45 and 1.74 milligrams per kilogram of body weight. This translates to about 20 milligrams per day for a typical person.

In other words, to achieve a minimum ability to effect gene expression of potential or already-formed cancer cells is 20 milligrams per day. A Harvard study found that 12 times this dose – equivalent to 240 milligrams per day – caused a significant amount of genetic expression results.

Other research established that 40 milligrams a day was enough to elicit a minimum effective dose (Ramírez-Garza *et al.* 2018).

From a safety standpoint, those versed in resveratrol supplementation have been recommending dosages that range from 20 milligrams to 100 milligrams per day of resveratrol supplements.

As a comparison, it would require 41 glasses of a typical red wine to achieve this minimally effective dose of 20 milligrams.

Foods such as red grapes, peanuts, cranberries, blueberries and bilberries all contain resveratrol. Like wine, their resveratrol content per serving tends to be far lower than the amount researchers have determined affects genetic expression.

However, these foods also contain numerous other compounds – nutrients and polyphenols – that work synergistically with resveratrol to produce its health benefits.

Ellagic Acid

Many plant foods contain a medicinal compound called ellagic acid. Turns out that this compound will help prevent heart disease and cancer.

Researchers from the University of Hong Kong's School of Chinese Medicine (Wang *et al.* 2012) have found that ellagic acid – a phytonutrient found in many fruits, vegetables and medicinal herbs – fights off the growth of breast cancer cells.

The researchers found ellagic acid interferes with a cancer's ability to expand through the process of creating blood vessels to feed its growth. This creation of blood vessels is called angiogenesis.

Cancer researchers have been experimenting with new pharmaceuticals in an effort to halt the process of angiogenesis among cancer cells. This new research found that a natural substance available in fruits, vegetables and herbal medicines can achieve the same purpose.

The research discovered that ellagic acid interferes with a receptor called VEGFR-2, which, when bound by vascular endothelial growth factor (VEGF), stimulates the growth of blood vessels among cancer cells.

The researchers tested ellagic acid among human breast cancer cells in the laboratory. They found that the ellagic acid *"significantly inhibited"* the growth of MDA-MB-231 breast cancer tumors, as well as blocked the ability of the tumor cells to expand and migrate – also called metastasizing. The researchers confirmed the findings using different experimental models.

The findings were published in this month's Breast cancer Researcher and Treatment Journal.

While ellagic acid is found in a large variety of fruits, vegetables and herbs, some of the highest levels are found among berry fruits and grapes. Strawberries, cranberries, blackberries, pomegranates, raspberries, blackberries and grapes have some of the highest amounts of ellagic acid. Walnuts and pecans also contain significant amounts. Ellagic acid is most known for its ability to neutralize free radicals – giving it a reputation of being a strong antioxidant.

Many foods with flavanols, which also help fight cancer, also tend to contain ellagic acid as well. Cumin also helps fight breast cancer according to other research. Hops also inhibits cancer growth according to other research.

Ellagic acid has also been shown in other research to slow and even reverse cancer growth. A previous study by the same researchers (Wang *et al.* 2012) found that an herbal medicine called *Sanguisorba officinalis* halted breast tumor progression. As they investigated the active compounds that produced this effect, they came upon the ellagic acid. They found that ellagic acid, along with gallic acid, reduced tumor size and inhibited the expansion of human breast cancer tumors.

Antioxidants

We've identified research confirming that cancer is related directly to oxidative stress. As expected, other research shows antioxidants reduce oxidative stress.

Research from the Brussels' Central Hospital, University of Charleroi, and the Hospital Vesale Experimental Medicine Laboratory at Free University of Brussels (Dequanter *et al.* 2013) tested 36 patients with head and neck squamous cell carcinomas.

This is one of the most lethal forms of skin cancer. Nine out of ten cancers on the head and neck are squamous cell carcinomas. About half of those with this cancer will die within five years.

The researchers collected the tumor tissues of the 36 patients along with close-by tissue without tumors.

They conducted an in-depth analysis of the tissues and tested them using capillary electrophoresis – testing that separates and breaks down tissues into their smaller components. The researchers also conducted oxidation testing and specifically determined the ratios between oxidized glutathione and reduced glutathione.

The ratio of oxidized glutathione to reduced glutathione in the tissues relates directly to the amount of oxidative stress in the tissues, as well as indicates the level of antioxidant activity. This is because glutathione is the leading scavenger of oxidation within the body.

The researchers found that the tumor tissues showed significantly higher variation in the glutathione GSH part of the ratio. This indicates that the free scavenging abilities of glutathione are reduced within skin cancer tissue.

This study confirms findings from the University of Oslo in Norway (Sakhi *et al.* 2009). This study compared 78 patients with head and neck squamous cell carcinoma together with 100 healthy people.

The scientists tested the tissues and blood of all the participants for levels of oxidative stress related to not only glutathione, but also hydroperoxides, gamma-glutamyl transpeptidase, prostagladin and oxidized/total ascorbic acid levels.

The researchers also tested for levels of antioxidants present in all the subjects – including total antioxidant capacity, glutathione redox potential, total glutathione levels and total cysteine levels.

They also tested all the subjects for dietary antioxidant levels - including six different carotenoids (carrots and tomatoes are high in carotenoids), four tocopherols (seeds, grains and oils are high in tocopherols, and ascorbic acid (fruits are high in ascorbic acid).

The study found that the patients with squamous cell carcinoma all had higher levels of oxidative stress biomarkers in their blood and tissues. The levels of total hydroperoxides were significantly higher in the skin cancer patients - indicating specifically that their bodies were under oxidative stress.

The researchers also found that these oxidative stress markers went up significantly when the cancer patients underwent radiation treatment.

The study also found that the skin cancer patients lower levels of the dietary antioxidants within their bloodstream as compared with the healthy control subjects. They also found that the levels of antioxidants fell dramatically as the patients were subjected to radiation treatment.

The researchers wrote in their conclusion:

"Biomarkers of antioxidants and oxidative stress are unfavorable in head and neck squamous cell carcinoma patients compared to healthy controls, and radiotherapy affects many of these biomarkers. Increasing levels of antioxidant biomarkers before radiotherapy and increasing oxidative stress during radiotherapy may improve survival indicating that different factors/mechanisms may be important for survival before and during radiotherapy in head and neck squamous cell carcinoma patients. Thus, the therapeutic potential of optimizing antioxidant status and oxidative stress should be explored further in these patients."

Okay, we get that: Antioxidants can help improve survival rates among patients with skin cancer, and help patients deal with radiation treatment.

But how about preventing cancer altogether by eating a healthy diet with lots of antioxidants, and reducing those lifestyle habits – such as smoking and alcohol consumption – that have been specifically linked with producing higher levels of oxidative stress in the body?

When we harvest a fresh plant-based food and eat it with minimal storage, processing and cooking, we are deriving significant benefits from the living organism that produced the food. Because living organisms defend themselves against toxins throughout their lives, by eating fresh whole foods or whole foods minimally cooked, our bodies can utilize the same elements the plant utilized to protect itself against toxins.

This in turn stimulates our immune systems, and also provides direct free radical protection. This is because antioxidants are designed to neutralize toxins.

As we've discussed, a plethora of research has confirmed that damage from free radicals is implicated in many health conditions. Free radicals from toxins damage cells, cell membranes, organs, blood vessel walls and airways—producing systemic inflammation—as the immune system responds to an overload of tissue damage.

Free radicals are produced by synthetic chemicals, pathogens, trans fats, fried foods, red meats, radiation, pollution and various intruders that destabilize within the body. Free radicals are molecules or ions that require stabilization. They reach stabilization by 'stealing' atoms from the cells or tissues of our body. This in turn destabilizes those cells and tissues—producing damage.

Antioxidants serve to stabilize free radicals before our cells and tissues are robbed—by donating their own atoms. A diet with plenty of fruits and vegetables supplies numerous antioxidants. Although antioxidants cannot be considered treatments for any disease, many studies have proved that increased antioxidant intake supports immune function and detoxification. These effects allow the immune system to respond with greater tolerance.

Antioxidant constituents in plant-based foods are known to significantly repeal free radicals, strengthen the immune system and help detoxify the system. These include *lecithin* and *octacosanol* from whole grains; *polyphenols* and *sterols* from vegetables; *lycopene* from tomatoes and watermelons; *quercetin* and *sulfur/allicin* from garlic, onions and peppers; *pectin* and *rutin* from apples and other fruits; *phytocyanidin flavonoids* such as *apigenin* and *luteolin* from various greenfoods; and *anthocyanins* from various fruits and oats.

Some sea-based botanicals like kelp also contain antioxidants as well. Consider a special polysaccharide compound from kelp called *fucoidan*. Fucoidan has been shown in animal studies to significantly reduce inflammation (Cardoso *et al.* 2009; Kuznetsova *et al.* 2004).

Procyanidins are found in apples, currants, cinnamon, bilberry and many other foods. The extract of *Vitis vinifera* seed (grapeseed) is one of the highest sources of bound antioxidant *proanthocyanidins* and *leucocyanidines* called *procyanidolic oligomers* or PCOs. Pycnogenol® also contains significant levels of these PCOs. Blueberries, parsley, green tea, black currant, some legumes and onions also contain PCOs and similar proanthocyanidins.

Research has demonstrated that PCOs have protective and strengthening effects on tissues by increasing enzyme conjugation (Seo *et al.* 2001). PCOs have also been shown to increase vascular wall strength (Robert *et al.* 2000).

Oxygenated carotenoids such as *lutein* and *astaxanthin* also have been shown to exhibit strong antioxidant activity. Astaxanthin is derived from the microalga *Haematococcus pluvialis,* and lutein is available from a number of foods, including spirulina.

Most of these phytonutrients specifically modulate the immune system. For example, the flavonoids *kaempferol* and *flavone* have been shown to block mast cell proliferation by over 80% (Alexandrakis *et al.* 2003). Sources of kaempferol include Brussels sprouts, broccoli, grapefruit and apples.

Furthermore, *resveratrol* from grapes and berries modulate nuclear factor-kappaB and transcription/Janus kinase pathways—which strengthens immunity. Good sources of resveratrol include peanuts, red grapes, cranberries and cocoa (wine is not advisable for cleansing as we'll discuss later).

Nearly every plant-food has some measure of phytonutrients discussed above and more. These phytonutrients alkalize the blood and increase the detoxification capabilities of the liver. They help clear the blood of toxins.

Foods that are particularly detoxifying and immunity-building include fresh pineapples, beets, cucumbers, apricots, apples, almonds, zucchini, artichokes, avocados, bananas, beans, collard greens, berries, casaba, celery, coconuts, cranberries, watercress, dandelion greens, grapes, raw honey, corn, kale, citrus fruits, watermelon, lettuce, mangoes, mushrooms, oats, broccoli, okra, onions, papayas, parsley, peas, whole grains, radishes, raisins, spinach, tomatoes, walnuts, and many others.

These plant-based foods are also our primary source of soluble and insoluble fiber. Diets with significant fiber help clear the blood and tissues of toxins, and lipid peroxidation-friendly LDL cholesterol. Fiber is also critical to a healthy digestive tract and intestinal barrier. Fiber in the diet should range from about 35 to 45 grams per day according to the recommendations of many diet experts. Six to ten servings of raw fruits and vegetables per day should accomplish this—which is even part of the USDA's recommendations. This means raw, fibrous foods should be present at every meal.

Good fibrous plant sources also contain healthy *lignans* and *phytoestrogens* that help balance hormone levels, and help the body make its own natural corticoids. Foods that contain these include peas, garbanzo beans, soybeans, kidney beans and lentils.

Plant-based foods provide these immune-stimulating factors because these vary same factors make up the plants' own immune systems. For example, the red, blue and green flavonoid pigments in plants and fruits help protect the plant from oxidative damage from radiation. The proanthocyanidins in grains like oats, for example, help protect the oat plant from crown rust caused by the *Puccinia coronata* fungus. So the same biochemicals that stimulate immunity in humans are part of plants' immune systems.

These same whole food phytonutrients also neutralize oxidative radicals in our bodies—the reason they are called antioxidants. How do we know this? Scientists can measure the ability of a particular food to neutralize free radicals with specific laboratory testing.

One such test is called the *Oxygen Radical Absorbance Capacity Test* (ORAC). This technical laboratory study is performed by a number of scientific organizations that include the USDA, as well as specialized labs such as Brunswick Laboratories in Massachusetts.

Research from the USDA's Jean Mayer Human Nutrition Research Center on Aging at Tufts University has suggested that a diet high in ORAC value may protect blood vessels and tissues from free radical damage that can result in inflammation (Sofic *et al.* 2001; Cao *et al.* 1998). These tissues, of course, include the airways. Research has confirmed that consuming 3,000 to 5,000 ORAC units per day can have protective benefits.

ORAC Values (100 grams) of Selected (raw) Fruits (USDA, 2007-2008)

Cranberry	9,382		Pomegranate	2,860
Plum	7,581		Orange	1,819
Blueberry	6,552		Tangerine	1,620
Blackberry	5,347		Grape (red)	1,260
Raspberry	4,882		Mango	1,002
Apple (Granny)	3,898		Kiwi	882
Strawberry	3,577		Banana	879
Cherry (sweet)	3,365		Tomato (plum)	389
Gooseberry	3,277		Pineapple	385
Pear	2,941		Watermelon	142

There is tremendous attention these days on two unique fruits from the Amazon rain forest and China called *açaí* and *goji berry* (or wolfberry) respectively. An ORAC test documented by Schauss *et al.* (2006) gives açaí a score of 102,700 and tests documented by Dr. Paul Gross gives goji berries a total ORAC of 30,300. However, subsequent tests done by Brunswick Laboratories, Inc. gave these two berries 53,600 (açaí) and 22,000 (goji) total-ORAC values.

In addition, we must remember that these are the dried berries being tested in the latter case, and a concentrate of acai being tested in the former case. The numbers in the chart above are for fresh fruits. Dried fruits will naturally have higher ORAC values, because the water is evaporated—giving more density and more antioxidants per 100 grams.

For example, in the USDA database, dried apples have a 6,681 total-ORAC value, while fresh apples range from 2,210 to 3,898 in total-ORAC value. This equates to a two-to-three times increase from fresh to dried. In another example, fresh red grapes have a 1,260 total-ORAC value, while raisins have a 3,037 total-ORAC value. This comes close to an increase of three times the ORAC value following dehydration.

Part of the equation, naturally, is cost. Dried fruit and concentrates are often more expensive than fresh fruit. High-ORAC dried fruits or concentrates from açaí or goji will also be substantially more expensive than most fruits grown domestically (especially for Americans and Europeans). Our conclusion is that local or in-country grown fresh fruits with high total-ORAC values produce the best value. Local fresh fruit offers great free radical scavenging ability, support for local farmers, and pollen proteins we are most likely more tolerant to.

By comparison, spinach—an incredibly wholesome vegetable with a tremendous amount of nutrition—has a fraction of the ORAC content of some of these fruits, at 1,515 total ORAC. Spinach, of course, contains many other nutrients, including proteins lacking in many high-ORAC fruits.

Dehydrated spices can have incredibly high ORAC values. For example, USDA's database lists ground Turmeric's total ORAC value at 159,277 and oregano's at 200,129. However, while we might only consume a few hundred milligrams of a spice per day, we can eat many grams—if not pounds—of sweet colorful fruit every day.

Chapter Five
Anticancer Herbs

For the purposes of organization, we are utilizing the herbalist's definition of herbs here. Literally, herbs would be plants. But we'll also include mushrooms (fungi) and seaweeds in this category due to their common use in herbalism.

Medicinal Mushrooms

Research proves that medicinal and culinary mushrooms fight cancer.

The Agaricus species is the most popular eating mushroom, and this species contains the button mushroom. But there are many, many others.

Biologists have cataloged some 50,000 mushrooms, and identified less than 20,000 different mushroom species. Some estimate there may be over 150,000 mushroom species within the Fungi kingdom, which likely encompasses more than 1.5 million total species. Biologists have described less than 5% of Fungi species.

Over 600 mushroom species have been documented to stimulate the immune system. However, the ones mentioned above have received the most attention. Research on these mushrooms have revealed their effects as being antimicrobial, cholesterol-lowering, anti-inflammatory, anti-oxidant, anti-mutagenic, anti-tumor, adaptogenic and immunostimulating.

Cancer has been a significant area of research. A number of these mushrooms have been shown to inhibit cancer cell line growth, for example. American researchers were awakened by Dr. Tetsuro Ikekawa's groundbreaking epidemiological study showing significantly lower cancer rates among Japanese mushroom growers between 1972 and 1986.

The research since then has shown significant anticarcinogenic properties among most of the mushrooms mentioned above. While most clinical research to date has been adjunctive to conventional therapies for ethical reasons, human studies have consistently confirmed animal and laboratory models. By September of 2030, there were 21,724 mushroom studies and scientific papers filed with the U.S. National Library of Medicine.

A immune-boosting compound called AHCC—Active Hexose Correlated Compound—has been is derived from Shiitake mushroom and their sub-species. This has been shown to stimulate the activity of white blood cells. Further research showed they stimulated interferon (IFN-y) and tumor necrosis factor (TNF-a) as well.

Much of the dramatic immunity effects of mushrooms are due to their polysaccharides and polysaccharide-protein complexes. Laboratory research has isolated multiple polysaccharide types within each species. Twenty-nine unique polysaccharides have been isolated in Maitake, for example.

Mushroom polysaccharides are primarily glucans with different glycosidic linkages, including 1->3 and 1->6 beta glucans, and 1->3 alpha glucans. The complex branching and even helical nature of mushroom glucans appears to be significant. Schizophyllan polysaccharides with (1,3)-b-glucans with 1,3-b-d-linked glucose with 1,6-b-d-glucosyl side groups have been described as "stiff triple-stranded" helices in laboratory research, for example. Schizophyllan (SPG) is an active macrophage stimulator, increasing T cell and NK cell activity and inhibiting various infective agents.

Various immunostimulatory effects have been also attributed to polysaccharide-protein complexes such as PSK (krestin), PSP, lentinan and others. While many varieties contain different levels of the various beta glucans, many researchers believe it is their unique protein sequencing that differentiates effects among species.

Medicinal mushrooms also contain a variety of nutrients. Many mushrooms contain significant amounts of protein. Shiitake can be as much as 17% protein while oyster mushrooms can be 30% protein by weight. Several also contain vitamin B complexes.

Most edible mushrooms also contain a variety of macro-minerals and trace elements. Shiitake also can contain as much as 126 mg of calcium, and 247 mg of magnesium per serving, for example. Reishi also contains magnesium, calcium, zinc, iron, copper and trace minerals. Many are good sources of selenium.

Maitake and a number of other mushrooms also contain ergosterols (provitamin D2), along with phosphatidylcholine and phosphatidylserine. Shiitake, Reishi and Maitake have been known to increase from less than 500 IU of D2 in indoor growing conditions to 46,000 IU, 2760 IU, and 31,900 IU respectively, following six to eight hours of sunlight exposure (Stamets 2005).

Various anti-oxidants have been isolated among popular mushroom varieties. Constituents such as ganoderic acid (*G. lucidum*), cordycepic acid (*C. sinensis*), linzhi (*G. frondosa*), agaric acid (several), sizofilan and sizofiran (*S. commune*), galactomannan (*C. sinesis*), and various triterpenoids (several) can actively reduce oxidative radicals and stimulate the immune system.

The density of these in mushrooms is quite incredible. Reishi has over 100 ethanol-soluble triterpenoids. Most of these are antioxidant, and many are anti-inflammatory agents.

Some of the mechanisms of mushrooms to safely stimulate the immune system and produce long-term cleansing benefits are quite complicated. For example, differently branched beta glucans have been observed stimulating immune cells in different ways.

For example, certain beta glucans from Maitake will stimulate T-cell production, while differently bonded-chain beta glucans from *Agaricus blazei* stimulate natural killer (NK) cells. Others stimulate B-cells, T-helper cells, lymphokine activated killer cells [LAK], macrophages; and the cytokines interferon gamma, interleukin-2, -12 and tumor necrosis factor [TNF].

Mushrooms significantly detoxify heavy metals inside our bodies, and in their natural environments. Their proteins will bind to certain heavy metals within the soil. These same metabolites become active within the body when eaten, and thus help chelate minerals in our bodies.

For this reason, Cordyceps, Reishi, *Agaricus blazei* and Maitake have been used in China to reduce effects of heavy metal and radiation poisoning.

Mushrooms can be eaten fresh, frozen, drank as teas, cooked with sauces or eaten as supplements. Parts used include the fruiting body (cap and stem) and the mycelia (colonizing rooting network).

While each form will stimulate our immune system, fresh or freeze-dried are preferable. Some supplements are hot-water extracted, and some are alcohol extracted. Hot water extracts likely retain more constituents, although alcohol can extract specific medicinal constituents as well.

Over four decades of laboratory and clinical research have established that a number of medicinal mushrooms work in a myriad of ways to help our bodies naturally fight cancer.

The science shows that medicinal mushrooms are not all alike. They each work a little differently. Nonetheless, the research does find that most of these medicinal mushrooms help boost the body's own immunity, along with working to kill or weaken cancer cells.

We should note that due to their care for patients, medical researchers are reluctant to test cancer patients by only treating them with mushroom extracts. Most of the research has therefore treated patients with mushroom therapy alongside conventional chemotherapy and/or radiotherapy (radiation).

This is logical, since chemotherapy and radiotherapy have received intensive research focus and have been dramatically improved over the past two decades. Survival rates have therefore increased for these therapies.

At the same time, these therapies are also still wrought with side effects. They also tend to severely depress the immune system. Both of these provide a segue for the use of mushroom therapy in cancer treatment alongside conventional therapy.

This is called adjunctive therapy.

At the same time, we should appreciate that mushroom therapy has come a long way over the past three decades. Not so long ago, treating cancer patients with mushroom extracts was unheard of by Western researchers. That left all the research on mushrooms mostly in the territory of laboratory research on human cancer cells or animals.

This preliminary research has yielded significant success. But as some of the research has moved to humans, it has been found that there is a definite place for mushroom therapy in cancer treatment.

But this is only the beginning of this human research. So much more is necessary. It behooves us to encourage medical researchers to put more focus on medicinal mushrooms and their extracts. Yes, it is difficult to patent a natural compound. But we're talking about helping people here, right? Isn't that the goal of medical science? Or at least, shouldn't it be?

Culinary Mushrooms

A number of studies have reported the anti-cancer effects of medicinal mushrooms. Many of these medicinal mushrooms are also culinary mushrooms. These include oyster mushrooms, button mushrooms, Shiitake mushrooms and others.

A large study from Japan's Tohoku University's School of Medicine (Zhang *et al.* 2019) followed 36,499 men for more than 13 years. During this time 1,204 of the men developed prostate cancer.

The researchers studied the diets of the men to determine the effect that eating mushrooms had on future prostate cancer risk. This study did not focus on other foods that may reduce prostate cancer risk – only looking at the effect of mushrooms on those who ate more or less of other food categories.

In the end, the researchers found those consuming culinary mushrooms three times a week or more experienced 17 percent lower incidence of prostate cancer compared to those who dined on mushrooms fewer than once a week.

Even eating mushrooms at least once a week seriously reduced prostate cancer incidence. Those who included mushrooms in their diet at least once a week had 8 percent less prostate cancer compared to those who ate mushrooms less than once a week.

There are several tasty mushrooms that are considered culinary. But we also know that every mushroom is also medicinal. Typical culinary mushrooms include:

> ➤ Shiitake mushrooms (*Lentinus edodes*)
> ➤ Oyster mushrooms (*Pleurotus ostreatus*)
> ➤ Button (white) mushrooms (*Agaricus bisporus*)
> ➤ Portobello mushrooms (also *Agaricus bisporus*)

Several studies have shown these mushrooms are anti-cancer. A review of research from the University of Pennsylvania (Xu *et al.* 2012) found that five common culinary mushrooms had significant effects of inhibiting cancer in laboratory and human studies. Studies have continued to confirm this finding since.

White Button Mushrooms

The American Cancer Society estimates there were 220,800 new cases of prostate cancer in the U.S. during 2015. And about 27,540 men died from prostate cancer in 2015.

Prostate cancer is the second leading cause of cancer deaths in men. It follows only lung cancer.

Yet the survival rates for prostate cancer are typically good, assuming the cancer remains in the prostate. If the cancer spreads to other parts of the body such as the lymphatic system or other organs, the five-year survival rate is only about 28 percent.

The issue for most men who've had prostate cancer is to prevent a progression and recurrence of the cancer. And prostate enlargement is linked specifically to prostate cancer, as well as recurrence.

Furthermore, for those men who have or have had prostate cancer, their cancer will often progress or recur as the prostate continues to become atypically enlarged. This is called continuous enlargement. An estimated 50,000 prostate cancer patients continue to have rising prostate enlargement. This is associated with a recurrence of the prostate cancer.

This means that strategies to reduce prostate enlargement can be of critical importance to just about any man at some point in our lives.

Prostate enlargement is medically called benign prostatic hyperplasia, or BPH. And prostate enlargement is measured by the prostate-specific antigen (PSA). This is a protein-enzyme produced by cells in the prostate gland, also called kallikrein-3.

We have discussed research of natural herbs and foods connected with BPH and PSA in this publication. Many of these have been shown to be preventative: They can help delay prostate rise in men or a slower rise in some men (even healthy men will also have some prostate enlargement as they age).

But a few of these natural products have been shown to help reduce or delay prostate enlargement. And there are even a few that have been shown to reverse enlargement.

Then again, there is prostate enlargement for a man who already has or has had prostate cancer. Can natural medicines provide any hope for men who now have an increased risk of recurrence due to continued prostate enlargement?

A phase I clinical trial has shown that a particular type of mushroom can reverse prostate enlargement.

The research comes from the Beckman Research Institute and the Department of Medical Oncology and Experimental Therapeutics at the City of Hope National Medical Center located in Duarte, California (Twardowski *et al.* 2015).

The researchers tested 36 men – who were patients and prostate cancer sufferers. The test subjects were divided into groups of six. Each group started off with 8 grams per day, and their doses were increased to up to 14 grams per day of a mushroom extract.

The therapy was given for three months, and the results were measured using a dose-dependent response. This means their results were compared to their levels of dosage.

The mushroom used was *Agaricus bisporus* – also referred to as white or button mushrooms. These are the common mushroom found at the supermarket or added to most dishes in restaurants. It is by far the most prolifically grown commercial mushroom.

The researchers found that over a third of the patients – or 36 percent – experienced reductions in their PSA levels during the three-month period. That is, their PSA levels were below the levels they had in the beginning of the study.

Some of the patients experienced what the researchers called a *"complete response."* This means their PSA levels went down so far that their PSA levels were "undetectable." Furthermore, these undetectable PSA levels continued for 30 months in one patient and 49 months in another patient.

Furthermore, those who experienced either a complete response or a partial response also saw increased immune strength. This is specific in interleukin-15 and myeloid-derived suppressor cells – both important in fighting prostate cancer or preventing its recurrence.

The researchers confirmed these effects in their conclusion:

"Therapy with white button mushrooms appears to both impact PSA levels and modulate the biology of biochemically recurrent prostate cancer by decreasing immunosuppressive factors."

Getting to a phase I clinical trial doesn't happen in a vacuum. For decades, researchers have found that Agaricus mushrooms stimulate the immune system. Some have found that Agaricus will boost anticancer cytokines.

Before they moved to a clinical trial, the researchers at the Beckman Research Institute (Adams *et al.* 2008) conducted laboratory research using Agaricus. Their research found positive results and found that one of the central components of Agaricus – conjugated linoleic acid – was effective in reducing PSA in the laboratory.

Another laboratory study from China's National Yang-Ming University (Yu *et al.* 2009) found that another Agaricus species – Agaricus blazei Murill – reduced prostate cancer growth in human cancer cells. They found this among both androgen-dependent and androgen-independent prostate cancer cells.

The researchers stated:

"We therefore suggest that A. blazei might have potential therapeutic use in the prevention and treatment of human prostate cancer."

In the clinical study and the laboratory studies, no adverse effects were found in the Agaricus mushroom treatments.

Oyster and Shiitake Mushrooms

For example, an international study (El-Deeb *et al.* 2019) found that fractions of oyster mushrooms inhibited the growth of breast and lung cancer cells and boosted immune system cytokines.

And a review of 12 years of research on Shiitake mushrooms (Zhang *et al.* 2018) found that significantly anti-cancer and boosted the effectiveness of chemotherapy during lung cancer treatment.

Much of the anti-cancer benefits of mushrooms come from their beta-glucan content.

What's the best way to cook mushrooms?

There are different ways to cook mushrooms. These include frying, grilling, boiling and even microwaving them. Taste is often the biggest consideration.

But that doesn't mean it doesn't matter how they are cooked. In fact, a study from Spanish researchers (Roncero-Ramos *et al.* 2016) tested the basic ways to cook several culinary mushrooms.

The food scientists determined that frying mushrooms seriously reduced their nutritional and antioxidant activities. They also found that boiling boosted their beta-glucan levels. But boiling also reduced their antioxidant levels. Microwaving and grilling were found to maintain antioxidant and general nutrient levels of culinary mushrooms by the researchers.

Another study tested the polyphenolic content of Shiitake mushrooms (Choia *et al.* 2006). They found that baking the mushrooms at 121 degrees Celsius for 30 minutes increased their free polyphenolic content by nearly double (1.9 times).

This would mean that mushrooms can be baked, microwaved and boiled to help maintain and even bring out some of their anti-cancer benefits.

Other research has shown that some mushrooms decrease prostate PSA levels.

Split-gill Mushroom (*Schizophyllum commune*)

Split gills grow throughout the world, often on decayed trees. But they are well known for their ability to fight cancer.

The Split-gill mushroom has been tested clinically and in the laboratory for decades. One of its main anti-cancer compounds is Hydrophobin SC3. In 2013, researchers from The Netherlands injected this compound into growing tumors in the laboratory.

The researchers found that after 12 days of daily injections, the compound suppressed the growth of the tumors. This was facilitated by the boosting of natural interleukin-10 and TNF-alpha levels, which naturally fight tumor growth.

Another anti-cancer compound from Split-gill is Schizophyllan. In one study, researchers from the Chinese Academy of Agricultural Sciences (Zhong *et al.* 2015) tested Schizophyllan against human breast cancer cells. They found the compound fights tumor growth for breast cancer.

Split-gill mushrooms have also been tested clinically. In another study, Tokyo's Cancer Institute Hospital (Shimizu *et al.* 1991) tested 40 patients, with 15 cervical cancer patients with benign tumors. Prior to surgery, they administered 20 milligrams of sizofiran, also called SPG – a schizophyllum glucan. After 8 days of injections, the researchers found the patients who received the injections had boosted immune markers such as helper-T cells and IL-2.

In a study from Japan's Kumamoto University School of Medicine (Miyazaki *et al.* 1995) 312 patients with cervical cancer were tested. In 90 patients given the SPG compound along with radiotherapy, their 5-year survival rates were significantly longer than those of a group of 82 patients treated with radiotherapy alone.

Furthermore, another 60 cervical cancer patients given the sizofiran along with chemotherapy had significantly better 5-year survival rates than those who had chemotherapy alone. And 244 cancer patients who were given the sizofiran compound showed boosted natural anticancer immunity such as CD8+ and CD4+ T-cells.

Patients with advanced uterine cervical cancer were treated (Yamamoto *et al.* 2001) with the split gill extract doxifluridine combined with radiotherapy and immunotherapy. Of the 37 patients, the effective response rate was 84.2% for those given 600 mg per day and 100% for those given 800 mg per day.

Researchers (Sekiguchi *et al.* 1990) gave 22 patients with uterine cervical cancers the split gill extract sizofilan with radiotherapy. They found CD3 levels and NK cell levels were significantly greater in those given sizofilan after radiotherapy.

Another clinical study (Hatae *et al.* 1998) tested 33 patients with uterine cervical cancer. They were separated into two groups. Chemotherapy and radiation therapy was combined with split gill extract. The research showed the combination therapy had a 69.7% response rate among those given the combination therapy.

Researchers (Nakano *et al.* 1996) treated 45 patients with stage II and III cervical cancer. Of these, 15 had their tumors injected with split gill extract, and another 20 patients received weak injections into their tumor. The weak injections boosted T-cell and langerhan cell infiltrations into cancer tissues compared to those given the full injections or received none.

Scientists (Fujimoto *et al.* 1991) of 386 Japanese patients with resected gastric cancer tested split gill extract Sizofiran. In 264 patients given Sizofiran adjunctively with other cancer treatment, had improved tumor size and prognosis compared to those not given the treatment. The extract was administered intramuscularly at 40mg per week.

Survival times were increased in two studies in the 90s. One tested 15 patients with head and neck cancer at the Yamagata University School of Medicine in Japan (Kimura *et al.* 1994). The five-year survival rate of patients given Sizofilan along with chemotherapy and radiation had better survival rates than the control group.

Another clinical study (Yoshida *et al.* 1997) tested patients with head and neck cancer with sizofiran in addition to other therapy. Those treated with the split gill extract had longer overall survival periods. Those in stages III and IV had particularly longer survival rates than the controls.

Huaier (*Trametes robiniophila*)

The Huaier mushroom has been used in Chinese Medicine for almost two thousand years. The mushroom has been found to help treat liver cancer, breast cancer, stomach cancer, ovarian cancer and others in laboratory research. Studies have shown it helps kill cancer cells, helps prevent tumors, helps inhibit tumor growth, reduces chemo side effects, and activates the immune system.

Researchers (Yang *et al.* 2018) have found that a water extract of Huaier inhibited human prostate cancer cell growth. In another study (Xu *et al.* 2017) researchers found Huaier significantly inhibited cancer growth on human stomach cancer cells. The researchers found it reduced MMP expression while boosting immune markers.

In another study, researchers (Hu *et al.* 2016) tested Huaier against human liver cancer cells. They found the extract inhibited tumor growth potential in this laboratory study.

Similarly, a study on human breast cancer cells (Ding *et al.* 2016) found Huaier extract inhibited tumor growth.

Yunzhi (*Coriolus versicolor*)

C. versicolor has been tested for more than three decades. Lab and clinical testing finds it boosts the body's natural immunity (including cytokines IL-1, IL-2, IL-6, IL-8, TNF-α, and TNF). It improves cancer survival.

In a 2017 study from the National Cancer Center in Singapore (Chay *et al.* 2017) researchers tested 15 acute liver cancer patients who were unable to receive other treatment. Those given the C. versicolor extract did not appear to reduce the disease progression of the patients. But it did significantly increase the quality of live for those patients. Those given the mushroom extract had reduced pain and less appetite loss as a result of the mushrooms. The researchers stated:

"Coriolus versicolor subjects generally had better Quality of Life on treatment compared to placebo subjects. The utility of this supplement in patients whose primary treatment goal is palliation should be further explored."

Other clinical studies have shown even better results. A 2003 study tested 34 patients with non-small cell lung cancer. Part of the group took a PSP extract from Coriolus versicolor for 28 days. The researchers found the extract improved symptoms and improved immune cell counts, along with boosted IgG and IgM. The mushroom extract patients also showed reduced symptoms of disease progression.

A clinical study (Wong *et al.* 2005) tested C. versicolor with 82 breast cancer patients for six months, following their conventional cancer treatment. The researchers found the PSP extract boosted anticancer immunity markers (such as CD4+, CD8_ and B-lymphocytes. They also decreased pro-cancer markers.

A clinical study on breast cancer patients (Wang *et al.* 2013) found that the PSP extract significantly boosted anticancer immune cells. It also downgraded tumor-boosting mechanisms among the cancer patients.

A study from Japan's Kyushu University (Sugimachi *et al.* 1997) tested 224 patients with stomach cancer after they received surgery to remove the cancer. The patients were split into two groups and one group received the PSP extract for a year.

The research found the PSP group had longer survival rates and decreased recurrence rates. They also had lower recurrence rates compared to those who didn't receive the PSP extract.

Maitake (*Grifola frondosa*)

Ancient Asian healers heralded Maitake mushroom for its ability to lengthen life. Maitake was used throughout Japan, Korea, Tibet and China to heal a myriad of disorders.

This ancient medicinal mushroom has been used for thousands of years and has undergone a tremendous amount of cancer research. It has been shown to stimulate anticancer macrophages, and boost the body's immunity against cancer. These include boosting leukocytes, IL-1, IL-6, and IL-8.

In a clinical study from New York's Memorial Sloan Kettering Cancer Center (Wesa *et al.* 2015) researchers tested 21 patients with MDS (Myelodysplastic syndromes). MDS are a group of bone marrow-related cancers.

The researchers found that the Maitake extract boosted basal neutrophils and improved monocyte function. The researchers found the treatment to be beneficial in this relatively short study.

In a 2010 study, researchers (Chen *et al.* 2010) tested 72 patients with polycystic ovary syndrome (PCOS). They gave the patients either a Maitake extract called MSX with or without chemo or the chemo therapy alone. The researchers found the mushroom extract boosted ovulation in a majority of the patients (77 percent and 93 percent), while the chemotherapy rates were much lower.

A study from the Memorial Sloan Kettering Cancer Center (Deng *et al.* 2009) tested 34 breast cancer patients in a safety and tolerance study. They were given Maitake liquid extract for three weeks. The researchers found the mushroom extract boosted immune function among the patients. Increasing doses increased some function while depressing other immune function. The researchers noted further testing was required to better understand the extract's effects.

In another study (Kodama *et al.* 2003) ten cancer patients were measured for numbers of CD4 and CD8 cells in peripheral blood, as well as NK cell activity with K-562 cells as target cells. Interleukin-2 receptor levels and tumor markers were determined in three and four patients respectively. Maitake D-fraction intake showed a suppression of metastatic progression and lessened tumor marker expression in all patients, and all patients showed increased NK cell activity. As measurement of NK cell activity is used as a indicator, Maitake D-fraction appears to inhibit cancer growth.

Another clinical study (Yang *et al.* 1999) tested 313 patients after being treated with bladder cancer. They were given either mitomycin treatment, Maitake extract, thiotepa chemo or served as controls. The patients were followed for up to 15 years. The researchers found that the control group had a 65 percent recurrence of the bladder cancer.

This was compared to only 34.9 percent in the Maitake group. Those in the mitomycin group had a slightly higher recurrence rate, while the thiotepa chemo group had a 42 percent recurrence rate. The Maitake recurrence rate was the lowest, and nearly half of the control group.

A similar study (Yang *et al.* 1994) from tested 146 bladder cancer patients, and found that tumor recurrence rates were 33.3 percent in the Maitake group, 34.3 percent in the conventional group and 65 percent in the control group.

In a 2002 series of case studies (Kodama *et al.* 2002), MD-fraction and whole Maitake combination powder were given to numerous cancer patients between the ages of 22 and 57 years old with various types of stage II-IV cancer.

Cancer regression or symptom improvement resulted in 58.3% of the liver patients, 68.8% of the breast cancer patients, and 62.5% of the lung cancer patients, although less then 10-20% improvement for leukemia, stomach and brain cancer patients.

When the combination powder was taken with chemotherapy, immune activity increased by 1.2-1.4 times as compared to chemo alone.

Reishi (*Ganoderma lucidum*)

The common name of Reishi mushroom in Chinese medicine means "immortal mushroom." It's common name Lingzhi in Japanese means "immortality plant."

A study from Italy's National Cancer Institute (Barbieri *et al.* 2017) tested Lingzhi mushroom against melanoma cancer cells and triple-negative breast cancer cells. They found that G. lucidum inhibited release of products these cells utilize to stay alive. The researchers also showed that Reishi helped prevent cancer cells from migrating.

The researchers concluded:

"Taken together, these results indicate the possible use of Ganoderma lucidum extract for the therapeutic management of melanoma and human triple-negative breast cancer."

A number of other studies have confirmed that Lingzhi inhibits a number of types of cancers.

Other studies have confirmed Lingzu's ability to boost liver health. In a study from the Fujian Academy of Agricultural Sciences (Wu *et al.* 2016) researchers found that the triterpenoids from Lingzhi – called Ganoderma triterpenoids – reduced ALT (alanine aminotransferase) enzymes by up to 51 percent, AST (aspartate aminotransferase) enzymes by as much as 33 percent.

They also found the Ganoderma triterpenoids reduced oxidative damage to liver cells. The researchers concluded:

"Our results showed that Ganoderma triterpenoids had potent cytoprotective effect against oxidative damage induced by t-BHP in HepG2 cells, thus suggesting their potential use as liver protectant."

A review from Taiwan's Tainan University of Technology (Weng *et al.* 2010) analyzed the research and found that Reishi inhibited cancer growth by affecting the following elements within cancer cells and tumor tissues:

- Activator protein-1(AP-1)
- Beta1-integrin (ITGB1)
- Interleukin (IL)
- Matrix metalloproteinase (MMP)
- Nitric oxide (NO)
- Nuclear factor-kappa B (NF-kappaB)
- Vascular endothelial growth factor (VEGF)
- Transforming growth factor (TGF)-beta1
- Urokinase plaminogen activator (uPA)
- uPA receptor (uPAR)

Agaricus blazei

We discussed other Agaricus species earlier, but *Agaricus blazei* or *Agaricus blazei* Murrill (also *Agaricus brasiliensis*) mushrooms deserve another discussion. These have been found to be significantly anticancer.

Agaricus yields 1,3-b-glucans and 1,6-b-glucans. Research has found that Agaricus and its b-1,3-Branched-b-1,6-glucans have antitumor activity in animals and humans.

Agaricus brasiliensis extract was studied (Ahn *et al.* 2004) on 100 cervical, ovarian and endometrial cancer patients. Patients received chemotherapy with or without A. brasiliensis extract. NK cell activity was significantly higher in the A. brasiliensis extract group compared to the placebo group.

The chemotherapy-related side effects including appetite loss, hair loss, emotional and general weakness were all reduced in the A. brasiliensis group.

In addition to this clinical study, Agaricus blazei has undergone numerous cancer studies with human cancer cell lines, rats and mice over three decades. These have consistently indicated that this mushroom seriously treats cancer.

Cordyceps sinensis

For more than two decades, Cordyceps has undergone numerous cancer cell and mice studies confirming its ability to inhibit the growth of a number of cancers. These include breast cancer, colorectal cancer and stomach cancer.

Indeed, many other laboratory and human studies have documented that Cordyceps boosts a number of cytokines, natural killer cells and other immune cells that have been shown to help prevent cancer cells from developing or proliferating.

A study from Korea's Bundang Jesaeng General Hospital (Kang *et al.* 2015) tested 79 healthy men for four weeks. Half were given Cordyceps extract and the other half were given a placebo.

The men given the Cordyceps had significant increases in cancer-fighting immune markers. These include natural killer cell activity and increased levels on the lymphocyte proliferation index. It also boosted levels of Th1 cytokines. This means the mushroom boosted immunity significantly among the men. The researchers concluded:

"C. militaris enhanced the NK cell activity and lymphocyte proliferation and partially increased Th1 cytokine secretion. Therefore, C. militaris is safe and effective for enhancing cell-mediated immunity of healthy male adults."

We should note that Cordyceps may not be so good for prostate cancer. A study from Peking University First Hospital (Ma *et al.* 2018) tested Cordyceps on prostate cancer cells and also in mice. They found the mushroom boosted the proliferation of prostate cancer cells.

Long Pepper

Several studies have confirmed that an Ayurvedic medicinal herb used for thousands of years has incredible cancer cell-killing potential, and may soon be employed by conventional medicine to treat cancer. The herb is called *Piper longum* – also called Long Pepper.

One of the mysteries of treating cancer with chemotherapy and radiation is that inserting chemicals and treatments that are unhealthy to most of the body can treat a growing cancer malignancy. This occurs through influencing a process called apoptosis, which is the process cells use to self-destruct.

By stimulating this process of self-destruction, primarily through a genetic switch called p53, cancer treatments can invoke the killing of cancer cells before the treatment kills off healthy cells.

The problem of chemotherapy and radiation has been this danger to healthy cells – and the potential negative side effects – of chemotherapy and radiation to the rest of the body. For this reason, many alternative health advocates have protested chemotherapy and radiation treatment.

Nobel Laureate Dr. James Watson published a paper (Watson 2013) showing that antioxidants – known for preventing cancer – will interfere in late-stage cancer treatment because they block the cell death process of chemotherapy and radiation.

At the same time, researchers and clinicians are becoming aware that many cancers are becoming resistant to many chemotherapy agents. This is because the cancer cells can communicate between each other ways to work around the chemotherapy.

Enter Ayurveda. A newly emerging anticancer therapy comes from a natural herb that may well be the answer to unhealthy chemotherapy: Piper longum.

The *Piper longum* herb has shown in a number of studies that it has the capability to kill cancer cells without damaging healthy cells.

In a study from Sweden's Uppsala University Medical College (Jarvius *et al.* 2013), a constituent of *Piper longum* called Piperlongumine was tested against cancer in the laboratory. They found that piperlongumine was able to stimulate death of cancer cells without harming healthy cells.

The process Long Pepper uses to stimulate cancer cell death has been proposed to be one of stimulating the increase in free radicals that damage the cancer cells. But the Swedish research showed that Piperlongumine is apparently more complex, in that it inhibits a genetic process called ubiquitin-proteasome system (UPS), and this apparently stimulates the cancer cell death process.

Another study, from Thailand's Chiang Mai University Medical School (Taka *et al.* 2012) has shown that *Piper longum* prevents cancer cells from resisting the killing effect of the herb by blocking the ability of cancer cells to talk with each other. The *Piper longum* was able to shut down telomerase activity – which stimulates the process of cellular communication through the cells' telomeres.

The researchers observed these effects in human lung cancer cells, proving that *Piper longum* can inhibit tumor malignancy – which requires the telomere communication. The researchers stated:

"In the long-term treatment of A549 lung cancer cells with sub-cytotoxic dose of these perylenes, telomere shortening, reduction of cell proliferation and tumorigenicity, and cell senescence were observed."

Yet another study found that another *Piper longum* constituent, called pipernonaline, stops the growth of prostate tumors. Researchers from Korean's Pusan National University found that pipernonaline stopped both the androgen-dependent and the androgen-independent prostate cancer cells from growing – or metastasizing.

The researchers concluded:

"This is the first report of pipernonaline toward the anticancer activity of prostate cancer cells, which provides a role for candidate agent as well as the molecular basis for human prostate cancer."

The scientific community first became aware of the anticancer potential of *Piper longum* in 2011, after Harvard researchers found in a series of laboratory and animal studies that the herb had the ability to stop cancer growth without hurting healthy cells. These effects were demonstrated among breast cancer tumors.

Piper longum has long been used by Ayurvedic practitioners for a variety of conditions, including bacterial and fungal infections, skin lesions, blood sugar problems, respiratory conditions, muscular pains, viral hepatitis and many others. It is known to stimulate the immune system and it has significant anti-inflammatory capabilities.

This newfound ability of *Piper longum* to stop cancer growth likely doesn't surprise those Ayurvedic clinicians who have seen *Piper longum's* array of healing potential in a variety of conditions.

Greater Burdock

Greater Burdock (*Arctium lappa L.*) blocks cancer growth and boosts cognition and memory. What a combination.

Greater Burdock seeds and roots have been utilized as a blood purification agent and for skin conditions in Chinese, Japanese and Korean traditional medicines. The root has also been part of herbal combinations for boosting immunity and even fighting colds and influenza.

Greater Burdock – Niu Bang Zi in Chinese Medicine – has been used for many centuries for medicinal and nutritional benefits. The roots and seeds are typically used, as they contain numerous medicinal compounds known to be anti-inflammatory.

Thus Greater Burdock is often used for lung infections and skin infections. It mucilage content is soothing to mucosal membranes while its arctigenin, arctiin aglycone, sulfur and acetylene compounds have been shown to be anti-viral and anti-inflammatory.

Burdock is also part of the Essiac anti-cancer tea formula.

Research from China and Japan has confirmed that Burdock and its constituents block the growth of cancer. In one study, researchers from China (Sun *et al.* 2018) tested two human liver cancer cell lines with Burdock. The research tested HepG2 and Hep3B cancer cell lines – taken from human tumors. The researchers also tested the Burdock extracts with animal cancer cases.

The researchers found that a constituent in Burdock called arctigenin halts the proliveration of cancer. It also prevents the migration of cancer cells to other parts of the body.

In addition, the researchers found that the Burdock extract halted the formation of tumors for the HepG2 cancer lines. The researchers stated:

"In the present study, we showed that arctigenin efficiently inhibited HCC growth, invasion, and metastasis in vitro. Arctigenin also decreased the levels of gankyrin in HepG2 and Hep3B cell lines. As gankyrin is overexpressed in human liver cancers…"

In a study from UCLA's David Gefen School of Medicine (Wang *et al.* 2017) the Burdock compound arctigenin was tested against human prostate cancer cell lines, LNCaP and LAPC-4. The researchers found that the arctigenin produced a genetic change in the cells that inhibited the proliferation of the cancer. The researchers also tested the compound with cancer mice and found the compound inhibited tumor growth by as much as 70 percent. Other tests showed the compound prevented the growth of prostate cancer cells by 75 percent.

The researchers noted that the combination of studies provided *"high promise in its translation to human application."*

Research, from Japan's Kagoshima University and University of the Ryukyus (Susanti *et al.* 2013) tested the constituent called Arctigenin from Greater Burdock (*Arctium lappa* L.) on lung cancer cells. Because Arctigenin has been shown in other cancer studies to be a potent anti-cancer constituent, the researchers delved into the mechanisms of its ability to knock down lung cancer cells.

The researchers exposed Arctigenin to human lung adenocarcinoma cells in the laboratory, and measured and analyzed its ability to produce cell death – apoptosis – among the cancer cells.

The study found that Arctigenin knocks out cancer cells with two simultaneous processes. The first is by inhibiting the cancer cells' production of particular proteins (NPAT proteins) – which effectively cripples the cancer's ability to reproduce.

Then Arctigenin performs a double-whammy by knocking out the cancer cell through its effect on the cell's intracellular glutathione metabolism – effectively weakening the cancer cell from the inside.

This 'smart' approach of this herbal constituent to cancer cells is typical among so many herbal medicines, that change cellular processes within the body to effect improved health and metabolism.

In a study from the School of Medicine from South Korea's Dongguk University (Maxwell *et al.* 2017) researchers tested the Burdock extract against human breast cancer cells lines.

Once against, the researchers found that the arctigenin compound significantly inhibited the metastasis of the cancer cells. They called the effect *"anti-metastatic effects."*

This study confirms another study done by researchers at Kagoshima University (Susanti *et al.* 2012). This research tested 364 herbal extracts for anti-cancer activity and found that Greater Burdock's Arctigenin had one of the highest levels among the other herbs.

The researchers found that Arctigenin killed human lung cancer cells, human liver cancer cells and human stomach cancer cells. The researchers wrote:

"In conclusion, this study found that arctigenin was one of cancer specific phytochemicals, and in part responsible for the tumor selective cytotoxicity of the herbal medicine."

Astragalus

Astragalus is a genus of plants and not an individual herb as often spoken of anecdotally. There are a few species of astragalus, however, that are known to inhibit some cancers. But some research has shown no benefit as we'll discuss.

An extract of *Astragalus saponins,* called AST, has been shown (Auyeung *et al.* 2016) to fight gastrointestinal cancers in some laboratory research.

A study from China's Fujian University of Traditional Chinese Medicine (Zhou *et al.* 2018) found that an alcohol extract of astragalus successfully inhibited the proliferation of human breast cancer cells.

Another study, from Second Clinical Medical College (Zhai *et al.* 2018) found that Astragalus polysaccharide extract significantly inhibited the proliferation of human cervical cancer cells. They also found that the extract increased the sensitivity of the cancer cells to the chemotherapy drug cisplatin.

The combination of the two killed even more cancer cells than either individually.

This combination therapy has gained traction. A 2020 study from China's College of Medicine at Chang Gung University (Hsieh *et al.*) enrolled 17 patients with advanced head and neck squamous cell cancer (HNSCC).

The patients were split into two groups. One group was given the cisplatin chemotherapy regimen (cisplatin/tegafur-uracil/leucovorin) with an injection of Astragalus polysaccharides extract or the chemotherapy alone.

The Astragalus group did not show any greater tumor response, but the Astragalus group did have fewer adverse events and less pain, greater appetite and better quality of life.

Another clinical study (Wang *et al.* 2015) tested an astragalus combination on 90 colorectal cancer patients.

After their surgery, half the group was given normal treatment while the other half was given *Astragalus membranaceus* with the TCM formula Jiaozhen.

The researchers found that the Astragalus group had recovery times and increased intestinal barrier protection after the surgery that closely matched the conventional treatment.

Bottom line on astragalus: More evidence is needed, but there is enough research that shows some astragalus species will boost immunity and possibly help inhibit cancer proliferation.

Ginseng

Panax ginseng is an immune stimulant with thousands of years of use. *Panax ginseng* will come in white forms and red forms. The color depends upon the aging or drying technique used.

When Ginseng is cultivated and steamed, it is called 'red root' or Hong Shen. Ginseng root will turn red when it is oxidized or processed with steaming. Some feel that red root is better than white, but this really depends upon its intended use, the age of the root, and how it was processed.

Soaking Ginseng in rock candy produces a white Ginseng that is called Bai shen. This soaking seems odd, but this has been known to increase some of its constituent levels such as superoxide and nitric oxide. When the root is simply dried, it is called 'dry root' or Sheng shaii shen. Korean Red Ginseng is soaked in a special herbal broth and then dried.

There are a number of species within the *Panax* genus, most of which also contain most of the same adaptogens, referred to as gensenosides. Most notable in the *Panex* genus is American Ginseng, *Panax quinquefolius.*

Ginseng contains camphor, mucilage, panaxosides, resins, saponins, gensenosides, arabinose and polysaccharides, among others.

Eleutherococcus senticosus, often called Siberian Ginseng, is actually not Ginseng. While it also contains adaptogens (eleutherosides), these are not the gensenoside adaptogens within Ginseng that have been observed for their ability to relieve hypersensitivity.

Research (Wang *et al.* 2016) has found that the ginsenosides that are more available in Panax significantly inhibits cancer cell proliferation.

In a clinical study from China's Guang'anmen Hospital (Zhang *et al.* 2018) studied 414 people suffering from non-small cell lung cancer. They treated half the group with conventional treatment alone and the other half with conventional treatment plus a Ginseng extract.

The survival rates among the Ginseng group were over 40 percent longer (12 months versus 8.46) than the conventional-only group. Side effects were also significantly milder in the Ginseng group.

Other clinical studies have shown cancer patients receiving Ginseng extracts with their cancer treatments had better quality of life and reduced fatigue compared to those not taking the Ginseng (Barton *et al.* 2013; Yennurajalingam *et al.* 2017; Kim *et al.* 2017).

Aloe vera

Research finds that aloe can prevent and treat skin cancer.

A number of new studies are showing that Aloe vera can both prevent and even treat melanoma.

Aloe-emodin is a compound found in Aloe. Turns out this compound can halt the growth of skin cancer cells.

Research from the University of Belgrade's School of Medicine (Popadic *et al.* 2013) confirmed what previous studies on aloe-emodin found. The biochemical inhibit the process of skin cancer growth – also called cancer cell proliferation.

The researchers tested Aloe-emodin on human skin cells called keratinocytes after being treated with radiation. Once radiated, keratinocytes will typically proliferate (expand) into skin cancer tumors.

The researchers found that the aloe-emodin significantly stopped the proliferation process. This confirmed Aloe's benefit in halting the progression of tumor formation after radiation by the sun.

A similar result was found by researchers from South Korea's Gachon University of Medicine and Science. They determined that aloe-emodin specifically halted the growth of human cancerous liver cells. The researchers found that Aloe-emodin stimulated a genetic change within the cancerous cells that not only halted their expansion, but induced cell death among the cancer cells.

Researchers from Sree Chitra Tirunal Institute for Medical Sciences and Technology found that aloe-emodin was able to inhibit the growth of colon cancer cells. The Aloe-emodin also induced cell death among the individual cancer cells.

These studies of human cells confirm similar findings in animal research – showing the application of Aloe vera gel onto the skin significantly inhibits the progression of skin cancer.

China Medical University researchers determined that another Aloe constituent called rhein also produced anticancer effects. They found that tumor progression was halted and cancer cell death occurred as a result of rhein.

While aloe has long been known for its skin irritation and wound healing abilities, science on its internal use is still emerging.

Aloe is now used for gastrointestinal health, immune support and cardio-vascular health, as well as the health of the skin and mucosal membranes.

Artemisia

Artemisia is a genus of a large collection of plant species. The most notable with respect to cancer is *A. absinthium*, also called Wormwood.

A flurry of research from around the world over the past few years has confirmed that Wormwood blocks the development of several types of cancer. These include colon cancer, breast cancer, lung cancer, pancreatic cancer, brain cancer, prostate cancer, leukemia and others.

Other research has found that several Artemisia species are antibiotic and anti-parasitic, as well as antiviral and antifungal.

Let's look at some of the research with regard to cancer.

Researchers from the Cancer Research Laboratory at the University of California at Berkeley (Steely *et al.* 2017) tested an extract of Artemisia against human prostate cancer cells of two different types. This 2017 study found the artemisnin extract interrupted the process of androgen reception among the prostate cancer cells. This effectively cuts off the process that prostate cancer cells utilize to expand.

Researchers from the medical school of Czech Republic's Masaryk University (Slezakova *et al.* 2017) found that several compounds in Artemisia, including dihydroartemisinin and artesunate, actively kill prostate cancer cells (cytotoxic).

Another 2017 study from China's Nanjing Medical University (Wang *et al.*) studied an extract of *Artemisia annua* called Artesunate. Like the Berkeley researchers, they found that Artesunate blocked androgen receptor proteins, which in turn suppressed tumor growth and resulted in cancer cell death.

In 2014, doctors at the St George's University of London (Krishna *et al.*) and the UK's St. George's Healthcare NHS Trust conducted a phase II clinical trial of the Artemisia extract Artesunate. This was a double-blind, placebo-controlled clinical trial.

The researchers tested 20 colorectal cancer patients. The patients were given either a placebo or 200 milligrams of oral Artesunate each day for fourteen days. After the treatment period, all the patients underwent surgery to remove the cancerous area of their colons.

The researchers found that a significant killing of tumor cells were found in two-thirds of the patients treated with the Artemisia extract. They also found an 89 to 92 percent reduction of colon cancer cells and increased CD31 expression – which helps the body kill cancer cells among these patients.

Then 42 months later, the researchers found there was only one recurrence of the colon cancer among those given the 14-day treatment. This compares to six patients that had recurrences among the placebo group.

The researchers concluded:

"Artesunate has anti-proliferative properties in colorectal cancer and is generally well tolerated."

In another study, medical researchers from Korea's Hannam University (Kim *et al.* 2017) found that Artemisia annua extract inhibited growth of human colon cancer cells. The extract did this using a number of different processes, including cotton off its ability to make DNA. The Artemisia also interrupted the cancer cells' immunity activities and metabolism tasks.

Several studies, including some of the above, have found that human breast cancer cells are inhibited and even killed with Artemisia treatment.

In a study from Germany's University of Heidelberg and Johannes Gutenberg University (von Hagens *et al.* 2018) 23 breast cancer patients were tested in a Phase I clinical study on the Artemisia extract Artesunate. A Phase I clinical study focuses on establishing safe doses for further clinical studies.

The researchers gave the patients either 100, 150 or 200 milligrams of Artesunate per day for -8 weeks. This was in addition to their ongoing cancer therapy.

The researchers found that 200 milligrams of Artesunate per day was safe and tolerated. They recommended 200 milligrams per day for future clinical study.

Another 2017 study (Mirkin *et al.*) tested Artemisia extract against K562 and HL-60 human leukemia cells. This study found the Artemisia extract killed the leukemia cells of both types within 48 hours of contact.

Researchers from Israel's Kaplan Medical Center obtained B chronic lymphocytic leukemia cells from seven leukemia patients. They were each at different stages of their disease.

The researchers found in this study *Artemisia absinthium* killed 75 percent of the leukemia cells, with 70 percent killed within the first 48 hours.

Researchers from Korea's Kyung Hee University (Jang *et al.* 2017) tested *Artemisia capillaris* extract against liver cancer cells. They found that the Artemisia extract blocked tumor growth by activating IL-6 cytokines. This blocked the transcription 3 signal pathway that these cancer cells use to form tumors.

Research from China's Yanbian University (Yuan *et al.* 2016) studied Artemisia extracts against liver cancer cells along with cervical cancer cells.

They also found the extract stimulated cancer inhibition among both of these cancer cell types.

The research has found that Artemisia seems to work quite well when combined with other treatments – even conventional chemotherapy. The research has found it to have a synergizing effect.

Dr. Thomas Efferth and associates from the Institute of Pharmacy and Biochemistry at Johannes Gutenberg University and his team also found that Artemisia annua extracts successfully inhibit cancer cells of different types.

In a 2017 paper, Dr. Efferth outlined a comprehensive methodology of combining Artemisia with drug therapies that have already shown success in inhibiting cancer and associated symptoms. His research found many of these conventional drugs to be synergistic with Artemisia.

Butchers Broom

Butchers Brook is a plant called *Ruscus aculeatus.* A set of compounds in this plant, called ruscogenins, have been found to inhibit cancer and tumor growth in a some laboratory studies.

One study (Song *et al.* 2020) found that a ruscogenin initiated the die off of pancreatic cancer among mice.

Cat's Claw

Cat's claw *(Uncaria tomentosa)* is an Amazon rainforest plant known to reduce inflammation. It also apparently inhibits the growth of precancerous squamous cells and may help improve quality of life for cancer patients.

A study from Italy (Cianu *et al.* 2018) tested Cat's Claw for squamous carcinoma cells. The study found that Cat's Claw caused cell death for developing cancer cells.

A study from Brazil (Kaiser *et al.* 2013) studied Cat's Claw against human bladder cancer cells. The researchers found that Cat's Claw extracts significantly inhibited the growth of the bladder cancer cells.

Another study (de Paula *et al.* 2015) tested Cat's Claw with 51 advanced cancer patients. They found that a daily dose of 300 milligrams of dried Cat's Claw improved quality of life for the cancer patients.

The Cat's Claw did not have a tumor response, however.

Other studies have found Cat's Claw had potential anticancer affects on leukemia, melanoma and breast cancer in laboratory studies.

Ginger

Ginger (*Zingiber officinale*) is one of the most versatile medicinal herbs and in Ayurveda—the oldest medicine still in use—Ginger is the most recommended medicine. According to the research of James Duke, Ph.D. of the U.S. Department of Agriculture and Norman Farnsworth, Ph.D., a research professor at the University of Illinois, Ginger contains at least 477 active constituents (Schulick 1996).

The most prominent of these include terpenes and phenolics. Terpenes in Ginger include zingiberene, bisabolene, farnesene, sesquiphellandrene and α-curcumene. Ginger's phenolic compounds include Gingerol, paradols, and shogaol.

One of these compounds, Gingerol, has been found to inhibit the growth of a variety of cancer types in laboratory studies. Multiple animal and human cancer cell studies have confirmed that Ginger inhibits gastric cancer, pancreatic cancer, liver cancer, colorectal cancer, and cholangiocarcinoma (Prasad and Tyagi 2015).

Some human research has also had favorable results.

Researchers from Emory University (Citronberg *et al.* 2013) tested 20 patients with colon cancer. They gave them either 2 grams of Ginger or a placebo each day for 4 weeks. And the end of the testing period, biopsies revealed that the Ginger group had significantly decreased proliferation among the colon crypts. Cancer cell death also was found. The researchers concluded:

"Ginger may reduce proliferation in the normal-appearing colorectal epithelium and increase apoptosis and differentiation relative to proliferation—especially in the differentiation zone of the crypts ..."

Ginger has also been found to reduce nausea and gastrointestinal upset for patients undergoing chemotherapy (de Lima *et al.* 2018; Bossi *et al.* 2017).

Euphorbia

Euphorbia hirta and related species of Euphorbia have been used as medicinal medicines around the world for thousands of years. Euphorbia treatments are included in Ayurvedic medicine, Kampo, Malaysian medicine, Polynesian medicines along with Thai, South African and Indonesian medicines.

The plant goes by various names. These include:

- ➢ Red spurge
- ➢ Snakeweed
- ➢ Pill-bearing spurge
- ➢ Mexican Shrubby Spurge
- ➢ Caribbean copper plant
- ➢ Asthma herb
- ➢ Bovi
- ➢ Dudhi

> ➤ Daun biji kacang
> ➤ Nelapalai
> ➤ Amampatchairaisi

Euphorbia is a short skinny tree with red leaves and branches. It is indigenous to many tropical regions, and is cultivated throughout the Southern United States among other regions.

It also grows throughout the world, including in Asia, Pacific Islands, Africa, Central America and South America.

Its beautiful red leaves are hardy in full sun or partial shade. The small branches contain a milky sap. The sap can irritate the eyes and skin for some, so testing is necessary before application.

Nonetheless, the sap, leaves and branches have been used as a remedy for several conditions. Here is a list of these, starting with those that have been confirmed in modern research:

Euphorbia has been found to inhibit several cancers.

A study from Pakistan's University of Karachi (Bano *et al.* 2017) found that Euphorbia herb species inhibited the growth of human lung cancer cells, human breast cancer cells, human prostate cancer cells and human cervical cancer cells.

Research from Africa's University of the Witwatersrand (Thafeni *et al.* 2012) found that extracts from Euphorbia fight lung cancer cells by inducing cell death. The researchers found cell death rates caused by the extracts were consistent with chemotherapy rates.

Researchers from the College of Pharmacy of Saudi Arabia's King Saud University (Marzouk *et al.* 2012) performed laboratory analyses on *Euphorbia cotinifolia*. The research determined that the plant's compounds were significant antioxidants. But the most significant finding was that the extracts inhibited the growth of human liver cancer cells – hepatocellular carcinoma cells.

About 2% of all cancers are liver cancer, but liver cancer is severe and not often diagnosed early. Only about a fifth of all liver cancer patients live past one year after diagnosis.

Hepatocellular cancer is the leading type of liver cancer. It often occurs when the liver is damaged from alcohol overuse, hepatitis, the overuse of pharmaceuticals, as well as a number of synthetic compounds such as vinyl chloride, herbicides and others.

A 2016 study from Malaysia's University Sains Malaysia showed that Euphorbia hirta also inhibited the growth of breast cancer cells.

Many other studies on Euphorbia species have shown anticancer effects.

Euphorbia contains many constituents, including at least a dozen of macrocyclic diterpenes and 17 different polyphenols.

Specific constituents include quercitrin, kaempferol, amyrin, heptacosane, gallic acid, protocatechuic acid, sitosterol, camphol, nonacosane, choline, quercitol, tinyatoxin, euphorbins (A, B, C, D), jatrophanes, euphopubescenol, methylenecycloartenol, euphomelliferene, myricitrin, afzelin, rutin and two ellagitannins.

This array of constituents – some of which have not been found elsewhere in nature – illustrates the complexity of this plant medicine.

Hopefully researchers will continue to test this complex medicinal herb.

Basil and Holy Basil

Basil (*Ocimom basilicum*) and Holy Basil (*Ocimom sanctum*) – also called Tulsi – have both been found to inhibit the growth of cancer.

A review of research from India's Father Muller Medical College (Baliga *et al.* 2013) analyzed a host of most laboratory studies and concluded:

"Tulsi and some of its phytochemicals eugenol, rosmarinic acid, apigenin, myretenal, luteolin, β-sitosterol, and carnosic acid prevented chemical-induced skin, liver, oral, and lung cancers and to mediate these effects by increasing the antioxidant activity, altering the gene expressions, inducing apoptosis, and inhibiting angiogenesis and metastasis."

Other research (Baliga *et al.* 2016) has found that Holy Basil helps protect the body from radiation-caused cancer.

Basil research has had similar results. A 2019 study from China's Guangzhou University of Chinese Medicine (Feng *et al.*) found that basil extract called BPS (basil polysaccharide) inhibited liver cancer genesis.

The researchers found that BPS stopped the progression of a liver cancer type called hepatocellular carcinoma. Interestingly, it halted a process called epithelial-mesenchymal transition. This is how many cancer cells metastasize.

Rosemary

Research has determined that Rosemary (*Salvia rosmarinus*) inhibits the growth of tumors and cancer cells. Laboratory studies have determined that Rosemary can suppress the growth of tumors in different organs, including the colon, breasts and stomach.

Studies have also found that melanoma and leukemia cells have been inhibited by Rosemary and its extracts (Ngo *et al.* 2011).

One of the major anticancer compounds in Rosemary is rosmarinic acid. In a study from Korea's Chungbuk National University (Jang *et al.* 2018) tested rosmarinic acid on human prostate cancer cells. The research found that the extract caused early cell death among the prostate cancer cells.

Laboratory studies (Sanchez *et al.* 2019) have found Rosemary extracts can inhibit the growth of colon cancer as well.

Red Raspberry Leaves

Researchers from Coatia's University of Zagreb (Durgo *et al.* 2012) determined that red raspberry leaves contain bioactive substances that kill colon cancer cells and produce significant antioxidant potential that helps prevent throat cancer.

The researchers tested raspberry leaves against human cancer cell lines for laryngeal carcinoma (throat cancer) and colon adenocarcinoma (colorectal cancer). They found that the raspberry leaves had a significant cytotoxic (cancer cell-killing) effect upon the colon cancer cells, and a "chemoprotective" antioxidant effect against throat cancer cells.

They analyzed the leaves and found them rich in a variety of polyphenols and antioxidants. To test their relative antioxidant effects, they treated the cells with hydrogen peroxide.

Red raspberry leaves – notably from the Meeker variety – are one of the few plants that contain an anti-carcinogenic substance called ellagitannins. As the ellagitannins are absorbed, the tannins are released, which releases highly absorbed ellagic acid. Other findings have confirmed anticancer research involving ellagic acid. Ellagic acid cleanses cells of oxidative radicals, and stimulates a cell death switch in cancer cells.

Red raspberries and their leaves also contain flavanols. We discuss research that confirms flavanols help prevent colon cancer elsewhere. Flavanols include anthocyanins. These help give raspberries their red color. Anthocyanins have been shown to be incredibly antioxidant as well as heart healthy. Anthocyanins also help the eyes due to their antioxidant abilities.

Red raspberries are native to North America. They grow profusely in nature, especially in the northwestern U.S. During the winter months they will lay bare. But when spring comes, they will spout hairy leaves that can be harvested as herbs.

The leaves can be dried and used as a dehydrated herb. Or they can be steeped in tea. Be sure to filter the tea well to prevent the stickers from getting in. The best form of the leaves is to extract them. raspberry leaf extract is available in some retail outlets.

Cardamom

The Cardamom spice (*Elettaria cardamomum*) can make a meal taste great, but it can also boost the immune system and inhibit cancer growth.

Research from Saudi Arabia's University of Hail (Qiblawi *et al.* 2015) found that Cardamom boosted the liver's production of glutathione-S-transferases, superoxide dismutase, glutathione peroxidase and catalase. As we discussed in the liver section, these are antioxidant and anti-inflammatory chemicals that help remove oxidative radicals before they can turn healthy cells into cancerous cells.

Indeed, researchers (Das *et al.* 2012) found that Cardamom protected mice against non-melanoma skin cancer.

A similar finding was established for skin cancer (Qiblawi *et al.* 2012).

Research from China's Xinxiang Medical University (Kong *et al.* 2019) found that a Cardamom extract called cardamonin produced cell death among human breast cancer cells.

Caraway

Multiple studies have confirmed that Caraway seeds (*Carum carvi*) can inhibit the growth of cancer.

Multiple studies (Allameh *et al*. 2013; Deeptha *et al*. 2006) have found that Caraway seed oil inhibited the growth of colon cancer in rats.

Other studies have found Caraway seeds exert anticancer effects on cancer cells (Naderi-Kalali *et al*. 2005). Other studies have seen similar findings with Caraway essential oil.

Indigo Herb

Herbs contain many medicinal compounds. Many of these inhibit the growth of cancer. Yes, nature has interwoven cancer fighting elements within plant compounds. A constituent of the herb Indigo (*Indigofera sumatrana*) has been found to do just that: Fight cancer.

Researchers from the Beckman Research Institute (Nam *et al*. 2012) determined that a constituent of the Indigo herb called indirubin prevents leukemia cells from growing.

The leukemia research, supported by the City of Hope Comprehensive Cancer Center's department of molecular medicine, applied indirubin to human chronic myelogenous leukemia tumor cells. They found that the indirubin blocked the cancer cells' signaling systems and their ability to regenerate their cell membranes—a process called autophosphorylation.

The mechanism revealed by the study involved blocking processes of particular genes within the tumor cells. Indirubin blocks the process of a protein called the Signal Transducer and Activator of Transcription 5 (STAT5) protein. In addition, a group of molecules called Src family kinases (SFKs) is blocked by indirubin, which prevents the cell from activating phosphorylation. This leads to cell death among the leukemia cells.

Another study from Korea's Chosun University (Yoon *et al*. 2012) has found that indirubin stops lung cancer cell growth. And a 2011 study from Ohio State University showed indirubin stops brain cancer cells from growing.

The lung cancer research found that indirubin also blocked phosphorylation activities, and reduced the polo-like kinase (PLK) activity, which also leads to the cell death of human lung cancer cells.

This is not the first study that has shown that indirubin shuts down cancer cells. A 2011 study (Williams *et al*.) showed that indirubin blocked the growth of brain cancer cells.

Indirubin is now seen as one of the most promising anti-cancer strategies available. Thanks to mother nature.

Indirubin was discovered well over a decade ago, when researchers were trying to isolate the compound within the Traditional Chinese Herbal formula called Danggui Longhui Wan that seemed to block leukemia cancer from growing. The Danggui Longhui Wan formula contains 11 different herbs, so, through the process of elimination, researchers have been able to gradually isolate which plant and which component the mechanism was coming from.

Eventually, the plant found to block cancer growth indigo, or Indigofera sumatrana, which is also called *Indigofera tinctoria*, and the active constituent was called indirubin.

It should be noted that whole plant herbs and herbal combinations are used in traditional medicine because the variety of multiple constituents help buffer the active ones, providing a higher level of safety and lower levels of side effects.

Saffron

We mentioned Saffron (*Crocus sativus*) in the carotenoids section earlier. Saffron contains a strong dose of several carotenoids, and these have been shown to inhibit the development and progression of tumors.

Not surprisingly, a number of studies have found that Saffron can specifically inhibit the progression of cancer (Zhang *et al.* 2013).

A review study from Italy (Colapietro *et al.* 2019) found 150 papers that documented Saffron's ability to inhibit cancer growth. These included the finding that two Saffron compounds, crocetin and crocin, specifically inhibit cell proliferation and cell differentiation among developing tumors.

Berberine Herbs

Berberine is an alkaloid contained in a number of plants, typically in their roots, stems and bark. Plants with considerable berberine content include:

- ➤ Barberry (*Berberis vulgaris*)
- ➤ Californian poppy (*Eschscholzia californica*)
- ➤ Chinese goldthread (*Coptis chinensis*)
- ➤ Goldenseal (*Hydrastis canadensis*)
- ➤ Oregon grape (*Mahonia aquifolium*)
- ➤ Yellow root (*Xanthorhiza simplicissima*)

A number of studies are confirming that berberine can inhibit the growth of various types of cancer.

Berberine has also been found in various studies to curb inflammation. Some have found it can curb inflammatory fat.

But berberine can do one further. It can stop the growth of cancer.

Research from the Nanjing Medical University in China (Liu *et al.* 2020) tested berberine and colon cancer. The researchers tested berberine on cell proliferation and lipogenesis in colon cancer cells.

They found that berberine inhibited cell proliferation of colon cancer cells. It did this by arresting the expressions of certain enzymes utilized by the cancer cells.

The researchers concluded:

"Together, our results suggest that berberine may serve as a candidate against tumor growth of colon cancer ..."

Research from China's Xiamen University Medical College (Ruan *et al.* 2017) tested colon cancer cells with barbering.

They initially found that inhibited the growth of intestinal polyps in animals and patients with hereditary adenomatous polyposis.

Their follow-up study found that berberine inhibits colon cancer polyps by down regulating beta-catenin signaling.

They also found that berberine suppresses the growth of human colon cancers directly.

In a study from the Shengjing Hospital of China Medical University (Wang and Zhang 2018), researchers tested endometrial cancer cells and berberine. They found that berberine was suppressed the growth of endometrial tumors.

The mechanism appeared to be berberine's effects on the COX-2/PGE2 pathways (cyclooxygenase-2/prostaglandin E2).

They suggested that berberine was *"a potential anticancer drug for treating endometrial cancer."*

Another study (Li Liu *et al.* 2019) found that berberine kills ovarian cancer cells. The researchers treated ovarian cancer cells (OVCAR3 and POCCLs) cells with berberine BBR with and without a chemotherapy drug cisplatin.

They found that berberine independently kills ovarian cancer cells. They also found that berberine in combination with the chemotherapy drug cisplatin kills ovarian cancer cells.

"Our results demonstrated that berberine significantly inhibited the proliferation of OVCAR3 and primary ovarian cancer cells in a dose- and time-dependent manner."

Pancreatic cancer is has become one of the deadliest forms of cancer around the world and has few effective treatments. People diagnosed with pancreatic cancer patients rarely live longer than a year after diagnosis.

Researchers from the Department of Microbiology and Immunology at the Brody School of Medicine at East Carolina University (Akula *et al.* 2019) studied berberine together with a consortium of researchers from universities around the world.

The researchers ran a number of tests that tested four human pancreatic cancer cell lines. They found that barbering inhibited proliferation of pancreatic cancer among these cell lines.

They also found that berberine possibly interfered with the effects of the drug metformin. Metformin has been linked with the development of pancreatic cancer in other research.

Research from the Department of Breast Surgery, Maternity and Child Health Care in Shandong, China (Sun *et al.* 2019) tested berberine in breast cancer patients. They found that berberine increased survival times among the breast cancer patients considerably.

The researchers compared survival times with cell studies and found that berberine apparently helps regulate levels of metadherin (MTDH) in breast cancer patients.

Higher metadherin levels is linked with faster proliferation of breast cancer in other studies.

A number of studies have confirmed that Helicobacter pylori is linked to gastric cancer worldwide. Some have estimated that as much as 90% of gastric cancers are linked to CagA-positive H. pylori.

Researchers from a Chinese medical university (Zhang *et al.* 2017) tested 612 people with H. pylori infections. They treated them with quadruple antibiotic therapy, but they treated half with berberine as well. The other half had bismuth treatment.

The researchers found the berberine treatment was effective in reducing H. pylori CagA-positive by 86 percent.

Berberine is a component of Goldenseal and Oregon Grape herbs.

Research from Italy (Ortiz *et al.* 2014) reviewed the various cancer cell studies showing berberine able to inhibit the growth of several types of cancer. The researchers stated, in their paper titled, *"Berberine, an epiphany against cancer":*

"In recent years, berberine has been reported to inhibit cell proliferation and to be cytotoxic towards cancer cells."

Kava Kava

Kava Kava (*Piper methysticum*) is a traditional herb with centuries of use among the islands of the Pacific. These include Fiji, Papua Guinea, Samoa, Solomon Islands and other Micronesia islands. These islanders consume Kava by simply mixing the whole powdered root with water. Often it is served in a coconut shell in a ceremonial social event.

The *P. methysticum* plant grows in the tropical jungle and lays down an impressive root system. This might be compared to the impressive roots of the Ginger or the Ginseng plants. Kava's roots are harvested and dried. They are then pulverized into powder. This root powder is typically consumed in whole form, though supplement companies will often produce extracts.

A 2019 study from the University of Melbourne (Celentano *et al.*) found that Kava helped protect people from developing a variety of cancers. Their study found 39 studies on kava and cancer. These included human cell studies and laboratory studies. Out of these 39 studies, 32 of them showed that kava helped prevent the proliferation of cancer. Other studies found that kava killed cancer cells.

The studies have found that several Kava components, such as Flavokawain B and Dihydromethysticin, reduce tumor growth and inhibit cancer (Sakai *et al.* 2012).

A study from the University of California at Irvine (Tang *et al.* 2010) illustrated that these Kava compounds kill and inhibit prostate cancer tumors.

A study from the University of Minnesota (Shaik *et al.* 2009) found that methysticin from *P. methysticum* significantly inhibited NF-kappaB activation, therapy halting lung tumor growth. A 2016 study from the same institution found that Dihydromethysticin from Kava blocks the development of lung cancer.

A study from the University of Hawaii (Pinner *et al.*) found that the Flavokawains A and B stimulate heat shock and antioxidant responses which kill liver cancer cells.

Yet another study from the University of California/Irvine (Tang *et al.* 2008) showed flavokawain A inhibited the growth of bladder cancer cells. The researchers concluded:

"This selectivity of flavokawain A for inducing a G(2)-M arrest in p53-defective cells deserves further investigation as a new mechanism for the prevention and treatment of bladder cancer."

Kava's central anti-anxiety constituents are kavalactones. In fact, this is why most kava is now standardized to kavalactone content. Constituents mentioned above include flavokawains and methysticin. Others include kawain, yangonin, dihydrokavain, desmethoxyyangonin, and dihydromethysticin. These all have different neurological effects, including MAO-B inhibition in the case of desmethoxyyangonin.

Kawain's effects are also sedative and tranquilizing, as well as anticonvulsant according to the literature.

Is Kava Harmful to the Liver?

Kava Kava's safety was stained a few years ago by a few case reports of liver toxicity. Let's clear this up right away: The evidence shows quite the opposite. It shows that P. methysticum is safe when taken properly, and the risk to the liver is little, if even at all. In fact, as shown in the cancer research, Kava is helpful for liver cells.

This is evidenced by the fact that in late 2015, two German courts lifted the ban on Kava. They found no good evidence to support the supposed risks of Kava.

A study from the University of Münster (Kuchta *et al.* 2015) that analyzed and reviewed the reports of risk of Kava concluded they were based on cases of mistaken identity and a lack of quality control on the part of those who administered them. The reality is that reports of liver issues were a few case reports, rather than any larger scale study.

Supporting this: In a large review of research from the University of Melbourne (Teschke *et al.* 2013) that included 24 clinical herbal studies, the researchers stated:

"Of the 435 clinical trial participants taking kava supplements in our review, some at high doses, no liver issues were reported. Therefore, the current review supports the conclusion that liver toxicity is indeed a rare side effect."

The researchers also analyzed the "few" reports of Kava's liver toxicity – the first of which was reported in 1998, well after many studies had been conducted – and stated:

"serious side effects may have occurred due to poor quality kava."

Furthermore, researchers from Germany's Goethe University of Frankfurt, the University of Melbourne and the Swinburne University of Technology in Australia (Teschke *et al.* 2013) have suggested that the reports of liver toxicity come not from ingesting Kava per se. Rather, they suggest that the evidence points to supplies of Kava that have become moldy.

They point to the type of liver toxicity that has resulted in the few cases of slight liver toxicity (mostly resulting in increased liver enzymes) actually being caused by fungal contamination of the Kava rather than the Kava roots themselves.

A paper from the University of Sydney's School of Pharmacy (Rowe *et al.* 2012) also revealed this possibility. While they weren't convinced they did admit that, *"background levels of aflatoxin have been detected in kava samples."*

The proposal – based on a thorough examination of the cases of Kava-liver issues as well as new research showing a lack of liver toxicity from properly prepared Kava – completely makes sense.

Why? Because for most of the history of the Kava industry, P. methysticum has been harvested and prepared by native populations among Pacific Islands where the plant is indigenous. The roots are often harvested in bulk and then stored in an exposed facility until preparation. As such, the handling and preparation of the dried Kava powder may easily become subjected to mold or any number of other contaminants as the roots are stored awaiting processing.

A lack of manufacturing protocols in *P. methysticum* production in the past has thus been largely been left to native harvesting groups, because this was the major source of Kava. Market buyers were in no position to begin dictating protocols.

Increasingly, many Kava suppliers harvest and process using international manufacturing standards such as ISO, GMP and others. Because of the restrictions by first world countries now on the importation of raw ingredients, these protocols are now stricter. Still, it often depends upon the particular importer of the product – whether or not they inspect and demand adherence to good manufacturing practices.

Another study – which analyzed the components of P. methysticum, found there to be no compound in the Kava that should cause liver toxicity. They concluded:

"To date, there remains no indisputable reason for the increased prevalence of kava-induced hepatotoxicity in Western countries."

Other evidence shows that in many of the reports of liver toxicity, alcohol consumption was involved and in some cases, pharmaceuticals that affect the liver were also involved. These of course include acetaminophen and many other over the counter drugs. After a review of most of the Kava liver toxicity cases (a little over 100), the researchers concluded:

"Alcohol is often co-ingested in kava hepatotoxicity cases."

In other words, there is enough evidence – the lack of toxicity among clinical studies, the potential for mold and other contamination of Kava root, and the ingestion of Kava with alcohol and/or other drugs – to make a case that the risk of liver toxicity from pure Kava when there is no alcohol or drugs consumed is minimal. And most of us know that both alcohol and many OTC drugs damage the liver. In fact, there are tens of thousands of liver toxicity cases every year in the U.S. alone.

Unless you are in Fiji at a Kava ceremony, you'll be taking Kava in supplement form or in imported root powder form. If you want to take Kava on a longer-term basis, you might consider a few simple measures:

1) Choose a reputable brand known for its focus on quality control.

2) Choose a product standardized to kavalactones.

3) Extracts are best because of their quality control. Non-alcohol liquid extracts are available.

4) Take only the amount as recommended by the manufacturer.

5) Take a day or two off for every four or five days used.

6) Do not consume alcohol or take any medications with Kava.

7) Do not consume Kava with other herbal medications.

8) Don't drive after you take Kava.

9) If you have sensitive skin, consider staying out of the sun after consuming Kava, as it has been known to cause photosensitivity among some sensitive people – as do other herbs such as St. Johns Wort.

Birch Bark

Bark from the Birch tree (*Betula* sp.) inhibits two kinds of cancers.

A study from Romania's Victor Babes University of Medicine and Pharmacy (Dehelean *et al.* 2012) found that a compound from Birch can inhibit cancer growth.

The finding confirms other research that have all found that Betulin, an extract from the bark of the Birch tree, stops the proliferation of certain cancerous cells into tumors.

The researchers tested the Betulin derivative betulinic acid against three types of human cancer cells in the laboratory. These included cervical cancer cells (HeLa cells), breast cancer cells (MCF7 cells) and skin cancer cells (epidermoid carcinoma A431 cells).

An MTT assay and the fluorescence double staining analysis were conducted on the cells after treatment with the Birch extract. The MTT assay measures the activity of cellular enzymes, which stimulate circulatory activity among cells.

This study found that the Birch tree extract blocked the ability of the cancerous cells from creating circulatory systems, which enable them to expand and become tumors.

This process of creating circulatory systems – typically through capillaries – is called angiogenesis: The creation of blood vessels among groups of cancer cells.

This study found the Birch bark extract was especially effective amongst the cervical cancer cells and the skin cancer cells.

The researchers found:

"Betulin induced the reduction of newly formed capillaries, especially in the mesenchyme."

The fact that the extract works in the mesenchyme is important because the mesenchyme are regions where cells develop into more specialized cells. To inhibit cancer growth among these regions is powerful because many cancers form from this region, as the unspecialized cells metastasize to specialized tumor regions.

This finding is critical in the comprehensive understanding of the ability of Birch tree bark to stop cancer growth. At least three previous studies have established that the Birch tree bark extract also stimulates the kill switch among cancer cells – also called apoptotic cell death.

One of the ways that cancer cells avoid the immune system is that they produce genetic changes that block the cells' normal kill-switch, which can be triggered by the immune system when the immune system senses that a cell has mutated.

Two studies – one from May of 2012 and another from 2006 from Poland's Curie-Sklodowska University – confirmed that Betulin was able to undo this genetic block, allowing cancer cells to be killed.

The earlier 2012 research found that Betulin was more powerful than its derivative, betulinic acid in promoting cell death among the cancer cells.

Betulin is classified as a pentacyclic triterpene. Birch bark contains a significant amount, as does the bark of the red alder (*Alnus rubra*) tree. Native American Indians used the bark of the red alder tree to treat a variety of inflammatory conditions, including poison oak and other inflammatory skin conditions, as well as tuberculosis.

Traditionally, the a tar or resin from the bark was prepared, and applied directly onto the skin. The researchers utilized extracts that were up to 50% bertulin content, from a raw extract of 3%.

Other plants also contain Betulin. The Malaysian plant *Phyllanthus watsonii* also contains betulin, and in June of 2012, Malaysian researchers tested the extract of this plant against colon cancer cells and cervical cancer cells.

Like the Romanian and Polish researchers, the Malaysian researchers found that the Betulin-containing plant induced the death of colon cancer and cervical cancer cells.

Magnolia Bark

A flurry of research has established that an extract of magnolia bark is a powerful anticancer agent.

The bark, cones and leaves from the magnolia tree (*Magnolia officinalis*) has been a part of traditional herbal medicine in Asia, but its relatives have also been used therapeutically in Europe and the Americas for centuries. Typically the bark, cones and leaves are cooked and boiled down to provide a natural syrupy extract.

It turns out this extract contains a compound called honokiol, which has been found to inhibit the growth of renal cancers, head and neck cancers, lung cell cancer and others. Let's look at some of this research.

Each year, more than 50,000 people in the U.S. are diagnosed with a head and neck cancer, according to the American Academy of Otolaryngology. The National Institute of Cancer estimates that some 20,000 Americans die every year will die from one of these cancers.

What is a head and neck cancer you say? The term is somewhat confusing because it does not include brain cancers, nervous system cancers or spinal cancers. Head and neck cancers are in tumors of the oral cavity, the pharynx and larynx (throat region); the sinuses and the salivary glands. To clarify the terminology, the term nasopharyngeal cancer is now progressively being used to describe these cancers.

Survival rates are quite low in head and neck cancers – at around 50 percent. This can also be seen in the ratio of diagnoses to deaths. This is not a very good ratio – with 20,000 deaths and 55,000 diagnosed each year die.

The leading causes of these types of cancers are alcohol and tobacco. Tobacco, in this case, refers to smoking and chewing tobacco.

A study from the University of Alabama (Prasad and Katiyar 2016) found that this magnolia herb extract called honokiol inhibits several types of head and neck cancers. The laboratory study utilized human cancer cell lines. These included oral cavity squamous tumor cells, and those from the larynx, tongue and pharynx.

The research team – working within the Veterans Administration system – found the honokiol extract inhibited the growth of each type of these cancer cells. This occurred as it induced cell death among the cancer cells.

The researchers, led by Dr. Santosh K. Katiyar, wrote in their paper:

"Conclusively, honokiol appears to be an attractive bioactive small molecule phytochemical for the management of head and neck cancer which can be used either alone or in combination with other available therapeutic drugs."

This honokiol extract has also been found to halt another invasive cancer – small-cell lung cancer.

About a fifth to a quarter of all lung cancers are small cell lung cancers. But this cancer is also more invasive and deadly – with from two-thirds to three-quarters of those who get this type of cancer suffering from invasive metastasis and many of those facing death from the disease.

In another study – this from the Chinese Academy of Medical Sciences and the Peking Union Medical College (Lv *et al.* 2015) studied small cell lung cancer cells in the laboratory. Once again, they found that the honokiol compound halted the growth of the tumor cells, and instigated the kill switch to kill the cells.

Researchers from China's Zhongshan Hospital and Fudan University (Yan and Peng 2015) studied gastric cancer cells with honokiol in the laboratory. Again, they found the compound halted the growth of the cancer cells – stimulating cell death among the tumor cells.

Renal cell cancers are cancers that affect the kidneys. Often the only thing a doctor can do to treat this type of cancer is to remove the affected kidney. The cancer is quite invasive and its incidence has been steadily growing over the years.

Researchers from Indiana University and California's Amitabha Medical Clinic and Healing Center (Cheng *et al.* 2016) tested renal cell cancer cells with honokiol in the laboratory. Once again, they found the extract inhibited the growth of the cancer cells. The researchers stated:

"Our results showed that honokiol significantly inhibited the invasion and colony formation of highly metastatic RCC cells 786-0 in a dose-dependent manner."

None of us should be reminded of the devastating and invasive qualities of breast cancer. Millions of women are diagnosed every year, and hundreds of thousands die from the disease every year.

Researchers from Johns Hopkins University School of Medicine (Avtanski *et al.* 2015) tested honokiol against leptin-stimulated breast cancer cells. They found the honokiol halted through growth and interfered with the cancer cells' ability to communicate. The researchers stated:

"Our results show that HNK significantly inhibits leptin-induced breast-cancer cell-growth, invasion, migration and leptin-induced breast-tumor-xenograft growth. Using a phospho-kinase screening array, we discover that HNK inhibits phosphorylation and activation of key molecules of leptin-signaling-network."

University of Mississippi researchers (Eastham *et al.* 2018) had similar findings when they tested the Magnolia compound on oral cancer cells.

The purified Magnolia extract has a chemical formula of chemical formula $C18-H18-O2$. This is just one compound in this complex herbal medicine. Magnolia is no different from other natural compounds – with hundreds of nature's blend of constituents. For this reason, magnolia and its extracts have been used in European, Japanese and Chinese medicine – typically for anxiety, but also for breathing conditions and others.

Hydrangea

A Hydrangea herb named *Dichroa febrifuga*, used for thousands of years for malaria and inflammation, has been the subject of focused cancer research. The research has so far shown the herb is effective for inhibiting cancer.

Dichroa febrifuga is also called Blue Evergreen Hydrangea or Chinese quinine. The traditional Chinese remedy name is Chang Shan (also changsang or chang-sang). The herb is known for its ability to combat even the toughest cases of malaria throughout Asia.

These effects are derived from the roots of the Hydrangea plant. The Hydrangea plant medicine has been in use for more than 2,000 years in Traditional Chinese Medicine, having been named Chang Shan.

Israeli researchers (Keller *et al.* 2012) found that halofuginone inhibited fibrosis when injected into the skin. Shortly thereafter, halofuginone was found to halt tumor growth in bladder cancer. Its anti-tumor effects appear to result from halofuginone's ability to inhibit the expression of the genetic factors collagen alpha1 and matrix metalloproteinase 2.

One of the most interesting issues is that when the plant's constituent febrifugine is extracted from the plant it produces some intense side effects, characterized by the researchers as "toxic." Yet the Chinese Medicine whole plant remedy from Dichroa febrifuga, Chang Shan has been prescribed safely by traditional herbalists for over two thousand years.

Once again, we find that like many other natural medicinal herbs, *Dichroa febrifuga* contains a whole array of constituents that serve to balance and buffer each other in the body. When a particular constituent is isolated from those other constituents, the constituent can produce side effects, including toxicity.

We've seen this effect with so many other plant isolates. A majority of today's drugs are based upon an isolated plant constituent, and about a third of the twenty top-selling drugs are derived from isolated plant constituents. So there is no question that plants render many medicinal effects. But their safety, however, lies in using whole plants or whole plant extracts as nature intended.

Turmeric

Turmeric helps prevent cancer and inhibits cancer cells from growing. This is the conclusion of hundreds of studies by researchers from around the world. Turmeric is the root of the plant, *Curcuma longa*.

Turmeric is a key ingredient in curry and is also in mustard. It is used to provide yellow food coloring to many other foods.

Turmeric has been shown to help treat viral infections.

But research on Turmeric and curcumin in cancer has surged over the past few years. With a resounding conclusion that Turmeric and its central compound curcumin, inhibits the growth of numerous types of cancers.

Here is a list of cancers that Turmeric and curcumin have been shown to block:

➢ Breast cancers
➢ Pancreatic cancers

- ➢ Bladder cancers
- ➢ Liver cancers
- ➢ Prostate cancer
- ➢ Bone cancers
- ➢ Cervical cancers
- ➢ Lymphatic cancers
- ➢ Human papillomavirus (HPV)
- ➢ Colorectal cancers
- ➢ Lung cancers
- ➢ Brain cancers
- ➢ Oral cancers
- ➢ Throat cancers
- ➢ Leukemia

Most of these studies have been laboratory studies. These include taking human cancer cell lines and exposing them to either Turmeric or curcumin. These studies have found that Turmeric and its phytochemical compound, curcumin, inhibit the growth of cancer cells.

Human cancer cell lines have been collected over the years from human cancer patients. Apoptosis is the death of a cell. In other words, the cancer cells were killed by the curcumin and the catechins. The mechanism observed by the researchers was the fragmentation of the cells' nucleus and the subsequent breakdown of their DNA. The ability to kill off certain cells is called cytotoxicity.

This doesn't mean there haven't been human studies on Turmeric and cancer patients. Most of these, however, have been what is called adjuvant therapy. This means the patients were also being treated with radiation, chemotherapy or other conventional cancer treatments.

For example, hospital researchers (Panahi *et al.* 2014) tested 80 cancer patients who underwent standard chemotherapy. Half the patients also took a Turmeric supplement in addition to their chemo treatments. The researchers found that the Turmeric supplement increased the quality of life for the chemo patients. They also helped patients suppress systemic inflammation - which in turn helped them fight their tumors.

In a study from the UK's University of Leicester (Irving *et al.* 2015) researchers treated 33 colorectal cancer patients who had inoperable liver tumors. Twelve of the patients received Turmeric in addition to chemotherapy, with doses up to two grams a day. The researchers found that the Turmeric increased the effectiveness of the chemotherapy. It also proved to be safe and tolerable when taken with the 5-fluorouracil and oxaliplatin chemotherapy.

In a study from France's University of Auvergne (Bayet-Robert *et al.* 2010) researchers gave 14 breast cancer patients curcumin doses in periodic cycles with their chemotherapy treatments (docetalel). They found that 6,000 milligrams per day for seven days in a row was the most effective dose. They found the curcumin dosing resulted in *"encouraging efficacy."*

There is ample evidence to conclude that Turmeric helps prevent cancer. But one of the most telling studies was a study from India's Chittaranjan National Cancer Institute. The research tested people in a region of West Bengal that were exposed to heightened levels of arsenic in the groundwater.

The researchers found that those who consumed more Turmeric over a three month period were significantly less likely to suffer from DNA damage, free radical damage, and lipid peroxidation compared to those who were not. DNA damage is a direct cause of mutation of the DNA, which sets up the right conditions for cancer cell production.

Free radicals can also damage the DNA, in turn producing mutations and cancer. Turmeric apparently inhibits these mechanisms. In addition to blocking the growth of cancer cells, Turmeric apparently helps prevent cancer cells in the first place.

Hops

About one in eight women in the U.S. will develop invasive breast cancer in their lifetime. According to the American Cancer Society, over 245,000 new cases of invasive breast cancer are expected among American women this year.

Breast cancer risk increases for a woman right about the age that estrogen levels begin to change. For this reason, we find that nature not only provides estrogenic remedies to help relieve menopause symptoms. Along with these, Nature also provides the active chemicals that help stop menopause-related cancers from developing.

Confirming this, studies from the University of Illinois and several other research institutions determined that Hops helps prevent and inhibit the growth and expansion of breast cancer.

The UIC researchers (Wang *et al.* 2016) have been testing Hops extracts for some time in the laboratory on breast cancer cells. With increasingly positive findings, they have discovered that another prenylnarigenin - 6-prenylnarigenin or 6-PN - activates a chemical pathway within the mammary cells that help prevent breast cancer cells from developing.

The research was led by Dr. Judy Bolton, a professor of medicinal chemistry and pharmacognosy at the UIC's College of Pharmacy. Dr. Bolton and fellow researchers applied the hops extract to multiple human breast cell lines.

They found that the 6-prenylnarigenin compound stimulated a cellular pathway that increased detoxification among those cells. This pathway had been found in other research to reduce the risk for breast cancer.

"We need to further explore this possibility, but our results suggest that 6-PN could have anti-cancer effects," Bolton said.

Compared to the 6-PN compound, 8-prenylnarigenin (8-PN) had weaker metabolic effects upon the breast cell lines, but it does increase anticancer metabolic activity in the breast cells.

The UIC researchers also tested other Hops extracted compounds such as isoxanthohumol and xanthohumol.

Other studies have also tested these two compounds from Hops, as well as tetrahydro-iso-alpha. The latter was found to antagonize the alpha estrogen receptor – which helps defer estrogen-related dysfunction.

Scientists from Poland's Wrocław University of Environmental and Life Science (Żołnierczyk *et al.* 2015) found that isoxanthohumol extracted from Hops prevented breast cancer and other cancer cells from proliferating:

"Isoxanthohumol exhibits an antiproliferative activity against human cell lines typical for breast cancer (MCF-7), ovarian cancer (A-2780), prostate cancer (DU145 and PC-3), and colon cancer (HT-29 and SW620) cells."

Researchers from South Korea's Konkuk University School of Medicine (Yoo *et al.* 2014) found that xanthohumol extracted from Hops also stopped the proliferation of breast cancer cells:

"Xanthohumol inhibited the proliferation of MDA-MB-231 cells through a mitochondria- and caspase-dependent apoptotic pathway. This result suggests that xanthohumol might serve as a novel therapeutic drug for breast cancer."

Remember that each of these compounds - the 6-prenylnarigenin, 8-prenylnarigenin, xanthohumol and isoxanthohumol - are individual compounds extracted from Hops, and tetrahydro-iso-alpha acids is a collection of compounds.

Studying the individual compounds extracted from Hops – as they are with most plants – are an attempt to find a single anti-cancer compound. The reason is that so many plant compounds have been isolated and found to inhibit cancer.

While these studies point out active compounds, it is the whole herb that typically provides the safety. The point is that these individual studies are telling us is what we have found repeatedly among nature's herbal medicines: The whole herb provides a synergistic combination of many different medicinal compounds. Together they form the ability to fight and prevent disease. Each of the compounds may have a single effect, but when they are together in the whole herb, the effect is synergized, and buffered.

The buffering effect of the multiple compounds in herbs is why whole medicinal herbs have a record of safety.

Breast cancer incidence has been to some degree tracking with hormone replacement therapy (HRT). HRT expanded during the 1980s and 1990s, as breast cancer incidence dramatically increased. Since 2002, after the Women's Health Initiative research linked HRT and breast cancer incidence, HRT prescriptions have fallen.

As hormone replacement therapy prescriptions have fallen, so have breast cancer rates.

This relationship between estrogen levels and breast cancer is reinforced by this research, as well as the research on the Hops plant.

There are a number of other plants that provide natural phytoestrogens. Others, such as Hops, modulate the estrogen receptors for the better.

Again we see the evidence that Nature takes care of itself. And if we let it, it can also care for our bodies too.

Cumin

Cumin is more than a common spice used in curry and other spice blends. Turns out that cumin also halts the growth of cancer.

Research from the University of Malaya's Medical School Faculty (Looi *et al.* 2013) has determined that a common spice used in Curry – not referring to Turmeric – stops the growth of breast cancer cells.

The researchers investigated the activity of the seeds often used to make curry spice often referred to as Cumin – with the botanical name *Centratherum anthelminticum*. While not the most common form of Cumin, this herb is also referred to in Ayurveda as Banjira and Jangali.

The researchers tested the cumin seeds against MCF-7 human breast cancer cells within the laboratory. They found that the cumin produced breast cancer cell death, along with a shrinking of cell size and deformed cellular structure among the cells.

The investigators then extracted the centratherum compound and produced six different fractions. These included dihydroxyoleic acid, vernodalin and others. The researchers then tested each fraction against the human breast cancer cells, and found that the vernodalin had the most ability to kill and halt the breast cancer growth.

The researchers concluded:

"Overall, our data suggest a potential therapeutic value of vernodalin to be further developed as new anti-cancer drug."

Part of the effect of Centratherum may be its ability to inhibit the tumor necrosis factor-alpha (TNF-a), as found in other research.

Other research has shown Centratherum to be a potent antifungal, an anti-inflammatory agent and an antioxidant in addition to its cancer-fighting potential.

Indian researchers (Singh *et al.* 2012) determined its antifungal qualities, while University of Malaya (Arya *et al.* 2012) scientists determined the seeds may have a rejuvenating effect upon pancreatic cells.

Cumin also contains carotenoids. Carotenoids have been found to inhibit cancer as well.

While Centratherum is often used to make the spice mix called Curry, another form of cumin, *Cuminum cyminum*, is also used to make Curry. *Cuminum cyminum* is a relative of parsley, with its own medicinal qualities. Curry's yellow color is due to its Turmeric content.

One way or another, adding Curry to our dinners is not such a bad spice choice.

Green Tea

Green tea is made from dried Camellia sinensis leaves. It is one of the most popular drinks in the world behind coffee.

Research from the U.S. National Institutes of Health showed that the biochemicals in green tea change a women's estrogen metabolism. This in turn reduces the risk of breast cancer.

The research team was led by Dr. Barbara Fuhrman (et al. 2013). The researchers tested the levels of urinary estrogens and metabolites among 181 healthy Japanese American women from California and Hawaii. Of the group, 72 of the women were postmenopausal. The remainder of the group was premenopausal.

The data was compiled using a combination of urinary testing along with personal interviews with each women. The woman's intake of not only green tea, but black tea, coffee (decaffeinated or not) and soda (decaffeinated or not) was also queried and recorded and measured, and the results were adjusted with respect to caffeine consumption. Considerations such as soy consumption, body mass index, age and others were also made and adjusted.

The research found that those postmenopausal women who drank green tea daily had 20% less urinary estrone and 40% less urinary estradiol levels, when compared to those levels of women who drank green tea less than one time per week.

These estrogen levels followed their categorization with regard to the estrogen metabolism pathway involved. This allowed the researchers to determine that these urinary estrogen differences were related to their estrogen metabolism and their future risk of breast cancer.

The primary estrogen pathway connected with breast cancer is the 16-hydroxylated estrogens. As for the 16-hydroxylated estrogen pathway, both estradiol and estrone markers were 40% lower among those women who drank green tea at least one time daily compared to those women who drank less than one cup of green tea a week.

Levels of caffeine consumption did not change these dynamics among the women. And black tea consumption did not produce these decreases in estrogen metabolites.

Furthermore, estrogen levels of premenopausal women did not respond to green tea consumption. This did not surprise the researchers, as previous research has found that postmenopausal women respond differently to medications such as tamoxifen and aromatase inhibitors.

Interestingly, the research also found that the average urinary estrogen levels of the entire postmenopausal Japanese-American group was about half of the levels that were found in a study of postmenopausal women from New York who were primarily Caucasian. The researchers could not determine the reason for the difference – stating that it could be related to differences in diet, lifestyle factors or others.

While other studies have shown some differences in urinary estrogen levels and green tea drinking among women, this is the first study that analyzed a broad range of estrogen metabolites among peri- and postmenopausal women.

Post-menopause follows one year after the stage of menopause, when a woman's ovaries halt egg production. During this period, estrogen and progesterone production is reduced.

During this period a woman may experience symptoms related to lower levels of estrogen production. These include hot flashes, night sweating, insomnia, headaches, mood swings and other physical symptoms.

Many doctors recommend halting caffeine consumption during post-menopause, to help with menopause symptoms. This may run some conflict to green tea consumption, as a cup of green tea will typically contain about 20 milligrams of caffeine – as compared to about 30 milligrams in black tea and many sodas, and about 80 milligrams in a cup of coffee.

Indeed, caffeine also changes estrogen levels in women.

However, there are forms of green tea that contain less and even no caffeine. Gyokuro and Sencha Green teas will contain about half the caffeine content. The Joujicha green tea, the Genmaicha tea (mix of Bancha and Genmai – rice grain), and the Bancha green tea can contain up to ten times less caffeine than standard green teas.

In addition, there are now several decaffeinated green tea products available. The Effervescence decaffeination process, which uses water and carbon dioxide will retain over 90% of the green tea's polyphenols. The other method, wherein ethyl acetate is used as a solvent, can lose as much as 70% of the green tea's polyphenols during decaffeination.

And of course, black tea has the most caffeine, and does not provide the same medicinal benefits. Even though black tea is made from the same plant – Camellia sinensis – black teas are dried and oxidized under intense heat and/or sun, during which they lose much of their medicinal constituents.

These constituents include polyphenols such as epigallocatechin, epicatechin, epigallocatechin gallate and epicatechin gallate. These catechins can comprise up to 30% of the dry weight of fresh tea leaves. These catechins have been shown to inhibit tumors in laboratory studies. The NIH researchers suggested that these polyphenols were the reason for the change in the estrogen metabolites:

"As a rich source of phytochemicals that can interact with and regulate xenobiotic metabolizing enzymes, green tea may modify metabolism or conjugation of estrogens and may thereby impact breast cancer risk."

Research from Italy's University of Parma (Negri *et al.* 2018) found that epigallocatechin gallate specifically regulates and inhibits cancer cell pathways through metalloproteinases (MMPs) that inhibit NF-kB. EGCG also modulates epithelial-mesenchimal transaction (EMT) and cellular invasion. They also found that EGCG works with DNA methyltransferases (DNMTs) and histone deacetylases (HDACs) to halt cancer progression.

Other foods containing catechins, such as olives, blackberries, raspberries, cherries, grapes, apples, papayas, mangoes among many others, also have shown anti-cancer effects. Many herbal teas also contain catechins.

Chamomile

Chamomile tea is likely the healthiest of the herbal teas commonly available at coffee shops and restaurants. But did you know that Chamomile tea helps prevent thyroid cancers and other thyroid conditions?

Okay so green tea has become the darling of research on medicinal plants. And it has lots of benefits due to its wealth of antioxidants and anti-cancer agents such as catechins. But green tea also has a considerable amount of caffeine – up to 70+ milligrams per cup – which can hype you up and interfere with sleep. Especially if its consumed too late in the day.

This isn't to take away from green tea, but green tea is after all derived from the same plant – Camellia sinensis – as black tea. The difference? Green tea is not as extensively dehydrated at higher temperatures as black teas are. As a result, green tea will often have less caffeine, but not by much.

Chamomile tea is the healthy decaf alternative. The reason I bring all this up is that tea drinkers may be looking for that no-caffeine solution that also provides outstanding healing benefits.

Not long ago we examined the ability of Chamomile tea to extend lifetime. A study of 1,677 men and women found that Chamomile tea was able to extend life by nearly a third for adults 65 years and older.

Now we find that regularly drinking Chamomile tea will reduce our risk of thyroid cancers and other thyroid disorders. How did they determine this?

The researchers, from the University of Athens (Riza *et al.* 2015) studied over 500 people, including 399 Greek patients who had been diagnosed with thyroid cancer or associated benign thyroid conditions. These included 113 people with thyroid cancer. Along with the thyroid cancer patients the researchers also tested 138 healthy subjects – who provided a control group.

The patients and healthy controls were extensively interviewed regarding their diet and other lifestyle habits. The interviews were conducted personally with trained interview technicians.

The researchers eliminated the effects of known thyroid condition associations including alcohol, smoking, coffee consumption, age and obesity.

The research – published in the European Journal of Public Health – found that drinking Chamomile tea regularly over a 30-year period reduced the risk of thyroid cancer by nearly 80 percent.

More specifically, those who drank Chamomile tea two to six times each week reduced their risk of any thyroid disease by 74 percent. Common thyroid disorders include hyperthyroidism, goiters and others.

Regularly drinking two other herbal teas – notably Greek mountain tea and herbal tea – also helped reduce thyroid conditions, but not nearly as much as the effect of drinking Chamomile tea.

One might wonder just how many of the test subjects drank Chamomile tea? Close to a third of the total subjects drank Chamomile tea regularly.

The significance of these numbers was enough for the researchers to write in their conclusion:

"Our findings suggest for the first time that drinking herbal teas, especially Chamomile, protects from thyroid cancer as well as other benign thyroid diseases."

Most of us refer to Chamomile as the common or Roman variety – *Chamaemelum nobile.* This species is also considered English Chamomile. Another species altogether is German Chamomile – or *Matricaria chamomilla.*

Both of these species are used in Chamomile tea – but they are different plants. Yes, they do have similar properties and have been used similarly. But the German variety has been used in traditional medicine for nerve pain in addition to other effects of Chamomile.

Among commercial brands we might find either – or even a combination of both of these species.

According to traditional texts (Potterton 1983, Weiss 1960) Common or Roman Chamomile, as well as German Chamomile, was used to treat gastrointestinal issues, inflammation, headaches, toothaches, earaches and a general tonic for aches and pains.

It was commonly used as a poultice – where it was applied to local injuries and inflammation. The oil derived from the flowers were applied to hard swellings and cramps. The tea was used to calm children down and tinctures were given to hypersensitivity.

A syrup from the stem and flower juice was also utilized in jaundice and dropsy – a traditional word used for edema – the swelling of the legs that can occur from heart conditions.

The effects of Chamomile have also been defined traditionally as antispasmodic, soothing, healing, tonic, carminative, anti-allergic among others.

Cloves

So you like the taste of Cloves as a spice? Turns out that Cloves have some fantastic effects when it comes to inflammation and cancer.

Cloves are dried flower buds from a plant named *Syzygium aromaticum L.*

Cloves have been used for centuries in several traditional medicines, including Ayurveda and Traditional Chinese Medicine. They have also been used in Indonesian, Thai and Kampo medicine of Japan for centuries.

This means that Cloves have been clinically used as a medicine on billions of people for thousands of years.

Cloves have been used for numerous types of infections, including those caused by bacteria, viruses and fungi. They also have a way of deadening pain, which is why they are often used for relieving teeth infections. Traditional therapies have used Cloves for gastrointestinal disorders, disorders of the kidneys and spleen, and for pain.

But because cancers are more of a modern disease, the use of medicinal herbs such as Cloves has been overlooked as anticancer agents. Nonetheless, over a third of today's anticancer agents are in fact based upon plant-derived pharmaceuticals.

As it turns out, Cloves are not simply antibacterial, antifungal, antiviral and carminative: Cloves are also potent anticancer agents.

This has been confirmed by research by scientists from the University of Minnesota, the University of Pittsburg and China's Capital Medical University (Liu *et al.* 2014) in a series of experiments.

The researchers tested a variety of human cancer cells in the laboratory using different whole clove extracts. The researchers tested SKOV-3 human ovarian cancer cells, human HeLa cervical epithelial cells, BEL-7402 human liver cancer cells, HT-29 human colon cancer cells, MCF-7 human breast cancer cells and PANC-1 human pancreatic cancer cells. They also tested normal colon wall cells and normal lung cells as controls.

The acronym names of the cancer cells above relate to a specific human cancer taken from a specific cancer sufferer. In other words, these are live human cancer cells that have been allowed to grow within the laboratory.

The researchers found that the clove extract halted the activity and growth of the colon cancer cells, the breast cancer cells, the ovarian cancer cells, the liver cancer and the colon cancer cells.

Meanwhile, the clove extract was not dangerous to the normal cells.

This of course means that the Cloves were smart. They stopped the growth of the cancer cells while allowing regular cells to grow.

Not only that, but they halted the cancer cells in a dose-dependent manner. This means that the more clove was applied, the greater the anticancer effect. This is considered the gold-standard of determining whether a particular compound is causing the effect.

The extract that proved the most efficacious was an ethanol extract. This means basically that the Cloves were soaked in alcohol and the resulting solution was used (don't self-medicate – talk to your doctor). More specifically, the Cloves were soaked in 95% alcohol for 72 hours at room temperature. The whole extract was then concentrated.

The extracting process had the effect of releasing the medicinal compounds from Cloves that may or may not be released when they are eaten. This is a common method used by herbalists for centuries. Today these are called tinctures.

Cloves have many different medicinal compounds. Some have been isolated while others have not. Those that have been isolated and identified include eugenol, β-caryophyllene, humulene, chavicol, methyl salicylate, α-ylangene, eugenone, eugenin, rhamnetin, kaempferol, eugenitin, oleanolic acid, stigmasterol, campesterol and others.

The variety of these compounds have been categorized as sesquiterpenes, flavonoids, triterpenoids and others.

This whole array of compounds within natural herbs provides the basis for the safety of many medicinal herbs. When compounds are isolated and prescribed without nature's blend of other constituents, the medicine often produces side effects. These other compounds provide a buffering effect.

That said, the two compounds that the researchers found provided critical anticancer potency were oleanolic acid and eugenol. The former is a triterpenic acid.

This is not the first time that oleanolic acid has been found to be a potent anticancer agent. A study from the Chinese Academy of Sciences (Wei *et al.* 2013) found that oleanolic acid was able to arrest and halt the cell cycle of human pancreatic cancer cells.

The researchers further found that oleanolic acid accomplished this using several different strategies, including interfering with the mitochondria of the cancer cells and altering the genes of the cancer cells.

Yes, this natural constituent of clove altered the cancer cells' DNA. Other anticancer plants we have discussed, such as red raspberry, Euphorbia herb and rainforest herbs also modulate DNA as well.

Seaweeds

Several international studies have illustrated that seaweeds and their extracts may have the capability of inhibiting and even treating cancer. Seaweed therapy may even outperform chemotherapy.

A study from Brazil's Federal University of Rio Grande do Norte (Dore *et al.* 2013) found that two fractionated polysaccharides from the seaweed species *Sargassum vulgare* inhibited the process of tumor angiogenesis – more specifically a tumor's development and maintenance of blood vessels in order to grow. They also found that the two constituents inhibited the growth of the HeLa human cancer cell line.

The HeLa is a cell line derived from Henrietta Lacks, a young woman who died with cervical cancer in 1951.

This result is boosted by another study from scientists from Malaysia's University Putra (Shamsabadi *et al.* 2013). This study utilized the edible red seaweed species *Eucheuma cottonii*. The researchers found that an extract of this seaweed was more effective at preventing the spread of breast cancer among rats than tamoxifen.

The treatment also resulted in no negative side effects and no toxicity to the liver or kidneys – only one of the negative side effects of chemotherapy drug tamoxifen.

Scientists from Japan's Red Cross Kyoto Daiichi Hospital (Okuyama *et al.* 2013) reported that zeaxanthin – along with other seaweed carotenoids – reduces colorectal cancer incidence among Japanese adults.

In this study 893 adults were tested along with having colorectal endoscopy. Men who had higher circulating levels of zeaxanthin had a third less incidence of colorectal cancer and half the incidence of polyps than those who had less zeaxanthin levels.

Among women, those who ate more seaweed had more than a 75% reduction in colorectal cancer incidence.

Research from Japan's Kyushu University (Zhang *et al.* 2013) confirmed that when human breast cancer cells (MDA-MB-231 cell line) were treated with fucoidan – a constituent of brown seaweeds – the cancer growth was inhibited through multiple processes.

Among these processes were the stimulation of caspase activity. Caspases are enzymes that are dormant until triggered into activity. When they are triggered, some can exert cell death among cancer cells, as took place following fucoidan treatment.

Another effect of fucoidan found in this study was its ability to alter the membranes of cancer cell mitochondria – changing the ion exchange through the membrane. This serves, along with the release of cytochrome c and Bcl-2 proteins, to contribute to cancer cell death as well.

Research from South Korea's College of Veterinary Medicine (Lee *et al.* 2012) found that fucoidan inhibited the metastasizing of the A549 human lung cancer cell line. The A549 human lung cancer cell line is one of the most aggressive forms of lung cancer. The mechanism seen in this study was that the fucoidan decreased the MMP-2 activity of the cancer cells. As MMP-2 activity is directly linked to caspase enzymes, this confirms the Kyushu University research noted above.

The researchers concluded:

"Fucoidan can be considered as a potential therapeutic reagent against the metastasis of invasive human lung cancer cells."

Other studies have shown that seaweeds and their extracts inhibit gastric cancer and several others. Research from the Science University of Tokyo (Wang *et al.* 2013) found seaweed extracts inhibited five different human cancer cell lines.

Research also confirms that seaweeds have incredible free radical scavenger abilities. A study from Denmark's National Food Institute and the Technical University of Denmark (Sabeena *et al.* 2013) tested extracts of 16 different seaweed species from the Danish coastlines for free radical scavenging, and found their phenolic content and sulphated polysaccharide content enabled them to produce significant antioxidation and radical-scavenging effects.

This has been confirmed by research from Hilo's College of Pharmacy at the University of Hawaii (Myobatake *et al.* 2012). The researchers are studying the anticancer effects of seaweeds, and finding that phenolic compounds such as phlorotannins and bromophenols, along with their fucoxanthin content contributes to an antioxidant effect that appears to help prevent different forms of cancer.

Kelps might be called seaweeds, but these phytonutrient powerhouses are anything but weeds. About 1,500 species of sea kelps flourish, many in the North Pacific and North Atlantic oceans.

Most kelps are stationary, and sustainably harvested in the wild. This means they must be allowed to regrow to guarantee future harvests. *Ascophyllum nodosum* kelp contains an impressive array of vitamins—more than many vegetables. They include over 60 essential minerals, amino acids and vitamins. They also contain growth promoters, according to kelp researchers.

Most kelps also contain fucoidan, a sulfated polysaccharide. Laboratory studies have indicated fucoidan has anti-tumor, anticoagulant and anti-angiogenic effects. It down-regulates Th2 (inhibiting allergic response), inhibits beta-amyloid formation (implicated in Alzheimer's), inhibits proteinuria in Heymann nephritis and decreases artery platelet deposits.

Other kelps include dulse, sargassi seaweed, *Undaria pinnatifida,* sea palm and others.

Chinese Herbal Medicine

Western medicine has been rejecting Chinese Herbal Medicine, Japanese Kampo medicine and Traditional Thai medicine for decades. It is not because these are unsubstantiated. It is not as if there isn't any scientific and clinical research being done on these traditional herbs.

The reality is that pharmaceutical medicine has been reluctant to embrace treatments that come plant medicines. Even though about two-thirds of all pharmaceuticals have been derived from isolated plant compounds.

Western doctors are not to blame. Most are focused upon caring for their patients. But the tools they receive from those that control the flow of medicines to prescribe are watching the dollars. And herbal therapies simply don't have the same potential for profits.

Nonetheless, these herbal medicines do have proven anticancer effects.

A large scale review of research from Australian and Chinese University scientists has proven with thousands of studies using hundreds of thousands of cancer patients that Chinese herbal medicine offers significant treatment for most types of cancers - including breast cancer.

The research comes from Australia's University of Western Sydney and the Beijing University of Chinese Medicine (Li *et al.* 2013). The researchers analyzed and reviewed 2,964 human clinical studies that involved 253,434 cancer patients. Among these were 2,385 randomized controlled studies and 579 non-randomized controlled studies.

These studies covered most of the cancer types, but the cancers most studied were lung cancer, liver cancer, stomach cancer, breast cancer, esophageal cancer, colorectal cancer and nasopharyngeal (throat and sinus) cancer. Yes, breast cancer was the fourth most-studied type of cancer among these thousands of clinical studies.

The researchers discovered that the overwhelming majority of studies – 90% of the clinical studies - utilized herbal medicine.

The researchers found that 72% of these studies applied Traditional Chinese Medicine alongside conventional treatment, but a full 28% applied Traditional Chinese Medicine separately to experimental groups.

In terms of cancer patients, about 64% were given both TCM and conventional medical treatments. The rest were given TCM therapy alone, but a little over half of them did not qualify whether the patient was given conventional treatment at some point in the past.

Because of the large number of studies, there were different types of results, depending upon the type of study, the type of treatment, and the outcome measures tested. Still, in a full 1,015 studies or 85% of those that reported on symptoms, TCM treatment resulted in improvement of cancer symptoms with many of those reporting reduced pain.

Another 883 studies – 70% – showed increased survival rates. Another 38% showed reduced tumor size, and 28% showed increased quality of life. Another 19% showed lower relapse rates and another 7% showed reduced complications.

The researchers also found that only a few studies tested TCM acupuncture treatment in cancer therapy. In their discussion they qualified that acupuncture treatment in cancer therapy to alleviate pain is quite popular in the U.S., but in Chinese cancer studies, herbal medicine therapy is the leading type of holistic treatment for cancer.

This study follows another extensive review of research published in on TCM cancer treatment. This study comes from Norway's National Research Center in Complementary and Alternative Medicine and the University of Tromsø, Norway, also with collaboration with the Beijing University of Chinese Medicine (Liu *et al.* 2011).

This earlier study reviewed significantly fewer studies, compiling 716 trials that included 1,198 cancer patients with either leukemia, stomach cancer, liver cancer or esophageal cancer.

Among these studies, 98.5% used herbal medicine, and again, acupuncture therapy was rare. In this study, symptom improvement was achieved in 85% of the patients that used the TCM therapy.

In yet another study - this one much larger than the second - 1,217 clinical studies between 1958 and 2011, involving 92,945 patients were analyzed and reviewed by researchers from the Beijing University of Chinese Medicine (Yang *et al.* 2012). Among these studies, 66% of the patients were treated with TCM therapy alone, while 34% of the patients were treated with a combination of TCM and conventional cancer therapy. Also, 82% of the patients were given herbal medicines orally.

Only 5% of the patients were given more than one type of TCM therapy. This means that 95% were treated with one type of TCM therapy.

This study found that among the studies treating cancer, symptom relief was the prominent result among 88% of the studies and among 88% of the patients tested with TCM therapy. Increased survival rates resulted in 73% of patients. Among all the rest of the studies, 96% of the trials resulted in symptom relief and 92% of the patients reported cancer symptom relief.

Did we get this right? Was that 88% and 92% symptom improvement or relief among thousands of studies and nearly 100,000 cancer patients? And 85% improvement of cancer symptoms among 716 clinical studies? And 85% symptom improvement among 1,015 clinical studies among a review involving over 250,000 cancer patients that tested the effectiveness of Chinese herbal medicine against cancer?

It sounds pretty solid that Chinese herbal medicine does indeed treat cancer and overwhelmingly results in the improvement or relief of symptoms as well as longer survival rates and reduced metastases.

Now why again is Western conventional medicine still refusing to at least consider herbal medicine therapy in cancer treatment? Could there be a profit motive involved? Could it have to do with the fact that herbal medicines cannot be patented? In other words, is Western conventional medicine ignoring inexpensive natural treatments that could help millions of cancer patients simply because of profits?

Australian Rainforest Herbs

Researchers have confirmed that three some rainforest herbs indigenous to Australia protect human cells against cancer and inhibit cancer growth among human cells.

Research from Australia's University of New South Wales (Sakulnarmrat *et al.* 2013) investigated three native Australian herbs: the Tasmania pepper leaf (*Tasmannia lanceolata*), Anise myrtle (*Syzygium anisatum*), and the Lemon myrtle (*Backhousia citriodora*). The researchers also tested these against a reference herb, the Bay leaf (*Laurus nobilis*).

The researchers applied whole extracts of the four herbs to cancerous human liver cells, cancerous human colon cells, cancerous human bladder cells, stomach cancer cells and human leukemia cells. The researchers then measured the proliferation of these cancer cells compared to the proliferation of similar cancer cells without the herbal extracts.

The scientists found that all three rainforest herbs significantly induced death among the liver cancer cells, the colon cancer cells, the stomach cancer cells and the bladder cancer cells.

In addition to their cancer cell-killing abilities, all three rainforest herbs were found to have superior antioxidant abilities. This allows them to help protect cells against the kind of oxidative radical damage that can produce the initial genetic damage that produces cancerous cells in the first place.

The mechanisms used by the three medicinal herbs to inhibit cancer growth includes genetic changes – changes that promote the death of cancer cells. Flow cytometry testing – measuring cell characteristics – found that the herbs altered the DNA of the leukemia and colon cancer cells, stimulating the increase of caspase-3 enzyme activity.

The caspase-3 enzyme activity prompts the cell's kill switch, killing off the cancer cells before they continue to proliferate. Decreased activity of the gene-regulator caspase proteins has been identified as one of the reasons cancerous cells proliferate into tumors.

The Tasmanian Pepper tree grows among the rainforests of Australia (Jensen *et al.* 2011). It contains a significant amount of chlorogenic acid – also a component of green coffee beans.

Research has shown chlorogenic acid can reduce glucose absorption and thus may have application for diabetes and even possibly weight loss. The leaves and berries of the plant are popular as spices, and it is used to flavor Japanese Wasabi. The spice has been shown to prevent spoilage due to its antimicrobial content.

The *Syzygium anisatum* or Australian Aniseed tree is differentiated from the true anise shrub. The tree can grow to over 100 feet tall, and bear white fragrant flowers. The myrtle aniseed tree contains antimicrobial anethole and methyl chavicol biochemicals, which also smell like licorice.

The *Backhousia citriodora* bush has also been shown in other research to inhibit cancer cells. A study (Hayes and Markovic 2002) tested it against human liver cancer cells and found it stimulated cell death of these in short order.

The crushed leaves of this tree have a strong lemon fragrance, and they contain a biochemical called citral – also known as the mosquito repellent citronella. *Backhousia citriodora* can contain up to 98% citral – the most of any other plant. The plant also contains geraniol and other constituents.

All three rainforest herbs have been used traditionally by Australians for a variety of infective and inflammatory disorders.

Chapter Six

Supplemental Cancer Fighters

Here we will discuss a few strategies that fall outside the realm of superfoods and herbs. Most can be taken as supplements, but some, like probiotics and yeasts, can be eaten in foods. Nonetheless, some of these may surprise you in their proven ability to fight cancer.

Probiotics

Probiotics work with the body to identify cancerous cells and help stimulate the body's immunity anticancer mechanisms. Let's look at some research confirming probiotics' amazing ability to counteract cancer growth.

A 2016 study from Ireland's University College Cork and Canada's Western University (Urbaniak *et al.*) analyzed the breast tissues from 81 women. Of the women tested, 58 had breast cancer and 23 were women with no history of breast cancer. Of the 58 women who had breast cancer, 13 had benign tumors.

The women who had breast cancer had increased colonies of *Escherichia coli* and *Staphylococcus epidermidis* in their breasts, along with reduced levels of *Lactobacillus* and *Streptococcus* species.

The healthy women, on the other hand, had increased colonies of *Lactobacillus* and *Streptococcus* species in their breast tissues. They also had reduced colonies of *E. coli* and *S. epidermidis*.

E. coli and *S. epidermidis* bacteria are implicated in cancer in other studies, specifically because their metabolites produce double-stranded DNA breaks among cells. The researchers wrote:

"Double-strand breaks are the most detrimental type of DNA damage and are caused by genotoxins, reactive oxygen species, and ionizing radiation."

Other genotoxins produced by pathogenic bacteria include beta-glucosidase, beta-glucuronidase and urease. These are associated with colorectal cancer and other digestive system cancers.

Researchers from University Hospital Gasthuisberg in Belgium (De Preter *et al.* 2008) found in study of 53 healthy volunteers, that probiotic combinations such as *Lactobacillus casei* Shirota, *Bifidobacterium breve* and *Saccharomyces boulardii* significantly reduce beta-glucuronidase activity in the colon.

Thirty-eight healthy volunteers were given either a placebo or a combination of *Lactobacillus rhamnosus* and *Propionibacterium freudenreichii* subsp. *shermanii* JS for four weeks (Hatakka *et al.* 2008). The probiotic group had significantly lower levels of beta-glucosidase activity and urease activity compared to the placebo group.

Researchers from the University of Tokyo (Aso *et al.* 1995) conducted a study of 138 patients with superficial transitional cell carcinoma of the bladder. They gave patients either *Lactobacillus casei* or a placebo. The probiotic groups showed significantly better results than the placebo group in all cases except for those with recurrent multiple tumors—where there was no significant difference. The researchers concluded that *L. casei "was thus safe and effective for preventing recurrence of superficial bladder cancer."*

In an earlier study from the University of Tokyo (Aso and Akazan 1992), 48 patients with bladder cancer were treated with *Lactobacillus casei* or placebo. Those treated with the probiotics had significantly lower cancer recurrence. Recurrence-free periods averaged 350 days, compared to the 195 days in the control (non-probiotic) group.

Scientists from Japan's Osaka University Medical School (Masuno *et al.* 1991) tested *L. casei* on 76 patients with malignant pleural effusions secondary to lung cancer. Response rates for treatment with intrapleural doxorubicin plus the probiotic was 73.7%, while response rates were 39.5% in the control group treated with doxorubicin alone.

The probiotic group also had a significantly longer survival rates than the control group. The probiotic group also had significantly greater improvement in symptoms such as chest pain, chest discomfort, and anorexia than the control group.

Researchers from the Graduate School of Medical Sciences at Japan's Kyushu University (Naito *et al.* 2008) studied 207 patients diagnosed with superficial bladder cancer who underwent transurethral resection, followed by treatment with the pharmaceutical epirubicin. One hundred of the patients were randomized to receive *L. casei* every day for one year in addition to the epirubicin treatment.

The lack of bladder cancer recurrence in three years was significantly higher among the probiotic group (74.6% versus 59.9%).

Japanese researchers (Matsumoto and Benno 2004) gave yogurt with *B. lactis* LKM512 or placebo to seven healthy adults for two weeks. The yogurt group had increased fecal spermidine levels (anticancer) and significantly reduced mutagenicity (less likelihood of tumors) compared to the placebo group (48% versus 79%).

Scientists from the Taipei Medical College Hospital and the College of Medicine at Taiwan's National University of Taiwan (Sheih *et al.* 2001) gave *Lactobacillus rhamnosus* HN001 in low-fat milk or lactose-hydrolyzed low-fat milk for 3 weeks to elderly adults with an average age of 64. PMN phagocytic activity increased among the two probiotic groups by 19% and 15%, respectively. NK cell tumor-killing activity increased by 71% and 147%. These declined after the supplement periods, but remained higher than before treatment.

Researchers from the School of Health Sciences and Nursing at the University of Tokyo (Ohashi *et al.* 2002) studied 180 cases of bladder cancer and 445 control subjects in a multi-center (7) study. Subjects given fermented milk products with *Lactobacillus casei* had a significantly reduced risk of bladder cancer, depending upon the frequency and dosage.

This Japanese study (Okamura *et al.* 1989) tested *L. casei* with and without mitomycin on patients with stomach cancer. The probiotic was given either alone or with the mitomycin C with 29 patients enrolled.

The positive response rate was 60% for the probiotic group and 70% for those given both the probiotic and mitomycin. The researchers concluded that this probiotic strain *"might be a useful therapeutic agent against carcinomatous peritonitis of gastric cancer whether used alone or in combination with mitomycin."*

Japanese researchers (Okawa *et al.* 1993) investigated a combined therapy of radiation with heat-killed *L. casei* on 228 patients with Stage IIIB cervical cancer.

They found that probiotic combination therapy significantly increased tumor regression, and prolonged survival rates. It also increased the relapse-free intervals of patients. In addition, they found that radiation-induced leukopenia was significantly less among the probiotic group.

Researchers from the Japan's Hyogo College of Medicine (Ishikawa *et al.* 2005) studied the association between fiber, probiotics and colorectal tumors. They gave 398 volunteers who were currently free from tumors but who had at least two colorectal tumors removed in the past either wheat bran, *L. casei*, a combination of both or neither.

The *L. casei* groups showed a significantly lower risk of atypia—cell abnormality—compared with the non-probiotic groups.

Researchers from the University of Wuerzburg's medical college (Bartram *et al.* 1994) concluded from several clinical studies that, *"diet-induced changes in the colonic microflora seem to play a role in colon carcinogenesis."*

Scientists from Sweden's Karolinska Institute (Rafter *et al.* 2007) examined probiotics' ability to inhibit colon cancer in a twelve-week study mentioned earlier. Thirty-seven colon cancer patients were given either a placebo or a combination of *Lactobacillus rhamnosus* GG and *Bifidobacterium lactis* Bb12 with FOS.

The probiotic group had significant changes in fecal flora. Fecal *Bifidobacterium* and *Lactobacillus* levels increased, while *Clostridium perfringens* levels decreased. The probiotic group also had significantly reduced colorectal proliferation; and fecal water from this group could better induce necrosis (killing) of tumor cells.

The probiotic group also had increased interleukin-2 production from peripheral blood mononuclear cells, and increased interferon gamma production among the cancer patients—all anticarcinogenic mechanisms.

German scientists (Roller *et al.* 2007) tested a combination of probiotics and prebiotics in colon cancer patients. Thirty-four colon cancer patients who underwent colon resection were given either a placebo or capsules with *Lactobacillus rhamnosus* GG and *B. lactis* Bb12 with inulin/FOS.

At six weeks and twelve weeks, researchers found that IL-2 cytokines from activated PBMCs increased significantly, IFN-gamma production capacity increased—both anticarcinogenic mechanisms.

Researchers from Japan's Nagoya University Graduate School of Medicine's Department of Surgery (Sugawara *et al.* 2006) studied 101 patients with liver/biliary cancer following liver surgery.

NK-cell activity and lymphocyte counts were significantly higher following surgery, and pro-inflammatory cytokine IL-6 decreased significantly in the probiotic group. C-reactive protein (another pro-inflammatory marker) also significantly decreased among the probiotic group. Postoperative infectious complications occurred in 30.0% of the placebo group and 12.1% of the probiotic group.

As babies, we get a good part of our innate probiotics colonies by playing in and even eating dirt. Soil bacteria also helps protect against melanoma.

Next time you are outside gardening, take a closer look at the soil you are digging into. Did you know that some bacteria in that soil may be protecting you against melanoma cancer?

This is precisely what science has found.

Further to nature's mysteries is how many species of bacteria are tuned into the human body. Many bacteria will protect the human body. Most often, this comes in the form of producing chemicals that fight off other pathogens or stimulate the immune system.

This is the case for many of the microbes we find within the body. This includes oral bacteria, gut bacteria, bacteria that live in other areas, such as the skin, eyes, ears and vagina. So many species of bacteria are helping to protect our body.

For example, certain gut bacteria help protect us from colon cancer.

That's because our body provides a home for these bacteria. Unlike the way humans treat our planet, long-term bacterial colonizers of our body will overtly protect our body from many threats, as I discuss in my book on probiotics.

Researchers from Oregon State University found that a species of bacteria called *Streptomyces bottropensis* produces a metabolite that kills melanoma cancer cells.

The researchers, led by Dr. Sandra Loesgen and Dr. Birte Plitzko, found that this metabolite called mensacarcin, attacks and kills melanoma cells. The compound destroys the mitochondria of the cancer cells.

Mitochondria are the energy plants of the cell. You take those out and the cell takes a dive.

Dr. Loesgen described how attacking mitochondrion was a great solution provided by nature:

"Mensacarcin has potent anticancer activity, with selectivity against melanoma cells. It shows powerful anti-proliferative effects in all tested cancer cell lines in the U.S. Cancer Institute's cell line panel, but inhibition of cell growth is accompanied by fast progression into cell death in only a small number of cell lines, such as melanoma cells."

In order to track the compound in living melanoma cells, the researchers utilized a probe of fluorescent material to monitor the compound's effects among the cancer cells. This illustrated that mensacarcin immediately interrupted the melanoma cells' energy production by changing mitochondria channels. Dr. Loesgen recalled:

"The probe was localized to mitochondria within 20 minutes of treatment. The localization together with mensacarcin's unusual metabolic effects in melanoma cells provide evidence that mensacarcin targets mitochondria."

The researchers also found that once mensacarcin altered the mitochondria, it activated the cell's programming to kick the bucket: programmed cell death.

The isolation of this compound from the bacteria was uncovered by German researchers in 2004. Research from the Institute of Organic and Biomolecular Chemistry at the George August University analyzed the substance and began immediately attempting to synthesize it.

This has proved difficult. Another study (Maier *et al.* 2015) showed that the compound was produced through a complex genetic process by the bacteria using a gene cluster. Yes, duplicating nature is often super hard.

Yeasts

Saccharomyces cerevisiae

Baking yeast and brewer's yeast are common yeasts that are primarily derived from an organism called *Saccharomyces cerevisiae*. In most applications, the yeast is not eaten alive, however. It is *heat-killed* prior to eating.

This simply means that it is cooked to a temperature that kills off the viable organisms. This doesn't mean that living *S. cerevisiae* organisms are toxic or anything. In reasonable colony sizes, they are perfectly docile, and even healthy to our bodies because they produce nutrients that our bodies use.

For baking, brewing and supplementation, the heat-killed version of this organism can be very healthy, because when it is alive, it produces a variety of nutrients and immune factors that are left behind in whatever food it was used to ferment.

Just before these yeasts die during heating or baking, they will release intense immune factors in an attempt to protect themselves. These immune factors also help protect our bodies, by stimulating our body's detoxification processes and boosting our immune system.

In addition, some of their nutrients, such as B-vitamins produced by yeasts, will donate methyl groups to our liver's glutathione radical-neutralizing processes.

Furthermore, because the biofactors that yeasts produce tend to be acidic, they will lend a tart flavor to the food. This of course lends the flavoring that we relish among our traditional probiotic foods such as cottage cheese, pickles, and so many other foods as we discussed above.

This is the case for sourdough bread, for example. Sourdough bread is not only delicious. It is healthy, even if it is made with white flour (for best results, try whole wheat sourdough bread). Fermented brews such as beer and wine Originally, all the fermented brews such as Ginger ale and root beer, were all made using probiotic fermentation.

Researchers from Iran's Urmia University (Abedi *et al.* 2018) studied Saccharomyces cerevisiae in rats with colorectal cancer. They fed the rats either a control diet, a diet enriched with selenium or a diet enriched with *Saccharomyces cerevisiae* and selenium.

The researchers found that the *Saccharomyces cerevisiae* group had significantly less colorectal cancer progression compared to the other groups.

One of the anticancer compounds in yeast is beta-glucan. As documented in research from University of Louisville School of Medicine (Geller *et al.* 2019), beta-glucan from yeast has a D-glucose backbone that inhibits cancer cell growth and boosts the immune system.

Animal and cell studies have shown this beta-glucan can stimulate the production of several anti-cancer immune cytokines. Other cancer cell studies have shown it can produce cancer cell death.

The beta-glucan from yeast also apparently suppresses what is called the tumor microenvironment. This is a collection of tumor cells and components that support the growth and progression of the tumor.

Among other cancers, beta-glucan from yeast has been found to inhibit bladder, breast and colon cancers.

Baking yeast and Brewer's yeast, Nutritional Yeast and EpiCor®, are all derived from *Saccharomyces cerevisiae.* This organism is used in brewing and baking. It is thus considered a healthy organism, and acts in a territorial manner to repel organisms and toxins that are seen as foreign to their territories.

For this reason, EpiCor®, Brewer's Yeast or Nutritional Yeast come in dehydrated forms. In other words, the yeast colonies are killed by heat. This heat-killing preserves their nutrients, yet prevents their overgrowth in the body. (However, a person who has mold allergies might still have a reaction to heat-killed yeast because those proteins are still present.)

So what is the difference between EpiCor®, Brewer's Yeast and Nutritional Yeast? The answer lies in their unique processes of fermentation.

Brewer's Yeast is a byproduct of the brewing industry, thus it typically does not have the higher levels of nutrients that the other two have. Brewer's yeast still has a variety of nutrients, including many trace elements (such as chromium and selenium), B vitamins (but typically not B12 as many assume), many antioxidants and proteins.

Nutritional Yeast will typically produce more of these same nutrients, because it has been prepared in such a way that both stresses the yeasts more, and preserves more of their nutrients. Nutritional yeast will contain chromium and selenium, as well as thiamin, riboflavin, niacin, vitamin B6, folate, vitamin B12, pantothenic acid, magnesium, zinc, and a number of amino acids. It is a great protein source, with 50% protein by weight.

EpiCor® is another yeast derivative that is produced using a proprietary method. EpiCor®, however, may have even more enhanced levels of certain nutrients, which include those mentioned above, along with nucleotides and possibly additional antioxidants and immune factors. The reason that Epi-Cor® may have additional immune factors is because during fermentation, the yeast is *stressed*. Like any organism, when it is stressed, it produces immune factors to protect itself.

After EpiCor® has been stressed, it is then heat-killed, dehydrated and powdered, rendering those immune factors and nutrients.

EpiCor® has been the subject of focused research, which has found that it significantly lowers systemic inflammation.

In one study (Robinson *et al.* 2009), 500 milligrams of EpiCor® or a placebo was given to 80 healthy volunteers with seasonal grass allergies during pollen season. After six and twelve weeks, the EpiCor® group experienced a significant reduction of allergy symptoms compared to the placebo group.

Other EpiCor® studies have shown that it increases salivary IgA (mucosal immunity), and reduces serum IgE (pro-allergy sensitivity).

Red Yeast Rice

The yeast *Monascus purpureus,* when fermented with rice, becomes what is known as red yeast rice. Red yeast rice has been shown in multiple studies to inhibit cancer growth.

Red yeast rice has been used in China for over a thousand years. However, red yeast rice use as a supplement has been questioned by the FDA and pharmaceutical industry.

This might have something to do with the fact that correctly fermented red yeast rice can be a significant source of the constituent monacolin K, the primary active ingredient of the statin drug lovastatin.

Researchers from the medical school at Japan's Kagoshima University (Kurokawa *et al.* 2017) studied *Monascus purpureus* on human stomach cancer cells. They found that the yeast caused cell death among the stomach cancer cells. They also found it to significantly scavenge oxidative free radicals from the mitochondria of the cancer cells.

Another study (Hsu and Pan 2012) found that *Monascus purpureus* and its metabolites were able to inhibit the progression of oral cancers. They stated:

"In several recent studies performed in our laboratory, these secondary metabolites have shown anti-inflammatory, anti-oxidative, and anti-tumor activities."

Fermented Wheat Germ

Fermented wheat germ is seriously good for you. In fact, research has confirmed that fermented wheat germ seriously inhibits the growth of cancer cells. This is also true for sourdough fermentation methods. Let's dig into the evidence a little.

Fermented wheat germ has been progressively studied for many years. For example, researchers from Florida's Lee Moffitt Cancer Center and Research Institute (Judson *et al.* 2012) found that fermented wheat germ extract significantly inhibited ovarian cancer cell lines. The researchers tested the fermented wheat germ against no less than 12 ovarian cell lines.

Clinical testing has also been done on fermented wheat germ. A phase II clinical trial of fermented wheat germ was done by researchers from Russia's N.N. Blokhin Cancer Research Center (Demidov *et al.* 2008 in conjunction with the Russian Academy of Medical Sciences.

The researchers gave a fermented wheat germ extract product (Avemar) together with conventional therapy to patients with stage III melanoma skin cancer. The patients were classified as "high-risk" in terms of survival rates.

The patients given the fermented wheat germ extract for one year, and all the patients were followed for seven years after the treatment. The researchers found that the average survival was 66 months among those who took the fermented wheat germ extract, while the average survival was nearly 45 months among the control group – given conventional treatment without the wheat germ product.

The researchers also found that the fermented wheat germ patients had significantly less progression of their cancers. They had an average of nearly 56 months of no progression of their cancers, while the conventional-treatment group had an average of 30 progression-free months.

At five years, survival rates improved by 50 percent among the fermented wheat germ extract group.

Research from Italy's University of Bari and Germany's Martin Luther University (Rizzello *et al.* 2013) screened over 40 fermenting bacteria types and tested wheat germ fermented using traditional sourdough methods against raw wheat germ.

The laboratory research then tested these against multiple human cancer cell lines. They found that while the raw wheat germ had no anticancer potential, the fermented wheat germs showed significant inhibition of cancer cell growth.

The researchers commented:

"These results are comparable to those found for other well-known pharmaceutical preparations..."

Research (Barabás *et al.* 2006) with oral cancer patients treated with surgery used fermented wheat germ extract (Avemar) daily for 12 months. Those taking the Avemar experienced an 85% reduced recurrence rate during the first year. At this point the patients stopped the Avemar supplementation. Five years later, their overall survival rate doubled compared to the control group.

Researchers from Hungary's Uzsoki Teaching Hospital (Jakab *et al.* 2000) tested fermented wheat-germ extract (Avemar) with 30 colorectal cancer patients. The 18 control patients received either chemotherapy or no therapy.

The 12 remaining patients received the Avemar with or without chemotherapy. The wheat germ patients had an 82% reduction in recurrence rates and a 67% reduction in metastatic tumor progression. This group also had a 62% lower mortality rate.

Research from the School of Medicine at Hungary's Semmelweis University (Garami *et al.* 2004) tested 22 children with febrile neutropenia in children being treated for pediatric solid tumors.

During their chemotherapy, half were treated with fermented wheat-germ extract (Avemar) and the other half received typical care. The researchers found after four years the that only 25 percent experienced episodes of febrile neutropenia while 43 percent of the control group did.

Yet another study (Marcsek *et al.* 2004) tested Avemar against breast cancer cells in the lab along with tamoxifen. The researchers found those treated with the fermented wheat germ extract had significantly greater cancer cell death.

Another study (Comin-Anduix *et al.* 2002) found that fermented wheat germ inhibited T-cell leukemia cells.

There was a variance between the extent of cancer inhibition among the types of cancer tested, which included ovarian cancer, colon cancer and germ cell tumors. The researchers found that the fermented wheat germs inhibited ovarian cancer cells the most between the three, but all three were inhibited by the fermented line.

The research also found that two of the bacteria used in fermentation – bacteria normally found among fermented wheat germ – were especially productive because they produced an enzyme called beta-glucosidase. The two highest beta-glucosidase producing fermentation processes utilized the bacteria species *Lactobacillus plantarum* and *Lactobacillus rossiae*.

Beta-glucosidase is an enzyme that breaks down glucose and other plant matter, releasing their beneficial phytonutrients.

A couple of the beneficial phytonutrients released by the fermentation process of wheat germ are methoxybenzoquinone and dimethoxybenzoquinone. These are also referred to by biochemists as quinones. Quinones of different types are used in the body for metabolic purposes. One of the most famous of these is ubiquinone, also known as Coenzyme Q10 – or CoQ10.

But these quinones are also benzoquinones, as they have a benzene ring. This means they can be toxic in some cases, but in this case, they are toxic against cancer cells.

This was described by the researchers:

"Quinones consist of a class of bioactive compounds with promising potential as components for anticancer chemotherapy drugs."

Besides the cancer cytotoxic effects of benzoquinones produced by the fermentation process, one of the potential mechanisms of fermented wheat germ relates to its ability to block the cancer cell's energy source – a process called glycolysis.

Glycolysis is a critical part of the process of converting glucose and oxygen into energy. To block this process among cancer cells means to smartly cut off their food source.

It should be noted that the bacteria used to ferment wheat germ – especially Lactobacillus plantarum – are normal inhabitants of healthy intestines. *Lactobacillus plantarum* and other species have also been used to ferment various other cultured foods over the centuries.

In other words, once again we find yet another indication of the wisdom of nature and our ancestors' use of fermentation. Nature's foods combined with probiotics – the process of fermentation which also takes place within a healthy gut – not only provides an array of readily available nutrients. They help prevent many of the diseases currently associated with our antimicrobial, overly-processed foods and lifestyles.

And in this case, fermented foods may well help treat the ravishes of cancer.

Homeopathy

Medical researchers from around the world have been investigating the ability of homeopathy to treat cancer. Yes, it is true that Western medicine has for the most part argued against homeopathy as a valid treatment option. This is despite a number of studies showing otherwise. Though to be fair, some research has shown mixed results, and some hasn't shown any success.

But let's not throw the baby out with the bath water.

Frankly, the question of homeopathy's usefulness as a medical treatment is tied up with issues relating to dosage and dilution. Classical Homeopathy utilizes a variety of dilution factors, which start from minimal dilutions to incredibly large dilutions.

Many argue that those larger dilutions that leave no discernible trace of the original substance will have little or no physiological effect. We discuss the science and mechanics of these incredible dilutions in my book on Homeopathy.

But those large dilutions that contain small, yet powerful traces of the substance have been shown to effect the immune system in large ways. Immunological research has shown that the immune system can indeed respond to very trace amounts of a substance, and develop antibody responses in kind.

With this in mind, let's discuss some scientific research showing that some Classical Homeopathy treatments can indeed kill cancer cells.

Researchers from India's University of Kalyani (Bishayee *et al.* 2015) studied a classical homeopathy treatment called Condurango against a broad spectrum of cancer cells in the laboratory. Condurango is an extract of the *Gonolobus condurango* vine, found in the mountain jungles of South America. Indigenous people used the Condurango plant for digestive ailments and inflammatory conditions.

The researchers tested an extract of Condurango against cervical cancer cells and prostate cancer cells. They found the extract was able to kill the cancer cells, with the cervical cancer cells being the most susceptible cells to the extract.

In the Cytogenetics and Molecular Biology Laboratory of Kalyani University (Sikdar *et al.* 2014) researchers tested two different homeopathy dilutions of Condurango – 6C and 30C – on lung cancer cells. A 6C solution is diluted to 1/100th of its original dilution multiplied (reduced) by 6 times. And 30C represents that the substance has been diluted to 1/100th of its original dilution multiplied by 30 times.

These two dilutions represent one above and one below the dilution level called Avogadro's limit. This means the substance lacks a theoretical molecule of the original substance.

The researchers found that both the 6C and the 30C effectively killed the cancer cells. The researchers found that body induced oxidative stress within the cancer cells, and depolarized MMP levels. This initiated what is called a pathway called caspase-3-mediated signaling – which has been shown in many other cancer studies (including chemo studies) to be involved in killing tumors.

Furthermore, the 30C dilution factor had a greater cancer cell killing effect than the 6C level did. This result confirms not only the ability of homeopathic Condurango to be anti-cancer. It also confirms the classical homeopathic method that teaches that larger dilutions can have greater effects for many conditions compared to smaller dilutions – those that exceed Avogadro's limit and thus theoretically have little or no remaining molecules of the original substance in the solution.

The researchers stated:

"Present findings would demonstrate that exposure of NSCLC- H460 cells to IC50 doses of both Condurango 6C and 30C for 48 hours resulted in apoptotic cell-death. Further, the effects of Condurango 30C, which actually was highly- diluted, caused relatively more palpable alterations in all parameters of this study than did Condurango 6C."

This phenomenon did not apparently follow the general pharmacological rule that the effect of a drug increases linearly with its concentration, but was in line with the claim of *"the higher the dilution, the stronger the effect"* as per homeopathic doctrine.

Researchers from India's Jaypee University of Information Technology (Jäger *et al.* 2015) conducted an experiment to test the ability of homeopathic medicines to alter cancer growth while controlling any apparent placebo effect.

The scientists utilized human cancer cell lines to test the effectiveness of homeopathic remedies that have been utilized by homeopathic practitioners for cancers. The researchers conducted a series of laboratory tests using four dilutions of three different homeopathic remedies on three different types of cancers.

The dilution rates used in the tests were 30C, 200C, 1M and 10M. Each of these dilution rates represents an ultra dilution. A 200C dilution is a 1/100 dilution multiplied by 200 times. A 1M dilution would represent 1,000 times the dilution of 1/100th, and 10M would represent that dilution multiplied by 10 times that dilution.

In other words, we are talking about very large dilutions, again exceeding Avogadro's limit – representing an ending solution having few if any physical molecules of the substance left in the dilution.

The researchers tested these dilutions of the homeopathic remedy Sarsaparilla (*Smilax regelii*) using the human cancer cell line for renal adenocarcinoma – kidney cancer.

Homeopathic dilutions of Sarsaparilla were also applied to canine kidney cancer cells – these were non-malignant cancer cells (MDCK).

The researchers then applied homeopathic dilutions of *Ruta graveolens* to human colon cancer cells (COLO-205).

And finally, thee researchers applied homeopathic dilutions of *Phytolacca decandra* to a human breast cancer cell line (MCF-7).

The tests conducted by the researchers utilized the conventional methods of gauging cancer cell cytotoxicity (cell death), using the MTT method (3-(4,5-dimethylthiazolyl-2)-2, 5-diphenyltetrazolium bromide), as well as a blue staining method using trypan, and a double-staining method using dyes ethidium bromide and acridine orange.

These procedures are typical among cancer drug research.

The researchers found that all three homeopathic remedies produced cancer cell death and significant reductions of proliferation among the human cancer cells. They found these effects were greatest among the higher dilution rates – the 1M and 10M dilutions.

The researchers noted that:

"hallmarks of apoptosis were evident including cell shrinkage, chromatin condensation and DNA fragmentation."

This said, the Sarsaparilla homeopathic remedy did not have any effect upon the canine non-malignant cancer cell line.

The researchers concluded their findings by saying:

"This study provides preliminary laboratory evidence indicating the ability of homeopathic medicines as anticancer agents. Further studies of the action of these homeopathic remedies are warranted."

Once again, this study also illustrated something that many in conventional medicine cannot accept: That decreasingly minute dilutions to the point where there is little if any physical molecule of the original substance left produce greater physical effects upon the body.

The fact that the greater dilutions (less original substance) had greater effects upon the cancer cells potentially illustrates what homeopathic provings and over two centuries of clinical use have possibly been indicating: That there is a potential residual energetic effect – an electromagnetic effect –

produced as the homeopathic remedy is diluted according to the methods of homeopathic medicine.

Homeopathy in cancer care – and in general – has been controversial to say the least. Some studies have been inconclusive. But there are ameliorating conditions because preparing a homeopathic medicine must be performed under strict rules according to Classical Homeopathy.

Reviews of homeopathic cancer studies have shown some studies with homeopathy had positive results. For example, researchers from France's University Claude Bernard (Cucherat *et al.* 2000) reviewed 16 clinical studies that tested 2,617 patients. The researchers concluded:

"There is some evidence that homeopathic treatments are more effective than placebo; however, the strength of this evidence is low because of the low methodological quality of the trials."

Other reviews, when lower quality studies were eliminated, showed a lack of effectiveness – such as one from the UK's University of Exeter and the University of Plymouth (Milazzo *et al.* 2006). Their review analyzed six clinical studies, and they concluded:

"Our analysis of published literature on homeopathy found insufficient evidence to support clinical efficacy of homeopathic therapy in cancer care."

But another review (Frenkel *et al.* 2015) analyzed 167 studies and came up with 84 studies that could be statistically analyzed. From these they found 29 studies that had the appropriate controls, and utilized dilution potencies that exceeded dilution levels of Avogadro's number.

The researchers found many studies showed effective for homeopathic medicines, though replication studies were recommended.

One of the problems here is what was also mentioned above. Classical Homeopathy requires strict dilution methods that some researchers do not believe are essential.

This means that some of the techniques utilized in many studies can eliminate the potential of success due to inadequate homeopathic potency preparation: For example, the swirling, shaking and tapping required in Classical Homeopathy. These methods have been a contention of many researchers that do not believe a dilution that exceeds the Avogadro number could ever be effective.

Thus we arrive at need for more clinical evidence, yet clear evidence indeed does exist that homeopathic medicines – depending upon the type and dilution – can indeed kill cancer cells.

The current situation is summarized nicely by Moshe Frenkel, M.D. from the University of Texas in Galveston and the founder of the integrative oncology clinic at the M.D. Anderson Cancer Center. Dr. Frenkel conducted an extensive review of the evidence, and concluded:

"Limited research has suggested that homeopathic remedies appear to cause cellular changes in some cancer cells. In animal models, several homeopathic remedies have had an inhibitory effect on certain tumor development. Some clinical studies of homeopathic remedies

combined with conventional care have shown that homeopathic remedies improve quality of life, reduce symptom burden, and possibly improve survival in patients with cancer.

The findings from several lab and clinical studies suggest that homeopathy might have some beneficial effect in cancer care; however, further large, comprehensive clinical studies are needed to determine these beneficial effects. Although additional studies are needed to confirm these findings, given the low cost, minimal risks, and the potential magnitude of homeopathy's effects, this use might be considered in certain situations as an additional tool to integrate into cancer care."

Anticancer Nutrients

Nicotinamide

A phase III study from the University of Sydney (Chen *et al.* 2015) studied 386 people with a history of skin cancer. The patients took nicotinamide supplements or placebo for a year.

The researchers found that those who took the nicotinamide supplements had a 23 percent reduced incidence of recurrent skin cancer compared to the placebo group.

The researchers also found that the nicotinamide supplements reduced pre-cancerous sun spots by 15 percent.

Nicotinamide is naturally made in the body from vitamin B3 (niacin). It is also made from tryptophan – an amino acid. Both of these nutrients are contained in many foods.

Practically any good protein source, such as beans, nuts, seeds, spirulina and leafy greens will contain a reasonable amount of tryptophan. Yogurt and other cultured dairy foods also contain considerable tryptophan.

In terms of niacin, lentils, lima beans, fava beans and other contain good measures of vitamin B3. So do many leafy greens and beets. Sunflower seeds and brewer's yeast are also good niacin sources.

Most multivitamins and fortified foods also contain a reasonable amount of niacin as well.

High-dose niacin or nicotinic acid is often used for cardiovascular health. Taking a high-dose flush niacin supplement can come with some side effects, including skin flushing. Best to talk to your doctor before doing this form of supplementation on an ongoing basis.

Supplemented nicotinic acid is different from nicotinamide supplements, however. Supplements of nicotinamide are available – and this is what the University of Sydney study used.

Vitamin C

The use of vitamin C for cancer has been controversial, but there is evidence that this vitamin is an anticancer agent. Because this text is not an anecdotal therapy rant, we will focus on the research. First, a little history.

Over a century ago. Dr. Linus Pauling, a two-time winner of the Nobel Prize, proposed doses of vitamin C over one gram per day would treat and prevent various ailments. Conventional medicine ignored this proposal, though more and more evidence is showing large dose vitamin C can help with colds and other conditions.

What about vitamin C for cancer? Vitamin C was proposed as a cancer treatment by Canadian Dr. William McCormick over a half-century ago. He found that many cancer patients had low blood levels of vitamin C. He proposed that vitamin C would lessen cancer growth through collagen synthesis.

In 1976, Dr. Ewan Cameron and Dr. Pauling undertook a case series of 100 terminal cancer patients. They gave them high-dose intravenous vitamin C and compared their survival times to 1,000 similar patients.

They found that the survival times were more than four times longer than the average survival time of those not doing the vitamin C. The survival times averaged 50 days for the 1,000 control patients, and 210 days for those doing the vitamin C therapy. In total, 22 percent of the vitamin C treated patients survived for more than a year, while less than 1/2 percent among the control patients. (Cameron and Pauling 1976).

A 1982 study from Japan (Murata *et al.*) did a similar study. They tested 99 patients with terminal cancer. There were 55 patients who were given the intravenious vitamin C and 44 patients were not given the vitamin C. The study found the vitamin C patients survived an average of 246 days, while the control group survived an average of 43 days.

These studies were criticized because they were not randomized or placebo controlled (Wilson *et al.* 2014).

A 1985 study by researchers from the Mayo Clinic also tested 100 patients. This was a placebo-controlled study where the patients had colorectal cancer. None had done chemotherapy. The researchers found that the vitamin C therapy had no advantage over the placebo group.

A 1979 study from some of the same researchers (Creagan *et al.* 1979) tested 123 patients with terminal cancer. They gave 60 10 grams of vitamin C per day. The others were given a placebo. Again, this study showed no better results for the vitamin C group.

What is the difference between these studies? The Pauling/ Cameron/ Murata studies utilized intravenous vitamin C. The two Mayo Clinic studies utilized oral vitamin C.

The Mayo Clinic studies also discontinued vitamin C in patients that had any tumor growth – and substituted chemotherapy. The Pauling/ Cameron/ Murata studies gave vitamin C intravenous throughout the duration of the study.

Later studies found that intravenous vitamin C boosts blood levels of vitamin C more than 25 times higher. Intestinal absorption decreases blood levels (Padayatty *et al.* 2004).

Later intravenous vitamin C research utilized 100 grams per day and found that to be safe (Monti *et al.* 2012).

So where does this leave vitamin C research on cancer?

A number of studies have followed the 2004 research. These were analyzed by researchers at Canada's Canadian College of Naturopathic Medicine (Fritz *et al.* 2014). The researchers compiled 37 studies, which included two randomized controlled trials, 15 uncontrolled studies and six observational studies. The data found a need for more clinical research, but there were other critical findings from the studies they analyzed:

"Based on 1 randomized controlled trial and data from uncontrolled human trials, intravenous vitamin C (IVC) may improve time to relapse and possibly enhance reductions in tumor mass and improve survival in combination with chemotherapy. IVC may improve quality of life, physical function, and toxicities associated with chemotherapy, including fatigue, nausea, insomnia, constipation, and depression. Case reports document several instances of tumor regression and long-term disease-free survival associated with use of IVC."

Another revew of research also found benefits, though again, not a provent treatment regimen in itself:

"The use of IV C is a safe supportive intervention to decrease inflammation in the patient and to improve symptoms related to antioxidant deficiency, disease processes, and side effects of standard cancer treatments."

Researchers from Auckland Hospital (Wilson *et al.* 2014) had a less positive spin after reviewing the research:

"The methodology exists to determine if there is a role for high-dose IV vitamin C in the treatment of cancer, but the limited understanding of its pharmacodynamic properties makes this challenging. Currently, the use of high-dose IV vitamin C cannot be recommended outside of a clinical trial."

Most studies have showed quality of life improvements for cancer patients. Vitamin C therapy reduces pain while protecting healthy tissues from chemotherapy toxicity. Vitamin C also has benefits when combined with radiation and chemotherapy.

Still, more research needs to be done. But for now, there is clear evidence of some benefit to cancer patients.

At the same time, vitamin C is a great free radical scavenger. Oral vitamin C remains an excellent strategy to reduce our risk of cancer.

Alpha Lipoic Acid

Alpha Lipoic Acid is compound found in most plants. Therefore, we can categorize it as a nutrient. Various studies have shown ALA is a free radical scavenger.

A few studies have also shown that ALA may inhibit the growth of cancers on a cellular level. A review of research on ALA and vitamin C combined from the UK's University of Sunderland (Attia *et al.* 2020) found that ALA helped deliver more vitamin C to cells, which they termed as "liposomal delivery." They considered ALA to be a type of nanocarrier of antioxidants to the cells.

Researchers from France's University of Lyon (Farhat and Lincet 2019) found that lipoic acid inhibits cancer proliferation and helps kill cancer cells in laboratory studies.

More study remains to be done on this nutrient.

Zinc and Iron

Researchers from medical schools, hospitals and government agencies in The Netherlands' (Muka *et al.* 2016) teased out a link between foods and cancer in a large, and lengthy study.

The researchers utilized the well-known Rotterdam Study, which has been analyzing the diets and ongoing health of 7,983 people living in Rotterdam for more than two decades.

The Rotterdam study began in 1990 and has continued to this day. The researchers have been periodically examining each of the subjects and following them over the years to associate their diseases with their diets and lifestyles.

This study has been utilizing food frequency questionnaires given periodically, and comparing them with cases of diseases.

Utilizing the data from this study, the researchers took the diets of the subjects and ran them through a nutritional database computation called Pearson's correlation coefficient. This susses out the nutrients from each particular food.

In this particular analysis, the 170-item food questionnaires were run through this for 5,435 people, to determine the mineral content of their diet.

In other words, certain foods are high in certain minerals. The minerals tested in this study included the big macro minerals, as well as some of the major trace (or micro) minerals. The minerals analyzed included calcium, copper, iron, magnesium, selenium and zinc. And the type of cancer the researchers focused on in this study was lung cancer.

Are any of these foods associated with a reduced risk of lung cancer?

Yes, the results of the study indicate. In a big way.

The research found that higher consumption of foods with zinc reduced the risk of lung cancer by 42 percent. And higher intakes of foods with iron reduced risk of lung cancer by 51 percent – but this effect was found only among men. Women saw no benefit with increased iron consumption in the diet. When men and women were averaged out, the decreased incidence overall also equaled 42 percent.

Because red and processed meat are associated with greater cancer incidence, and because some minerals – especially iron - can be found in red and processed meat, the researchers eliminated red and processed meat from the final analysis for minerals and cancer.

This means that the relationship between the zinc and iron and lung cancer included plant-based foods and dairy.

Zinc is one of the most important trace minerals for immunity and well-being. It is used by the cells for various functions. It is a component used in catalyzing activities of some 100 enzymes. It is involved in wound healing and DNA synthesis. Zinc also utilized in insulin production. It is also an important component within the immune system.

Foods high in zinc: The U.S. recommended daily allowance (RDA) for adults is 8 milligrams per day.

The research correlated dairy (.45 grams per day), whole grain foods (.42 grams per day) and nuts (.23 grams per day). But we also find specific foods are rich in zinc, including cashews (1.6 milligrams per serving, 11% DV), chickpeas or garbanzos (1.3 mg per serving), oatmeal (1.1 mg per serving), almonds (0.9 mg per serving) and kidney beans (0.9 mg per serving).

Other foods rich in zinc include tofu (2 mg per ½ cup), pinto beans (.8 mg per half cup), lentils (1.1 mg per 1.2 cup), walnuts, pistachios, pecans, peanuts, sunflower seeds, corn, wheat germ and chia seeds.

Foods high in iron: Recommended daily intake of iron changes with age and gender. Adult men need 8 milligrams a day according to the U.S. Food and Nutrition Board. Adult women, however, need 18 milligrams a day until the age of 50. After 50, they need 8 milligrams a day according to this nutritional panel.

When people hear iron, they might think red meat. But many foods have more iron than red meat. For example, spinach has 15.5 milligrams of iron per 100 milligrams (6.4 mg per cup) – more than 15 times the iron in a sirloin steak.

Ahead of even spinach are lentils (6.6 mg per cup), molasses (7.2 mg per 2 Tbsp) and soybeans (8.8 mg per cup cooked). Other foods rich in iron include chickpeas (4.7 mg per cup), lima beans (4.5 mg per cup), black-eye peas (4.3 mg per cup), Swiss chard (4.0 mg per cup) and kidney beans (3.9 mg per cup). Black and pinto beans both have 3.6 mg per cup. And one large potato has 3.2 milligrams of iron.

Selenium

A considerable amount of research has illustrated that selenium deficiencies are common among those who have muscle fatigue, thyroid issues, reproductive issues, lung disorders, immune disorders and cognitive issues. While many diets might be lacking in selenium, it should be noted that selenium deficiency is dramatically *more common* among those with these issues than the general population.

Significant research confirms that selenium deficiency relates directly to systemic inflammation:

Researchers from the University of Alabama's School of Public Health (Stone *et al.* 2010) reviewed the association between low levels of selenium and higher rates of AIDS, HIV infections and other immune diseases. They found that HIV-infected persons who have low selenium levels have a faster progression of their disease to AIDS, and higher rates of mortality.

Selenium is a key ingredient in the liver's production of glutathione peroxidase. Glutathione peroxidase neutralizes toxins and free radicals, especially those relating to lipid peroxides.

In one of the early studies that established this link, researchers from Stockholm's Karolinska Institute (Hasselmark *et al.* 1993) gave 24 intrinsic asthma patients either placebo or 100 micrograms of sodium selenite per day for two weeks. The selenium group had higher glutathione levels and activity, and their asthma significantly improved as compared with the placebo group.

Researchers from Slovakia's Institute of Preventive and Clinical Medicine (Jahnova *et al.* 2002) also gave 20 asthmatic adults either a placebo or 200 micrograms of selenium per day for six months, in addition to inhaled corticosteroids and beta-agonists. They found that the selenium blocked IFN-gamma adhesion molecules, reducing inflammation.

Researchers from Britain's Imperial College (Shaheen *et al.* 2007) tested 197 patients with 100 micrograms of a selenium-yeast formula or a placebo for 24 weeks. Quality of life increased among the selenium patients but in this study, there was little difference between the selenium group and the placebo (yeast only) group.

It should be noted, however, that the patients were all taking regular steroid medication and this study only used 100 micrograms of a blend of selenium and yeast. So the selenium dosage was substantially (less than half) the dosage of the studies that showed reductions in inflammation symptoms and improvement in lung function.

The recommended daily allowance for selenium is 55 micrograms. The studies above illustrated that those with inflammation require more like 200 micrograms for a therapeutic effect.

The critical component in this mystery is glutathione peroxidase—an enzyme produced in the liver. Glutathione peroxidase is the leading enzyme responsible for the breakdown and removal of lipid hydroperoxides. Lipid hydroperoxides are oxidized fats that damage cell membranes.

As they do this, they create pores in the cell. The resulting damage eventually kills most cells. Lipid hydroperoxides are one of the most damaging molecules within the body. They are responsible for many deadly metabolic diseases, including heart disease, artery disease, Alzheimer's disease and many others.

When lipid hydroperoxides accumulate in the body, they can also damage the cells of the airways, causing irritation and inflammation. The damage from lipid hydroperoxides stimulates an inflammatory response.

Researchers have called the initial signal from the cell that initiates this inflammatory response *lipid peroxidation/LOOH-mediated stress signaling*. In other words, the cells are stressed by lipid peroxidation, and this initiates a distress signal to the immune system.

This distress signal stimulates the contraction of the smooth bronchial muscles while stimulating leukotriene activity—which delivers cytotoxic (cell-destroying) T-cells and eosinophils into the region. This stimulates the production of more mucous, which drowns the cilia and restricts breathing.

The production of more mucous is intended to clear out the damaged cells. In other words, much of the increased mucous that drowns the cilia and produces wheezing is caused by the influx of dead cell matter from lipid hydroperoxide damage.

By virtue of removing lipid hydroperoxides, glutathione peroxidase—not to be confused with glutathione reductase—regulates pro-inflammatory arachidonic acid metabolism. In other words, glutathione regulates the release and populations of those pro-inflammatory mediators, the leukotrienes.

Leukotriene activity is directly associated with the damage created by lipid hydroperoxides. Thus, when lipid hydroperoxide levels are reduced by glutathione peroxidase, leukotriene density is reduced.

Selenium is required for glutathione peroxidase production. Should the body be overloaded with lipid hydroperoxides, more glutathione is required to clear out the damage. As more glutathione is produced, more selenium is utilized, which runs selenium levels down.

This issue was illustrated by research from Britain's South Manchester University Hospital (Hassan 2008). The researchers studied 13 aspirin-induced asthmatics and a healthy matched control group. They found that the asthmatics maintained higher levels of selenium in the bloodstream—especially among blood platelets.

This high selenium content in the bloodstream correlated with higher glutathione peroxidase activity. The research illustrated how selenium is used up faster in by those with inflammation through this glutathione peroxidase process.

Minerals

Several of the compounds discussed above are classified as either trace minerals or macro minerals. Minerals provide so many metabolic benefits it would fill another book. Every enzyme and protein in the body utilizes minerals. Every metabolic process – including those that remove free radicals – utilize minerals.

Certainly, food-sources of minerals provide the most balanced form. This is confirmed by the above study, which eliminated supplemented minerals from its calculations.

When it comes to vitamins, food sources are best. This is because vitamins are not single compounds. They are a collection of cofactors and provitamins, which allows the body to utilize them within hormonal and energetic functions.

Yet minerals can more easily be supplemented, especially when the supplement is from natural sources. Many supplement minerals are derived from natural sources, and thus are good candidates for supplementing if our diet is low in these anticancer minerals.

This said, it is my personal opinion that the best mineral supplements will have a full spectrum of trace and macro minerals. This will avoid an unnatural overload of some minerals over others. Sources for full-spectrum mineral supplements include greenfood blends and Himalayan or other salt-mine crystal salts.

Chapter Seven

The Anticancer Lifestyle

This chapter is a big one. Sorry about that. This could be divided into foods, herbs and lifestyle strategies. One problem is that so

Hydration

Very few people will argue that we don't need to drink at least 6-8 glasses of water a day. The science is solid. Water is necessary for practically all of our body's metabolic functions. The body can survive for months without food. Water is a more urgent need. There are many symptoms of dehydration. Many of these are sub-clinical - they aren't readily observed. Many symptoms of dehydration are also misdiagnosed.

A 1999 Harvard study of 47,909 health professionals showed that six cups of water per day reduced the risk of bladder cancer by over 50%. A 2009 study of 58 children showed that those who drank more water performed better on cognitive tests. And there's more.

In 2004, the National Academy of Sciences released a study showing that the average woman needs about 91 ounces of water per day and the average man needs about 125 ounces per day. The report indicated that about 20% of hydration can come from a typical diet, leaving 73 ounces of water for the average adult woman and 100 ounces of water for the average adult man. That's a lot more water than the adage of 6-8 glasses a day (48-64 oz).

Dr. Jethro Kloss studied water use and fluid loss in the 1930's. He found that every day the average person loses about 550 cubic centimeters of water through the skin, 440 cc through the lungs, 1550 through the urine, and another 150 cc through the stool. This adds up to 2650 cc per day in fluid loss, equivalent to a little over two and a half quarts (about 85 fluid ounces). He wasn't too far off.

Learn more about water and hydration in my book, *"Pure Water."*

Sunshine

We discussed in the causes chapter how adequate sun exposure reduces the risk of many types of cancer. Some of this relates to vitamin D, but it also relates to healing effects of the sun's rays.

Research has illustrated that many cancers can be prevented or improved by therapeutic sunlight and/or vitamin D. These include prostate cancer, lung cancer, colon cancer, ovary cancer, kidney disease, uterine cancer, stomach cancer, kidney cancer, lymphoma, pancreatic cancer, ovarian cancer.

Healthy exposure to the sun depends upon the melanin content of our skin. The darker our body is, the less exposure our melanocytes have to UVB rays, and the less vitamin D our body will produce. At the same time, darker skin will allow more time in the sun without burning, so it can balance out.

We know now with certainty that the active and most therapeutic version of vitamin D is 1,25-dihydroxyvitamin D₃ produced through the conversion of sunlight. It is also thought that the availability of 1,25-dihydroxyvitamin D in the tissues and bloodstream is raised – and possibly somewhat regulated – by the levels of isoflavones in the body. Isoflavones are nutrients available in various plant foods, with higher levels in grains and beans (Wietrzyk 2007).

Not many foods contain vitamin D. It is found in various dairy products such as cheese, butter, and cream, and in some fish and oysters, but the sun or supplements are the most reliable sources. The average American diet will only provide about 100-300 IU at the most. Dr. Grant reports that 2,000 to 4,000 IU is required for significant cancer rate reduction (i.e., with a poor diet).

Researchers at University of California (Garland *et al.* 2007) estimated that vitamin D levels of 52 nanograms per milliliter of serum (ng/ml) (equivalent to 4000 IU dosage) had 50% less risk of breast cancer than those with less than 13 ng/ml per day (equivalent to 1000 IU dosage). Minimally protective benefits were seen at 24 ng/ml (1845 IU dosage).

Leading vitamin D researcher Dr. Michael Holick recommends maintaining serum levels of no less than 20 ng/ml. This is equivalent to approximately a 1530 IU dose per day. Others have suggested that anything below 50 ng/ml is insufficient or deficient, while anything greater than 100 ng/ml is maximal.

Sunlight exposure at over 2500 lux with UV-B radiation produces sufficient vitamin D through the summer and parts of the spring and fall through most of the United States.

This is less for northern states. Just twelve to twenty minutes of sunlight on the arms, legs, hands and face – with the sun at a 45-degree angle or more – will produce from 400 IU to 1000 IU of vitamin D for the average skin type, depending upon the health and metabolism of the person. A few hours of summer sun in a bathing suit until the skin is pink (not advisable) can produce as much as 20,000 IU.

A day in the tropics could easily result in 100,000 IU/day. Although the RDA is 200-700 IU (700 for elderly adults), many nutritionists believe that 1,000 to 4,000 IU per day is optimal.

Exposure to enough sun to produce vitamin D is insufficient above latitude 42 degrees north (Azimuth) for six months of the year (November through February) (Cranney *et al.* 2007). This is about at the northern border of California on the west coast and Boston on the east coast.

Below latitude 34 north, sun exposure is enough for year-round vitamin D production (Holick 2006). Between latitudes 34 and 42, the exposure is proportional. For northern latitudes, summertime vitamin D production generally takes place between about 11 a.m. and 1 p.m. Using the 45-degree sun angle is a good approximation. If your shadow is shorter than you, you are probably able to make vitamin D.

Cloud cover can reduce vitamin D production by about 50%, and smog can reduce it as much as 60% (Wharton *et al.* 2003). Vitamin D production does not occur from sun shining through a window, because UV-B does not penetrate glass (Holick 2005).

Therefore, some have suggested that it is better to be above the 50 degree north Azimuth, given city atmospheric conditions, clouds or haze. The web will provide the sun's azimuth charts for your area. Look up the times where the Azimuth is above 45 degrees for clear, sunny weather, or 50 degrees during cloudy or hazy weather. The times will suggest the periods we can expose our skin to receive the maximal UV-B exposure and vitamin D production.

There has been some debate whether vitamin D is produced inside the epidermis or on top of the skin, within the sebum (fat) produced within the epidermis. While vitamin D3 can be obtained from the lanolin and fat within the skin of sheep – often used to make vitamin D supplements – this does not mean that vitamin D is produced on the skin. As shown by Dr. Hollick's research, vitamin D3 is produced within the epidermis, as the sebum was removed from the skin surface in these experiments. This should illustrate the production within the skin.

As the conjecture goes, some of that vitamin D3 may still remain on top of the dermis (skin surface) requiring a day or two to fully be absorbed into the skin. The conjecture thus suggests not showering or soaping off in order to conserve the vitamin D3.

It must be emphasized that there is no evidence to indicate this. Still, it may be possible that some of the vitamin D3 produced in the epidermal region may indeed be secreted to the surface, along with sebum and other waste as the body cleanses itself of toxins through the skin.

But refraining from cleaning the skin for two days would allow the potential of bacteria build up on the skin. Yes, the skin produces its own mucosal membrane that can control these colonies. But one sniff of skin that has been unwashed for two days will reveal unhealthy bacteria buildup.

One argument made to the hypothesis is that Hawaiian surfers tend to have lower vitamin D levels than lifeguards, and this is supposedly proving that the water is washing off the vitamin D. This, however, is a weak assumption, because Hawaiian surfers receive less sun exposure than lifeguards due to their legs being under water while they wait for waves.

This assumption that vitamin D is produced on top of the skin also contradicts the repeated research showing significantly high blood vitamin D levels are produced with sun exposure. None required the participants to avoid showering for two days.

The bottom line is that we know from direct evidence that vitamin D is produced within the epidermis. And yes, some may be secreted onto the skin with sebum. That means we may wash off some of the vitamin D. But this in no way discounts that we can produce and absorb healthy levels and still take a shower.

The more concerning issue is sunscreen. Sunscreen is robbing us of our necessary vitamin D, and the other tremendous benefits of the sun. An SPF-8 sunscreen will block about 95% of vitamin D synthesis, while possibly not even blocking damaging UV-A rays (Wolpowitz and Gilchrest 2006).

This later point brings up another speculative discourse, and that is that morning sun and evening sun will produce a higher risk of cancer because they contain more UV-A rays and fewer UV-B rays. This again, is speculative. The fact is, when the sun is lower in the sky, more UV-A and UV-B levels are being blocked.

This is why it is less bright during these hours of the day. It is still important to receive sunlight during these hours of the day because of the effect that light in general has upon our pineal glands, and our production of melatonin and other important hormones.

This doesn't mean that we overdo it either. Getting sun in the early morning and late evening does little for our vitamin D levels, but these times are important for our exposure to the sun for other reasons, as we've discussed extensively in this book.

This brings us to the possibility that tanning beds offer a solution for vitamin D deficiency. To some degree, they might. A 2008 Boston University Medical School study noted that tanning beds produce therapeutic levels of 1,25-dihydroxyvitamin D_3. However, studies have also reported higher incidence of melanoma among tanning bed users. In one study of 551 persons, those who used tanning beds more than 20 minutes per session had significantly higher rates of malignant melanoma (Ting *et al.* 2007).

One of the issues to consider with tanning beds is that the UV-A/UV-B proportion can be extremely high. This high proportion may allow increased exposure without visible burning, hiding skin damage. New suntanning beds have come out that produce a more balance of rays.

These may be beneficial for increasing vitamin D production for high latitude winters. While they can increase our vitamin D levels, their use should accompany caution and research. Nonetheless, they will not replace the sun's rays in general, so even when using tanning beds, it is advisable to spend considerable time outside in the sun.

Hypervitaminosis-D (high vitamin D levels) can be a consideration with supplementation. Some research has illustrated liver or kidney issues and even bone loss might result from extremely high serum levels of vitamin D. This has led researchers to conclude that extreme vitamin D doses may cause toxicity. Vitamin D from sun exposure is ameliorated by melanin production – nature's sunscreen.

Caution should accompany going from no sun to a tropical location or summer and spending too much time in the sun too soon. The best scenario is to slowly graduate our exposure to the sun as our body produces more melanin. In other words, we gradually increase our sun exposure as we begin to tan.

Most of the benefits of the sun occur through the stratum corneum of the epidermis. This is the outer layer of the skin. Research has attempted to quantify the dose needed for health benefit – referred to as the *minimal erythema dose* (ME dose or MED). This minimal effective dose is considered the minimum dose required to produce a slight reddening of the skin.

However, the amount of sun required to accomplish this dose is different for each skin type. A darker-skinned person, for example, will require several times the amount of sun than a fairer-skinned person might. A dark African American may require from ten or twenty times the amount of sunlight a Caucasian might to achieve the same vitamin D production. However, multiple studies have indicated that possibly, African Americans require slightly lower levels of vitamin D than Caucasians to maintain health.

There are six basic skin types. They range from the fairest skin type at number one to the darkest skin with the number six. While the number one skin type might quickly burn and require only about 10 minutes of mid-day summer sun to establish an ME dose, a number six skin type will take about four times longer or 40 minutes, with little chance of burning. Most Caucasian people fall into the number three skin type, which might require about 20-30 minutes before establishing the minimum dose level.

This minimal dose might even be too much for someone not accustomed to the sun – at least until some tolerance is developed. Sunlight studies from Russia have indicated that about 30% to 60% of the ME dose levels are advisable until this tolerance is built up among the skin cells. This tolerance comes from a build up of melanin in the skin cells as mentioned. Melanin effectively shields the skin from UV over-exposure. With gradual exposure, melanin levels rise. ME dose can increase with increased melanin.

When humans lived primarily out-of-doors, the build-up of melanin was typical, and naturally protected us from these longer waves throughout life. Occasional sunlight – such as vacation exposure – exposes skin without melanin protection. Melanin protects skin cells in other ways, preserving their (anti-cancer) folate content and protecting the cell from other radical damage.

In the beginning, a fair-skinned person (type 1-2) should receive about ten minutes of arm-leg-face overhead sun in the summer, or better yet, about 30-45 minutes in the early evening or mid-morning sun to achieve a therapeutic dose of sun (lat. 34-42 degrees). A medium-skinned person (type 2-4) with more melanin should get about 15 minutes of overhead sun or better 45-60 minutes of morning or early-evening sun in the beginning. This increases to 20 minutes overhead or 75 minutes early/late sun for darker-skinned people (type 3-5) and 30 minutes overhead sun and 90 minutes of early/late sun for darker skin types (5-7) each day to achieve ME.

It will take longer to achieve a therapeutic dose at latitudes north of 42, and these should be focused upon the middle of the day. During the wintertime, the focus should also be upon the mid-day for those who live south of latitude 42. For those who live north of latitude 42, wintertime will not deliver vitamin D production (exceptions at high altitudes). Spending time outside during the day is still critical for the other reasons mentioned in this book.

For those living north of latitude 42, vacationing in a tropical place a couple of times during the winter is a good idea for vitamin D production, because we do store vitamin D (research has indicated a month or more) long after a trip to the tropics. This, in addition to vitamin D_3 supplementation, is not a bad idea. Getting outside into whatever sun is available is necessary at any rate.

Periodic Fasting

Fasting can quickly reduce our toxic burden and systemic inflammation, because it allows the body's liver, kidneys and immune system to clear waste with a lower dietary workload. This means that periodic fasting can help prevent cancer from developing or growing. Research has also shown that periodic fasting can enhance the effectiveness of chemotherapy.

Cancer researchers from The Netherlands' Leiden University Medical Center (de Groot *et al.* 2019) analyzed the research evidence to date. They found clear evidence that short-term fasting (24 hours to 60 hours) slowed tumor growth during chemotherapy. It also helps protect healthy cells against the toxicity of chemotherapy. The researchers stated:

"Therefore, short-term fasting is a promising strategy to enhance the efficacy and tolerability of chemotherapy in cancer patients, especially as short-term fasting is an affordable and accessible approach and is potentially effective in a wide variety of tumors. However, patients with severe weight loss, sarcopenia, cachexia or malnutrition are probably not good candidates for a short-term fasting intervention."

Fasting must be done cautiously. Fasting too aggressively may stimulate too much detoxification too fast, which can overload the bloodstream with toxin byproducts as the tissues clear waste. For this reason, it may be safer to do short, one-day fasts once or twice a week, or fast with soups, juices or fruits.

Fasting with healthy but limited food selections also allows the liver, kidneys and immune system to do a deep cleanse, yet adds some energy nutrients to sustain blood sugar levels.

A systematic approach to fasting is recommended. Here are a few optional approaches to consider:

➢ Fast for one afternoon with lemon juice.

➢ Water fast from morning until dinner time once or twice a week

➢ Fast for one day with only vegetable soups and fresh juices of carrot and celery.

Any of these fasts should be accompanied by the following:

➢ Increased water consumption: 3/4-ounce per pound of weight.

> ➤ Increased relaxation and rest (days off work are suggested).
> ➤ Only light exercise, such as walking or swimming.
> ➤ Peaceful environments (no parties or shouting matches).

Liver Health

The liver is the primary organ involved in removing toxins before they turn into free radicals that cause healthy cells to mutate to cancerous cells.

A healthy liver reduces the risk of cancer. And a diseased liver boosts the risk of cancer.

This was illustrated in research from Italy's University of Turin (Marengo *et al.* 2016). Here scientists reviewed the research connecting obesity and nonalcoholic fatty liver disease (NAFLD) to hepatocellular carcinoma (liver cancer). The stated:

"Systemic and hepatic molecular mechanisms involved in obesity- and NAFLD-induced hepatocarcinogenesis as well as potential early markers of HCC are being extensively investigated."

In other words, liver health is crucial. The liver produces a number of enzymes that help break down toxins and endotoxins (waste material from microorganisms). The liver also filters blood through its hepatocytes to remove toxins, while breaking apart pathogens using its kuppfer cells.

There are several strategies we can utilize to increase the liver's health. Here are a few:

> ➤ Reducing or eliminating alcohol consumption from our lifestyle.
> ➤ Reducing or eliminating our intake of chemical preservatives, food dyes and synthetic sweeteners. All of these require the liver's resources to break them down.
> ➤ Reducing or eliminating our exposure to formaldehydes, cleaning chemicals, pesticides, herbicides, benzenes, VOCs and other harsh chemicals that the liver must work hard to break down once absorbed into the skin or lungs.
> ➤ Drinking enough water (as outlined earlier). Water nourishes and helps the liver flush and detoxify the blood and lymph.
> ➤ Eliminating unnecessary pharmaceuticals, as pharmaceuticals are typically rough on the liver. (This requires that we work closely with those doctors who have prescribed our pharmaceuticals.)
> ➤ Reducing saturated fats and increasing intake of monounsaturates, polyunsaturates (to a degree) along with omega-3 fats. High levels of the wrong fats can put a strain on the liver. In terms of DHA: In a study by researchers from The Netherlands' Wageningen University Toxicology Research Center (van Beelen *et al.* 2007), all three species of commercially produced algal oil showed equivalency with fish oil in their inhibition of cancer cell growth.

> Keeping our cholesterol levels in balance through wise dietary choices. Foods that produce high levels of low-density lipoproteins (such as fried foods, saturated fats, grilled meats and so on) will strain the liver as it seeks to balance cholesterol and reduce lipid peroxidation.

> Liver strengthening foods include beets, carrots, turnips, radishes, onions, leafy-green vegetables, spirulina, chlorella, squash, celery and other plant-based foods.

> Liver restoring herbs include Milk Thistle, Turmeric, Garlic, Dandelion, Goldenseal, Ginger, Bupleurum and Guduchi.

> Healthy probiotic colonies are critical for liver health. Consider these studies:

Researchers from Russia's Northern State Medical University (Kirpich *et al.* 2008) studied 66 adult Russian males admitted to a psychiatric hospital with a diagnosis of alcoholic psychosis. They gave the patients standard therapy (abstinence plus vitamins) with *Bifidobacterium bifidum* and *Lactobacillus plantarum* 8PA3 or standard therapy alone without probiotics for five days. Stool cultures and liver enzymes were examined and compared with 24 healthy, matched non-drinker controls.

The alcoholic patients had significantly fewer bifidobacteria, lactobacilli, and enterococci than did the healthy non-drinkers. The average starting levels of liver enzymes alanine aminotransferase (ALT), aspartate aminotransferase (AST), and gamma-glutamyl transpeptidase (GGT) were significantly greater in the alcoholic group compared to the healthy non-drinkers.

After 5 days of daily probiotics, alcoholic patients had significantly more bifidobacteria and lactobacilli populations compared to the control group. The probiotic group also had significantly lower AST and ALT levels at the end of treatment than the standard therapy control group.

Of the 26 patients with mild alcoholic hepatitis, probiotic therapy significantly reduced liver enzymes ALT, AST, GGT, lactate dehydrogenase and total bilirubin. The researchers concluded that:

"Short-term oral supplementation with B. bifidum and L. plantarum 8PA3 was associated with restoration of the bowel flora and greater improvement in alcohol-induced liver injury than standard therapy alone."

Scientists from Italy's University of Catania (Malaguarnera *et al.* 2007) gave 60 cirrhotic patients *Bifidobacterium longum* plus fructo-oligosaccharides (FOS) or placebo. After 90 days, fasting NH(4) serum levels significantly decreased among the probiotic patients. Other liver tests, including MMSE, Trail Making Test-A and Test-B also significantly improved among the probiotic group as compared with the placebo group.

Researchers from the Liver Failure Group and The Institute of Hepatology at the University College London's Medical School (Stadlbauer *et al.* 2008) studied neutrophil function and cytokine responses in alcoholic cirrhosis patients in an open-label study. Twenty patients with alcoholic cirrhosis were treated with a placebo or *Lactobacillus casei* Shirota for 4 weeks.

The data were also compared to 13 healthy control subjects who did not receive probiotics. The cirrhosis patients' starting neutrophil phagocytic capacity was significantly lower than healthy controls (73% versus 98%) before probiotic treatment. After the probiotics treatments, neutrophil levels increased while the placebo group's neutrophil capacity did not change. In addition, endotoxin-stimulated TNF-receptor-1, TNFR-2 and interleukin IL10 levels were significantly lower among the probiotic group.

China's Capital University of Medical Sciences and the Beijing Friendship Hospital (Zhao *et al.* 2004) studied fifty patients with liver cirrhosis. They tested and graded the entire group for intestinal probiotic content and severity of liver disease. The researchers found that the cirrhosis was directly associated with intestinal probiotic content.

The more severe the cirrhosis, the more imbalanced the intestinal probiotic content was. The patients were randomized and given *Bifidobacterium*, *Lactobacillus acidophilus* and *Enterococcus faecium;* or *Bacillus subtilis* and *Enterococcus faecium* for 14 days. Fecal flora, pH and ammonia content, and plasma endotoxin levels were tested before and after.

All levels improved after both probiotic treatments. In addition, those given *B. subtilis* and *E. faecium* showed a reduction in endotoxin levels among endotoxemia cirrhosis cases.

Researchers from the Department of Surgery at Japan's Nagoya University Graduate School of Medicine (Kanazawa *et al.* 2005) investigated the effects of *L. casei* with 54 patients following hepatectomy. Infection complications were 19% in the probiotic group and 52% in the placebo group.

Juicing and Smoothies

We described a number of superfoods known to inhibit cancer growth. One of the best way to get anticancer superfoods into our diet is with juicing or smoothies.

Personally, I think smoothies are healthier. Let me tell you why.

Juicing has been advocated for many years by a number of health experts and nutritionists. Many have promoted juicing for detoxification and cleansing.

However, juicing is a suboptimal way to glean the benefits of fruits and vegetables. This is because it is the combination of the antioxidant nutrients and the soluble and insoluble fibers in fruits and vegetables that give them their true anticancer benefits. Especially when it comes to reducing the risk of colorectal cancers.

The moral here is that natural fiber with antioxidants renders more cleansing benefits than do antioxidants alone. While antioxidants do attach and bind to toxins and neutralize radicals such as lipid peroxides, fiber attaches to LDL cholesterol in the intestines, which prevents them from becoming lipid peroxides in the first place. Fibers also attach to numerous other radicals and toxins within the intestines, flushing them out through the colon. *This prevents their entry into the bloodstream.*

While juicing is somewhat practical for hard fiber vegetables like carrots, the best strategy for most other fruits and vegetables is to make smoothies. This is basically putting the whole fruit or vegetable into a blender (after peeling in the case of oranges and the like, although orange peels are also a great cleansing nutrient), mixing with some water, a greenfood powder, and perhaps some kefir or yogurt, and then blending them up into a fruit/vegetable smoothie. For thinner consistency, simply add more water, and for thicker consistency, less water.

While juice can also be added to our smoothies, juices are not recommended in the living cleanse diet. This is because juices have been separated from their fibers, and this makes the juice not wholesome.

Furthermore, many commercial juices are pasteurized or flash-pasteurized, rendering many of the enzymes and antioxidants useless, and often denatured. Furthermore, the sugars in pasteurized juices can turn to more simplified versions, rendering them unstable and acidic upon consumption and subject to becoming radicals within the body.

This denaturing can easily be observed. Simply pour some pasteurized filtered orange juice into a glass. Now peel an orange and put into the blender. Pour that into a glass next to the juice glass.

Now take a gulp of the juice, and then take a gulp of the orange smoothie. You will taste the difference. As you let the juice slide past your throat, take an extra swallow and see if you do not sense the acidification of the juice on the epithelia of the throat/esophagus. Now do the same with the smoothie. The smoothie will go down, uh, okay, *smoother.*

Colonics and Enemas

As Dr. John Harvey Kellogg pointed out a century ago, the colon of practically every adult on a Western diet is significantly putrefied. This means there is a thick crusty layer of putrefied pathogenic bacteria lining the colon. For some colons, only a small opening allows waste to move out. The rest of the colon is clogged with crusted old waste products.

These waste products include histamines, ketones, ammonia, microorganism endotoxins and various other toxic materials that leak back into our bloodstream. Research has shown these contribute to systemic inflammation, as they produce radical oxygen species (free radicals).

Polyps often develop as a result, followed sometimes by colon cancer.

The best strategy for anyone with systemic inflammation and/or toxicity is to periodically cleanse the colon. This can be done with periodic enemas, or more deeply and effectively, with a colonic.

Enemas can be done quite easily in the privacy of ones bathroom:

➢ The enema bag can be filled with warm water or herbal tea—anti-inflammatory herbs listed earlier can be used.

➢ Hang the bag up, with the tubing clamped.

➢ Insert the tubing nozzle into the rectum about 3-4 inches. A small amount of castor bean oil or vegetable oil can be put on the nozzle to help its entry.

➢ Unclamp the tubing.

➢ The water/herbal tea should begin moving up into the colon, slightly extending the lower abdomen. Maintain the filling until the colon begins to feel full.

➢ Reclamp the tubing and remove from the rectum.

➢ There will soon be a tremendous urge for a bowel movement. Try to resist this urge for two or three minutes.

➢ Lightly massage the lower abdomen before bowel movement.

➢ The bowel movement will flush the water and waste out.

An enema can be done fairly regularly, but it is important not to overdo enemas, because they can lead to undisciplined bowel movements. After doing one per day for two or three days, once a week is probably sufficient. Consultation with a health professional is suggested.

Colonics are performed by professionals who graduate from schools that teach and certify what is called *colon hydrotherapy*. The colonic is typically done with a sanitary machine that flushes water through the colon, while vacuuming out the waste. A colonic is significantly better and cleanses more deeply than an enema—or even many enemas.

Hydrotherapists typically recommend a colonic at least twice a year if not more. For someone with toxicity and/or inflammation, three colonics per year is considered minimal. Consult a colon hydrotherapist for more information, and as always, discuss with your doctor as well, especially if polyps have developed.

Stress

Does stress cause cancer? Well, a growing body of evidence shows that psychosocial stress increases the incidence of cancer, and worsens outcomes for those who contract it.

Researchers from the Department of Epidemiology and Public Health at the University College London (Chida *et al.* 2008) analyzed hundreds of studies that tested these hypotheses.

They found that 165 studies concluded that stress is associated with more incidence of cancer among healthy populations. And 330 studies found that stress contributed to more deaths among cancer patients.

The body must be equipped to immediately respond to cancerous cells. This response requires a coordinated attack between the immune system, the liver and the adrenals.

For this reason, it is important to reduce our mental stress levels. Mental stress can artificially produce the fight or flight response in the body. This is not good, because it takes our body's focus away from correcting cancer creation.

The adrenal glands respond to stress initially by signaling between the hypothalamus and pituitary gland. One of the primary signals comes in the form of adrenocorticotropic hormone (or ACTH). This master hormone signals nerve centers, and stimulates the adrenal glands to produce cortisol and other glucocorticoids. This is called the *hypothalamic-pituitary-adrenal axis stress response.*

Remember that the adrenals are critical to the production of cortisol, and it is cortisol and other glucocorticoids that control inflammation. Therefore, the adrenals are necessary to balance inflammation and detoxification. This is why cortisone is used for inflammation: It blocks and controls the inflammatory response by interrupting the interleukin-1 and IL-2 cytokine communications.

However, cortisone medications over longer periods also depress adrenal function. Because they provide corticoids directly, the adrenal gland begins to switch off its corticoid production. This adrenal switching off has been linked to adrenal insufficiency and systemic inflammation (Polito *et al.* 2007).

For this very reason, withdrawing from or reducing cortisone medications after their long-term use can result in a dramatic rise in uninhibited inflammation throughout the body. This is because inflammatory cytokines such as the interleukins are allowed to act without adequate corticoid control.

This can be compounded by a situation called adrenal exhaustion. Under stressful situations, the healthy adrenal gland is stimulated to produce cortisol. This trigger effect is natural and supports our ability to respond to dire circumstances. However, should we become stressed too often, this automatic adrenal response begins the wear out the adrenals. They become exhausted because they have been over-stimulated.

In other words, healthy adrenals should be balancing inflammatory responses by supplying natural corticoids. In the case of adrenal exhaustion and in the absence of sufficient natural corticoids (and/or inflammatory episodes that have gone way out of control) physicians prescribe synthetic cortisone to achieve what our body's adrenal glands should have: Shutting down inflammation before it got out of control.

Relaxation is critical to the adrenal glands. As the system relaxes more, the adrenal glands are allowed some time to refresh, enabling them to better respond to small inflammatory episodes—before they get out of control.

But what about adrenal glands that are already exhausted? Can we do anything to rebuild and strengthen them? Absolutely.

In fact, many of the strategies we have outlined in this chapter, including many of the herbs, foods, detoxification and exercises will directly or indirectly strengthen the adrenal glands. This is accomplished because they can:

> ➢ Reduce inflammation—unburdening the adrenal glands.
> ➢ Stimulate relaxation—allowing the adrenals to recuperate.
> ➢ Directly stimulate healthy adrenal activity.
> ➢ Supply adrenals with the raw materials to produce corticoids and androgens.

With regard to the latter point, the adrenal glands do more than simply produce cortisol. They also produce androgens, glucocorticoids and many other hormones that stabilize and balance the body's metabolism.

Without a strong and active adrenal complex, the body's hormone and steroid system becomes unbalanced and out of whack. This encourages inflammatory responses to become uncontrolled, producing a number of possible symptoms.

What are some of the more immediate ways to increase adrenal capacity? Here are a few of the many that either unburden or strengthen the adrenals:

> ➢ Decreased toxin consumption, and detoxification efforts.
> ➢ Greenfoods, fruits and vegetables that provide adrenal gland stimulating antioxidants.
> ➢ Plenty of water, as discussed earlier.
> ➢ Relaxation: Letting things roll off the back, so to speak. Not sweating inconsequential things. This is particularly important for those who drive everyday. Driving is highly stressful. It can help, therefore, to listen to soothing music while driving. Or take public transportation.
> ➢ Deep breathing: This is important for relaxation, as we discussed above. Breathing not only nourishes the adrenals with oxygen and alkalinity: It also stimulates the VNO nerves.
> ➢ Visual imagery: Looking at scenes of nature, or imagining natural settings. Multiple studies have shown that those who live near green spaces, those who walk in forests or on beaches have significantly reduced stress and increased immunity.
> ➢ Humor and comedy: A number of studies have shown that humor and comedy can significantly reduce stress and boost the immune system. We can integrate humor or comedy into our lifestyles by choosing people to be with that see the funny side of life. Those who laugh generously are dead giveaways for those we would want to be with. We can also accelerate humor and comedy in our lives by choosing comedy shows over horror and other stress-inducing entertainment.
> ➢ Higher sounds: Consider what we hear. Are we hearing a lot of chatter about what other people are stressed about? (This includes television.) Hearing stressful language can stimulate our adrenals. A dramatic movie or TV program has been shown to stimulate the adrenals and increase cortisol levels. This may be okay periodically, but not constantly. For those with already

over-stimulated adrenals, being around uplifting sounds and discussions is a better strategy.

➤ Foods particularly good for the adrenals include onions, garlic, peppers, papaya, mango, apricots, squash and broccoli.

➤ Herbs that help strengthen and revitalize the adrenals include Shizandra, Tylophora, Astragalus, Dandelion and Licorice.

We might add that the Licorice mentioned here should not be deglycyrrhized licorice, as in the DGL used primarily for stomach ulcers. This is because glycyrrhizin and its triterpenoid, glycyrrhizinic acid, are considered primary adrenal-restorative constituents.

This said, a 2003 European Commission suggested that a person should not consume more than 100 milligrams of glycyrrhizinic acid per day. Note, however, that even concentrated extracts of licorice herb will contain only 4-25% glycyrrhizinic acid.

This means that 400-500 mg a day of *raw, unconcentrated* licorice root will contain far less than the maximum levels documented by the European Commission. Natural licorice root, in fact, has been used safely by Western and Eastern traditional herbalists for many centuries.

Reducing Carcinogen Exposure

By reducing our toxin exposure, we can dramatically lighten the burden on our immune systems, allowing our body's own detoxification systems to work more effectively. While this is not the total solution, reducing toxin exposure should not be overlooked. Below are some strategies to reduce our incoming toxins.

Know Your Carcinogens

One of the first things we can do is find out precisely what toxins are in our immediate environment. This means inspecting tags, reading labels and in general getting to know that materials that surround us in our home and work environments.

We should understand what is in our local drinking water. If on a municipal water supply, our local water district will likely list the results of their periodic tests. The EPA mandates that municipalities make this information available to the public, so there should be a website for our local water district that reveals what is in the water.

We should also investigate the makeup and levels of our local air pollution levels are important. We might also find out what times of day the smog levels are higher and lower. Coordinating our exercise times and outdoor activities with lower smog periods is not a bad idea. An internet search will usually reveal local pollution contents, levels and comparison to averages.

Keeping abreast of local news is also a good idea, in order to be alerted to the locations of toxic spills, hazardous waste sites, or other toxic sites that may have been categorized as an NPL site: The National Priorities List.

➤ Notifications of water quality issues.

> ➢ Sites of oil, natural gas or other mining operations nearby.
> ➢ Any toxic releases in area.
> ➢ Any sites subject to Superfund, Brownfields or other cleanup projects.
> ➢ Sites that have been subject to environmental enforcement nearby.

Fresh Air

The best recommendation we find in some texts is simply to shut all the windows as much as possible. Is this really a solution? As we mentioned earlier, research has confirmed that indoor pollution is generally worse than outdoor pollution. What are we to do, then?

Living around or at least visiting a natural setting such as a forest or beach has many advantages. For example, researchers from Japan's Chiba University (Park *et al.* 2010) conducted 24 field experiments using 280 subjects among 24 forests throughout Japan.

In each of the tests, six subjects walked through a forest, while another six walked through a city. The next day the six that walked the city would walk the forest and vice versa. The research concluded that forest environments reduce stress-related cortisol levels, lower heart rate, reduce blood pressure, lower anxiety and increase reaction time.

The researchers concluded that: *"These results will contribute to the development of a research field dedicated to forest medicine, which may be used as a strategy for preventive medicine."*

Other studies have confirmed these results. One study found that people living in natural environments had lower levels of stress than those living in urban environments (Ulrich *et al.* 1991). Another, from Emory University, found that natural environments improve health conditions (Frumkin 2001).

City Versus Rural Living

There is little doubt that city living increases toxicity. For example, a study done by the Arizona Health Care Cost Containment System (Smith *et al.* 2010) found that among 3,013 people, urban residents had a 55% greater likelihood of respiratory disorders than did rural residents.

As much as we may want to, not everyone can pick up and move away from the city. In this case, focus can turn towards reducing immediate air pollutant exposure. We can make logical choices to reduce our exposure.

This doesn't mean staying inside and closing all the windows either. It is important that we get enough sunshine and "fresh" air, and this requires us to go outside. We can simply use some common sense. For example, we can *avoid* the following:

> ➢ Running, walking or biking next to a freeway where soot and carbon monoxide levels are greatest.
> ➢ Hanging out downwind of a smokestack of an industrial plant known to throw toxins into the air.

> ➤ Sitting or standing downwind, or next to, an outdoor fire or gas stove for an extended period.
> ➤ Standing, sitting or walking next to someone spraying pesticides, herbicides or other chemicals.
> ➤ Frequenting tobacco-filled bars or other smoky places.
> ➤ Avoiding dusty areas such as construction sites, runways, racetracks, rodeos and other events that stir up lots of airborne particulates.

In addition, there are a number of proactive things we can do to reduce our airborne toxins. As discussed earlier, breathing in through the nose helps to filter out some particulates and other foreigners. This also warms the air. As we discussed, cold air can dry the mucous membranes, and thinned mucous membranes expose our airways to more airborne toxins.

If we live in an urban area with poor air quality we might consider exercising or getting outside during the morning, when the air quality is typically better. As temperatures rise, immediate ozone levels increase. We might also consider exercising near a lake, river, or ocean. Polluted air around water tends to disperse more quickly in the presence of wind, humidity, pressure gradients, and temperature differences around the water.

Wearing a face mask may also be a good idea, to filter out some of the larger particles. More subtle strategies include wearing a scarf during winter months, and covering our mouth and nose with it when outside. In colder climates, a fleece ski mask could also help filter out some particulates.

These are but a few ways to prevent burdening our immune system with airborne toxins—but again, these cannot be our only strategy. We must also undertake reducing the *other, more controllable* immune system burdens to the greatest degree possible.

Home Pollution Strategies

Americans spend over 90% of their lives indoors, and indoor air pollution averages double to five times worse than outdoor pollution levels. In some cases, indoor pollution can be tens, even hundreds of times higher than outdoor pollutant levels.

The issue here is ventilation. While older homes might exchange all the air in the house every couple of hours—even up to twice an hour—modern energy-efficient homes exchange air well over five times slower. The average, in fact, is about .25 times per hour, meaning that it would take four hours to exchange all the air in the home. This problem has been termed the *tight building syndrome.*

Tight building syndrome can result in sick building syndrome if it is not properly ventilated, or ventilated with a clean ventilation system. In comfortable weather, this can be mitigated by keeping windows open throughout the house. Winters are more of a challenge in this regard. At least a crack in key windows can bring in lots of fresh air when it is cold outside.

Air Filtration

A good ventilation system will circulate air while sending it through a filter. A good filter can reduce indoor air pollution is caused by fungi-laden basements, formaldehydes, asbestos, fire retardants, household chemicals, volatile organic compounds, smoking, moldy ventilation systems, moldy dust-mite ridden carpets, and so on.

Air purifiers: These can significantly remove toxins from the air, as they draw air through a filter and then push the air out. Studies have shown that air purifiers can significantly increase the quality of life among asthmatics (Brodtkorb *et al.* 2010).

The concern here is changing the filters. High-Efficiency Particular Arresting (HEPA) filters are recommended, and these should be changed periodically depending upon use.

A HEPA filter is a good strategy for removing dust, dander and other particulates. HEPA filters are designed to pick up over 99.9% of particulate sized .3 micron in size. Putting a HEPA filter on a simple air ducting system with a fan or heater will thus do wonders for removing dust, dander, and allergens.

Electric ion generating machines generate negative ions. Ionizers have been reputed to remove dust and bacteria, yet this remains controversial. While dust and soot may be attracted to negative ions, they are likely to remain airborne, or possibly end up on floors or furniture to be picked up again.

The amount of ions generated by these machines may also be of concern. While outdoor air may range from 500 to 5,000 negative ions per cubic centimeter, and indoor air may only have a couple hundred per cubic centimeter, negative ion generators can easily pump out from ten thousand to ten million negative ions per cubic centimeter.

At these higher levels—especially over a million—negative ions can become irritating to mucous membranes. They can irritate the throat, the eyes, and the lungs. Quite simply, our bodies were not designed for this level of negative ions.

This may require further investigation, but a Cochrane review (Blackhall *et al.* 2003) of six good quality studies concluded that ionizers exerted no significant effects upon respiratory health.

Ozone generators appear to be more effective at removing bacteria and mold, because these require oxygen to live, and ozone depletes their oxygen levels. Ozone generators also produce positive ions apparently decrease dust particles and other pollutants from their air.

Multiple studies have tested gaseous ozone generation in storage facilities to decrease mycotoxins such as aflatoxin molds. One study (Trombete *et al.* 2016) found total aflatoxins were reduced by 48 percent by using an ozone generator. Fungal counts in general were also significantly reduced.

Another study (Piemontese *et al.* 2018) found that gaseous ozone treatment in wheat storage facilities reduced a number of other contaminants:

"This study reports the efficacy of gaseous ozone treatments in reducing deoxynivalenol, DON-3-Glc, bacteria, fungi and yeasts in naturally contaminated durum wheat."

For this reason, a good ozone generator will often create a fresher smelling indoor environment. While ozone is not the same as smog, which has carbon or sulphur molecules connected to the molecules, ozone is an atmospheric response to smog, as ozone helps stabilize oxygen levels and clear out other molecules.

At the same time, higher ozone levels may also result in lung irritation and allergic response. As mentioned earlier, the FDA limits ozone generating machines in medical devices (used in hospitals and clinics) to emit no more than 50 parts per billion.

A 2017 study from Brazil (Cestonaro *et al.*) tested ozone with rats and found no negative effects. But a 2005 study (Hubbard *et al.*) tested ozone generators in apartments and houses in Texas. They found increased levels of particles when household cleaners were used together with ozone machines. The concerning compounds were terpenes – which come from pine oil-based cleaners.

Given these studies, experts recommend ozone generators are used when there are no humans in the room. They can be used to help clear the air in between room occupation.

The bottom line with both ionizers and ozone generators is that the atmosphere contains a fragile balance of components: It is not a random mixture. The level of ozone present in outdoor pollution reflects the atmosphere's cleansing process.

Electrostatic air filters for forced air systems can be a good choice. These HEPA filters typically filter between ninety and a hundred percent of dander, mold, mites, dust, soot, and bacteria. Many of these filters come with the ability to clean and reuse, allowing us to clean them as often as needed—which should be at least monthly if use is constant.

Environmental filters are good alternatives, especially for cold urban environments. These draw in, filter and heat outdoor air. This maximizes circulation, ventilation and temperature control: The best of all worlds.

Pillowcase filters: This air filtration device is designed to filter the nighttime air through the pillowcase. One study (Stillerman *et al.* 2010) tested this with 35 adults who had allergic rhinoconjunctivitis and sensitivities to either dander or dust mites. The device was found to reduce 99.99% of allergen particulates greater than .3 microns within the patients' breathing zones. The patient group using the filtration device was found to have significantly fewer symptoms and better quality of lie than the placebo group.

Choosing to use household products with natural ingredients free as possible from chemicals will reduce our carcinogen exposure. This means using natural flooring and furniture, natural fragrance-free soaps and cosmetics, and cotton clothing. This also means buying fewer plastic household goods and more natural fiber goods. Should we change our purchasing behavior, we may also alter the behavior of those companies manufacturing these items.

When it comes to freshening up stale indoor air, pressurized aerosol air fresheners are not the way to go. They may contain various synthetic fragrances, benzyl ethanols, naphthalene, and formaldehydes among other undesirables. Various micro-particles are also created by these aerosols.

As mentioned in the trigger chapter, many aerosols and pump sprays also contain noxious propellants—many of which are also volatile organic compounds (VOCs). These include butane and propane. Despite their demand in the marketplace, aerosols are not required for survival: Humankind did just fine without them for thousands of years. An effective disbursing method is a simple spray bottle. An active ingredient—say lemon juice—can be diluted with water and lightly sprayed through a room to freshen it up nicely. There are, of course, many other uses for such a common spray bottle—effectively replacing propellant aerosols.

Beware of perfumes and colognes that may reside in the bathroom or on family members. And be careful of fashion magazines and men's magazines that insert fragrances into their pages and advertisements. These perfumes might smell nice, but they can also contain toxins that can burden the immune system.

Candles may smell nice, but they are often made with synthetic fragrances, hydrocarbon-based paraffin waxes, and lead or other heavy metal wicks. The combination often releases unhealthy black soot into our air. Beeswax candles with essential oils can provide good alternatives for the candle-loving household, combined, of course, with fresh air.

Healthy alternatives to toxic household cleaners include lemon, vinegar, borax and/or baking soda. Borax is a great scrubbing detergent for heavy household and yard cleaning jobs. Olive oil, lemon oil or beeswax make for good natural furniture polishes.

Cleaning surfaces with these will also significantly freshen indoor air as well. Rotting food and unclean surfaces create mildew and bacteria quite quickly. Fresh air is quite easy to achieve with clean surfaces. Dusting and wiping down flooring and walls with vinegar can be a good strategy. A small cup of vinegar or a box of baking soda placed in a corner can also absorb odors and airborne toxins. Non-septic friendly chlorine bleach or rubbing alcohol can be used sparingly to remove mold or other microorganisms.

As far as pests, there now lots of organic or natural alternatives. These include clove oil, mints, orange oil, borax and others. Many pest control companies will now apply natural pesticide alternatives upon request.

House Plants

A house full of indoor plants will do wonders for improving our indoor air quality. Placing between two and five plants in a hundred square foot room—depending upon the outside air—can significantly remove carbon and raise oxygen levels. Research from the *Mississippi Stennis Space Center* concluded that indoor plants absorbed and broke down formaldehydes, trichloroethylenes, benzenes and zylenes.

Better performing plants included the lady palm, the rubber plant, English ivy, and the areca palm plants. Toxin removal rates can range from 1,000 to 1,800 micrograms per hour. One study done in Norway (Fjeld *et al.* 1998) found 23% fewer complaints of fatigue and sinus congestion among workers working around plants.

Studies performed in Texas and at Washington State University found that cognition response and problem-solving were also significantly higher among people working around plants (Wolverton 1997).

It should be noted that potting soils of indoor plants can also harbor some molds, so care can be taken to dry out the soil between waterings, and keep some sunlight on the soil surface.

We can also create forests around our homes. This means planting and maintaining indigenous trees that provide oxygen, shade and soil health: Soils without good plant life and rooting systems become loose and dusty. Nearby outdoor plants can significantly decrease the carbon and toxins in our immediate circulating environment. This also means instead of tearing out trees and paving our courtyards, we can leave the trees or replant them. Living in a space surrounded by trees can also render more privacy, allowing us to keep our windows open more often.

Indoor Materials

Using nature's materials for floors, walls and furniture is also a good strategy. This means using stone, ceramic, wood, wool, cotton and so on. Practically every synthetic piece of furniture, wall covering or floor covering contains a host of chemicals, including formaldehyde, VOCs, insecticides, asbestos and fire retardants.

Retarding fires is certainly commendable, but these chemicals can also make us sick in the worst case, and add to our toxin load in the best case. Besides, stone can be a pretty good fire retardant.

Stone, ceramic tile or wooden floors can also be easily cleaned with vinegar and baking soda to safely eliminate dust and allergens. Wood can also be polished and cleaned with olive oil. Nowadays, most walls are sheet rock, which often contains chalks and asbestos that can slowly build up in the airways. Replacing them with wood siding is a possible strategy.

Outgassing

Outgassing (or off-gassing) any new materials we buy is a good idea, regardless. To outgas a material, we can simply set it in the sun for a day before using it. This is a good idea for any new piece of furniture, wall covering, and anything else that may have been coated in VOCs or formaldehydes during manufacturing. Plastics may also be outgassed, but outgassing plastic in direct sunlight can also release additional monomer plasticizers.

Outgassing a new car might also be considered. That "new car smell" is more than just a nice smell. Leave the car in the sun for a few days or weeks with the windows open. For best results, always keep car windows cracked.

Work and School Strategies

Work and school environments are toxin traps. Why? Because they bring people and limited ventilation systems together under the same roof. They also host a number of toxins in building materials, carpets, desks, chairs, production materials, manufacturing exhaust, and whatever anyone brings in to work or school. This of course includes animal dander, dust mites, micro-organisms and mold attached to people's clothing, hair and skin as they venture into the building.

This was illustrated in the New Zealand research discussed earlier, where cat allergens were found throughout schools, workplaces, theaters and airplanes.

While there is no way to eliminate these potential toxins, we can certainly take measures to lower our exposure, since as a whole, toxins from the workplace and school do contribute to our overall toxic load and burden upon our immune system. Furthermore, exposure to workplace toxicity in the form of manufacturing wastes, cleaners, gases and other chemical toxins can single-handedly make a person downright sick.

A number of policies and strategies that can reduce our toxin exposure among workplaces and schools:

Hazardous Materials: Workplaces and schools typically utilize various chemicals and cleaning materials. Some workplaces use hazardous materials on a daily basis. These should be handled with care, to make sure that exposures are minimized.

According to United States Occupational Safety Code, *Manufacturer's Safety Data Sheets* (MSDS) are required for every chemical used by consumers, workers or cleaning professionals. These should be carefully read over to make sure that the material is being used in accordance with the MSDS.

HVAC: Our school and workplace should have a heating, ventilating and air conditioning system (also called HVAC) that is adequate for the population, space and environmental conditions. The more people, space and toxins present, the better the HVAC system needs to be. In the United States, these are typically determined by local, state or county building codes. When a building is designed, its HVAC must comply with the building code in place.

The standard codes are determined by The *American Society of Heating, Refrigerating and Air Conditions Engineers* (ASHRAE), who have developed the standards that most municipalities abide by. For example, the 1989 standards (6.2-1989) called for 15-20 cubic feet of fresh air to be brought in per minute (CFM) and per person occupying an indoor space. This means, for example, that an office with 10 people must have a system that pumps in 150-200 cubic feet of fresh air per minute.

This same calculation can be done for any school or other space.

In addition, building codes have changed over the years with respect to insulation. This means that if the building has been built in the past few decades, the building codes are tighter, and there will be likely less ventilation in general. This puts an extra strain on the HVAC system.

Windows are certainly a form of ventilation, but they should not be included in this calculation, because during cold or hot weather, the windows are often closed (though they should not be).

Any building needs to be checked with current code to make sure that the HVAC system matches the use and occupancy of the building. The building specifications designed by the architect before the building was built can easily be different from the building's current use. There may be many more workers or children in the building than originally specified for example.

Or if the HVAC was designed for office space, but the building is now used as manufacturing space, for example, the HVAC requirements will be different—depending upon what is being produced, and the municipality. So the company owners or school administrators must be reminded to assure their workers or parents that the workplace's/school's HVAC systems are compliant with current codes. This should also be reviewed for any apartment or condominium.

HVAC systems also should also be periodically cleaned. This includes the drip pans and ducting. These can build up with molds and other microorganisms, and infect their occupants. As we discussed earlier, cases have shown that extreme weather changes (from cold to warm or wet) can dramatically affect the HVAC system ducting in terms of mold and microorganisms—significantly infecting the building's occupants.

Flooring: Carpeting in workplaces and schools is particularly problematic. This is because they attract bacteria, molds, dander, allergens and other toxins quickly. Cleaning carpets is typically expensive and difficult. Wood, stone or concrete floors clean easier and can be disinfected more easily, as we've discussed.

Furniture: Chairs and sofas in the work place are susceptible to mold, toxin and allergen build-up as they age, and formaldehydes when newer. Therefore, they need to be periodically cleaned or replaced. Wooden furniture or furniture with cleanable surfaces and moisture barriers are preferred.

Windows: From an individual perspective, sitting or working close to an openable window is suggested in any workplace or school classroom. Any time there is an offensive odor or concern about indoor air quality, the window should be opened and left open until the risk has subsided. Hotel rooms can also be checked for openable windows before they are reserved. A closed-in room with a dirty HVAC system can practically produce illness in itself.

Keeping the house on the dry side. Water feeds molds and fungi. Look for leaks into the windowsills, basements and house corners.

Chemicals: Our houses and work places are best clear of pesticides, fragrances, incense, and other chemicals. If bugs are a problem, try borax or traps.

Household and workplace cleaners should be natural. These include baking soda, vinegar, lemon and borax. These are all, to relative degrees, also antimicrobial.

Tubs and bathrooms should be cleaned of molds and fungi frequently, before mold forms. Mold grows in moist, dark places, so those areas of the bathroom should be cleaned more frequently than areas exposed to sunshine.

Fans: Fans are a valuable and inexpensive addition to any room. These can help blow offensive air out the door or window, for example. Fans, in fact, are better strategies than air conditioning, because they do not artificially cool the body down—as we've discussed. In the opinion of this author, every workplace and school should be equipped with fans.

Carbon monoxide and NO$_2$ strategies include venting any gas appliance to the outdoors, making sure there are no leaks, using the right fuels for each appliance; using an exhaust fan over a gas appliance; using certified wood stoves; having stoves inspected and cleaned; opening fireplace flues (vents to the outside); and opening the garage door before starting the car.

Air purifiers: Small air purifiers can significant help a person working in a workplace with questionable air. These can be placed right on the desk. These can significantly help remove particulates, mold and allergens from our immediate breathing airspace.

Regular Cleaning: This is a requisite for any workplace, school or apartment building. Common areas should be cleaned at least weekly. Floors and walls should be sanitized. Good natural cleaners include vinegar, lemon, borax and baking soda. Chlorine or rubbing alcohol can be used sparingly to disinfect. Furniture requires regular dusting and sanitization, and HVAC systems and ducts require regular cleaning.

Wearing a mask when we are using any chemical that might contain VOCs or other breathable toxins. Best strategy is to not use these types of chemicals at all, but sometimes we might have to. The mask should have an outside rubber seal. Paper masks do very little to prevent breathing in toxins.

Exercise

A plethora of research has shown that sedentary lifestyles dramatically increase the risk of systemic inflammation and cancer.

A review of research from the U.S. National Institutes of Health (Stout *et al.* 2017) reviewed 302 studies on the topic. They found:

"Moderate-to-vigorous exercise is the best level of exercise intensity to improve physical function and mitigate cancer-related impairments. Therapeutic exercises are beneficial to manage treatment side effects, may enhance tolerance to cancer treatments, and improve functional outcomes. Supervised exercise yielded superior benefits versus unsupervised. Serious adverse events were not common."

A study from Canada (Lynch *et al.* 2011) found that more sitting increases the risk of breast cancer among women. This study, led by researchers from the Alberta Health Services of Calgary, Canada, used the U.S. National Health and Nutrition Examination Survey of 2003-2006 to analyze the lifestyles of 1,024 elderly women.

They followed the activity levels of the women together with their length of sitting. They found that breast cancer incidence was highest amongst those women who sat the most each day, and that light physical exercise such as walking significantly decreased breast cancer incidence.

Other cancers are also caused by sedentary lifestyles. Researchers presenting at the Annual Research Conference on Food, Nutrition, Physical Activity and Cancer in Washington, have estimated that inactivity causes nearly 100,000 cancer cases each year in the United States.

This notion is strengthened by a study published last year in the American Journal of Epidemiology by researchers from the American Cancer Society's Epidemiology Research Program (Patel *et al.* 2010). This study followed 53,440 U.S. men and 69,776 U.S. women for fourteen years, and analyzed their daily sitting and physical activity times through questionnaire. During the fourteen years, 11,307 of the men died and 7,923 women died.

After removing being overweight, smoking and other lifestyle and diet factors, the researchers found that death incidence was 94% higher among women and 48% greater among men who sat for more than or equal to six hours per day combined with lower levels of physical activity.

Another review of research showed that exercise for cancer patients increases the availability of immune cells to tumor sites. This, as identified in research from Denmark's Center for Cancer Immune Therapy (Idorn and Straten 2017), has been shown to reduce tumor size by as much as 60 percent.

This kind of immune cell boost is partially based on the fact that exercise increases circulation and detoxification, stimulates the immune system, pumps the lymphatic system and increases lung capacity. Exercise is one of the most assured ways to strengthen the immune system and thus increase tolerance.

When we exercise, we contract muscles. Muscle contraction is what circulates (or pumps) lymph around the body through the lymph vessels. This is because the lymphatic system does not have a heart like the circulatory system has. The lymphatic system relies on muscle contraction for circulation.

Lymph circulation is critical for systemic inflammation because immune cells circulating through the blood and lymph break down and carry out of the body those broken-down toxins and cell parts.

And of course, exercise also circulates oxygen and nutrients throughout the body. Exercise also stimulates the thymus gland, and speeds up healing of the intestinal cell walls. In all, exercise is one of the best and cheapest therapies available to boost immunity and tolerance.

All of these effects and more are produced by daily exercise and activity. And as mentioned in the NIH research, supervised activity has shown to be more successful than unsupervised. This means working out with someone who knows what they are doing, and can help monitor the quality and quantity of the exercise.

Sleep

A review of research (Chen *et al.* 2018) analyzed 65 studies that followed more than 1,550,000 people. They found that short sleep increased the risk of all cancers by 36 percent. They also found that long sleep increased the risk of colorectal cancer by 21 percent.

A large study from China's First Hospital of China Medical University (Lu *et al.* 2017) analyzed 10 studies that followed over 415,000 people. They found that increased sleep beyond 7 hours increased the risk of breast cancer.

These and other studies show that the right amount of sleep is critical to our immune system and our ability to purge toxins. This is especially true when it comes to deep sleep and REM-stage cycles.

When we sleep, our immune system moves into overdrive. Like microscopic elves, our probiotics become more active, taking out pathogenic microorganisms and breaking down toxins. Our T- and B-cells help coordinate the process, and participate in breaking down pathogens and toxins.

Our liver will produce more antioxidant enzymes during sleep. The body's purification systems all move into overdrive. When we sleep deeply, we also breathe deeper, which removes more toxins from the lungs and the airway mucosal membranes. Our intestinal probiotics switch into high gear, and our cells dump more toxins into intercellular fluids.

This was illustrated by researchers from Chicago's Rush University Medical Center (Ranjbaran *et al.* 2007), who studied sleep abnormalities and their association with *"chronic inflammatory conditions (CIC)."* They found that changes in the *"sleep-wake cycle"* stimulate an increased systemic inflammation response. Their research also showed that slow wave (deep) sleep can curb inflammation and strengthen immunity.

They also found that sleep disturbances can cause greater levels of inflammatory pain and fatigue, while reducing quality of life. This scenario is often seen amongst those with toxemia. The researchers commented that the underlying mechanism causing a lack of sleep to spurn systemic inflammation relates to the *"dysregulation of the immune system."*

A key strategy for deep sleep is to spend time outside everyday. This helps regulate our light-dark cycles. This means getting outside early in the daytime to stimulate the pineal gland and the SCN cells. Then as the night proceeds towards bedtime, we should turn the lights low and then off. This will regulate the circulation of melatonin and cortisol, allowing us to fall asleep at the right time of the cortisol-melatonin cycle—allowing us to sleep deeper through the night.

If we are consistently tired during the day, we can have someone watch us sleep, looking for irregular breathing, stopping breathing for a short period and/or partial wakening while sleeping. These may be signs of sleep apnea. If someone close says that they see some of these symptoms, we should see a sleep specialist.

For more information on sleep, including many lifestyle, dietary and herbal strategies that promote deep sleep, please refer to the author's book, *Natural Sleep - Insomnia Solutions*.

Music

Music may not be able to cure or treat cancer in itself, but it may help significantly improve quality of life during cancer treatment.

A study from Case Western Reserve University (Palmer *et al.* 2015) tested 207 breast cancer patients who were treated with surgery. They were divided into three groups. One group listened to music selected by therapists before the surgery. Another group listened to the music during the surgery. And the other group listened to music after the surgery.

The researchers found the music helped all the groups in their recoveries. However, the group that listened to music before their surgery had the shortest recovery times compared to the other two groups.

Other studies have found that music therapy during cancer treatment can significantly reduce anxiety, depression and pain, and improve quality of life (Gramaglia *et al.* 2019).

Hospital or Home

Certainly, the hospital is where we can receive the most urgent cancer treatments. But cancer treatments do vary from hospital to hospital, depending upon the oncologist. Therefore it is wise to get second and even third opinions on treatment protocols.

Sometimes a newly-diagnosed cancer patient will ask me what natural cancer treatments they should do. I always steer them to discuss these with their oncologist, especially before trying to self-treat. This is because natural therapies for cancer can also interfere with certain chemotherapy or radiation programs.

It is thus very important to discuss with your doctor any natural therapies being considered. Chemotherapy and radiation have specific objectives, to obliterate tumors before they proliferate. A natural therapy can actually have the effect of interfering with this process, and may even feed a tumor. Therefore it is always best to ask your doctor.

This said, there are now a number of integrative cancer treatment centers located throughout the U.S. and other countries around the world. These treatment centers are often staffed both with conventional oncologists alongside natural health experts. They can work together to provide treatments that do not conflict or interfere.

At least in the U.S., these integrative cancer centers are typically licensed and staffed with high quality professionals.

When it comes to cancer treatment in the hospital, there are other considerations to consider, especially for terminal cancer patients.

A large multi-hospital study followed 2,069 cancer patients from Japan (Hamano *et al.* 2016). They had terminal cancer and were expected to die soon. Of these, 1,582 patients stayed in the hospital and received the focused care of doctors and nurses. The remaining 487 cancer patients remained at home and received home-based care. There was no difference regarding the seriousness of their cancers.

The researchers found that those patients who stayed at home lived significantly longer than the patients who stayed at the hospital. This was after adjusting for any other factors that may have contributed to their longevity.

Those with a worse prognosis lived 30 percent longer when they stayed at home. Across the board: After calculating the hazard analysis based on survival rates, the research found that staying at home results in a 14 percent increased risk of survival. That is, compared to staying at the hospital.

The study was conducted in conjunction with cancer treatment centers at several major hospitals. It was published in the American Cancer Society's journal Cancer.

Lead researcher Jun Hamano, MD of Japan's University of Tsukuba commented:

"The cancer patient and family tend to be concerned that the quality of medical treatment provided at home will be inferior to that given in a hospital and that survival might be shortened; however, our finding—that home death does not actually have a negative influence on the survival of cancer patients at all, and rather may have a positive influence— could suggest that the patient and family can choose the place of death in terms of their preference and values," said Dr. Hamano. "Patients, families, and clinicians should be reassured that good home hospice care does not shorten patient life, and even may achieve longer survival."

This study may not include a major issue that takes place among many U.S. hospitals – superbug infections. That is, that many people will die in the hospital because they are infected with a hospital-acquired infection.

According to the Centers for Disease Control, about 772,000 people were infected during a visit to an acute care hospital in 2011. And some 75,000 people died of a hospital-acquired infection during that year.

This is not to say that there has been significant efforts to decrease these outrageous statistics. The CDC also reports decreases among hospital infections. MRSA (methicillin-resistant Staphylococcus aureus) infections fell by 13 percent between 2011 and 2014. And *Clostridium difficile* infections dropped by 8 percent during this time. And surgical site infections and others have dropped in recent years. That's the good news.

The bad news is that many of these hospital-acquired infections have gotten harder to control with antibiotics. Those superbugs have become more super. So fewer antibiotics are able to treat them.

Another consideration is medical errors that occur in hospitals.

A 2010 study (Levinson *et al.*) published in the *New England Journal of Medicine* studied this at length. They investigated admissions between 2001 and 2007 at 10 hospitals in North Carolina. They found that out of 2,341 patients, there were 588 medical errors that caused harm. This equated to 25 harmful medical errors out of every 100 patient admissions.

Of these mistakes, 186 were related to procedures, 162 were related to medications, 87 were related to hospital-acquired infections, 59 were related to therapies, and 7 were related to diagnoses.

Of these 588 medical errors, 245 required further treatment. And 251 required extended hospitalization. Worse, 50 of these were life-threatening, and 14 caused the death of the patient. And 17 of the harms – or about 3% – caused permanent injury.

A full 63 percent of these medical errors were classified as preventable by the researchers.

A 2010 report from the U.S. Department of Health and Human Services found that in one in seven people experienced an adverse event in the hospital. This equated to 13.5 percent of every hospital visit: And 134,000 adverse events in just one month.

This means 1.6 million people each year have an adverse event in the hospital.

They also found that 1.5 percent of Medicare patients experienced an adverse event in the hospital that contributed to their death. This calculated to a full 15,000 patient deaths in a month – or 180,000 deaths each year in the United States. This is where an event occurring in the hospital contributed to the death of a patient.

Hospitals are Not Bad

Yes, there are risks, but hospitals are also important for critical care and intensive care. Sometimes cancer patients will need this sort of care at some point.

Doctors and nurses work hard at hospitals throughout the world, and care tremendously for their patients. Countless patients have survived illnesses and injuries by visiting the hospital. They receive surgeries and medications that extend their lives. So let's not miss the benefits of hospitalization. We are grateful for their hard work and dedication. And grateful for the some of the technologies hospitals offer.

But when we don't absolutely have to be in the hospital, let's open a bed for someone who needs it worse. Recovering at home by using out-patient care and home nursing care can not only be cheaper: It may extend our life or the life of a family member a little. And it might allow for some respite and spiritual awakening that perhaps the sterile surroundings of a hospital may not support.

Conclusion

Cancer is not a foreign condition. All of us get cancer throughout our lives. But nature was designed for our bodies to be able to fight cancer before it can take the body down. That is, if we work with nature.

To date, we've been failing that effort. Today we are working against nature in so many ways. We are producing cancer-causing toxins that we mix into our air and into our foods and other consumer goods. So now we have an uphill battle on our hands. Can we work with nature to beat cancer?

The question is whether our bodies are fit enough to counteract the invasion of free radicals to begin with. And should a cell turn cancerous, whether our immune system is tuned up well enough to kill that cell and dispose of it before it proliferates and spreads.

This means keeping our body's antioxidation processes, such as the liver and the lymphatic system, are working to their full potential. It also means eating a diet with enough antioxidants to counteract the oxidation potential that our environment and diet brings into our body.

This also means trying to reduce those toxins from entering our body.

It also means getting the right amount of sleep, exercise, water consumption and sunlight. It means being a responsible consumer in terms of reducing our toxin load.

And finally, it means incorporating those dietary habits, superfoods, herbs, supplements and probiotics that directly help our body fight cancer.

In terms of prevention, the older we get, the more attentive we will have to be with regard to incorporating these elements into our lifestyles.

Why? Because human research (Valgimigli *et al.* 2014) has shown that each year, our body loses about one percent of its natural antioxidant capacity. That means we have to continually increase our ingestion of antioxidants, herbs and other immunity boosting elements.

All this requires work. Reading labels, and understanding which things increase our bodies' toxin levels.

Yes, fighting or preventing cancer requires knowledge and work. I hope this book has brought you a good amount of that knowledge. Now the work is left up to you. And me. All of us. This is the lesson that cancer presents to us in the long term: Are we ready as a society and as individuals to take responsibility for our body's long-term health and join nature in its fight against cancer?

References and Bibliography

Abaskharoun R, Depew W, Vanner S. Changes in renal function following administration of oral sodium phosphate or polyethylene glycol for colon cleansing before colonoscopy. Can J Gastroenterol. 2007 Apr;21(4):227-31.

Abdou AM, Higashiguchi S, Horie K, Kim M, Hatta H, Yokogoshi H. Relaxation and immunity enhancement effects of gamma-aminobutyric acid GABA. Biofactors. 2006;26(3):201-8.

Abdureyim S, Amat N, Umar A, Upur H, Berke B, Moore N. Anti-inflammatory, immunomodulatory, and heme oxygenase-1 inhibitory activities of ravan napas, a formulation of uighur traditional medicine, in a rat model of allergic asthma. Evid Based Complement Alternat Med. 2011;2011. pii: 725926.

Abedi J, Saatloo MV, Nejati V, Hobbenaghi R, Tukmechi A, Nami Y, Khosroushahi AY. Selenium-Enriched Saccharomyces cerevisiae Reduces the Progression of Colorectal Cancer. Biol Trace Elem Res. 2018 Oct;185(2):424-432. doi: 10.1007/s12011-018-1270-9. Epub 2018 Feb 21. PMID: 29468612.

Abrams SL, Follo MY, Steelman LS, Lertpiriyapong K, Cocco L, Ratti S, Martelli AM, Candido S, Libra M, Murata RM, Rosalen PL, Montalto G, Cervello M, Gizak A, Rakus D, Mao W, Lombardi P, McCubrey JA. Abilities of berberine and chemically modified berberines to inhibit proliferation of pancreatic cancer cells. Adv Biol Regul. 2019 Jan;71:172-182. doi: 10.1016/j.jbior.2018.10.003.

Ackerman D. A Natural History of the Senses. New York: Vintage, 1991.

Adams LS, Phung S, Wu X, Ki L, Chen S. White button mushroom (Agaricus bisporus) exhibits antiproliferative and proapoptotic properties and inhibits prostate tumor growth in athymic mice. Nutr Cancer. 2008;60(6):744-56. doi: 10.1080/01635580802192866.

Adoga AS, Otene AA, Yiltok SJ, Adekwu A, Nwaorgu OG. Cervical necrotizing fasciitis: case series and review of literature. Niger J Med. 2009 Apr-Jun;18(2):203-7.

Agache I, Ciobanu C. Risk factors and asthma phenotypes in children and adults with seasonal allergic rhinitis. Phys Sportsmed. 2010 Dec;38(4):81-6.

Agarwal KN, Bhasin SK, Faridi MM, Mathur M, Gupta S. Lactobacillus casei in the control of acute diarrhea—a pilot study. Indian Pediatr. 2001 Aug;38(8):905-10.

Agarwal SK, Singh SS, Verma S. Antifungal principle of sesquiterpene lactones from Anamirta cocculus. Indian Drugs. 1999;36:754-5.

Agerholm-Larsen L, Raben A, Haulrik N, Hansen AS, Manders M, Astrup A. Effect of 8 week intake of probiotic milk products on risk factors for cardiovascular diseases. Eur J Clin Nutr. 2000 Apr;54(4):288-97.

Aggarwal BB, Harikumar KB. Potential therapeutic effects of curcumin, the anti-inflammatory agent, against neurodegenerative, cardiovascular, pulmonary, metabolic, autoimmune and neoplastic diseases. Int J Biochem Cell Biol. 2009 Jan;41(1):40-59.

Aggarwal BB, Sung B. Pharmacological basis for the role of curcumin in chronic diseases: an age-old spice with modern targets. Trends Pharmacol Sci. 2009 Feb;30(2):85-94.

Agune D, Keum N, Giovannucci E, Fadnes LT, Boffetta P, Greenwood DC, Tonstad S, Vatten LJ, Riboli E, Norat T. Nut consumption and risk of cardiovascular disease,total cancer, all-cause and cause-specific mortality: a systematic review and dose-response meta-analysis of prospective studies. BMC Med. 2016 Dec 5;14(1):207.

Agustina R, Lukito W, Firmansyah A, Suhardjo HN, Murniati D, Bindels J. The effect of early nutritional supplementation with a mixture of probiotic, prebiotic, fiber and micronutrients in infants with acute diarrhea in Indonesia. Asia Pac J Clin Nutr. 2007;16(3):435-42.

Ahmed M, Prasad J, Gill H, Stevenson L, Gopal P. Impact of consumption of different levels of Bifidobacterium lactis HN019 on the intestinal microflora of elderly human subjects. J Nutr Health Aging. 2007 Jan-Feb;11(1):26-31.

Ahmed, AA, McCarthy RD, Porter GA. Effectof of milk constituents on hepatic cholesterogenesis. Atherosclerosis. 1979;32:347-57.

Ahn WS, Kim DJ, Chae GT, Lee JM, Bae SM, Sin JI, Kim YW, Namkoong SE, Lee IP. 2004. Natural killer cell activity and quality of life were improved by consumption of a mushroom extract, Agaricus blazei Murill Kyowa, in gynecological cancer patients undergoing chemotherapy. Int J Gynecol Cancer, 14(4), 589-94.

Aho K, Koskenvuo M, Tuominen J, Kaprio J. Occurrence of rheumatoid arthritis in a nationwide series of twins. J Rheumatol. 1986 Oct;13(5):899-902.

Ahola AJ, Yli-Knuuttila H, Suomalainen T, Poussa T, Ahlström A, Meurman JH, Korpela R. Short-term consumption of probiotic-containing cheese and its effect on dental caries risk factors. Arch Oral Biol. 2002 Nov;47(11):799-804.

Aihara K, Kajimoto O, Hirata H, Takahashi R, Nakamura Y. Effect of powdered fermented milk with Lactobacillus helveticus on subjects with high-normal blood pressure or mild hypertension. J Am Coll Nutr. 2005 Aug;24(4):257-65.

Ainsleigh HG. Beneficial effects of sun exposure on cancer mortality. Prev Med. 1992;22:132-40.

Airola P. How to Get Well. Phoenix, AZ: Health Plus, 1974.

Akanbi MH, Post E, van Putten SM, de Vries L, Smisterova J, Meter-Arkema AH, Wösten HA, Rink R, Scholtmeijer K. The antitumor activity of hydrophobin SC3, a fungal protein. Appl Microbiol Biotechnol. 2013 May;97(10):4385-92. doi: 10.1007/s00253-012-4311-x.

Akbar-Khanzadeh F, Bitovski DK. Exposure of school employees to extremely low frequency magnetic fields. Can J Public Health. 2000 Jan-Feb;91(1):21-4.

Akbar-Khanzadeh F, Bitovski DK. Exposure of school employees to extremely low frequency magnetic fields. Can J Public Health. 2000 Jan-Feb;91(1):21-4.

Akil I, Yilmaz O, Kurutepe S, Degerli K, Kavukcu S. Influence of oral intake of Saccharomyces boulardii on Escherichia coli in enteric flora. Pediatr Nephrol. 2006 Jun;21(6):807-10.

Akinbami LJ, Moorman JE, Garbe PL, Sondik EJ. Status of childhood asthma in the United States, 1980-2007. Pediatrics. 2009;123:S131-45.

Akula SM, Candido S, Libra M, Abrams SL, Steelman LS, Lertpiriyapong K, Ramazzotti G, Ratti S, Follo MY, Martelli AM, Murata RM, Rosalen PL, Bueno-Silva B, Matias de Alencar S, Montalto G, Cervello M, Gizak A, Rakus D, Mao W, Lin HL, Lombardi P, McCubrey JA. Abilities of berberine and chemically modified berberines to interact with metformin and inhibit proliferation of pancreatic cancer cells. Adv Biol Regul. 2019 Aug;73:100633. doi: 10.1016/j.jbior.2019.04.003.

Albrechtsen O. The influence of small atmospheric ions on human well-being and mental performance. Intern. J. of Biometeorology. 1978;22(4): 249-262.

Aldinucci C, Bellussi L, Monciatti G, Passàli GC, Salerni L, Passàli D, Bocci V. Effects of dietary yoghurt on immunological and clinical parameters of rhinopathic patients. Eur J Clin Nutr. 2002 Dec;56(12):1155-61.

Alexander DD, Cabana MD. Partially hydrolyzed 100% whey protein infant formula and reduced risk of atopic dermatitis: a meta-analysis. J Pediatr Gastroenterol Nutr. 2010 Apr;50(4):422-30.

Alexandrakis M, Letourneau R, Kempuraj D, Kandere-Grzybowska K, Huang M, Christodoulou S, Boucher W, Seretakis D, Theoharides TC. Flavones inhibit proliferation and increase mediator content in human leukemic mast cells (HMC-1). Eur J Haematol. 2003 Dec;71(6):448-54.

Alexandre P, Darmanyan D, Yushen G, Jenks W, Burel L, Eloy D, Jardon P. Quenching of Singlet Oxygen by Oxygen- and Sulfur-Centered Radicals: Evidence for Energy Transfer to Peroxyl Radicals in Solution. J. Am. Chem. Soc., 120 (2), 396 -403, 1998.

Al-Harrasi A, Al-Saidi S. Phytochemical analysis of the essential oil from botanically certified oleogum resin of Boswellia sacra (Omani Luban). Molecules. 2008 Sep 16;13(9):2181-9.

Allen SJ, Okoko B, Martinez E, Gregorio G, Dans LF. Probiotics for treating infectious diarrhea. The Cochrane Library. 2004;3. Chichester, UK: John Wiley & Sons, Ltd.

Alleva R, Tomasetti M, Bompadre S, Littarru GP. Oxidation of LDL and their subfractions: kinetic aspects and CoQ10 content. Mol Aspects Med. 1997;18 Suppl:S105-12.

Al-Yasiri AY, Khoobchandani M, Cutler CS, Watkinson L, Carmack T, Smith CJ, Kuchuk M, Loyalka SK, Lugão AB, Katti KV. Mangiferin in prostate tumor therapy: green nanotechnology for production, in vivo tumor retention and evaluation of therapeutic efficacy. Dalton Trans. 2017 Oct 31;46(42):14561-14571. doi:10.1039/c7dt00383h

Amassian VE, Cracco RQ, Maccabee PJ, Cracco JB, Rudell A, Eberle L. Suppression of visual perception by magnetic coil stimulation of human occipital cortex. Electroencephalogr Clin Neurophysiol. 1989 Nov-Dec;74(6):458-62.

Amassian VE, Cracco RQ, Maccabee PJ. A sense of movement elicited in paralyzed distal arm by focal magnetic coil stimulation of human motor cortex. Brain Res. 1989 Feb 13;479(2):355-60.

Amato R, Pinelli M, Monticelli A, Miele G, Cocozza S. Schizophrenia and Vitamin D Related Genes Could Have Been Subject to Latitude-driven Adaptation. BMC Evol Biol. 2010 Nov 11;10(1):351.

Amenta M, Cascio MT, Di Fiore P, Venturini I. Diet and chronic constipation. Benefits of oral supplementation with symbiotic zir fos (Bifidobacterium longum W11 + FOS Actilight). Acta Biomed. 2006 Dec;77(3):157-62.

American Cancer Society. What are the key statistics about prostate cancer? Accessed Feb. 15, 2016.

American Conference of Governmental Industrial Hygienists. Threshold limit values for chemical substances and physical agents in the work environment. Cincinnati, OH: ACGIH, 1986.

American Dietetic Association; Dietitians of Canada. Position of the American Dietetic Association and Dietitians of Canada: vegetarian diets. Can J Diet Pract Res. 2003 Summer;64(2):62-81.

American Public Health Association. Opposition to Hormone Growth Promoters in Beef and Dairy Cattle Production. Policy Date: 11/10/2009. Policy Number: 20098. Ted Strickland, Governor, State of Ohio. Executive Order 2008-03S.

Ammon HP. Boswellic acids (components of frankincense) as the active principle in treatment of chronic inflammatory diseases. Wien Med Wochenschr. 2002;152(15-16):373-8.

Ammon HP. Boswellic acids in chronic inflammatory diseases. Planta Med. 2006 Oct;72(12):1100-16.

Ammor MS, Michaelidis C, Nychas GJ. Insights into the role of quorum sensing in food spoilage. J Food Prot. 2008 Jul;71(7):1510-25.

Anand P, Thomas SG, Kunnumakkara AB, Sundaram C, Harikumar KB, Sung B, Tharakan ST, Misra K, Priyadarsini IK, Rajasekharan KN, Aggarwal BB. Biological activities of curcumin and its analogues (Congeners) made by man and Mother Nature. Biochem Pharmacol. 2008 Dec 1;76(11):1590-611.

Anderson DR, Huston AC, Schmitt KL, Linebarger DL, Wright JC. Early childhood television viewing and adolescent behavior: the recontact study. Monogr Soc Res Child Dev. 2001;66(1):I-VIII, 1-147.

Anderson GC, Moore E, Hepworth J, Bergman N. Early skin-to-skin contact for mothers and their healthy newborn infants. Cochrane Database Syst Rev. 2003;(2):CD003519.

Anderson JL, May HT, Horne BD, Bair TL, Hall NL, Carlquist JF, Lappé DL, Muhlestein JB; Intermountain Heart Collaborative (IHC) Study Group. Relation of vitamin D deficiency to cardiovascular risk factors, disease status, and incident events in a general healthcare population. Am J Cardiol. 2010 Oct 1;106(7):963-8.

Anderson JW, Gilliland SE. Effect of fermented milk (yogurt) containing Lactobacillus acidophilus L1 on serum cholesterol in hypercholesterolemic humans. J Am Coll Nutr. 1999 Feb;18(1):43-50.

Anderson M., Grissom C. Increasing the Heavy Atom Effect of Xenon by Adsorption to Zeolites: Photolysis of 2,3-Diazabicyclo[2.2.2]oct-2-ene. J. Am. Chem. Soc. 1996;118:9552-9556.

Anderson RC, Anderson JH. Acute respiratory effects of diaper emissions. Arch Environ Health. 1999 Sep-Oct;54(5):353-8.

Anderson RC, Anderson JH. Acute toxic effects of fragrance products. Arch Environ Health. 1998 Mar-Apr;53(2):138-46.

Anderson RC, Anderson JH. Respiratory toxicity in mice exposed to mattress covers. Arch Environ Health. 1999 May-Jun;54(3):202-9.

Anderson RC, Anderson JH. Respiratory toxicity of fabric softener emissions. J Toxicol Environ Health. 2000 May 26;60(2):121-36.

Anderson RC, Anderson JH. Respiratory toxicity of mattress emissions in mice. Arch Environ Health. 2000 Jan-Feb;55(1):38-43.

Anderson RC, Anderson JH. Sensory irritation and multiple chemical sensitivity. Toxicol Ind Health. 1999 Apr-Jun;15(3-4):339-45.

Anderson RC, Anderson JH. Toxic effects of air freshener emissions. Arch Environ Health. 1997 Nov-Dec;52(6):433-41.

Anderson SD, Charlton B, Weiler JM, Nichols S, Spector SL, Pearlman DS; A305 Study Group. Comparison of mannitol and methacholine to predict exercise-induced bronchoconstriction and a clinical diagnosis of asthma. Respir Res. 2009 Jan 23;10:4.

Anim-Nyame N, Sooranna SR, Johnson MR, Gamble J, Steer PJ. Garlic supplementation increases peripheral blood flow: a role for interleukin-6? J Nutr Biochem. 2004 Jan;15(1):30-6.

Annweiler C, Schott AM, Berrut G, Chauviré V, Le Gall D, Inzitari M, Beauchet O. Vitamin D and ageing: neurological issues. Neuropsychobiology. 2010 Aug;62(3):139-50.

Anonymous. Cimetidine inhibits the hepatic hydroxylation of vitamin D. Nutr Rev. 1985;43:184-5.

Antczak A, Nowak D, Shariati B, Król M, Piasecka G, Kurmanowska Z. Increased hydrogen peroxide and thiobarbituric acid-reactive products in expired breath condensate of asthmatic patients. Eur Respir J. 1997 Jun;10(6):1235-41.

Anthony J. Bazzan, Andrew B. Newberg, William C. Cho, and Daniel A. Monti, "Diet and Nutrition in Cancer Survivorship and Palliative Care," Evidence-Based Complementary and Alternative Medicine, vol. 2013, Article ID 917647, 12 pages, 2013. doi:10.1155/2013/917647.

Anukam K, Osazuwa E, Ahonkhai I, Ngwu M, Osemene G, Bruce AW, Reid G. Augmentation of antimicrobial metronidazole therapy of bacterial vaginosis with oral probiotic Lactobacillus rhamnosus GR-1 and Lactobacillus reuteri RC-14: randomized, double-blind, placebo controlled trial. Microbes Infect. 2006 May;8(6):1450-4.

Anukam KC, Osazuwa E, Osemene GI, Ehigiagbe F, Bruce AW, Reid G. Clinical study comparing probiotic Lactobacillus GR-1 and RC-14 with metronidazole vaginal gel to treat symptomatic bacterial vaginosis. Microbes Infect. 2006 Oct;8(12-13):2772-6.

Anukam KC, Osazuwa EO, Osadolor HB, Bruce AW, Reid G. Yogurt containing probiotic Lactobacillus rhamnosus GR-1 and L. reuteri RC-14 helps resolve moderate diarrhea and increases CD4 count in HIV/AIDS patients. J Clin Gastroenterol. 2008 Mar;42(3):239-43.

Aoki T, Usuda Y, Miyakoshi H, Tamura K, Herberman RB. Low natural killer syndrome: clinical and immunologic features. Nat Immun Cell Growth Regul. 1987;6(3):116-28.

Apáti P, Houghton PJ, Kite G, Steventon GB, Kéry A. In-vitro effect of flavonoids from Solidago canadensis extract on glutathione S-transferase. J Pharm Pharmacol. 2006 Feb;58(2):251-6.

APHA (American Public Health Association). Opposition to the Use of Hormone Growth Promoters in Beef and Dairy Cattle Production. Policy Date: 11/10/2009. Policy Number: 20098. http://www.apha.org/advocacy/policy/id=1379. Accessed Nov. 24, 2010.

Apperley FL. The relation of solar radiation to cancer mortality in North America. Cancer Res. 1941;1:191-96.

Araki K, Shinozaki T, Irie Y, Miyazawa Y. Trial of oral administration of Bifidobacterium breve for the prevention of rotavirus infections. Kansenshogaku Zasshi. 1999 Apr;73(4):305-10.

Araujo AC, Aprile LR, Dantas RO, Terra-Filho J, Vianna EO. Bronchial responsiveness during esophageal acid infusion. Lung. 2008 Mar-Apr;186(2):123-8. 2008 Feb 23.

Argento A, Tiraferri E, Marzaloni M. Oral anticoagulants and medicinal plants. An emerging interaction. Ann Ital Med Int. 2000 Apr-Jun;15(2):139-43.

Arif AA, Delclos GL, Colmer-Hamood J. Association between asthma, asthma symptoms and C-reactive protein in US adults: data from the National Health and Nutrition Examination Survey, 1999-2002. Respirology. 2007 Sep;12(5):675-82. .

Arif AA, Shah SM. Association between personal exposure to volatile organic compounds and asthma among US adult population. Int Arch Occup Environ Health. 2007 Aug;80(8):711-9.

Armas LA, Hollis BW, Heaney RP. Vitamin D2 is much less effective than vitamin D3 in humans. J Clin Endocrinol Metab. 2004 Nov;89(11):5387-91.

Armstrong B, Thériault G, Guénel P, Deadman J, Goldberg M, Héroux P. Association between exposure to pulsed electromagnetic fields and cancer in electric utility workers in Quebec, Canada, and France. Am J Epidemiol. 1994 Nov 1;140(9):805-20.

Armstrong BK, Kricker A. Sun exposure and non-Hodgkin lymphoma. Cancer Epidemiol Biomarkers Prev. 2007 Mar;16(3):396-400.

Armstrong BK. Absorption of vitamin B12 from the human colon. Am J Clin Nutr. 1968;21:298-9.

Armuzzi A, Cremonini F, Bartolozzi F, Canducci F, Candelli M, Ojetti V, Cammarota G, Anti M, De Lorenzo A, Pola P, Gasbarrini G, Gasbarrini A. The effect of oral administration of Lactobacillus GG on antibiotic-associated gastrointestinal side-effects during Helicobacter pylori eradication therapy. Aliment Pharmacol Ther. 2001 Feb;15(2):163-9.

Arora S, Aggarwal A, Singla P, Jyoti S, Tandon S. Anti-proliferative effects of homeopathic medicines on human kidney, colon and breast cancer cells. Homeopathy. 2013 Oct;102(4):274-82. doi: 10.1016/j.homp.2013.06.001.

Arrigo A, D'Angelo A. Achromycin and anaphylactic shock. Riv Patol Clin. 1959 Oct;14:719-22.

Arslanoglu S, Moro GE, Schmitt J, Tandoi L, Rizzardi S, Boehm G. Early dietary intervention with a mixture of prebiotic oligosaccharides reduces the incidence of allergic manifestations and infections during the first two years of life. J Nutr. 2008 Jun;138(6):1091-5.

Arterburn LM, Oken HA, Bailey Hall E, Hamersley J, Kuratko CN, Hoffman JP. Algal-oil capsules and cooked salmon: nutritionally equivalent sources of docosahexaenoic acid. J Am Diet Assoc. 2008 Jul;108(7):1204-9.

Arterburn LM, Oken HA, Hoffman JP, Bailey-Hall E, Chung G, Rom D, Hamersley J, McCarthy D. Bio-equivalence of Docosahexaenoic acid from different algal oils in capsules and in a DHA-fortified food. Lipids. 2007 Nov;42(11):1011-24.

Arunachalam K, Gill HS, Chandra RK. Enhancement of natural immune function by dietary consumption of Bifidobacterium lactis (HN019). Eur J Clin Nutr. 2000 Mar;54(3):263-7.

Arvola T, Laiho K, Torkkeli S, Mykkänen H, Salminen S, Maunula L, Isolauri E. Prophylactic Lactobacillus GG reduces antibiotic-associated diarrhea in children with respiratory infections: a randomized study. Pediatrics. 1999 Nov;104(5):e64.

Arya A, Achoui M, Cheah SC, Abdelwahab SI, Narrima P, Mohan S, Mustafa MR, Mohd MA. Chloroform Fraction of Centratherum anthelminticum (L.) Seed Inhibits Tumor Necrosis Factor Alpha and Exhibits Pleotropic Bioactivities: Inhibitory Role in Human Tumor Cells. Evid Based Complement Alternat Med. 2012;2012:627256.

Arya A, Cheah SC, Looi CY, Taha H, Mustafa MR, Mohd MA. The methanolic fraction of Centratherum anthelminticum seed downregulates pro-inflammatory cytokines, oxidative stress, and hyperglycemia in STZ-nicotinamide-induced type 2 diabetic rats. Food Chem Toxicol. 2012 Nov;50(11):4209-20.

Arya A, Looi CY, Cheah SC, Mustafa MR, Mohd MA. Anti-diabetic effects of Centratherum anthelminticum seeds methanolic fraction on pancreatic cells, β-TC6 and its alleviating role in type 2 diabetic rats. J Ethnopharmacol. 2012 Oct 31;144(1):22-32.

Asakawa Y, Ludwiczuk A, Harinantenaina L, Toyota M, Nishiki M, Bardon A, Nii K. Distribution of dri-mane sesquiterpenoids and tocopherols in liverworts, ferns and higher plants: Polygonaceae, Canellaceae and Winteraceae species. Nat Prod Commun. 2012 Jun;7(6):685-92.

Ashok P, Koti BC, Thippeswamy AH, Tikare VP, Dabadi P, Viswanathaswamy AH. Evaluation of Antiin-flammatory Activity of Centratherum anthelminticum (L) Kuntze Seed. Indian J Pharm Sci. 2010 Nov;72(6):697-703.

Ashrafi K, Chang FY, Watts JL, Fraser AG, Kamath RS, Ahringer J, Ruvkun G. Genome-wide RNAi analysis of Caenorhabditis elegans fat regulatory genes. Nature. 2003 Jan 16;421(6920):268-72.

Asimov I. The Chemicals of Life. New York: Signet, 1954.

Askeland D. The Science and Engineering of Materials. Boston: PWS, 1994.

Aso Y, Akaza H, Kotake T, Tsukamoto T, Imai K, Naito S. Preventive effect of a Lactobacillus casei preparation on the recurrence of superficial bladder cancer in a double-blind trial. The BLP Study Group. Eur Urol. 1995;27(2):104-9.

Aso Y, Akazan H. Prophylactic effect of a Lactobacillus casei preparation on the recurrence of superficial bladder cancer. BLP Study Group. Urol Int. 1992;49(3):125-9.

Aspect A, Grangier P, Roger G. Experimental Realization of Einstein-Podolsky-Rosen-Bohm Gedankenexperiment: A New Violation of Bell's Inequalities. Physical Review Letters. 1982;49(2): 91-94.

Ataie-Jafari A, Larijani B, Alavi Majd H, Tahbaz F. Cholesterol-lowering effect of probiotic yogurt in comparison with ordinary yogurt in mildly to moderately hypercholesterolemic subjects. Ann Nutr Metab. 2009;54(1):22-7.

Atkinson W, Harris J, Mills P, Moffat S, White C, Lynch O, Jones M, Cullinan P, Newman Taylor AJ. Domestic aeroallergen exposures among infants in an English town. Eur Respir J. 1999 Mar;13(3):583-9.

Aton SJ, Colwell CS, Harmar AJ, Waschek J, Herzog ED. Vasoactive intestinal polypeptide mediates circadian rhythmicity and synchrony in mammalian clock neurons. Nat Neurosci. 2005 Apr;8(4):476-83.

Atsumi T, Tonosaki K. Smelling lavender and rosemary increases free radical scavenging activity and decreases cortisol level in saliva. Psychiatry Res. 2007 Feb 28;150(1):89-96.

Attia M, Essa EA, Zaki RM, Elkordy AA. An Overview of the Antioxidant Effects of Ascorbic Acid and Alpha Lipoic Acid (in Liposomal Forms) as Adjuvant in Cancer Treatment. Antioxidants (Basel). 2020 Apr 25;9(5):359. doi: 10.3390/antiox9050359.

Autier P, Boniol M, Pizot C, Mullie P. Vitamin D status and ill health: A systematic review. Lancet Diab Endo. 2014; 2(1):76-89 doi:10.1016/S2213-8587(13)70165-7

Autier P, Gandini S, Mullie P. A systematic review: influence of vitamin D supplementation on serum 25-hydroxyvitamin D concentration. J Clin Endocrinol Metab. 2012 Aug;97(8):2606-13. doi: 10.1210/jc.2012-1238.

Autier P, Gandini S. Vitamin D supplementation and total mortality: a meta-analysis of randomized controlled trials. Arch Intern Med. 2007 Sep 10;167(16):1730-7.

Auyeung KK, Han QB, Ko JK. Astragalus membranaceus: A Review of its Protection Against Inflammation and Gastrointestinal Cancers. Am J Chin Med. 2016;44(1):1-22. doi: 10.1142/S0192415X16500014. PMID: 26916911.

Avtanski DB, Nagalingam A, Kuppusamy P, Bonner MY, Arbiser JL, Saxena NK, Sharma D. Honokiol abrogates leptin-induced tumor progression by inhibiting Wnt1-MTA1-β-catenin signaling axis in a microRNA-34a dependent manner. Oncotarget. 2015 Apr 15.

Axelson M. 25-Hydroxyvitamin D3 3-sulphate is a major circulating form of vitamin D in man. FEBS Lett. 1985 Oct 28;191(2):171-5.

Aydin S, Bacanli M, Taner G, Sahin T, Basaran A, Basaran N. Protective effects of resveratrol on sepsis-induced DNA damage in the lymphocytes of rats. Hum Exp Toxicol. 2012 Nov 15.

Azar JA, Conroy T. Measuring the effectiveness of horticultural therapy at a veterans administration medical center: experimental design issues. In Relf, D. (ed) The Role of Horticulture in Human Well-Being and Social Development: A National Symposium. Portland: Timber Press. 1992:169-171.

Azar JA, Conroy T. Measuring the effectiveness of horticultural therapy at a veterans administration medical center: experimental design issues. In Relf, D. (ed) The Role of Horticulture in Human Well-Being and Social Development: A National Symposium. Portland: Timber Press. 1992:169-171.

Bachmann KA, Sullivan TJ, Jauregui L, Reese J, Miller K, Levine L. Drug interactions of H2-receptor antagonists. Scand J Gastroenterol Suppl. 1994;206:14-9.

Bacopoulou F, Veltsista A, Vassi I, Gika A, Lekea V, Priftis K, Bakoula C. Can we be optimistic about asthma in childhood? A Greek cohort study. J Asthma. 2009 Mar;46(2):171-4.

Badar VA, Thawani VR, Wakode PT, Shrivastava MP, Gharpure KJ, Hingorani LL, Khiyani RM. Efficacy of Tinospora cordifolia in allergic rhinitis. J Ethnopharmacol. 2005 Jan 15;96(3):445-9.

Bae GS, Kim MS, Jung WS, Seo SW, Yun SW, Kim SG, Park RK, Kim EC, Song HJ, Park SJ. Inhibition of lipopolysaccharide-induced inflammatory responses by piperine. Eur J Pharmacol. 2010 Sep 10;642(1-3):154-62.

Bae JM, Kim EH. Dietary intakes of citrus fruit and risk of gastric cancer incidence: an adaptive meta-analysis of cohort studies. Epidemiol Health. 2016 Jul 25;38:e2016034.

Baginski C. Organic dairy industry wins battle against Ohio labeling rule. Newhope360. 2011 Nov 1

Bai AP, Ouyang Q, Xiao XR, Li SF. Probiotics modulate inflammatory cytokine secretion from inflamed mucosa in active ulcerative colitis. Int J Clin Pract. 2006 Mar;60(3):284-8.

Bai H, Yu P, Yu M. Effect of electroacununcture on sex hormone levels in patients with Sjogren's syndrome. Zhen Ci Yan Jiu. 2007;32(3):203-6.

Baik HW. Nutritional therapy in gastrointestinal disease. Korean J Gastroenterol. 2004 Jun;43(6):331-40.

Bailey DP, Locke CD. Breaking up prolonged sitting with light-intensity walking improves postprandial glycemia, but breaking up sitting with standing does not. J Sci Med Sport. 2015 May;18(3):294-8. doi: 10.1016/j.jsams.2014.03.008.

Baker DW. An introduction to the theory and practice of German electroacupuncture and accompanying medications. Am J Acupunct. 1984;12:327-332.

Baker SM. Detoxification and Healing. Chicago: Contemporary Books, 2004.

Balch P, Balch J. Prescription for Nutritional Healing. New York: Avery, 2000.

Baliga MS, Jimmy R, Thilakchand KR, Sunitha V, Bhat NR, Saldanha E, Rao S, Rao P, Arora R, Palatty PL. Ocimum sanctum L (Holy Basil or Tulsi) and its phytochemicals in the prevention and treatment of cancer. Nutr Cancer. 2013;65 Suppl 1:26-35. doi: 10.1080/01635581.2013.785010.

Baliga MS, Rao S, Rai MP, D'souza P. Radio protective effects of the Ayurvedic medicinal plant Ocimum sanctum Linn. (Holy Basil): A memoir. J Cancer Res Ther. 2016 Jan-Mar;12(1):20-7. doi: 10.4103/0973-1482.151422. PMID: 27072205.

Balimane P, Yong-Haen H, Chong S. Current Industrial Practices of Assessing Permeability and P-Glycoprotein Interaction. J AAPS 2006; 8(1).

Ballentine R. Diet & Nutrition: A holistic approach. Honesdale, PA: Himalayan Int., 1978.

Ballentine R. Radical Healing. New York: Harmony Books, 1999.

Balli F, Bertolani P, Giberti G, Amarri S. High-dose oral bacteria-therapy for chronic non-specific diarrhea of infancy. Pediatr Med Chir. 1992 Jan-Feb;14(1):13-5.

Bamford JT, Ray S, Musekiwa A, van Gool C, Humphreys R, Ernst E. Oral evening primrose oil and borage oil for eczema. Cochrane Database Syst Rev. 2013 Apr 30;(4):CD004416. doi: 10.1002/14651858.CD004416.pub2.

Banno N, Akihisa T, Yasukawa K, Tokuda H, Tabata K, Nakamura Y, Nishimura R, Kimura Y, Suzuki T. Anti-inflammatory activities of the triterpene acids from the resin of Boswellia carteri. J Ethnopharmacol. 2006 Sep 19;107(2):249-53.

Bano S, Siddiqui BS, Farooq AD, Begum S, Siddiqui F, Kashif M, Azhar M. In vitro growth inhibition and cytotoxicity of Euphorbia caducifolia against four human cancer cell lines and its phytochemical characterisation. Nat Prod Res. 2017 Apr 1-5. doi: 10.1080/14786419.2017.1305380.

Bant A, Kruszewski J. Increased sensitization prevalence to common inhalant and food allergens in young adult Polish males. Ann Agric Environ Med. 2008 Jun;15(1):21-7.

Banyo T. The role of electrical neuromodulation in the therapy of chronic lower urinary tract dysfunction. Ideggyogy Sz. 2003 Jan 20;56(1-2):68-71.

Bao P-P, Shu X-O, Zheng Y, Cai H, Ruan Z-X, et al.: Fruit, vegetable, and animal food intake and breast cancer risk by hormone receptor status. Nutr Cancer 64, 806–819, 2012.

Bao Y, Hu FB, Giovannucci EL, Wolpin BM, Stampfer MJ, Willett WC, Fuchs CS. Nut consumption and risk of pancreatic cancer in women. Br J Cancer. 2013 Oct 22. doi: 10.1038/bjc.2013.665.

Barabás J, Németh Z. A Magyar Arc-, Allcsont. Recommendation of the Hungarian Society for Face, Mandible and Oral Surgery in the indication of supportive therapy with Avemar. Orv Hetil. 2006 Sep 3;147(35):1709-11.

Baran D, Apostol I. Signification of biorhythms for human performance assessment. Rev Med Chir Soc Med Nat Iasi. 2007 Jan-Mar;111(1):295-302.

Baranauskas G, Nistri A. Sensitization of pain pathways in the spinal cord: cellular mechanisms. Prog Neurobiol. 1998 Feb;54(3):349-65.

Barbeito CG, Ortega HH, Matiller V, Gimeno EJ, Salvetti NR. Lectin-binding pattern in ovarian structures of rats with experimental polycystic ovaries. Reprod Domest Anim. 2013 Oct;48(5):850-7. doi: 10.1111/rda.12174.

Barbieri A, Quagliariello V, Del Vecchio V, Falco M, Luciano A, Amruthraj NJ, Nasti G, Ottaiano A, Berretta M, Iaffaioli RV, Arra C. Anticancer and Anti-Inflammatory Properties of Ganoderma lucidum Extract Effects on Melanoma and Triple-Negative Breast cancer Treatment. Nutrients. 2017 Feb 28;9(3). pii: E210. doi: 10.3390/nu9030210.

Barnett AG, Williams GM, Schwartz J, Neller AH, Best TL, Petroeschevsky AL, Simpson RW. Air pollution and child respiratory health: a case-crossover study in Australia and New Zealand. Am J Respir Crit Care Med. 2005 Jun 1;171(11):1272-8.

Baron M. A patented strain of Bacillus coagulans increased immune response to viral challenge. Postgrad Med. 2009 Mar;121(2):114-8.

Baron RA. Effects of negative ions on interpersonal attraction: evidence for intensification. J Pers Soc Psychol. 1987 Mar;52(3):547-53.

Barone A, Giusti A, Pioli G, Girasole G, Razzano M, Pizzonia M, Palummeri E, Bianchi G. Secondary hyperparathyroidism due to hypovitaminosis D affects bone mineral density response to alendronate in elderly women with osteoporosis. J Am Geriatr Soc. 2007 May;55(5):752-7.

REFERENCES AND BIBLIOGRAPHY

Barrager E, Veltmann JR Jr, Schauss AG, Schiller RN. A multicentered, open-label trial on the safety and efficacy of methylsulfonylmethane in the treatment of seasonal allergic rhinitis. J Altern Complement Med. 2002 Apr;8(2):167-73.

Barron M. Light exposure, melatonin secretion, and menstrual cycle parameters: an integrative review. Biol Res Nurs. 2007 Jul;9(1):49-69.

Barton DL, Liu H, Dakhil SR, Linquist B, Sloan JA, Nichols CR, McGinn TW, Stella PJ, Seeger GR, Sood A, Loprinzi CL. Wisconsin Ginseng (Panax quinquefolius) to improve cancer-related fatigue: a randomized, double-blind trial, N07C2. J Natl Cancer Inst. 2013 Aug 21;105(16):1230-8. doi: 10.1093/jnci/djt181.

Bartram HP, Scheppach W, Gerlach S, Ruckdeschel G, Kelber E, Kasper H. Does yogurt enriched with Bifidobacterium longum affect colonic microbiology and fecal metabolites in health subjects? Am J Clin Nutr. 1994 Feb;59(2):428-32.

Bastide M, Doucet-Jaboeuf M, Daurat V. Activity and chronopharmacology of very low doses of physiological immune inducers. Immun Today. 1985;6: 234-235.

Bastide M. Immunological examples on ultra high dilution research. In: Endler P, Schulte J (eds.): Ultra High Dilution. Physiology and Physics. Dordrech: Kluwer Academic Publishers, 1994:27-34.

Basu A, Devaraj S, Jialal I. Dietary factors that promote or retard inflammation. Arterioscler Thromb Vasc Biol. 2006 May;26(5):995-1001.

Basu S, Chatterjee M, Ganguly S, Chandra PK. Effect of Lactobacillus rhamnosus GG in persistent diarrhea in Indian children: a randomized controlled trial. J Clin Gastroenterol. 2007 Sep;41(8):756-60.

Basu S, Chatterjee M, Ganguly S, Chandra PK. Efficacy of Lactobacillus rhamnosus GG in acute watery diarrhoea of Indian children: a randomised controlled trial. J Paediatr Child Health. 2007 Dec;43(12):837-42.

Bateman B, Warner JO, Hutchinson E, Dean T, Rowlandson P, Gant C, Grundy J, Fitzgerald C, Stevenson J. The effects of a double blind, placebo controlled, artificial food colourings and benzoate preservative challenge on hyperactivity in a general population sample of preschool children. Arch Dis Child. 2004 Jun;89(6):506-11.

Bates DW, Cullen DJ, Laird N, Petersen LA, Small SD, Servi D, Laffel G, Sweitzer BJ, Shea BF, Hallisey R, et al. Incidence of adverse drug events and potential adverse drug events. Implications for prevention. ADE Prevention Study Group. JAMA. 1995 Jul 5;274(1):29-34.

Batmanghelidj F. Neurotransmitter histamine: an alternative view point, Science in Medicine Simplified. Falls Church, VA: Foundation for the Simple in Medicine, 1990.

Batmanghelidj F. Pain: a need for paradigm change. Anticancer Res. 1987 Sep-Oct;7(5B):971-89.

Batmanghelidj F. Your Body's Many Cries for Water. 2nd Ed. Vienna, VA: Global Health, 1997.

Baudry J, Assmann KE, Touvier M, Allès B, Seconda L, Latino-Martel P, Ezzedine K, Galan P, Hercberg S, Lairon D, Kesse-Guyot E. Association of Frequency of Organic Food Consumption With Cancer Risk Findings From the NutriNet-Santé Prospective Cohort Study. JAMA Intern Med. Published online October 22, 2018. doi:10.1001/jamainternmed.2018.4357.

Baur JA, Pearson KJ, Price NL, Jamieson HA, Lerin C, Kalra A, Prabhu VV, Allard JS, Lopez-Lluch G, Lewis K, Pistell PJ, Poosala S, Becker KG, Boss O, Gwinn D, Wang M, Ramaswamy S, Fishbein KW, Spencer RG, Lakatta EG, Le Couteur D, Shaw RJ, Navas P, Puigserver P, Ingram DK, de Cabo R, Sinclair DA. Resveratrol improves health and survival of mice on a high-calorie diet. Nature. 2006 Nov 16;444(7117):337-42.

Bayet-Robert M, Kwiatkowski F, Leheurteur M, Gachon F, Planchat E, Abrial C, Mouret-Reynier MA, Durando X, Barthomeuf C, Chollet P. Phase I dose escalation trial of docetaxel plus curcumin in patients with advanced and metastatic breast cancer. Cancer Biol Ther. 2010 Jan;9(1):8-14.

Beasley R, Clayton T, Crane J, von Mutius E, Lai CK, Montefort S, Stewart A; ISAAC Phase Three Study Group. Association between paracetamol use in infancy and childhood, and risk of asthma, rhinoconjunctivitis, and eczema in children aged 6-7 years: analysis from Phase Three of the ISAAC programme. Lancet. 2008 Sep. 20;372(9643):1039-48.

Beaulieu A, Fessele K. Agent Orange: management of patients exposed in Vietnam. Clin J Oncol Nurs. 2003 May-Jun;7(3):320-3.

Beausoleil M, Fortier N, Guénette S, L'ecuyer A, Savoie M, Franco M, Lachaine J, Weiss K. Effect of a fermented milk combining Lactobacillus acidophilus Cl1285 and Lactobacillus casei in the prevention of antibiotic-associated diarrhea: a randomized, double-blind, placebo-controlled trial. Can J Gastroenterol. 2007 Nov;21(11):732-6.

Beaver LM, Löhr CV, Clarke JD, Glasser ST, Watson GW, Wong CP, Zhang Z, Williams DE, Dashwood RH, Shannon J, Thuillier P, Ho E. Broccoli Sprouts Delay Prostate Cancer Formation and Decrease Prostate Cancer Severity with a Concurrent Decrease in HDAC3 Protein Expression in Transgenic Adenocarcinoma of the Mouse Prostate (TRAMP) Mice. Curr Dev Nutr. 2017 Dec 26;2(3):nzy002. doi: 10.1093/cdn/nzy002.

Becker KG, Simon RM, Bailey-Wilson JE, Freidlin B, Biddison WE, McFarland HF, Trent JM. Clustering of non-major histocompatibility complex susceptibility candidate loci in human autoimmune diseases. Proc Natl Acad Sci U S A. 1998 Aug 18;95(17):9979-84.

Becker R. Cross Currents. Los Angeles: Tarcher, 1990.

Becker R. The Body Electric. New York: Morrow, Inc., 1985.

Beckerman H, Becher J, Lankhorst GJ. The effectiveness of vibratory stimulation in anejaculatory men with spinal cord injury. Paraplegia. 1993 Nov;31(11):689-99.

Beddoe AF. Biologic Ionization as Applied to Human Nutrition. Warsaw: Wendell Whitman, 2002.

Beecher GR. Phytonutrients' role in metabolism: effects on resistance to degenerative processes. Nutr Rev. 1999 Sep;57(9 Pt 2):S3-6.

Beekwilder J, Hall RD, de Vos CH. Identification and dietary relevance of antioxidants from raspberry. Biofactors. 2005;23(4):197-205.

Beeson, C. The moon and plant growth. Nature. 1946;158:572–3.

Behin A, Hoang-Xuan K, Carpentier AF, Delattre JY. Primary brain tumours in adults. Lancet. 2003 Jan 25;361(9354):323-31.

Belcaro G, Cesarone MR, Errichi S, Zulli C, Errichi BM, Vinciguerra G, Ledda A, Di Renzo A, Stuard S, Dugall M, Pellegrini L, Gizzi G, Ippolito E, Ricci A, Cacchio M, Cipollone G, Ruffini I, Fano F, Hosoi M, Rohdewald P. Variations in C-reactive protein, plasma free radicals and fibrinogen values in patients with osteoarthritis treated with Pycnogenol. Redox Rep. 2008;13(6):271-6.

Bell B, Defouw R. Concerning a lunar modulation of geomagnetic activity. J Geophys Res. 1964;69:3169-3174.

Bell IR, Baldwin CM, Schwartz GE, Illness from low levels of environmental chemicals: relevance to chronic fatigue syndrome and fibromyalgia. Am J Med. 1998;105 (suppl 3A).:74-82. S.

Ben, X.M., Zhou, X.Y., Zhao, W.H., Yu, W.L., Pan, W., Zhang, W.L., Wu, S.M., Van Beusekom, C.M., Schaafsma, A. (2004) Supplementation of milk formula with galactooligosaccharides improves intestinal micro-flora and fermentation in term infants. Chin Med J. 117(6):927-931, 2004.

Benatuil L, Apitz-Castro R, Romano E. Ajoene inhibits the activation of human endothelial cells induced by porcine cells: implications for xenotransplantation. Xenotransplantation. 2003 Jul;10(4):368-73.

Benedetti F, Radaelli D, Bernasconi A, Dallaspezia S, Falini A, Scotti G, Lorenzi C, Colombo C, Smeraldi E. Clock genes beyond the clock: CLOCK genotype biases neural correlates of moral valence decision in depressed patients. Genes Brain Behav. 2007 Mar 26.

Bengmark S. Curcumin, an atoxic antioxidant and natural NFkappaB, cyclooxygenase-2, lipooxygenase, and inducible nitric oxide synthase inhibitor: a shield against acute and chronic diseases. JPEN J Parenter Enteral Nutr. 2006 Jan-Feb;30(1):45-51.

Bengmark S. Immunonutrition: role of biosurfactants, fiber, and probiotic bacteria. Nutrition. 1998 Jul-Aug;14(7-8):585-94.

Bennet LW, Cardone S, Jarczyk J. Effects of therapeutic camping program on addiction recovery. Journal of Substance Abuse Treatment. 1998;15(5):469-474.

Bennett GJ, Update on the neurophysiology of pain transmission and modulation: focus on the NMDA-receptor. J Pain Symptom Manage. 2000;19 (suppl 1):S.:2-6.

Bennett WD, Zeman KL, Jarabek AM. Nasal contribution to breathing and fine particle deposition in children versus adults. J Toxicol Environ Health A. 2008;71(3):227-37.

Benor D. Healing Research. Volume 1. Munich, Germany: Helix Verlag, 1992.

Bensky D, Gable A, Kaptchuk T (transl.). Chinese Herbal Medicine Materia Medica. Seattle: Eastland Press, 1986.

Bensky D, Gable A, Kaptchuk T (transl.). Chinese Herbal Medicine Materia Medica. Seattle: Eastland Press, 1986.

Benson VS, Pirie K, Schüz J, Reeves GK, Beral V, Green J; Million Women Study Collaborators. Mobile phone use and risk of brain neoplasms and other cancers: prospective study. Int J Epidemiol. 2013 Jun;42(3):792-802. doi:10.1093/ije/dyt072.

Bentley E. Awareness: Biorhythms, Sleep and Dreaming. London: Routledge, 2000.

Benveniste J. Meta-analysis of homoeopathy trials. Lancet. 1998 Jan 31;351(9099):367.

Bergman M, Levin GS, Bessler H, Djaldetti M, Salman H. Resveratrol affects the cross talk between immune and colon cancer cells. Biomed Pharmacother. 2012 Nov 15.

Bergner P. The Healing Power of Garlic. Prima Publishing, Rocklin CA 1996.

Berin MC, Yang PC, Ciok L, Waserman S, Perdue MH. Role for IL-4 in macromolecular transport across human intestinal epithelium. Am J Physiol. 1999 May;276(5 Pt 1):C1046-52.

Berk M, Dodd S, Henry M. Do ambient electromagnetic fields affect behaviour? A demonstration of the relationship between geomagnetic storm activity and suicide. Bioelectromagnetics. 2006 Feb;27(2):151-5.

Berk M, Dodd S, Henry M. Do ambient electromagnetic fields affect behaviour? A demonstration of the relationship between geomagnetic storm activity and suicide. Bioelectromagnetics. 2006 Feb;27(2):151-5.

Berkow R., (Ed.) The Merck Manual of Diagnosis and Therapy. 16th Edition. Rahway, N.J.: Merck Research Labs, 1992.

Berman S, Fein G, Jewett D, Ashford F. Luminance-controlled pupil size affects Landolt C task performance. J Illumin Engng Soc. 1993;22:150-165.

Berman S, Jewett D, Fein G, Saika G, Ashford F. Photopic luminance does not always predict perceived room brightness. Light Resch and Techn. 1990;22:37-41.

Bernardi D, Dini FL, Azzarelli A, Giaconi A, Volterrani C, Lunardi M. Sudden cardiac death rate in an area characterized by high incidence of coronary artery disease and low hardness of drinking water. Angiology. 1995;46:145-149.

Berry J. Work efficiency and mood states of electronic assembly workers exposed to full-spectrum and conventional fluorescent illumination. Diss Abstr Internl. 1983;44:635B.

Berseth CL, Mitmesser SH, Ziegler EE, Marunycz JD, Vanderhoof J. Tolerance of a standard intact protein formula versus a partially hydrolyzed formula in healthy, term infants. Nutr J. 2009 Jun 19;8:27.

Berteau O and Mulloy B. 2003. Sulfated fucans, fresh perspectives: structures, functions, and biological properties of sulfated fucans and an overview of enzymes active toward this class of polysaccharide. Glycobiology. Jun;13(6):29R-40R.

Bertin G. Spiral Structure in Galaxies: A Density Wave Theory. Cambridge: MIT Press, 1996.

Besset A, Espa F, Dauvilliers Y, Billiard M, de Seze R. No effect on cognitive function from daily mobile phone use. Bioelectromagnetics. 2005 Feb;26(2):102-8.

Bevan R, Young C, Holmes P, Fortunato L, Slack R, Rushton L; British Occupational Cancer Burden Study Group. Occupational cancer in Britain. Gastrointestinal cancers: liver, oesophagus, pancreas and stomach. Br J Cancer. 2012 Jun 19;107 Suppl 1:S33-40. doi: 10.1038/bjc.2012.116.

Bhattacharjee C, Bradley P, Smith M, Scally A, Wilson B. Do animals bite more during a full moon? BMJ. 2000 December 23; 321(7276): 1559-1561.

Bickham DS, Rich M. Is television viewing associated with social isolation? Roles of exposure time, viewing context, and violent content. Arch Pediatr Adolesc Med. 2006 Apr;160(4):387-92.

Bindslev-Jensen C, Skov PS, Roggen EL, Hvass P, Brinch DS. Investigation on possible allergenicity of 19 different commercial enzymes used in the food industry. Food Chem Toxicol. 2006 Nov;44(11):1909-15.

Binkley N, Wiebe D. Clinical controversies in vitamin D: 25(OH)D measurement, target concentration, and supplementation. J Clin Densitom. 2013 Oct-Dec;16(4):402-8. doi: 10.1016/j.jocd.2013.08.006.Grad B. A telekinetic effect on plant growth: II. Experiments involving treatment of saline in stoppered bottles. Internl J Parapsychol. 1964;6:473-478, 484-488.

Bin-Nun A, Bromiker R, Wilschanski M, Kaplan M, Rudensky B, Caplan M, Hammerman C. Oral probiotics prevent necrotizing enterocolitis in very low birth weight neonates. J Pediatr. 2005 Aug;147(2):192-6.

Birch EE, Khoury JC, Berseth CL, Castañeda YS, Couch JM, Bean J, Tamer R, Harris CL, Mitmesser SH, Scalabrin DM. The impact of early nutrition on incidence of allergic manifestations and common respiratory illnesses in children. J Pediatr. 2010 Jun;156(6):902-6, 906.e1. 2010 Mar 15.

Biro FM, Galvez MP, Greenspan LC, Succop PA, Vangeepuram N, Pinney SM, Teitelbaum S, Windham GC, Kushi LH, Wolff MS. Pubertal assessment method and baseline characteristics in a mixed longitudinal study of girls. Pediatrics. 2010 Sep;126(3):e583-90.

Bishayee K, Mondal J, Sikdar S, Khuda-Bukhsh AR. Condurango (Gonolobus condurango) Extract Activates Fas Receptor and Depolarizes Mitochondrial Membrane Potential to Induce ROS-dependent Apoptosis in Cancer Cells in vitro: CE-treatment on HeLa: a ROS-dependent mechanism. J Pharmacopuncture. 2015 Sep;18(3):32-41. doi: 10.3831/KPI.2015.18.022.

Bishop B. Pain: its physiology and rationale for management. Part III. Consequences of current concepts of pain mechanisms related to pain management. Phys Ther. 1980 Jan;60(1):24-37.

Bishop ID, Rohrmann B. Subjective responses to simulated and real environments: a comparison. Landscape and Urban Planning. 2003;65(4):261-277.

Bishop KS, Kao CH, Xu Y, Glucina MP, Paterson RR, Ferguson LR. Ganoderma lucidum recent developments in nutraceuticals. Phytochemistry. 2015 Jun;114:56-65. doi: 10.1016/j.phytochem.2015.02.015.

Bisset N.. Herbal Drugs and Phytopharmaceuticals. Stuttgart: CRC, 1994.

Biswas J, Sinha D, Mukherjee S, Roy S, Siddiqi M, Roy M. Curcumin protects DNA damage in a chronically arsenic-exposed population of West Bengal. Hum Exp Toxicol. 2010 Jun;29(6):513-24. doi: 10.1177/0960327109359020.

Bitbol M, Luisi PL. Autopoiesis with or without cognition: defining life at its edge. J R Soc Interface. 2004 Nov 22;1(1):99-107.

Bjarnason I, MacPherson A, Hollander D. Intestinal permeability: an overview. Gastroenterology. 1995 May;108(5):1566-81.

Black HS. Influence of dietary factors on actinically-induced skin cancer. Mut Res. 1998 Nov 9;422(1):185-90.

Blackhall K, Appleton S, Cates FJ. Ionisers for chronic asthma. Cochrane Database Syst Rev 2003;(3):CD002986.

Blackley, CH. Experimental Researchers on the Causes and Nature of Catarrhus Aestivus (Hay Fever or Hay-Asthma). London, 1873.

Blackman CF, Benane SG, House DE, Pollock MM. Action of 50 Hz magnetic fields on neurite outgrowth in pheochromocytoma cells. Bioelectromagnetics. 1993;14(3):273-86.

Blanquer-Rosselló MM, Oliver J, Valle A, Roca P. Effect of xanthohumol and 8-prenylnaringenin on MCF-7 breast cancer cells oxidative stress and mitochondrial complexes expression. J Cell Biochem. 2013 Dec;114(12):2785-94. doi: 10.1002/jcb.24627.

Bliakher MS, Fedorova IM, Lopatina TK, Arkhipov SN, Kapustin IV, Ramazanova ZK, Karpova NV, Ivanov VA, Sharapov NV. Acilact and improvement of the health status of sickly children. Vestn Ross Akad Med Nauk. 2005;(12):32-5.

Blood AJ, Zatorre RJ, Bermudez P, Evans AC. Emotional responses to pleasant and unpleasant music correlate with activity in paralimbic brain regions. Nat Neurosci. 1999;2:382-7.

Blumenthal M (ed.) The Complete German Commission E Monographs. Boston: Amer Botan Council, 1998.

Blumenthal M, Brinckmann J, Goldberg A (eds). Herbal Medicine: Expanded Commission E Monographs. Newton, MA: Integrative Med., 2000.

Bobe G, Sansbury LB, Albert PS, Cross AJ, Kahle L, Ashby J, Slattery ML, Caan B, Paskett E, Iber F, Kikendall JW, Lance P, Daston C, Marshall JR, Schatzkin A, Lanza E. Dietary flavonoids and colorectal adenoma recurrence in the Polyp Prevention Trial. Cancer Epidemiol Biomarkers Prev. 2008 Jun;17(6):1344-53.

Bockemühl, J. Towards a Phenomenology of the Etheric World. New York: Anthroposophical Press, 1985.

Bode C, Bode JC. Effect of alcohol consumption on the gut. Best Pract Res Clin Gastroenterol. 2003 Aug;17(4):575-92.

Bodinier M, Legoux MA, Pineau F, Triballeau S, Segain JP, Brossard C, Denery-Papini S. Intestinal translocation capabilities of wheat allergens using the Caco-2 cell line. J Agric Food Chem. 2007 May 30;55(11):4576-83.

Bodnar L, Simhan H. The prevalence of preterm birth varies by season of last menstrual period. Am J Obst and Gyn. 2003;195(6):S211-S211.

Boehm, G., Lidestri, M., Casetta, P., Jelinek, J., Negretti, F., Stahl, B., Martini, A. (2002) Supplementation of a bovine milk formula with an oligosaccharide mixture increases counts of faecal bifidobacteria in preterm infants. Arch Dis Child Fetal Neonatal Ed. 86: F178-F181

Bogdanich W and McGinty JC. Medicare Claims Show Overuse for CT Scanning. NY Times. June 7, 2011.

Bohay RN, Bencak J, Kavaliers M, Maclean D. A survey of magnetic fields in the dental operatory. J Can Dent Assoc. 1994 Sep;60(9):835-40.

Boivin DB, Czeisler CA. Resetting of circadian melatonin and cortisol rhythms in humans by ordinary room light. Neuroreport. 1998 Mar 30;9(5):779-82.

Boivin DB, Duffy JF, Kronauer RE, Czeisler CA. Dose-response relationships for resetting of human circadian clock by light. Nature. 1996 Feb 8;379(6565):540-2.

Bonfils P, Halimi P, Malinvaud D. Adrenal suppression and osteoporosis after treatment of nasal polyposis. Acta Otolaryngol. 2006 Dec;126(11):1195-200.

Bongaerts GP, Severijnen RS. Preventive and curative effects of probiotics in atopic patients. Med Hypotheses. 2005;64(6):1089-92.

Bongartz D, Hesse A. Selective extraction of quercetrin in vegetable drugs and urine by off-line coupling of boronic acid affinity chromatography and high-performance liquid chromatography. J Chromatogr B Biomed Appl. 1995 Nov 17;673(2):223-30.

Bonsignore MR, La Grutta S, Cibella F, Scichilone N, Cuttitta G, Interrante A, Marchese M, Veca M, Virzi' M, Bonanno A, Profita M, Morici G. Effects of exercise training and montelukast in children with mild asthma. Med Sci Sports Exerc. 2008 Mar;40(3):405-12.

Boray P, Gifford R, Rosenblood L. Effects of warm white, cool white and full-spectrum fluorescent lighting on simple cognitive performance, mood and ratings of others. J Environl Psychol. 1989;9:297-308.

Borchers AT, Hackman RM, Keen CL, Stern JS, Gershwin ME. Complementary medicine: a review of immunomodulatory effects of Chinese herbal medicines. Am J Clin Nutr. 1997 Dec;66(6):1303-12.

Borchert VE, Czyborra P, Fetscher C, Goepel M, Michel MC. Extracts from Rhois aromatica and Solidaginis virgaurea inhibit rat and human bladder contraction. Naunyn Schmiedebergs Arch Pharmacol. 2004 Mar;369(3):281-6.

Borresen EC, Brown DG, Harbison G, Taylor L, Fairbanks A, O'Malia J, Bazan M, Rao S, Bailey SM, Wdowik M, Weir TL, Brown RJ, Ryan EP. A Randomized Controlled Trial to Increase Navy Bean or Rice Bran Consumption in Colorectal Cancer Survivors. Nutr Cancer. 2016 Nov-Dec;68(8):1269-1280.

Boscoe FP, Schymura MJ. Solar ultraviolet-B exposure and cancer incidence and mortality in the United States, 1993-2002. BMC Cancer. 2006 Nov 10;6:264.

Bose J. Response in the Living and Non-Living. New York: Longmans, Green & Co., 1902.

Bossi P, Cortinovis D, Fatigoni S, Cossu Rocca M, Fabi A, Seminara P, Ripamonti C, Alfieri S, Granata R, Bergamini C, Agustoni F, Bidoli P, Nolè F, Pessi MA, Macchi F, Michellini L, Montanaro F, Roila F. A randomized, double-blind, placebo-controlled, multicenter study of a Ginger extract in the management of chemotherapy-induced nausea and vomiting (CINV) in patients receiving high-dose cisplatin. Ann Oncol. 2017 Oct 1;28(10):2547-2551. doi: 10.1093/annonc/mdx315.

Bottorff JL. The use and meaning of touch in caring for patients with cancer. Oncol Nurs Forum. 1993 Nov-Dec;20(10):1531-8.

Bouchez-Mahiout I, Pecquet C, Kerre S, Snégaroff J, Raison-Peyron N, Laurière M. High molecular weight entities in industrial wheat protein hydrolysates are immunoreactive with IgE from allergic patients. J Agric Food Chem. 2010 Apr 14;58(7):4207-15.

Bougault V, Turmel J, Boulet LP. Bronchial challenges and respiratory symptoms in elite swimmers and winter sport athletes: Airway hyperresponsiveness in asthma: its measurement and clinical significance. Chest. 2010 Aug;138(2 Suppl):31S-37S. 2010 Apr 2.

Bouvard V, Loomis D, Guyton KZ, Grosse Y, Ghissassi FE, Benbrahim-Tallaa L, Guha N, Mattock H, Straif K; International Agency for Research on Cancer Monograph Working Group. Carcinogenicity of consumption of red and processed meat. Lancet Oncol. 2015 Dec;16(16):1599-600. doi: 10.1016/S1470-2045(15)00444-1.

Boyce P, Rea M. A field evaluation of full-spectrum, polarized lighting. Paper presented at the 1993 Annual Convention of the Illuminating Engineering Society of North America, Houston, TX. 1993 Aug.

Boyce P. Investigations of the subjective balance between illuminance and lamp colour properties. Light Resch and Technol. 1977;9:11-24.

Boylan R, Li Y, Simeonova L, Sherwin G, Kreismann J, Craig RG, Ship JA, McCutcheon JA. Reduction in bacterial contamination of toothbrushes using the Violight ultraviolet light activated toothbrush sanitizer. Am J Dent. 2008 Oct;21(5):313-7.

Bråbäck L, Breborowicz A, Julge K, Knutsson A, Riikjärv MA, Vasar M, Björkstén B. Risk factors for respiratory symptoms and atopic sensitisation in the Baltic area. Arch Dis Child. 1995 Jun;72(6):487-93.

Bradette-Hébert ME, Legault J, Lavoie S, Pichette A. A new labdane diterpene from the flowers of Solidago canadensis. Chem Pharm Bull. 2008 Jan;56(1):82-4.

Brainard GC, Kavet R, Kheifets LI. The relationship between electromagnetic field and light exposures to melatonin and breast cancer risk: a review of the relevant literature. J Pineal Res. 1999 Mar;26(2):65-100.

Brandtzaeg P. The mucosal immune system and its integration with the mammary glands. J Pediatr. 2010 Feb;156(2 Suppl):S8-15.

Brasseur JG, Nicosia MA, Pal A, Miller LS. Function of longitudinal vs circular muscle fibers in esophageal peristalsis, deduced with mathematical modeling. World J Gastroenterol. 2007 Mar 7;13(9):1335-46.

Brauer, M. et al. 2016. "Ambient Air Pollution Exposure Estimation for the Global Burden of Disease 2013." Environmental Science & Technology 50, no. 1: 79–88. (The World Bank. PM2.5 air pollution, mean annual exposure (micrograms per cubic meter).

Braunstein G, Labat C, Brunelleschi S, Benveniste J, Marsac J, Brink C. Evidence that the histamine sensitivity and responsiveness of guinea-pig isolated trachea are modulated by epithelial prostaglandin E2 production. Br J Pharmacol. 1988 Sep;95(1):300-8.

Brenner D, Hall E. Computed Tomography — An Increasing Source of Radiation Exposure. NE J Med. 2007;357(22):2277-2284.

Breslow RA, Chen CM, Graubard BI, Mukamal KJ. Prospective Study of Alcohol Consumption Quantity and Cancer-Specific Mortality in the US Population. Am J Epidemiol. 2011 Nov 1;174(9):1044-53

Breton ME, Montzka DP. Empiric limits of rod photocurrent component underlying a-wave response in the electroretinogram. Doc Ophthalmol. 1992;79(4):337-61.

Breton ME, Montzka DP. Empiric limits of rod photocurrent component underlying a-wave response in the electroretinogram. Doc Ophthalmol. 1992;79(4):337-61.

Brighenti F, Valtueña S, Pellegrini N, Ardigò D, Del Rio D, Salvatore S, Piatti P, Serafini M, Zavaroni I. Total antioxidant capacity of the diet is inversely and independently related to plasma concentration of high-sensitivity C-reactive protein in adult Italian subjects. Br J Nutr. 2005 May;93(5):619-25.

Brillaud E, Piotrowski A, de Seze R. Effect of an acute 900MHz GSM exposure on glia in the rat brain: a time-dependent study. Toxicology. 2007 Aug 16;238(1):23-33.

Brink Y, Louw QA. A systematic review of the relationship between sitting and upper quadrant musculoskeletal pain in children and adolescents. Man Ther. 2013 Aug;18(4):281-8. doi: 10.1016/j.math.2012.11.003.

NATURAL CANCER SCIENCE

Brisman J, Torén K, Lillienberg L, Karlsson G, Ahlstedt S. Nasal symptoms and indices of nasal inflammation in flour-dust-exposed bakers. Int Arch Occup Environ Health. 1998 Nov;71(8):525-32.

Britt R. Hole Drilled to Bottom of Earth's Crust, Breakthrough to Mantle Looms. LiveScience. 2005. 07 Apr. http://www.livescience.com/ technology/050407_earth_drill.html. Acc. 2006 Nov.

Brodeur P. Currents of Death. New York: Simon and Schuster, 1989.

Brodtkorb TH, Zetterström O, Tinghög G. Cost-effectiveness of clean air administered to the breathing zone in allergic asthma. Clin Respir J. 2010 Apr;4(2):104-10.

Broekhuizen BD, Sachs AP, Hoes AW, Moons KG, van den Berg JW, Dalinghaus WH, Lammers E, Verheij TJ. Undetected chronic obstructive pulmonary disease and asthma in people over 50 years with persistent cough. Br J Gen Pract. 2010 Jul;60(576):489-94.

Brosseau LU, Pelland LU, Casimiro LY, Robinson VI, Tugwell PE, Wells GE. Electrical stimulation for the treatment of rheumatoid arthritis. Cochrane Database Syst Rev. 2002;(2):CD003687.

Brostoff J, Gamlin L, Brostoff J. Food Allergies and Food Intolerance: The Complete Guide to Their Identification and Treatment. Rochester, VT: Healing Arts, 2000.

Brownstein D. Salt: Your Way to Health. West Bloomfield, MI: Medical Alternatives, 2006.

Brown-Whitehorn TF, Spergel JM. The link between allergies and eosinophilic esophagitis: implications for management strategies. Expert Rev Clin Immunol. 2010 Jan;6(1):101-9.

Bruneton J. Pharmacognosy, Phytochemistry, Medicinal Plants. Paris: Lavoisier, 1995.

Bruton A, Lewith GT. The Buteyko breathing technique for asthma: a review. Complement Ther Med. 2005 Mar;13(1):41-6. 2005 Apr 18.

Bu LN, Chang MH, Ni YH, Chen HL, Cheng CC. Lactobacillus casei rhamnosus Lcr35 in children with chronic constipation. Pediatr Int. 2007 Aug;49(4):485-90.

Buchanan TW, Lutz K, Mirzazade S, Specht K, Shah NJ, Zilles K, et al. Recognition of emotional prosody and verbal components of spoken language: an fMRI study. Cogn Brain Res. 2000;9:227-38.

Buckley NA, Whyte IM, Dawson AH. There are days ... and moons. Self-poisoning is not lunacy. Med J Aust. 1993 Dec 6-20;159(11-12):786-9.

Budzianowski J. Coumarins, caffeoyltartaric acids and their artifactual methyl esters from Taraxacum officinale leaves. Planta Med. 1997 Jun;63(3):288.

Buijs RM, Scheer FA, Kreier F, Yi C, Bos N, Goncharuk VD, Kalsbeek A. Organization of circadian functions: interaction with the body. Prog Brain Res. 2006;153:341-60.

Bulsing PJ, Smeets MA, van den Hout MA. Positive Implicit Attitudes toward Odor Words. Chem Senses. 2007 May 7.

Bundy R, Walker AF, Middleton RW, Booth J. Turmeric extract may improve irritable bowel syndrome symptomology in otherwise healthy adults: a pilot study. J Altern Complement Med. 2004 Dec;10(6):1015-8.

Burdge GC, Jones AE, Wootton SA. Eicosapentaenoic and docosapentaenoic acids are the principal products of alpha-linolenic acid metabolism in young men. B J Nutr. 2002 Oct;88(4):355-63.

Buret AG. How stress induces intestinal hypersensitivity. Am J Pathol. 2006 Jan;168(1):3-5.

Burgess CD, Bremner P, Thomson CD, Crane J, Siebers RW, Beasley R. Nebulized beta 2-adrenoceptor agonists do not affect plasma selenium or glutathione peroxidase activity in patients with asthma. Int J Clin Pharmacol Ther. 1994 Jun;32(6):290-2.

Burikov AA, Bereshpolova YuI. The activity of thalamus and cerebral cortex neurons in rabbits during "slow wave-spindle" EEG complexes. Neurosci Behav Physiol. 1999 Mar-Apr;29(2):143-9.

Burks W, Jones SM, Berseth CL, Harris C, Sampson HA, Scalabrin DM. Hypoallergenicity and effects on growth and tolerance of a new amino acid-based formula with docosahexaenoic acid and arachidonic acid. J Pediatr. 2008 Aug;153(2):266-71.

Burney PG, Luczynska C, Chinn S, Jarvis D. The European Community Respiratory Health Survey. Eur Respir J. 1994;7: 954-960.

Burnham K, Andersson D. Model Selection and Inference. A Practical Information-Theoretic Approach. New York: Springer, 1998

Burns WR. East meets West: how China almost cured malaria. Endeavour. 2008 Sep;32(3):101-6.

Burr H, Hovland C. Bio-Electric Potential Gradients in the Chick. Yale Journal of Biology & Medicine. 1937;9:247-258

Burr H, Lane C, Nims L. A Vacuum Tube Microvoltmeter for the Measurement of Bioelectric Phenomena. Yale Journal of Biology & Medicine. 1936;10:65-76.

Burr H, Smith G, Strong L. Bio-electric Properties of Cancer-Resistant and Cancer-Susceptible Mice. American Journal of Cancer. 1938;32:240-248

Burr H. The Fields of Life. New York: Ballantine, 1972.

Burr ML, Butland BK, King S, Vaughan-Williams E. Changes in asthma prevalence: two surveys 15 years apart. Arch Dis Child. 1989;64:1452-1456.

Buscemi N, Vandermeer B, Pandya R, Hooton N, Tjosvold L, Hartling L, Baker G, Vohra S, Klassen T. Melatonin for treatment of sleep disorders. Evid Rep Technol Assess. 2004 Nov;(108):1-7.

Bustamante-Rengifo JA, Matta AJ, Pazos AJ, Bravo LE. CagA EPIYA motif in Helicobacter pylori strains. World J Gastroenterol. 2017 Mar 21;23(11):1980-1989. doi: 10.3748/wjg.v23.i11.1980.

Buzsaki G. Theta rhythm of navigation: link between path integration and landmark navigation, episodic and semantic memory. Hippocampus. 2005;15(7):827-40.

Buzsaki G. Theta rhythm of navigation: link between path integration and landmark navigation, episodic and semantic memory. Hippocampus. 2005;15(7):827-40.

Cabanillas B, Pedrosa MM, Rodríguez J, González A, Muzquiz M, Cuadrado C, Crespo JF, Burbano C. Effects of enzymatic hydrolysis on lentil allergenicity. Mol Nutr Food Res. 2010 Mar 19.

Caglar E, Cildir SK, Ergeneli S, Sandalli N, Twetman S. Salivary mutans streptococci and lactobacilli levels after ingestion of the probiotic bacterium Lactobacillus reuteri ATCC 55730 by straws or tablets. Acta Odontol Scand. 2006 Oct;64(5):314-8.

Caglar E, Kavaloglu SC, Kuscu OO, Sandalli N, Holgerson PL, Twetman S. Effect of chewing gums containing xylitol or probiotic bacteria on salivary mutans streptococci and lactobacilli. Clin Oral Investig. 2007 Dec;11(4):425-9.

Caglar E, Kuscu OO, Cildir SK, Kuvvetli SS, Sandalli N. A probiotic lozenge administered medical device and its effect on salivary mutans streptococci and lactobacilli. Int J Paediatr Dent. 2008 Jan;18(1):35-9.

Caglar E, Kuscu OO, Selvi Kuvvetli S, Kavaloglu Cildir S, Sandalli N, Twetman S. Short-term effect of ice-cream containing Bifidobacterium lactis Bb-12 on the number of salivary mutans streptococci and lactobacilli. Acta Odontol Scand. 2008 Jun;66(3):154-8.

Cahill RT. A New Light-Speed Anisotropy Experiment: Absolute Motion and Gravitational Waves Detected. Progress in Physics. 2006; (4).

Cahn J, Borzeix MG. Administration of procyanidolic oligomers in rats. Observed effects on changes in the permeability of the blood-brain barrier. Sem Hop. 1983 Jul 7;59(27-28):2031-4.

Cai L, Mu LN, Lu H, Lu QY, You NC, Yu SZ, Le AD, Zhao J, Zhou XF, Marshall J, Heber D, Zhang ZF. Dietary selenium intake and genetic polymorphisms of the GSTP1 and p53 genes on the risk of esophageal squamous cell carcinoma. Cancer Epidemiol Biomarkers Prev. 2006 Feb;15(2):294-300.

Cajochen C, Zeitzer JM, Czeisler CA, Dijk DJ. Dose-response relationship for light intensity and ocular and electroencephalographic correlates of human alertness. Behav Brain Res. 2000 Oct;115(1):75-83.

Calastretti A, Gatti G, Lucini V, Dugnani S, Canti G, Scaglione F, Bevilacqua A. Melatonin Analogue Anti-proliferative and Cytotoxic Effects on Human Prostate Cancer Cells. Int J Mol Sci. 2018 May 18;19(5). pii: E1505. doi:10.3390/ijms19051505.

Calder PC. Dietary modification of inflammation with lipids. Proc Nutr Soc. 2002 Aug;61(3):345-58.

Caldwell MM, Bornman JF, Ballare CL, Flint SD, Kulandaivelu G. Terrestrial ecosystems, increased solar ultraviolet radiation, and interactions with other climate change factors. Photochem Photobiol Sci. 2007 Mar;6(3):252-66.

Callender ST, Spray GH. Latent pernicious anemia. Br J Haematol 1962;8:230-240.

Calvin W. The Handbook of Brain Theory and Neural Networks. Boston: MIT Press, 1995.

Cameron E, Pauling L. Experimental studies designed to evaluate the management of patients with incurable cancer. Proc Natl Acad Sci U S A. 1978 Dec;75(12):6252. doi: 10.1073/pnas.75.12.6252.

Cameron E, Pauling L. Supplemental ascorbate in the supportive treatment of cancer: Prolongation of survival times in terminal human cancer. Proc Natl Acad Sci U S A. 1976 Oct;73(10):3685-9. doi: 10.1073/pnas.73.10.3685

Campbell A. The role of aluminum and copper on neuroinflammation and Alzheimer's disease. J Alzheimers Dis. 2006 Nov;10(2-3):165-72.

Campbell TC, Campbell TM. The China Study. Dallas, TX: Benbella Books, 2006.

Campieri C, Campieri M, Bertuzzi V, Swennen E, Matteuzzi D, Stefoni S, Pirovano F, Centi C, Ulisse S, Famularo G, De Simone C. Reduction of oxaluria after an oral course of lactic acid bacteria at high concentration. Kidney Int. 2001 Sep;60(3):1097-105.

Canakcioglu S, Tahamiler R, Saritzali G, Alimoglu Y, Isildak H, Guvenc MG, Acar GO, Inci E. Evaluation of nasal cytology in subjects with chronic rhinitis: a 7-year study. Am J Otolaryngol. 2009 Sep-Oct;30(5):312-7.

Canali R, Comitato R, Schonlau F, Virgili F. The anti-inflammatory pharmacology of Pycnogenol in humans involves COX-2 and 5-LOX mRNA expression in leukocytes. Int Immunopharmacol. 2009 Sep;9(10):1145-9.

Canani RB, Cirillo P, Terrin G, Cesarano L, Spagnuolo MI, De Vincenzo A, Albano F, Passariello A, De Marco G, Manguso F, Guarino A. Probiotics for treatment of acute diarrhoea in children: randomised clinical trial of five different preparations. BMJ. 2007 Aug 18;335(7615):340.

Canducci F, Armuzzi A, Cremonini F, Cammarota G, Bartolozzi F, Pola P, Gasbarrini G, Gasbarrini A. A lyophilized and inactivated culture of Lactobacillus acidophilus increases Helicobacter pylori eradication rates. Aliment Pharmacol Ther. 2000 Dec;14(12):1625-9.

Canducci F, Cremonini F, Armuzzi A, Di Caro S, Gabrielli M, Santarelli L, Nista E, Lupascu A, De Martini D, Gasbarrini A. Probiotics and Helicobacter pylori eradication. Dig Liver Dis. 2002 Sep;34 Suppl 2:S81-3.

Cantor KP, Stewart PA, Brinton LA, Dosemeci M. Occupational exposures and female breast cancer mortality in the United States. J Occup Environ Med. 1995 Mar;37(3):336-48.

Cao G, Alessio HM, Cutler RG. Oxygen-radical absorbance capacity assay for antioxidants. Free Radic Biol Med. 1993 Mar;14(3):303-11.

Cao G, Shukitt-Hale B, Bickford PC, Joseph JA, McEwen J, Prior RL. Hyperoxia-induced changes in antioxidant capacity and the effect of dietary antioxidants. J Appl Physiol. 1999 Jun;86(6):1817-22.

Capasso R, Laudato M, Borrelli F. Meeting report: First National Meeting on Aloe, April 20-21, 2013, Isernia, Italy. New perspectives in Aloe research: from basic science to clinical application. Nat Prod Commun. 2013 Sep;8(9):1333-4.

Caramia G. The essential fatty acids omega-6 and omega-3: from their discovery to their use in therapy. Minerva Pediatr. 2008 Apr;60(2):219-33.

Carey DG, Aase KA, Pliego GJ. The acute effect of cold air exercise in determination of exercise-induced bronchospasm in apparently healthy athletes. J Strength Cond Res. 2010 Aug;24(8):2172-8.

Carlberg M, Hardell L. Evaluation of Mobile Phone and Cordless Phone Use and Glioma Risk Using the Bradford Hill Viewpoints from 1965 on Association or Causation. Biomed Res Int. 2017;2017:9218486. doi: 10.1155/2017/9218486.

Carlberg M, Söderqvist F, Hansson Mild K, Hardell L. Meningioma patients diagnosed 2007–2009 and the association with use of mobile and cordless phones: a case–control study. Environ Health. 2013 Jul 19;12(1):60.

Carlsen E, Olsson C, Petersen JH, Andersson AM, Skakkebaek NE. Diurnal rhythm in serum levels of inhibin B in normal men: relation to testicular steroids and gonadotropins. J Clin Endocrinol Metab. 1999 May;84(5):1664-9.

Carlsen E, Olsson C, Petersen JH, Andersson AM, Skakkebaek NE. Diurnal rhythm in serum levels of inhibin B in normal men: relation to testicular steroids and gonadotropins. J Clin Endocrinol Metab. 1999 May;84(5):1664-9.

Carpita N. C., Kanabus J., Housley T. L. Linkage structure of fructans and fructan oligomers from Triticum aestivum and Festuca arundinacea leaves. J. Plant Physiol. 1989;134:162-168

Carroll D. The Complete Book of Natural Medicines. New York: Summit, 1980.

Caruso M, Frasca G, Di Giuseppe PL, Pennisi A, Tringali G, Bonina FP. Effects of a new nutraceutical ingredient on allergen-induced sulphidoleukotrienes production and CD63 expression in allergic subjects. Int Immunopharmacol. 2008 Dec 20;8(13-14):1781-6.

Carvalho AM, Miranda AM, Santos FA, Loureiro AP, Fisberg RM, Marchioni DM. High intake of heterocyclic amines from meat is associated with oxidative stress. Br J Nutr. 2015 Apr 28;113(8):1301-7. doi: 10.1017/S0007114515000628.

Carvalho M, Ferreira PJ, Mendes VS, Silva R, Pereira JA, Jerónimo C, Silva BM. Human cancer cell antiproliferative and antioxidant activities of Juglans regia L. Food Chem Toxicol. 2010 Jan;48(1):441-7. doi: 10.1016/j.fct.2009.10.043.

Castellarin M, Warren RL, Freeman JD, Dreolini L, Krzywinski M, Strauss J, Barnes R, Watson P, Allen-Vercoe E, Moore RA, Holt RA. Fusobacterium nucleatum prevalent in human colorectal carcinoma. Genome Res. 2011 Oct 18.

Cats A, Kuipers EJ, Bosschaert MA, Pot RG, Vandenbroucke-Grauls CM, Kusters JG. Effect of frequent consumption of a Lactobacillus casei-containing milk drink in Helicobacter pylori-colonized subjects. Aliment Pharmacol Ther. 2003 Feb;17(3):429-35.

Caughey AB, Nicholson JM, Cheng YW, Lyell DJ, Washington AE. Induction of labor and Cesarean delivery by gestational age. Am J Obstet Gynecol. 2006 Sep;195(3):700-5.

Cavalli-Sforza L, Feldman M. Cultural Transmission and Evolution: A quantitative approach. Princeton: Princeton UP, 1981.

CDC. Healthcare-associated infections: HAI Data and Statistics. Accessed Mar 30, 2016

Cejas, P., Casado, E., Belda-Iniesta, C. et al. Implications of Oxidative Stress and Cell Membrane Lipid Peroxidation in Human Cancer (Spain). Cancer Causes Control 15, 707–719 (2004).

Celec P, Ostaniková D, Skoknová M, Hodosy J, Putz Z, Kúdela M. Salivary sex hormones during the menstrual cycle. Endocr J. 2009 Jun;56(3):521-3.

Celec P, Ostatníková D, Hodosy J, Putz Z, Kúdela M. Increased one week soybean consumption affects spatial abilities but not sex hormone status in men. Int J Food Sci Nutr. 2007 Sep;58(6):424-8.

Celec P, Ostatníková D, Hodosy J, Skoknová M, Putz Z, Kúdela M. Infradian rhythmic variations of salivary estradiol and progesterone in healthy men. Biol Res. 2006;37(1): 37-44.

Celec P, Ostatníková D, Putz Z, Hodosy J, Burský P, Stárka L, Hampl R, Kúdela M. Circatrigintan Cycle of Salivary Testosterone in Human Male. Biol Rhythm Res. 2003;34(3): 305-315.

Celec P, Ostatnikova D, Putz Z, Kudela M. The circalunar cycle of salivary testosterone and the visual-spatial performance. Bratisl Lek Listy. 2002;103(2):59-69.

Celec P. Analysis of rhythmic variance - ANORVA. A new simple method for detecting rhythms in biological time series. Biol Res. 2004;37:777-782.

Celentano A, Tran A, Testa C, *et al.* The protective effects of Kava (Piper Methysticum) constituents in cancers: A systematic review. J Oral Pathol Med. 2019;48(7):510-529. doi:10.1111/jop.12900

Centers for Disease Control and Prevention (CDC). Obesity prevalence among low-income, preschool-aged children - United States, 1998-2008. MMWR Morb Mortal Wkly Rep. 2009 Jul 24;58(28):769-73.

Centers for Disease Control and Prevention (CDC). Vital signs: nonsmokers' exposure to secondhand smoke - United States, 1999-2008. MMWR Morb Mortal Wkly Rep. 2010 Sep 10;59(35):1141-6.

Cereijido M, Contreras RG, Flores-Benítez D, Flores-Maldonado C, Larre I, Ruiz A, Shoshani L. New diseases derived or associated with the tight junction. Arch Med Res. 2007 Jul;38(5):465-78.

Cerimele JM, Katon WJ. Associations between health risk behaviors and symptoms of schizophrenia and bipolar disorder: a systematic review. Gen Hosp Psychiatry. 2013 Jan-Feb;35(1):16-22. doi: 10.1016/j.genhosppsych.2012.08.001.

Cestonaro LV, Marcolan AM, Rossato-Grando LG, Anzolin AP, Goethel G, Vilani A, Garcia SC, Bertol CD. Ozone generated by air purifier in low concentrations: friend or foe? Environ Sci Pollut Res Int. 2017 Oct;24(28):22673-22678. doi: 10.1007/s11356-017-9887-3. Epub 2017 Aug 16. PMID: 28812184.

Chafen JJ, Newberry SJ, Riedl MA, Bravata DM, Maglione M, Suttorp MJ, Sundaram V, Paige NM, Towfigh A, Hulley BJ, Shekelle PG. Diagnosing and managing common food allergies: a systematic review. JAMA. 2010 May 12;303(18):1848-56.

Chahine BG, Bahna SL. The role of the gut mucosal immunity in the development of tolerance versus development of allergy to food. Curr Opin Allergy Clin Immunol. 2010 Aug;10(4):394-9.

Chaitow L. Conquer Pain the Natural Way. San Francisco: Chronicle Books, 2002.

Chakŭrski I, Matev M, Koĭchev A, Angelova I, Stefanov G. Treatment of chronic colitis with an herbal combination of Taraxacum officinale, Hipericum perforatum, Melissa officinaliss, Calendula officinalis and Foeniculum vulgare. Vutr Boles. 1981;20(6):51-4.

Challier B, Perarnau J-M, and Viel J-F: Garlic, onion and cereal fibre as protective factors for breast cancer: a French case-control study. Eur J Epidemiol 14, 737–747, 1998.

Cham, B. Solasodine glycosides as anti-cancer agents: Pre-clinical and Clinical studies. Asia Pac J Pharmac. 1994;9:113-118.

Chan YS, Xia L, Ng TB. White kidney bean lectin exerts anti-proliferative and apoptotic effects on cancer cells. Int J Biol Macromol. 2016 Apr;85:335-45. doi: 10.1016/j.ijbiomac.2015.12.094.

Chaney M, Ross M. Nutrition. New York: Houghton Mifflin, 1971.

Chang HT, Tseng LJ, Hung TJ, Kao BT, Lin WY, Fan TC, Chang MD, Pai TW. Inhibition of the interactions between eosinophil cationic protein and airway epithelial cells by traditional Chinese herbs. BMC Syst Biol. 2010 Sep 13;4 Suppl 2:S8.

Chang TT, Huang CC, Hsu CH. Clinical evaluation of the Chinese herbal medicine formula STA-1 in the treatment of allergic asthma. Phytother Res. 2006;20:342-7.

Chang TT, Huang CC, Hsu CH. Inhibition of mite-induced immunoglobulin E synthesis, airway inflammation, and hyperreactivity by herbal medicine STA-1. Immunopharmacol Immunotoxicol. 2006;28:683-95.

Chao A, Thun MJ, Connell CJ, McCullough ML, Jacobs EJ, Flanders WD, Rodriguez C, Sinha R, Calle EE. Meat consumption and risk of colorectal cancer. JAMA. 2005 Jan 12;293(2):172-82.

Chapat L, Chemin K, Dubois B, Bourdet-Sicard R, Kaiserlian D. Lactobacillus casei reduces CD8+ T cell-mediated skin inflammation. Eur J Immunol. 2004 Sep;34(9):2520-8.

Chapidze G, Kapanadze S, Dolidze N, Bachutashvili Z, Latsabidze N. Prevention of coronary atherosclerosis by the use of combination therapy with antioxidant coenzyme q10 and statins. Georgian Med News. 2005 Jan;(1):20-5.

Chapman S, Morrell S. Barking mad? another lunatic hypothesis bites the dust. BMJ. 2000 Dec 23-30;321(7276):1561-3.

Chapman, S. Fear of frying: power lines and cancer. BMJ 2001;322:682.

Characterization and quantitation of Antioxidant Constituents of Sweet Pepper (Capsicum annuum - Cayenne). J Agric Food Chem. 2004 Jun 16;52(12):3861-9.

Chatzi L, Apostolaki G, Bibakis I, Skypala I, Bibaki-Liakou V, Tzanakis N, Kogevinas M, Cullinan P. Protective effect of fruits, vegetables and the Mediterranean diet on asthma and allergies among children in Crete. Thorax. 2007 Aug;62(8):677-83.

Chatzi L, Torrent M, Romieu I, Garcia-Esteban R, Ferrer C, Vioque J, Kogevinas M, Sunyer J. Mediterranean diet in pregnancy is protective for wheeze and atopy in childhood. Thorax. 2008 Jun;63(6):507-13.

Chaves TC, de Andrade e Silva TS, Monteiro SA, Watanabe PC, Oliveira AS, Grossi DB. Craniocervical posture and hyoid bone position in children with mild and moderate asthma and mouth breathing. Int J Pediatr Otorhinolaryngol. 2010 Sep;74(9):1021-7.

Chay WY, Tham CK, Toh HC, Lim HY, Tan CK, Lim C, Wang WW, Choo SP. Coriolus versicolor (Yunzhi) Use as Therapy in Advanced Hepatocellular Carcinoma Patients with Poor Liver Function or Who Are Unfit for Standard Therapy. J Altern Complement Med. 2017 Aug;23(8):648-652. doi: 10.1089/acm.2016.0136.

Chellini E, Talassi F, Corbo G, Berti G, De Sario M, Rusconi F, Piffer S, Caranci N, Petronio MG, Sestini P, Dell'Orco V, Bonci E, Armenio L, La Grutta S; Gruppo Collaborativo SIDRIA-2. Environmental, social and demographic characteristics of children and adolescents, resident in different Italian areas. Epidemiol Prev. 2005 Mar-Apr;29(2 Suppl):14-23.

Chen AC, Martin AJ, Choy B, Fernández-Peñas P, Dalziell RA, McKenzie CA, Scolyer RA, Dhillon HM, Vardy JL, Kricker A, St George G, Chinniah N, Halliday GM, Damian DL.A Phase 3 Randomized Trial of Nicotinamide for Skin-Cancer Chemoprevention. N Engl J Med. 2015 Oct 22;373(17):1618-26. doi: 10.1056/NEJMoa1506197.

Chen C, Ono M, Takeshima M, Nakano S. Antiproliferative and apoptosis-inducing activity of nobiletin against human breast cancer cell lines. Anticancer Res. 2014 Apr;34(4):1785-92.

Chen CY, Wang FY, Wan HJ, Jin XX, Wei J, Wang ZK, Liu C, Lu H, Shi H, Li DH, Liu J. Amino acid polymorphisms flanking the EPIYA-A motif of Helicobacter pylori CagA C-terminal region is associated with gastric cancer in East China. J Dig Dis. 2013 Mar 21.

Chen HJ, Shih CK, Hsu HY, Chiang W. Mast cell-dependent allergic responses are inhibited by ethanolic extract of adlay (Coix lachryma-jobi L. var. ma-yuen Stapf) testa. J Agric Food Chem. 2010 Feb 24;58(4):2596-601.

Chen HY, Shi Y, Ng CS, Chan SM, Yung KK, Zhang QL. Auricular acupuncture treatment for insomnia: a systematic review. J Altern Complement Med. 2007 Jul-Aug;13(6):669-76.

Chen J, Creed A, Chen AY, Huang H, Li Z, Rankin GO, Ye X, Xu G, Chen YC. Nobiletin suppresses cell viability through AKT pathways in PC-3 and DU-145 prostate cancer cells. BMC Pharmacol Toxicol. 2014 Oct 24;15:59. doi: 10.1186/2050-6511-15-59.

Chen JT, Tominaga K, Sato Y, Anzai H, Matsuoka R. Maitake mushroom (Grifola frondosa) extract induces ovulation in patients with polycystic ovary syndrome: a possible monotherapy and a combination therapy after failure with first-line clomiphene citrate. J Altern Complement Med. 2010 Dec;16(12):1295-9. doi: 10.1089/acm.2009.0696.

Chen JX, Ji B, Lu ZL, Hu LS. Effects of chai hu (radix burpleuri) containing formulation on plasma beta-endorphin, epinephrine and dopamine on patients. Am J Chin Med. 2005;33(5):737-45.

Chen Y, Blaser MJ. Helicobacter pylori colonization is inversely associated with childhood asthma. J Infect Dis. 2008 Aug 15;198(4):553-60.

Chen Y, Tan F, Wei L, Li X, Lyu Z, Feng X, Wen Y, Guo L, He J, Dai M, Li N. Sleep duration and the risk of cancer: a systematic review and meta-analysis including dose-response relationship. BMC Cancer. 2018 Nov 21;18(1):1149. doi: 10.1186/s12885-018-5025-y.

Cheney G, Waxler SH, Miller IJ. Vitamin U therapy of peptic ulcer; experience at San Quentin Prison. Calif Med. 1956 Jan;84(1):39-42.

Cheng S, Castillo V, Eliaz I, Sliva D. Honokiol suppresses metastasis of renal cell carcinoma by targeting KISS1/KISS1R signaling. Int J Oncol. 2015 Jun;46(6):2293-8. doi: 10.3892/ijo.2015.2950.

Chen-Goodspeed M, Cheng Chi Lee. Tumor suppression and circadian function. J Biol Rhythms. 2007 Aug;22(4):291-8.

Chevallier A. Encyclopedia of Medicinal Plants. New York, NY: DK Publishing; 1996.

Chevrier MR, Ryan AE, Lee DY, Zhongze M, Wu-Yan Z, Via CS. Boswellia carterii extract inhibits TH1 cytokines and promotes TH2 cytokines in vitro. Clin Diagn Lab Immunol. 2005 May;12(5):575-80.

Chiang BL, Sheih YH, Wang LH, Liao CK, Gill HS. Enhancing immunity by dietary consumption of a probiotic lactic acid bacterium (Bifidobacterium lactis HN019): optimization and definition of cellular immune responses. Eur J Clin Nutr. 2000 Nov;54(11):849-55.

Chilton F, Tucker L. Win the War Within. New York: Rodale, 2006.

Chilton FH, Rudel LL, Parks JS, Arm JP, Seeds MC. Mechanisms by which botanical lipids affect inflammatory disorders. Am J Clin Nutr. 2008 Feb;87(2):498S-503S.

Chin A Paw MJ, de Jong N, Pallast EG, Kloek GC, Schouten EG, Kok FJ. Immunity in frail elderly: a randomized controlled trial of exercise and enriched foods. Med Sci Sports Exerc. 2000 Dec;32(12):2005-11.

Chirkova E. Mathematical methods of detection of biological and heliogeophysical rhythms in the light of developments in modern heliobiology: A platform for discussion. Cybernet Sys. 2000;31(6):903-918.

Chirkova EN, Suslov LS, Avramenko MM, Krivoruchko GE. Monthly and daily biorhythms of amylase in the blood of healthy men and their relation with the rhythms in the external environment. Lab Delo. 1990;(4):40-4.

Chiu HF, Fu HY, Lu YY, Han YC, Shen YC, Venkatakrishnan K, Golovinskaia O, Wang CK. Triterpenoids and polysaccharide peptides-enriched Ganoderma lucidum: a randomized, double-blind placebo-controlled crossover study of its antioxidation and hepatoprotective efficacy in healthy volunteers. Pharm Biol. 2017 Dec;55(1):1041-1046. doi: 10.1080/13880209.2017.1288750.

Chiurillo MA, Moran Y, Cañas M, Valderrama E, Granda N, Sayegh M, Ramírez JL. Genotyping of Helicobacter pylori virulence-associated genes shows high diversity of strains infecting patients in western Venezuela. Int J Infect Dis. 2013 Apr 20.

Cho JH, Jeon YJ, Park SM, Shin JC, Lee TH, Jung S, Park H, Ryu J, Chen H, Dong Z, Shim JH, Chae JI. Multifunctional effects of honokiol as an anti-inflammatory and anti-cancer drug in human oral squamous cancer cells and xenograft. Biomaterials. 2015 Jun;53:274-84. doi: 10.1016/j.biomaterials.2015.02.091.

Choia Y, Leea SM, Chunb J, Leea HB, Lee J. Influence of heat treatment on the antioxidant activities and polyphenolic compounds of Shiitake (Lentinus edodes) mushroom. Food Chem. 2006, 99;2, Pages 381-387

Chong AS, Boussy IA, Jiang XL, Lamas M, Graf LH Jr. CD54/ICAM-1 is acostimulator of NK cell-mediated cytotoxicity. Cell Immunol. 1994 Aug;157(1):92-105.

Chong Neto HJ, Rosário NA; Grupo EISL Curitiba (Estudio Internacional de Sibilancias en Lactantes). Risk factors for wheezing in the first year of life. J Pediatr. 2008 Nov-Dec;84(6):495-502.

Chong NW, Codd V, Chan D, Samani NJ. Circadian clock genes cause activation of the human PAI-1 gene promoter with 4G/5G allelic preference. FEBS Lett. 2006 Aug 7;580(18):4469-72.

Chopra RN, Chopra IC, Handa KL, Kapur LD. Calcutta, India: Academic Publishers; 1994. Indigenous drugs of India

Chopra RN, Nayar SL, Chopra IC, eds. Glossary of Indian Medicinal plants. New Delhi: CSIR, 1956.

Choudhry S, Seibold MA, Borrell LN, Tang H, Serebrisky D, Chapela R, Rodriguez-Santana JR, Avila PC, Ziv E, Rodriguez-Cintron W, Risch NJ, Burchard EG. Dissecting complex diseases in complex populations: asthma in latino americans. Proc Am Thorac Soc. 2007 Jul;4(3):226-33.

Chouraqui JP, Grathwohl D, Labaune JM, Hascoet JM, de Montgolfier I, Leclaire M, Giarre M, Steenhout P. Assessment of the safety, tolerance, and protective effect against diarrhea of infant formulas containing mixtures of probiotics or probiotics and prebiotics in a randomized controlled trial. Am J Clin Nutr. 2008 May;87(5):1365-73.

Christensen LP. Bioactive Polyacetylenes of Carrots in Cancer Prevention. Bioactive Dietary Factors and Plant Extracts in Dermatology. Humana, 2012.

Christopher JR. School of Natural Healing. Springville UT: Christopher Publ, 1976.

Christophersen, A. G., Jun, H., Jørgensen, K., and Skibsted, L. H. Photobleaching of astaxanthin and canthaxanthin: quantum-yields dependence of solvent, temperature, and wavelength of irradiation in relation to packaging and storage of carotenoid pigmented salmonoids. Z. Lebensm. Unters. Forsch., 1991;192:433-439.

Chu Q, Wang L, Liu GZ. Clinical observation on acupuncture for treatment of diabetic nephropathy. Zhongguo Zhen Jiu. 2007 Jul;27(7):488-90.

Chu YF, Liu RH. Cranberries inhibit LDL oxidation and induce LDL receptor expression in hepatocytes. Life Sci. 2005;77(15):1892-1901.

Chung SY, Butts CL, Maleki SJ, Champagne ET Linking peanut allergenicity to the processes of maturation, curing, and roasting. J Agric Food Chem. 2003;51: 4273-4277.

Churchill G, Doerge R. Empirical threshold values for quantitative trait mapping. Genetics 1994;138:963-971.

Chwirot B, Kowalska M, Plóciennik N, Piwinski M, Michniewicz Z, Chwirot S. Variability of spectra of laser-induced fluorescence of colonic mucosa: Its significance for fluorescence detection of colonic neoplasia. Indian J Exp. Biol. 2003;41(5):500-510.

Chwirot WB, Popp F. White-light-induced luminescence and mitotic activity of yeast cells. Folia Histochemica et Cytobiologica. 1991;29(4):155.

Cianci A, Giordano R, Delia A, Grasso E, Amodeo A, De Leo V, Caccamo F. Efficacy of Lactobacillus rhamnosus GR-1 and of Lactobacillus reuteri RC-14 in the treatment and prevention of vaginoses and bacterial vaginitis relapses. Minerva Ginecol. 2008 Oct;60(5):369-76.

Ciani F, Tafuri S, Troiano A, Cimmino A, Fioretto BS, Guarino AM, Pollice A, Vivo M, Evidente A, Carotenuto D, Calabrò V. Anti-proliferative and pro-apoptotic effects of Uncaria tomentosa aqueous extract in squamous carcinoma cells. J Ethnopharmacol. 2018 Jan 30;211:285-294. doi: 10.1016/j.jep.2017.09.031.

Cibella F, Cuttitta G. Nocturnal asthma and gastroesophageal reflux. Am J Med. 2001 Dec 3;111 Suppl 8A:31S-36S.

Cingi C, Demirbas D, Songu M. Allergic rhinitis caused by food allergies. Eur Arch Otorhinolaryngol. 2010 Sep;267(9):1327-35.

Ciprandi G, De Amici M, Negrini S, Marseglia G, Tosca MA. TGF-beta and IL-17 serum levels and specific immunotherapy. Int Immunopharmacol. 2009 Sep;9(10):1247-9.

Cisneros C, García-Río F, Romera D, Villasante C, Girón R, Ancochea J. Bronchial reactivity indices are determinants of health-related quality of life in patients with stable asthma. Thorax. 2010 Sep;65(9):795-800.

Citro M, Endler PC, Pongratz W, Vinattieri C, Smith CW, Schulte J. Hormone effects by electronic transmission. FASEB J. 1995:Abstract 12161.

Citro M, Smith CW, Scott-Morley A, Pongratz W, Endler PC. Transfer of information from molecules by means of electronic amplification, in P.C. Endler, J. Schulte (eds.): Ultra High Dilution. Physiology and Physics. Dordrecht: Kluwer Academic Publishers. 1994;209-214.

Citronberg J, Bostick R, Ahearn T, Turgeon DK, Ruffin MT, Djuric Z, Sen A, Brenner DE, Zick SM. Effects of Ginger supplementation on cell-cycle biomarkers in the normal-appearing colonic mucosa of patients at increased risk for colorectal cancer: results from a pilot, randomized, and controlled trial. Cancer Prev Res (Phila). 2013 Apr;6(4):271-81. doi: 10.1158/1940-6207.CAPR-12-0327. Epub 2013 Jan 9. PMID: 23303903; PMCID: PMC3618532.

Clark D. The use of electrical current in the treatment of nonunions. Vet Clin North Am Small Anim Pract. 1987 Jul;17(4):793-8.

Clement YN, Williams AF, Aranda D, Chase R, Watson N, Mohammed R, Stubbs O, Williamson D. Medicinal herb use among asthmatic patients attending a specialty care facility in Trinidad. BMC Complement Altern Med. 2005 Feb 15;5:3.

Clerici M, Balotta C, Meroni L, Ferrario E, Riva C, Trabattoni D, Ridolfo A,Villa M, Shearer GM, Moroni M, Galli M. Type 1 cytokine production and low prevalence of viral isolation correlate with long-term nonprogression in HIV infection. AIDS Res Hum Retroviruses. 1996 Jul 20;12(11):1053-61.

Clifton PM. Protein and coronary heart disease: the role of different protein sources. Curr Atheroscler Rep. 2011 Dec;13(6):493-8.

Cobo Sanz JM, Mateos JA, Muñoz Conejo A. Effect of Lactobacillus casei on the incidence of infectious conditions in children. Nutr Hosp. 2006 Jul-Aug;21(4):547-51.

Cogliano VJ, Baan R, Straif K, Grosse Y, Lauby-Secretan B, El Ghissassi F, Bouvard V, Benbrahim-Tallaa L, Guha N, Freeman C, Galichet L, Wild CP. Preventable exposures associated with human cancers. J Natl Cancer Inst. 2011 Dec 21;103(24):1827-39. doi: 10.1093/jnci/djr483.

Colapietro A, Mancini A, D'Alessandro AM, Festuccia C. Crocetin and Crocin from Saffron in Cancer Chemotherapy and Chemoprevention. Anticancer Agents Med Chem. 2019;19(1):38-47. doi: 10.2174/1871520619666181231112453.

Colecchia A, Vestito A, La Rocca A, Pasqui F, Nikiforaki A, Festi D; Symbiotic Study Group. Effect of a symbiotic preparation on the clinical manifestations of irritable bowel syndrome, constipation-variant. Results of an open, uncontrolled multicenter study. Minerva Gastroenterol Dietol. 2006 Dec;52(4):349-58.

Coles JA, Yamane S. Effects of adapting lights on the time course of the receptor potential of the anuran retinal rod. J Physiol. 1975 May;247(1):189-207.

Coll AP, Farooqi IS, O'Rahilly S. The hormonal control of food intake. Cell. 2007 Apr 20;129(2):251-62.

Collado Mateo D, Pazzi F, Domínguez Muñoz FJ, Martín Martínez JP, Olivares PR, Gusi N, Adsuar JC. Ganoderma Lucidum improves physical fitness in women with fibromyalgia. Nutr Hosp. 2015 Nov 1;32(5):2126-35. doi: 10.3305/nh.2015.32.5.9601.

Collins RL, Elliott MN, Berry SH, Kanouse DE, Kunkel D, Hunter SB, Miu A. Watching sex on television predicts adolescent initiation of sexual behavior. Pediatrics. 2004 Sep;114(3):e280-9.

Colodner R, Edelstein H, Chazan B, Raz R. Vaginal colonization by orally administered Lactobacillus rhamnosus GG. Isr Med Assoc J. 2003 Nov;5(11):767-9.

Colorectal Cancer Statistics. Centers for Disease Control and Prevention.

Colquhoun DM, Moores D, Somerset SM, Humphries JA. Comparison of the effects on lipoproteins and apolipoproteins of a diet high in monounsaturated fatty acids, enriched with avocado, and a high-carbohydrate diet. Am J Clin Nutr. 1992 Oct;56(4):671-7.

Comin-Anduix B, Boros LG, Marin S, Boren J, Callol-Massot C, Centelles JJ, Torres JL, Agell N, Bassilian S, Cascante M. Fermented wheat germ extract inhibits glycolysis/pentose cycle enzymes and induces apoptosis through poly(ADP-ribose) polymerase activation in Jurkat T-cell leukemia tumor cells. J Biol Chem. 2002 Nov 29;277(48):46408-14. doi: 10.1074/jbc.M206150200.

Conquer JA, Holub BJ. Dietary docosahexaenoic acid as a source of eicosapentaenoic acid in vegetarians and omnivores. Lipids. 1997 Mar;32(3):341-5.

Consumer Reports. Probiotics: Are enough in your diet? Cons Rpts Mag. 2005:34-35.

Conti S, Vexler A, Hagoel L, Kalich-Philosoph L, Corn BW, Honig N, Shtraus N, Meir Y, Ron I, Eliaz I, Lev-Ari S. Modified Citrus Pectin as a Potential Sensitizer for Radiotherapy in Prostate Cancer. Integr Cancer Ther. 2018 Dec;17(4):1225-1234. doi: 10.1177/1534735418790382.

Contreras D, Steriade M. Cellular basis of EEG slow rhythms: a study of dynamic corticothalamic relationships. J Neurosci. 1995 Jan;15(1 Pt 2):604-22.

Conway PL, Gorbach SL, Goldin BR. Survival of lactic acid bacteria in the human stomach and adhesion to intestinal cells. J Dairy Sci. 1987 Jan;70(1):1-12.

Cook J, The Therapeutic Use of Music. Nursing Forum. 1981;20:3: 253-66.

Cook N, Freeman S. Report of 19 cases of photoallergic contact dermatitis to sunscreens seen at the Skin and Cancer Foundation. Australas J Dermatol. 2001 Nov;42(4):257-9.

Cooper GS, Miller FW, Germolec DR: Occupational exposures and autoimmune diseases. Int Immunopharm 2002, 2:303-313.

Cooper K. The Aerobics Program for Total Well-Being. New York: Evans, 1980.

Corbe C, Boissin JP, Siou A. Light vision and chorioretinal circulation. Study of the effect of procyanidolic oligomers (Endotelon). J Fr Ophtalmol. 1988;11(5):453-60.

Corbe C, Boissin JP, Siou A. Light vision and chorioretinal circulation. Study of the effect of procyanidolic oligomers (Endotelon). J Fr Ophtalmol. 1988;11(5):453-60.

Corbo GM, Forastiere F, De Sario M, Brunetti L, Bonci E, Bugiani M, Chellini E, La Grutta S, Migliore E, Pistelli R, Rusconi F, Russo A, Simoni M, Talassi F, Galassi C; Sidria-2 Collaborative Group. Wheeze and asthma in children: associations with body mass index, sports, television viewing, and diet. Epidemiology. 2008 Sep;19(5):747-55.

Corkin S, Amaral DG, González RG, et al: H. M.'s medial temporal lobe lesion: findings from magnetic resonance imaging. J Neurosci. 1997;17:3964-3979.

Corrêa NB, Péret Filho LA, Penna FJ, Lima FM, Nicoli JR. A randomized formula controlled trial of Bifidobacterium lactis and Streptococcus thermophilus for prevention of antibiotic-associated diarrhea in infants. J Clin Gastroenterol. 2005 May-Jun;39(5):385-9.

Cory S, Ussery-Hall A, Griffin-Blake S, Easton A, Vigeant J, Balluz L, Garvin W, Greenlund K; Centers for Disease Control and Prevention (CDC). Prevalence of selected risk behaviors and chronic diseases and conditions-steps communities, United States, 2006-2007. MMWR Surveill Summ. 2010 Sep 24;59(8):1-37.

Cosmetic Ingredient Review Expert Panel. Final report on the safety assessment of Aloe … Int J Toxicol. 2007;26 Suppl 2:1-50.

Council Recommendation on the Limitation of Exposure of the General Public to Electromagnetic Fields (0 Hz to 300 GHz). Official Journal of the European Communities. 1999. July 12.

Coureau G, Bouvier G, Lebailly P, Fabbro-Peray P, Gruber A, Leffondre K, Guillamo JS, Loiseau H, Mathoulin-Pélissier S, Salamon R, Baldi I. Mobile phone use and brain tumours in the CERENAT case-control study. Occup Environ Med. 2014 Jul;71(7):514-22. doi: 10.1136/oemed-2013-101754.

Courtney R, Cohen M. Investigating the claims of Konstantin Buteyko, M.D., Ph.D.: the relationship of breath holding time to end tidal CO_2 and other proposed measures of dysfunctional breathing. J Altern Complement Med. 2008 Mar;14(2):115-23.

Couto E, Boffetta P, Lagiou P, Ferrari P, Buckland G, Overvad K, Dahm CC, Tjønneland A, Olsen A, Clavel-Chapelon F, Boutron-Ruault MC, Cottet V, Trichopoulos D, Naska A, Benetou V, Kaaks R, Rohrmann S, Boeing H, von Ruesten A, Panico S, Pala V, Vineis P, Palli D, Tumino R, May A, Peeters PH, Bueno-de-Mesquita HB, Büchner FL, Lund E, Skeie G, Engeset D, Gonzalez CA, Navarro C, Rodríguez L, Sánchez MJ, Amiano P, Barricarte A, Hallmans G, Johansson I, Manjer J, Wirfärt E, Allen NE, Crowe F, Khaw KT, Wareham N, Moskal A, Slimani N, Jenab M, Romaguera D, Mouw T, Norat T, Riboli E, Trichopoulou A. Mediterranean dietary pattern and cancer risk in the EPIC cohort. Br J Cancer. 2011 Apr 26;104(9):1493-9.

Couzy F, Kastenmayer P, Vigo M, Clough J, Munoz-Box R, Barclay DV. Calcium bioavailability from a calcium- and sulfate-rich mineral water, compared with milk, in young adult women. Am J Clin Nutr. 1995 Dec;62(6):1239-44.

Cragg GM, Newman DJ. Plants as a source of anti-cancer agents. J Ethnopharmacol. 2005 Aug 22;100(1-2):72-9. doi: 10.1016/j.jep.2005.05.011.

Cranney A, Horsley T, O'Donnell S, Weiler H, Puil L, Ooi D, Atkinson S, Ward L, Moher D, Hanley D, Fang M, Yazdi F, Garritty C, Sampson M, Barrowman N, Tsertsvadze A, Mamaladze V. Effectiveness and safety of vitamin D in relation to bone health. Evid Rep Technol Assess. 2007 Aug;(158):1-235.

Cranney A, Horsley T, O'Donnell S, Weiler H, Puil L, Ooi D, Atkinson S, Ward L, Moher D, Hanley D, Fang M, Yazdi F, Garritty C, Sampson M, Barrowman N, Tsertsvadze A, Mamaladze V. Effectiveness and safety of vitamin D in relation to bone health. Evid Rep Technol Assess. 2007 Aug;(158):1-235.

Crawley J. The Biorhythm Book. Boston: Journey Editions, 1996.

Crawley J. The Biorhythm Book. Boston: Journey Editions, 1996.

Creagan ET, Moertel CG, O'Fallon JR, Schutt AJ, O'Connell MJ, Rubin J, Frytak S. Failure of high-dose vitamin C (ascorbic acid) therapy to benefit patients with advanced cancer. A controlled trial. N Engl J Med. 1979 Sep 27;301(13):687-90. doi: 10.1056/NEJM197909273011303.

Creinin MD, Keverline S, Meyn LA. How regular is regular? An analysis of menstrual cycle regularity. Contraception. 2004 Oct;70(4):289-92.

Crescente M, Jessen G, Momi S, Höltje HD, Gresele P, Cerletti C, de Gaetano G. Interactions of gallic acid, resveratrol, quercetin and aspirin at the platelet cyclooxygenase-1 level. Functional and modelling studies. Thromb Haemost. 2009 Aug;102(2):336-46.

Crinnion WJ. Toxic effects of the easily avoidable phthalates and parabens. Altern Med Rev. 2010 Sep;15(3):190-6.

Crofford LJ. Neuroendocrine abnormalities in fibromyalgia and related disorders. Am J Med Sci. 1998;315:359-66.

Crönlein T, Langguth B, Geisler P, Hajak G. Tinnitus and insomnia. Prog Brain Res. 2007;166:227-33.

Cruccu G, Aziz TZ, Garcia-Larrea L, Hansson P, Jensen TS, Lefaucheur JP, Simpson BA, Taylor RS. EFNS guidelines on neurostimulation therapy for neuropathic pain. Eur J Neurol. 2007 Sep;14(9):952-70.

Cserhati E. Current view on the etiology of childhood bronchial asthma. Orv Hetil. 2000;141:759-760.

Cucherat M, Haugh MC, Gooch M, Boissel JP. Evidence of clinical efficacy of homeopathy. A meta-analysis of clinical trials. HMRAG. Homeopathic Medicines Research Advisory Group. Eur J Clin Pharmacol. 2000 Apr;56(1):27-33.

Cummings M. Human Heredity: Principles and Issues. St. Paul, MN: West, 1988.

Cuppari L, Garcia-Lopes MG. Hypovitaminosis D in chronic kidney disease patients: prevalence and treatment. J Ren Nutr. 2009 Jan;19(1):38-43.

Cuppari L, Garcia-Lopes MG. Hypovitaminosis D in chronic kidney disease patients: prevalence and treatment. J Ren Nutr. 2009 Jan;19(1):38-43.

Cuthbert SC, Goodheart GJ Jr. On the reliability and validity of manual muscle testing: a literature review. Chiropr Osteopat. 2007 Mar 6;15:4.

Cutolo M, Straub RH. Circadian rhythms in arthritis: hormonal effects on the immune/inflammatory reaction. Autoimmun Rev. 2008 Jan;7(3):223-8.

Cvjetićanin T, Stojanović I, Timotijević G, Stosić-Grujicić S, Miljković D. T cells cooperate with palmitic acid in induction of beta cell apoptosis. BMC Immunol. 2009 May 22;10:29. doi: 10.1186/1471-2172-10-29.

D'Ambrosio SM, Han C, Pan L, Kinghorn AD, Ding H. Aliphatic acetogenin constituents of avocado fruits inhibit human oral cancer cell proliferation by targeting the EGFR/RAS/RAF/MEK/ERK1/2 pathway. Biochem Biophys Res Commun. 2011 Jun 10;409(3):465-9. doi: 10.1016/j.bbrc.2011.05.027.

D'Anneo RW, Bruno ME, Falagiani P. Sublingual allergoid immunotherapy: a new 4-day induction phase in patients allergic to house dust mites. Int J Immunopathol Pharmacol. 2010 Apr-Jun;23(2):553-60.

D'Orazio N, Ficoneri C, Riccioni G, Conti P, Theoharides TC, Bollea MR. Conjugated linoleic acid: a functional food? Int J Immunopathol Pharmacol. 2003 Sep-Dec;16(3):215-20.

D'Orazio N, Gemello E, Gammone MA, de Girolamo M, Ficoneri C, Riccioni G. Fucoxantin: a treasure from the sea. Mar Drugs. 2012 Mar;10(3):604-16.

Da C, Liu Y, Zhan Y, Liu K, Wang R. Nobiletin inhibits epithelial-mesenchymal transition of human non-small cell lung cancer cells by antagonizing the TGF-β1/Smad3 signaling pathway. Oncol Rep. 2016;35(5):2767-2774. doi:10.3892/or.2016.4661

Dalaly BK, Eitenmiller RR, Friend BA, Shahani KM. Human milk ribonuclease. Biochim Biophys Acta. 1980 Oct;615(2):381-91.

Dalaly BK, Eitenmiller RR, Vakil JR, Shahani KM. Simultaneous isolation of human milk ribonuclease and lysozyme. Anal Biochem. 1970 Sep;37(1):208-11.

Dalmose A, Bjarkam C, Vuckovic A, Sorensen JC, Hansen J. Electrostimulation: a future treatment option for patients with neurogenic urodynamic disorders? APMIS Suppl. 2003;(109):45-51.

Dam Marie K, Hvidtfeldt Ulla A, Tjønneland Anne, Overvad Kim, Grønbæk Morten, Tolstrup Janne S et al. Five year change in alcohol intake and risk of breast cancer and coronary heart disease among post-menopausal women: prospective cohort study BMJ 2016; 353 :i2314

D'Angelo S, Ingrosso D, Migliardi V, Sorrentino A, Donnarumma G, Baroni A, Masella L, Tufano MA, Zappia M, Galletti P. Hydroxytyrosol, a natural antioxidant from olive oil, prevents protein damage induced by long-wave ultraviolet radiation in melanoma cells. Fr Rad Bio Med. 2005 Apr 1;38(7):908-19.

Darby S, Hill D, Auvinen A, Barros-Dios JM, Baysson H, Bochicchio F, Doll R, et al. Radon in homes and risk of lung cancer: collaborative analysis of individual data from 13 European case-control studies. BMJ. 2005 Jan 29;330(7485):223.

Darby S, Hill D, Auvinen A, Bochicchio F, et al. Radon in homes and risk of lung cancer: collaborative analysis of individual data from 13 European case-control studies. BMJ. 2005 Jan 29;330(7485):223.

Das I, Acharya A, Berry DL, Sen S, Williams E, Permaul E, Sengupta A, Bhattacharya S, Saha T. Antioxidative effects of the spice cardamom against non-melanoma skin cancer by modulating nuclear factor erythroid-2-related factor 2 and NF-κB signaling pathways. Br J Nutr. 2012 Sep 28;108(6):984-97. doi: 10.1017/S0007114511006283.

Davidson T. Rhinology: The Collected Writings of Maurice H. Cottle, M.D. San Diego, CA: American Rhinologic Society, 1987.

Davies G. Timetables of Medicine. New York: Black Dog & Leventhal, 2000.

Davin JC, Forget P, Mahieu PR. Increased intestinal permeability to (51 Cr) EDTA is correlated with IgA immune complex-plasma levels in children with IgA-associated nephropathies. Acta Paediatr Scand. 1988 Jan;77(1):118-24.

DaVinci L. (Dickens E. ed.) The Da Vinci Notebooks. London: Profile, 2005.

Davis DL, Kesari S, Soskolne CL, Miller AB, Stein Y. Swedish review strengthens grounds for concluding that radiation from cellular and cordless phones is a probable human carcinogen. Pathophysiology. 2013 Apr;20(2):123-9. doi: 10.1016/j.pathophys.2013.03.001.

Davis GE Jr, Lowell WE. Chaotic solar cycles modulate the incidence and severity of mental illness. Med Hypotheses. 2004;62(2):207-14.

Davis GE Jr, Lowell WE. Solar cycles and their relationship to human disease and adaptability. Med Hypothe-ses. 2006;67(3):447-61.

Davis GE Jr, Lowell WE. The Sun determines human longevity: teratogenic effects of chaotic solar radia-tion. Med Hypotheses. 2004;63(4):574-81.

Davis RL, Mostofi FK. Cluster of testicular cancer in police officers exposed to hand-held radar. Am J Ind Med. 1993 Aug;24(2):231-3.

Davis S, Kaune WT, Mirick DK, Chen C, Stevens RG. Residential magnetic fields, light-at-night, and noc-turnal urinary 6-sulfatoxymelatonin concentration in women. Am J Epidem. 2001 Oct 1;154(7):591-600.

Davis S, Mirick DK, Stevens RG. Night shift work, light at night, and risk of breast cancer. J Natl Cancer Inst. 2001 Oct 17;93(20):1557-62.

Davis-Berman J, Berman DS. The widlerness therapy program: an empirical study of its effects with adoles-cents in an outpatient setting. Journal of Contemporary Psychotherapy. 1989;19 (4):271-281.

de Groot AC, Maibach HI. Does allergic contact dermatitis from formaldehyde in clothes treated with durable-press chemical finishes exist in the USA? Contact Dermatitis. 2010 Mar;62(3):127-36. doi: 10.1111/j.1600-0536.2009.01581.x.

de Groot S, Pijl H, van der Hoeven JJM, Kroep JR. Effects of short-term fasting on cancer treatment. J Exp Clin Cancer Res. 2019 May 22;38(1):209. doi: 10.1186/s13046-019-1189-9. PMID: 31113478; PMCID: PMC6530042.

de Lima RMT, Dos Reis AC, de Menezes APM, Santos JVO, Filho JWGO, Ferreira JRO, de Alencar MVOB, da Mata AMOF, Khan IN, Islam A, Uddin SJ, Ali ES, Islam MT, Tripathi S, Mishra SK, Mubarak MS, Melo-Cavalcante AAC. Protective and therapeutic potential of Ginger (Zingiber offici-nale) extract and [6]-Gingerol in cancer: A comprehensive review. Phytother Res. 2018 Oct;32(10):1885-1907. doi: 10.1002/ptr.6134.

De Lucca AJ, Bland JM, Vigo CB, Cushion M, Selitrennikoff CP, Peter J, Walsh TJ. CAY-I, a fungicidal saponin from Capsicum sp. fruit. Med Mycol. 2002 Apr;40(2):131-7.

de Paula LC, Fonseca F, Perazzo F, Cruz FM, Cubero D, Trufelli DC, Martins SP, Santi PX, da Silva EA, Del Giglio A. Uncaria tomentosa (cat's claw) improves quality of life in patients with advanced solid tumors. J Altern Complement Med. 2015 Jan;21(1):22-30. doi: 10.1089/acm.2014.0127.

De Preter V, Raemen H, Cloetens L, Houben E, Rutgeerts P, Verbeke K. Effect of dietary intervention with different pre- and probiotics on intestinal bacterial enzyme activities. Eur J Clin Nutr. 2008 Feb;62(2):225-31.

De Simone C, Ciardi A, Grassi A, Lambert Gardini S, Tzantzoglou S, Trinchieri V, Moretti S, Jirillo E. Effect of Bifidobacterium bifidum and Lactobacillus acidophilus on gut mucosa and peripheral blood B lymphocytes. Immunopharmacol Immunotoxicol. 1992;14(1-2):331-40.

De Smet PA. Herbal remedies. N Engl J Med. 2002;347:2046-2056.

de Vrese M, Rautenberg P, Laue C, Koopmans M, Herremans T, Schrezenmeir J. Probiotic bacteria stimu-late virus-specific neutralizing antibodies following a booster polio vaccination. Eur J Nutr. 2005 Oct;44(7):406-13.

de Vrese M, Winkler P, Rautenberg P, Harder T, Noah C, Laue C, Ott S, Hampe J, Schreiber S, Heller K, Schrezenmeir J. Effect of Lactobacillus gasseri PA 16/8, Bifidobacterium longum SP 07/3, B. bifidum MF 20/5 on common cold episodes: a double blind, randomized, controlled trial. Clin Nutr. 2005 Aug;24(4):481-91.

de Vries E, Coebergh JW, van der Rhee H. Trends, causes, approach and consequences related to the skin-cancer epidemic in the Netherlands and Europe. Ned Tijdschr Geneeskd. 2006 May 20;150(20):1108-15.

Dean AM, Secrest AM, Powell DL. Contact Urticaria From Occupational Exposure to Formaldehyde. Dermatitis. 2016 Jul-Aug;27(4):232. doi: 10.1097/DER.0000000000000194.

Dean C. Death by Modern Medicine. Belleville, ON: Matrix Verite-Media, 2005.

Dean E, Mihalasky J, Ostrander S, Schroeder L. Executive ESP. Englewood Cliffs, NJ: Prentice-Hall, 1974.

Dean E. Infrared measurements of healer-treated water. In: Roll W, Beloff J, White R (Eds.): Research in parapsychology 1982. Metuchen, NJ: Scarecrow Press, 1983:100-101.

Debley JS, Carter ER, Redding GJ. Prevalence and impact of gastroesophageal reflux in adolescents with asthma: a population-based study. Pediatr Pulmonol. 2006 May;41(5):475-81.

Debras C, Chazelas E, Srour B, Kesse-Guyot E, Julia C, Zelek L, Agaësse C, Druesne-Pecollo N, Galan P, Hercberg S, Latino-Martel P, Deschasaux M, Touvier M. Total and added sugar intakes, sugar types, and cancer risk: results from the prospective NutriNet-Santé cohort. Am J Clin Nutr. 2020 Sep 16. doi: 10.1093/ajcn/nqaa246.

Deeptha K, Kamaleeswari M, Sengottuvelan M, Nalini N. Dose dependent inhibitory effect of dietary caraway on 1,2-dimethylhydrazine induced colonic aberrant crypt foci and bacterial enzyme activity in rats. Invest New Drugs. 2006 Nov;24(6):479-88. doi: 10.1007/s10637-006-6801-0.

Defrin R, Ohry A, Blumen N, Urca G. Sensory determinants of thermal pain. Brain. 2002 Mar;125(Pt 3):501-10.

Dehelean CA, Feflea S, Molnár J, Zupko I, Soica C. Betulin as an antitumor agent tested in vitro on A431, HeLa and MCF7, and as an angiogenic inhibitor in vivo in the CAM assay. Nat Prod Commun. 2012 Aug;7(8):981-5.

Deitel M. Applications of electrical pacing in the body. Obes Surg. 2004 Sep;14 Suppl 1:S3-8.

DeKoven JG, Warshaw EM, Belsito DV, Sasseville D, Maibach HI, Taylor JS, Marks JG, Fowler JF Jr, Mathias CG, DeLeo VA, Pratt MD, Zirwas MJ, Zug KA. North American Contact Dermatitis Group Patch Test Results: 2013-2014. Dermatitis. 2016 Oct 21.

Del Giudice E, Preparata G, Vitiello G. Water as a free electric dipole laser. Phys Rev Lett. 1988;61:1085-1088.

Del Giudice E. Is the 'memory of water' a physical impossibility?, in P.C. Endler, J. Schulte (eds.): Ultra High Dilution. Physiology and Physics. Dordrecht: Kluwer Academic Publishers, 1994:117-120.

Delacourt C. Bronchial changes in untreated asthma. Arch Pediatr. 2004 Jun;11 Suppl 2:71s-73s.

Delcomyn F. Foundations of Neurobiology. New York: W.H. Freeman and Co., 1998.

Delia A, Morgante G, Rago G, Musacchio MC, Petraglia F, De Leo V. Effectiveness of oral administration of Lactobacillus paracasei subsp. paracasei F19 in association with vaginal suppositories of Lactobacillus acidofilus in the treatment of vaginosis and in the prevention of recurrent vaginitis. Minerva Ginecol. 2006 Jun;58(3):227-31.

Delmanto, R. D.; de Lima, P. L. A.; Sugui, M. M.; da Eira, A. F.; Salvadori, D. M. F.; Speit, G.; Ribeiro, L. R. 2001. Antimutagenic effect of Agaricus blazei Murrill mushroom on the genotoxicity induced by cyclophosphamide. Mutation Research, 496(1-2), 15-21.

Delyukov A, Didyk L. The effects of extra-low-frequency atmospheric pressure oscillations on human mental activity. Int J Biometeorol. 1999 Jul;43(1):31-7.

DeMan, JC, Rogosa M, Sharpe ME. A medium for the cultivation of lactobacilli. J Bacteriol. 1960:23;130.

Dement W, Vaughan C. The Promise of Sleep. New York: Dell, 1999.

Demers PA, Thomas DB, Rosenblatt KA, Jimenez LM, McTiernan A, Stalsberg H, Stemhagen A, Thompson WD, Curnen MG, Satariano W, et al. Occupational exposure to electromagnetic fields and breast cancer in men. Am J Epidemiol. 1991 Aug 15;134(4):340-7.

Demidov LV, Manziuk LV, Kharkevitch GY, Pirogova NA, Artamonova EV. Adjuvant fermented wheat germ extract (Avemar) nutraceutical improves survival of high-risk skin melanoma patients: a randomized, pilot, phase II clinical study with a 7-year follow-up. Cancer Biother Radiopharm. 2008 Aug;23(4):477-82. doi: 10.1089/cbr.2008.0486. Erratum in: Cancer Biother Radiopharm. 2008 Oct;23(5):669.

Demidov LV, Manziuk LV, Kharkevitch GY, Pirogova NA, Artamonova EV. Adjuvant fermented wheat germ extract improves melanoma patient survival: a randomized, pilot, phase II clinical study with a 7-year follow-up. Cancer Biother Radiopharm. 2008 Aug;23(4):477-82. doi:10.1089/cbr.2008.0486.

Demonty I, Ras RT, van der Knaap HC, Duchateau GS, Meijer L, Zock PL, Geleijnse JM, Trautwein EA. Continuous dose-response relationship of the LDL-cholesterol-lowering effect of phytosterol intake. J Nutr. 2009 Feb;139(2):271-84. doi: 10.3945/jn.108.095125.

Deneo-Pellegrini H, Ronco AL, De Stefani E. Meat consumption and risk of squamous cell carcinoma of the lung: a case-control study in Uruguayan men. Nutr Cancer. 2015;67(1):82-8. doi: 10.1080/01635581.2015.970290.

Deng G, Lin H, Seidman A, Fornier M, D'Andrea G, Wesa K, Yeung S, Cunningham-Rundles S, Vickers AJ, Cassileth B. A phase I/II trial of a polysaccharide extract from Grifola frondosa (Maitake mushroom) in breast cancer patients: immunological effects. J Cancer Res Clin Oncol. 2009 Sep;135(9):1215-21. doi: 10.1007/s00432-009-0562-z.

Deng Q, Tian YX, Liang J. Mangiferin inhibits cell migration and invasion through Rac1/WAVE2 signalling in breast cancer. Cytotechnology. 2018 Apr;70(2):593-601. doi: 10.1007/s10616-017-0140-1.

Dengate S, Ruben A. Controlled trial of cumulative behavioural effects of a common bread preservative. J Paediatr Child Health. 2002 Aug;38(4):373-6.

Denys GA, Koch KM, Dowzicky MJ. Distribution of resistant gram-positive organisms across the census regions of the United States and in vitro activity of tigecycline, a new glycylcycline antimicrobial. Am J Infect Control. 2007 Oct;35(8):521-6.

Deorah S, Lynch CF, Sibenaller ZA, Ryken TC. Trends in brain cancer incidence and survival in the US: Surveillance, Epidemiology, and End Results, 1973 to 2001. Neurosrg Foc. 2006 Apr 15;20(4):E1.

Depeint F, Tzortzis G, Vulevic J, I'anson K, Gibson GR. Prebiotic evaluation of a novel galactooligosaccharide mixture produced by the enzymatic activity of Bifidobacterium bifidum NCIMB 41171, in healthy humans: a randomized, double-blind, crossover, placebo-controlled intervention study. Am J Clin Nutr. 2008 Mar;87(3):785-91.

Depue BE, Banich MT, Curran T. Suppression of emotional and nonemotional content in memory: effects of repetition on cognitive control. Psychol Sci. 2006 May;17(5):441-7.

Depypere HT, Comhaire FH. Herbal preparations for the menopause: beyond isoflavones and black cohosh. Maturitas. 2014 Feb;77(2):191-4. doi: 10.1016/j.maturitas.2013.11.001.

Dequanter D, Van de Velde M, Nuyens V, Nagy N, Van Antwerpen P, Vanhamme L, Zouaoui Boudjeltia K, Vanhaeverbeek M, Brohée D, Lothaire P. Assessment of oxidative stress in tumors and histologically normal mucosa from patients with head and neck squamous cell carcinoma: a preliminary study. Eur J Cancer Prev. 2013 Mar 12.

Dere E, Kart-Teke E, Huston JP, De Souza Silva MA. The case for episodic memory in animals. Neurosci Biobehav Rev. 2006;30(8):1206-24.

Desai G, Schelske-Santos M, Nazario CM, Rosario-Rosado RV, Mansilla-Rivera I, Ramírez-Marrero F, Nie J, Myneni AA, Zhang ZF, Freudenheim JL, Mu L. Onion and Garlic Intake and Breast cancer, a Case-Control Study in Puerto Rico. Nutr Cancer. 2019 Aug 12:1-10. doi: 10.1080/01635581.2019.1651349.

Desbonnet L, Garrett L, Clarke G, Bienenstock J, Dinan TG. The probiotic Bifidobacteria infantis: An assessment of potential antidepressant properties in the rat. J Psychiatr Res. 2008 Dec;43(2):164-74.

Desjeux JF, Heyman M. Milk proteins, cytokines and intestinal epithelial functions in children. Acta Paediatr Jpn. 1994 Oct;36(5):592-6.

Deutsche Gesellschaft für Ernährung. Drink distilled water? Med. Mo. Pharm. 1993;16:146.

Devaraj TL. Speaking of Ayurvedic Remedies for Common Diseases. New Delhi: Sterling, 1985.

Devirgiliis C, Zalewski PD, Perozzi G, Murgia C. Zinc fluxes and zinc transporter genes in chronic diseases. Mutat Res. 2007 Sep 1;622(1-2):84-93. 2007 Feb 17.

Devulder J, Crombez E, Mortier E. Central pain: an overview. Acta Neurol Belg. 2002 Sep;102(3):97-103.

DeWitt RC, Kudsk KA. The gut's role in metabolism, mucosal barrier function, and gut immunology. Infect Dis Clin North Am. 1999 Jun;13(2):465-81.

Dharmage SC, Erbas B, Jarvis D, Wjst M, Raherison C, Norbäck D, Heinrich J, Sunyer J, Svanes C. Do childhood respiratory infections continue to influence adult respiratory morbidity? Eur Respir J. 2009 Feb;33(2):237-44.

Dhond RP, Kettner N, Napadow V. Neuroimaging acupuncture effects in the human brain. J Altern Complement Med. 2007 Jul-Aug;13(6):603-16.

Di Gioacchino M, Cavallucci E, Di Stefano F, Paolini F, Ramondo S, Di Sciascio MB, Ciuffreda S, Riccioni G, Della Vecchia R, Romano A, Boscolo P. Effect of natural allergen exposure on non-specific bronchial reactivity in asthmatic farmers. Sci Total Environ. 2001 Apr 10;270(1-3):43-8.

Di Marzio L, Centi C, Cinque B, Masci S, Giuliani M, Arcieri A, Zicari L, De Simone C, Cifone MG. Effect of the lactic acid bacterium Streptococcus thermophilus on stratum corneum ceramide levels and signs and symptoms of atopic dermatitis patients. Exp Dermatol. 2003 Oct;12(5):615-20.

Diamond WJ, Cowden WL, Goldberg B. Cancer Diagnosis: What to Do Next. Tiburon, CA: AlternMed, 2000.

Dierksen KP, Moore CJ, Inglis M, Wescombe PA, Tagg JR. The effect of ingestion of milk supplemented with salivaricin A-producing Streptococcus salivarius on the bacteriocin-like inhibitory activity of streptococcal populations on the tongue. FEMS Microbiol Ecol. 2007 Mar;59(3):584-91.

Diğrak M, Ilçim A, Hakki Alma M. Antimicrobial activities of several parts of Pinus brutia, Juniperus oxycedrus, Abies cilicia, Cedrus libani and Pinus nigra. Phytother Res. 1999 Nov;13(7):584-7.

DiMango E, Holbrook JT, Simpson E, Reibman J, Richter J, Narula S, Prusakowski N, Mastronarde JG, Wise RA; American Lung Association Asthma Clinical Research Centers. Effects of asymptomatic proximal and distal gastroesophageal reflux on asthma severity. Am J Respir Crit Care Med. 2009 Nov 1;180(9):809-16. 2009 Aug 6.

Dimbylow PJ, Mann SM. SAR calculations in an anatomically realistic model of the head for mobile communication transceivers at 900 MHz and 1.8 GHz. Phys Med Biol. 1994 Oct;39(10):1537-53.

Dimitonova SP, Danova ST, Serkedjieva JP, Bakalov BV. Antimicrobial activity and protective properties of vaginal lactobacilli from healthy Bulgarian women. Anaerobe. 2007 Oct-Dec;13(5-6):178-84.

Dimitriadis GD, Raptis SA. Thyroid hormone excess and glucose intolerance. Exp Clin Endocrinol Diabetes. 2001;109 Suppl 2:S225-39.

Din FV, Theodoratou E, Farrington SM, Tenesa A, Barnetson RA, Cetnarskyj R, Stark L, Porteous ME, Campbell H, Dunlop MG. Effect of aspirin and NSAIDs on risk and survival from colorectal cancer. Gut. 2010 Dec;59(12):1670-9.

Ding X, Yang Q, Kong X, Haffty BG, Gao S, Moran MS. Radiosensitization effect of Huaier on breast cancer cells. Oncol Rep. 2016 May;35(5):2843-50. doi: 10.3892/or.2016.4630.

Dinleyici EC, Eren M, Yargic ZA, Dogan N, Vandenplas Y. Clinical efficacy of Saccharomyces boulardii and metronidazole compared to metronidazole alone in children with acute bloody diarrhea caused by amebiasis: a prospective, randomized, open label study. Am J Trop Med Hyg. 2009 Jun;80(6):953-5.

Dinu M, Abbate R, Gensini GF, Casini A, Sofi F. Vegetarian, vegan diets and multiple health outcomes: a systematic review with meta-analysis of observational studies. Crit Rev Food Sci Nutr. 2016 Feb 6:0.

Diop L, Guillou S, Durand H. Probiotic food supplement reduces stress-induced gastrointestinal symptoms in volunteers: a double-blind, placebo-controlled, randomized trial. Nutr Res. 2008 Jan;28(1):1-5.

Dirt-dwelling microbe ... anti-melanoma weapon. Oregon State University. January 4, 2018.

Dixon AE, Kaminsky DA, Holbrook JT, Wise RA, Shade DM, Irvin CG. Allergic rhinitis and sinusitis in asthma: differential effects on symptoms and pulmonary function. Chest. 2006 Aug;130(2):429-35.

do Prado SBR, Shiga TM, Harazono Y, Hogan VA, Raz A, Carpita NC, Fabi JP. Migration and proliferation of cancer cells in culture are differentially affected by molecular size of modified citrus pectin. Carbohydr Polym. 2019 May 1;211:141-151. doi: 10.1016/j.carbpol.2019.02.010.

Dobrowolski J, Ezzahir A, Knapik M. Possibilities of chemiluminescence application in comparative studies of animal and cancer cells with special attention to leucemic blood cells. In: Jezowska-Trzebiatowska, B., et al. (eds.). Photon Emission from Biological Systems. Singapore: World Scientific Publ, 1987:170-183.

Dolcos F, LaBar KS, Cabeza R. Interaction between the amygdala and the medial temporal lobe memory system predicts better memory for emotional events. Neuron. 2004 Jun 10;42(5):855-63.

Dona A, Arvanitoyannis IS. Health risks of genetically modified foods. Crit Rev Food Sci Nutr. 2009 Feb;49(2):164-75.

Donato F, Monarca S, Premi S., and Gelatti, U. Drinking water hardness and chronic degenerative diseases. Part III. Tumors, urolithiasis, fetal malformations, deterioration of the cognitive function in the aged and atopic eczema. Ann. Ig. 2003;15:57-70.

Dong Y, Cao A, Shi J, Yin P, Wang L, Ji G, Xie J, Wu D. Tangeretin, a citrus polymethoxyflavonoid, induces apoptosis of human gastric cancer AGS cells through extrinsic and intrinsic signaling pathways. Oncol Rep. 2014 Apr;31(4):1788-94.

Donovan S. NZ tests find formaldehyde in Chinese-made clothes. ABC News. Aug. 2007.

Dooley, M.A. and Hogan S.L. Environmental epidemiology and risk factors for autoimmune disease. Curr Opin Rheum. 2003;15(2):99-103.

Dorant E, van den Brandt PA, Goldbohm RA. Allium vegetable consumption, garlic supplement intake, and female breast carcinoma incidence. Breast cancer Res Treat. 1995;33(2):163-70.

Dore CM, Alves MG, Santos ND, Cruz AK, Câmara RB, Castro AJ, Alves LG, Nader HB, Leite EL. Antiangiogenic activity and direct antitumor effect from sulfated polysaccharide isolated from seaweed. Microvasc Res. 2013 Mar 15.

dos Santos LH, Ribeiro IO, Sánchez PG, Hetzel JL, Felicetti JC, Cardoso PF. Evaluation of pantoprazol treatment response of patients with asthma and gastroesophageal reflux: a randomized prospective double-blind placebo-controlled study. J Bras Pneumol. 2007 Apr;33(2):119-27.

Dotolo Institute. The Study of Colon Hydrotherapy. Pinellas Park, FL: Dotolo, 2003.

Dove MS, Dockery DW, Connolly GN. Smoke-free air laws and asthma prevalence, symptoms, and severity among nonsmoking youth. Pediatrics. 2011 Jan;127(1):102-9. 2010 Dec 13.

Dowd JB, Zajacova A, Aiello A. Early origins of health disparities: burden of infection, health, and socioeconomic status in U.S. children. Soc Sci Med. 2009 Feb;68(4):699-707. 2009 Jan 17.

Draelos ZD. A pilot study investigating the efficacy of botanical anti-inflammatory agents in an OTC eczema therapy. J Cosmet Dermatol. 2016 Jun;15(2):117-9. doi: 10.1111/jocd.12199.

Drago L, De Vecchi E, Nicola L, Zucchetti E, Gismondo MR, Vicariotto F. Activity of a Lactobacillus acidophilus-based douche for the treatment of bacterial vaginosis. J Altern Complement Med. 2007 May;13(4):435-8.

Drouault-Holowacz S, Bieuvelet S, Burckel A, Cazaubiel M, Dray X, Marteau P. A double blind randomized controlled trial of a probiotic combination in 100 patients with irritable bowel syndrome. Gastroenterol Clin Biol. 2008 Feb;32(2):147-52.

Drubaix I, Maraval M, Robert L, Robert AM. Hyaluronic acid (hyaluronan) levels in pathological human saphenous veins. Effects of procyanidol oligomers, Pathol Biol. 1997 Jan;45(1):86-91.

Drubaix I, Robert L, Maraval M, Robert AM. Synthesis of glycoconjugates by human diseased veins: modulation by procyanidolic oligomers. Int J Exp Pathol. 1997 Apr;78(2):117-21.

Ducrotté P. Irritable bowel syndrome: from the gut to the brain-gut. Gastroenterol Clin Biol. 2009 Aug-Sep;33(8-9):703-12.

Duke J. CRC Handbook of Medicinal Herbs. Boca Raton: CRC; 1989.

Duke J. The Green Pharmacy. New York: St. Martins, 1997.

Duke M. Acupuncture. New York: Pyramid, 1973.

Dunlop KA, Carson DJ, Shields MD. Hypoglycemia due to adrenal suppression secondary to high-dose nebulized corticosteroid. Pediatr Pulmonol. 2002 Jul;34(1):85-6.

Dunne B, Jahn R, Nelson R. Precognitive Remote Perception. Princeton Engineering Anomalies Res Lab Rep. Princeton. 1983 Aug.

Dupont C, Barau E, Molkhou P. Intestinal permeability disorders in children. Allerg Immunol. 1991 Mar;23(3):95-103.

Dupuy P, Cassé M, André F, Dhivert-Donnadieu H, Pinton J, Hernandez-Pion C. Low-salt water reduces intestinal permeability in atopic patients. Dermatology. 1999;198(2):153-5.

Duran-Tauleria E, Vignati G, Guedan MJ, Petersson CJ. The utility of specific immunoglobulin E measurements in primary care. Allergy. 2004 Aug;59 Suppl 78:35-41.

Durgo K, Belšćak-Cvitanović A, Stančić A, Franekić J, Komes D. The Bioactive Potential of Red Raspberry (Rubus idaeus L.) Leaves in Exhibiting Cytotoxic and Cytoprotective Activity on Human Laryngeal Carcinoma and Colon Adenocarcinoma. J Med Food. 2012 Mar;15(3):258-68.

Durlach J, Bara M, Guiet-Bara A. Magnesium level in drinking water: its importance in cardiovascular risk. In: Itokawa Y, Durlach J: Magnesium in Health and Disease. London: J.Libbey, 1989:173-182.

Duwiejua M, Zeitlin IJ, Waterman PG, Chapman J, Mhango GJ, Provan GJ. Anti-inflammatory activity of resins from some species of the plant family Burseraceae. Planta Med. 1993 Feb;59(1):12-6.

Dwivedi S, Agarwal MP. Antianginal and cardioprotective effects of Terminalia arjuna, an indigenous drug, in coronary artery disease. J Assoc Physicians India. 1994 Apr;42(4):287-9.

Eastham EJ, Walker WA. Effect of cow's milk on the gastrointestinal tract: a persistent dilemma for the pediatrician. Pediatrics. 1977 Oct;60(4):477-81.

Eastham LL, Howard CM, Balachandran P, Pasco DS, Claudio PP. Eating Green: Shining Light on the Use of Dietary Phytochemicals as a Modern Approach in the Prevention and Treatment of Head and Neck Cancers. Curr Top Med Chem. 2018;18(3):182-191. doi: 10.2174/1568026618666180112160713.

Eaton KK, Howard M, Howard JM. Gut permeability measured by polyethylene glycol absorption in abnormal gut fermentation as compared with food intolerance. J R Soc Med. 1995 Feb;88(2):63-6.

Ebbesen F, Agati G, Pratesi R. Phototherapy with turquoise versus blue light. Arch Dis Child Fetal Neonatal Ed. 2003 Sep;88(5):F430-1.

Ebers GC, Kukay K, Bulman DE, Sadovnick AD, Rice G, Anderson C, Armstrong H, Cousin K, Bell RB, Hader W, Paty DW, Hashimoto S, Oger J, Duquette P, Warren S, Gray T, O'Connor P, Nath A, Auty A, Metz L, Francis G, Paulseth JE, Murray TJ, Pryse-Phillips W, Nelson R, Freedman M, Brunet D, Bouchard JP, Hinds D, Risch N. A full genome search in multiple sclerosis. Nat Genet. 1996 Aug;13(4):472-6.

Ebina, Takusaburo; Fujimiya, Yoshiaki. 1998. Antitumor effect of a peptide-glucan preparation extracted from Agaricus blazei in a double-grafted tumor system in mice. Biotherapy, 11(4), 259-265.

Eccles R. Menthol and related cooling compounds. J Pharm Pharmacol. 1994 Aug;46(8):618-30.

ECRHS (2002) The European Community Respiratory Health Survey II. Eur Respir J. 20: 1071-1079.

Eden D, Feinstein D. Energy Medicine. New York: Penguin Putnam, 1998.

Edgecombe K, Latter S, Peters S, Roberts G. Health experiences of adolescents with uncontrolled severe asthma. Arch Dis Child. 2010 Dec;95(12):985-91. 2010 Jul 30.

Edgell PG. The psychology of asthma. Can Med Assoc J. 1952 Aug;67(2):121-5.

Edwards B. Drawing on the Right Side of the Brain. Los Angeles, CA: Tarcher, 1979.

Edwards R, Ibison M, Jessel-Kenyon J, Taylor R. Light emission from the human body. Comple Med Res. 1989;3(2):16-19.

Edwards R, Ibison M, Jessel-Kenyon J, Taylor R. Measurements of human bioluminescence. Acup Elect Res, Intl Jnl, 1990;15:85-94.

Edwards, L. The Vortex of Life, Nature's Patterns in Space and Time. Floris Press, 1993.

Efferth T. Cancer combination therapies with artemisinin-type drugs. Biochem Pharmacol. 2017 Sep 1;139:56-70. doi: 10.1016/j.bcp.2017.03.019.

Efferth T. From ancient herb to modern drug: Artemisia annua and artemisinin for cancer therapy. Semin Cancer Biol. 2017 Oct;46:65-83. doi: 10.1016/j.semcancer.2017.02.009.

Egan KM, Sosman JA, Blot WJ. Sunlight and reduced risk of cancer: is the real story vitamin D? J Natl Cancer Inst. 2005 Feb 2;97(3):161-3.

Egashira Y, Nagano H. A multicenter clinical trial of TJ-96 in patients with steroid-dependent bronchial asthma. A comparison of groups allocated by the envelope method. Ann N Y Acad Sci. 1993 Jun 23;685:580-3.

Ege MJ, Frei R, Bieli C, Schram-Bijkerk D, Waser M, Benz MR, Weiss G, Nyberg F, van Hage M, Pershagen G, Brunekreef B, Riedler J, Lauener R, Braun-Fahrländer C, von Mutius E; PARSIFAL Study team.

Not all farming environments protect against the development of asthma and wheeze in children. J Allergy Clin Immunol. 2007 May;119(5):1140-7.

Egon G, Chartier-Kastler E, Denys P, Ruffion A. Spinal cord injury patient and Brindley neurostimulation. Prog Urol. 2007 May;17(3):535-9.

Ehling S, Hengel M, and Shibamoto T. Formation of acrylamide from lipids. Adv Exp Med Biol 2005, 561:223-233.

Ehren J, Morón B, Martin E, Bethune MT, Gray GM, Khosla C. A food-grade enzyme preparation with modest gluten detoxification properties. PLoS One. 2009 Jul 21;4(7):e6313.

Eijkemans M, Mommers M, de Vries SI, van Buuren S, Stafleu A, Bakker I, Thijs C. Asthmatic symptoms, physical activity, and overweight in young children: a cohort study. Pediatrics. 2008 Mar;121(3):e666-72.

Einbonda LS, Negrinb A, Kulakowskib DM, Wud HA, Antonettib V, Jaleesb F, Lawa W, Rollere M, Redentib S, Kennellyb EJ, Balicka MJ. Traditional preparations of kava (Piper methysticum) inhibit the growth of human colon cancer cells in vitro. Phytomedicine. Volume 24, 15 January 2017, Pages 1–13.

Ekström AM, Serafini M, Nyrén O, Hansson LE, Ye W, Wolk A. Dietary antioxidant intake and the risk of cardia cancer and noncardia cancer of the intestinal and diffuse types: a population-based case-control study in Sweden. Int J Cancer. 2000;87:133–140.

El-Deeb NM, El-Adawi HI, El-Wahab AEA, Haddad AM, El Enshasy HA, He YW, Davis KR. Modulation of NKG2D, KIR2DL and Cytokine Production by Pleurotus ostreatus Glucan Enhances Natural Killer Cell Cytotoxicity Toward Cancer Cells. Front Cell Dev Biol. 2019 Aug 13;7:165. doi: 10.3389/fcell.2019.00165.

Electromagnetic fields: the biological evidence. Science. 1990;249:1378-1381.

el-Ghazaly M, Khayyal MT, Okpanyi SN, Arens-Corell M. Study of the anti-inflammatory activity of Populus tremula, Solidago virgaurea and Fraxinus excelsior. Arzneimittelforschung. 1992 Mar;42(3):333-6.

Elias S, van Noord P, Peeters P, den Tonkelaar I, Kaaks R, Grobbee D. Menstruation during and after caloric restriction: The 1944-1945 Dutch famine. Fertil Steril. 2007 Jun 1.

Eliassen AH, Liao X, Rosner B, Tamimi RM, Tworoger SS, Hankinson SE. Plasma carotenoids and risk of breast cancer over 20 y of follow-up. Am J Clin Nutr. 2015 Jun;101(6):1197-205. doi: 10.3945/ajcn.114.105080.

Eliaz I, Weil E, Schwarzbach J, Wilk B. Modified Citrus Pectin / Alginate Dietary Supplement Increased Fecal Excretion of Uranium: A Family. Altern Ther Health Med. 2019 Jul;25(4):20-24.

Elkin M, Ariel I, Miao HQ, Nagler A, Pines M, de-Groot N, Hochberg A, Vlodavsky I. Inhibition of bladder carcinoma angiogenesis, stromal support, and tumor growth by halofuginone. Cancer Res. 1999 Aug 15;59(16):4111-8.

Ellingwood F. American Materia Medica, Therapeutics and Pharmacognosy. Portland: Eclectic Medical Publ., 1983.

Elliott RB, Harris DP, Hill JP, Bibby NJ, Wasmuth HE. Type I (insulin-dependent) diabetes mellitus and cow milk: casein variant consumption. Diabetologia. 1999 Mar;42(3):292-6.

Elmer GW, McFarland LV, Surawicz CM, Danko L, Greenberg RN. Behaviour of Saccharomyces boulardii in recurrent Clostridium difficile disease patients. Aliment Pharmacol Ther. 1999 Dec;13(12):1663-8.

Eltiti S, Wallace D, Ridgewell A, Zougkou K, Russo R, Sepulveda F, et al. Does Short-Term Exposure to Mobile Phone Base Station Signals Increase Symptoms in Individuals who Report Sensitivity to Electromagnetic Fields? Environ Health Perspect. 2007;115(11):1603-1608.

Elwood PC. Epidemiology and trace elements. Clin Endocrinol Metab. 1985 Aug;14(3):617-28.

Emberlin JC, Lewis RA. Pollen challenge study of a phototherapy device for reducing the symptoms of hay fever. Curr Med Res Opin. 2009 Jul;25(7):1635-44.

EN 50360. Product Standard to Demonstrate the Compliance of Mobile Phones with the Basic Restrictions Related to Human Exposure to Electromagnetic Fields (300 MHz 3GHz). Brussels: CENELEC, 2001.

Endler PC, Schulte, J. Ultra High Dilution. Physiology and Physics. Dordrecht: Kluwer Academic Publ, 1994.

Environmental Working Group. Human Toxome Project. ewg.org Accessed: 2020 Sep.

EPA. A Brief Guide to Mold, Moisture and Your Home. Environmental Protection Agency, Office of Air and Radiation/Indoor Environments Division. EPA 2002;402-K-02-003.

Epplein M, Zheng W, Li H, et al. Diet, Helicobacter pylori strain-specific infection, and gastric cancer risk among Chinese men. Nutr Cancer. 2014;66(4):550-557. doi:10.1080/01635581.2014.894096

Epstein GN, Halper JP, Barrett EA, Birdsall C, McGee M, Baron KP, Lowenstein S. A pilot study of mind-body changes in adults with asthma who practice mental imagery. Altern Ther Health Med. 2004 Jul-Aug;10(4):66-71.

Erdelyi R. MHD waves and oscillations in the solar plasma. Introduction. Philos Transact A Math Phys Eng Sci. 2006 Feb 15;364(1839):289-96.

Ernst E. Frankincense: systematic review. BMJ. 2008 Dec 17;337:a2813.

Eschenhagen T, Zimmermann WH. Engineering myocardial tissue. Circ Res. 2005 Dec 9;97(12):1220-31.

REFERENCES AND BIBLIOGRAPHY

EuroPrevall. WP 1.1 Birth Cohort Update. 1st Quarter 2006. Berlin, Germany: Charité University Medical Centre.

Evans P, Forte D, Jacobs C, Fredhoi C, Aitchison E, Hucklebridge F, Clow A. Cortisol secretory activity in older people in relation to positive and negative well-being. Psychoneuroendocrinology. 2007 Aug 7.

Everhart JE. Digestive Diseases in the United States. Darby, PA: Diane Pub, 1994.

Ezzo JM, Richardson MA, Vickers A, Allen C, Dibble SL, Issell BF, Lao L, Pearl M, Ramirez G, Roscoe J, Shen J, Shivnan JC, Streitberger K, Treish I, Zhang G. Acupuncture-point stimulation for chemotherapy-induced nausea or vomiting. Cochrane Database Syst Rev. 2006 Apr 19;(2):CD002285.

Fabian E, Elmadfa I. Influence of daily consumption of probiotic and conventional yoghurt on the plasma lipid profile in young healthy women. Ann Nutr Metab. 2006;50(4):387-93.

Fabian E, Majchrzak D, Dieminger B, Meyer E, Elmadfa I. Influence of probiotic and conventional yoghurt on the status of vitamins B1, B2 and B6 in young healthy women. Ann Nutr Metab. 2008;52(1):29-36.

Fadelu T, et al. Nut consumption and survival in colon cancer patients: Results from CALGB 89803 (Alliance). J Clin Oncol 35, 2017 (suppl; abstr 3517).

Fairchild SS, Shannon K, Kwan E, Mishell RI. T cell-derived glucosteroid response-modifying factor (GRMFT): a unique lymphokine made by normal T lymphocytes and a T cell hybridoma. J Immunol. 1984 Feb;132(2):821-7.

Fallahzadeh H, Jalali A, Momayyezi M, Bazm S. Effect of Carrot Intake in the Prevention of Gastric Cancer: A Meta-Analysis. J Gastric Cancer. 2015 Dec;15(4):256-61. doi: 10.5230/jgc.2015.15.4.256.

Fallen EL, Kamath MV, Tougas G, Upton A. Afferent vagal modulation. Clinical studies of visceral sensory input. Auton Neurosci. 2001 Jul 20;90(1-2):35-40.

Fan AY, Lao L, Zhang RX, Zhou AN, Wang LB, Moudgil KD, Lee DY, Ma ZZ, Zhang WY, Berman BM. Effects of an acetone extract of Boswellia carterii Birdw. (Burseraceae) gum resin on adjuvant-induced arthritis in lewis rats. J Ethnopharmacol. 2005 Oct 3;101(1-3):104-9.

Fan X, Zhang D, Zheng J, Gu N, Ding A, Jia X, Qing H, Jin L, Wan M, Li Q. Preparation and characterization of magnetic nano-particles with radiofrequency-induced hyperthermia for cancer treatment. Sheng Wu Yi Xue Gong Cheng Xue Za Zhi. 2006 Aug;23(4):809-13.

Fanaro S, Marten B, Bagna R, Vigi V, Fabris C, Peña-Quintana, Argüelles F, Scholz-Ahrens KE, Sawatzki G, Zelenka R, Schrezenmeir J, de Vrese M and Bertino E. Galacto-oligosaccharides are bifidogenic and safe at weaning: A double-blind Randomized Multicenter study. J Pediatr Gastroent Nutr. 2009 48; 82-88

Fang H, Elina T, Heikki A, Seppo S. Modulation of humoral immune response through probiotic intake. FEMS Immunol Med Microbiol. 2000 Sep;29(1):47-52.

Fang SP, Tanaka T, Tago F, Okamoto T, Kojima S. Immunomodulatory effects of gyokuheifusan on INF-gamma/IL-4 (Th1/Th2) balance in ovalbumin (OVA)-induced asthma model mice. Biol Pharm Bull. 2005;28:829-33.

Fang T, Liu DD, Ning HM, Dan Liu, Sun JY, Huang XJ, Dong Y, Geng MY, Yun SF, Yan J, Huang RM. Modified citrus pectin inhibited bladder tumor growth through downregulation of galectin-3. Acta Pharmacol Sin. 2018 May 16. doi:10.1038/s41401-018-0004-z.

Fanigliulo L, Comparato G, Aragona G, Cavallaro L, Iori V, Maino M, Cavestro GM, Soliani P, Sianesi M, Franzè A, Di Mario F. Role of gut microflora and probiotic effects in the irritable bowel syndrome. Acta Biomed. 2006 Aug;77(2):85-9.

FAO/WHO Expert Committee. Fats and Oils in Human Nutrition. Food and Nutrition Paper. 1994;(57).

Farber JE, Ross J, Stephens G. Antibiotic anaphylaxis. Calif Med. 1954 Jul;81(1):9-11.

Farber JE, Ross J. Antibiotic anaphylaxis; a note on the treatment and prevention of severe reactions to penicillin, streptomycin and dihydrostreptomycin. Med Times. 1952 Jan;80(1):28-30.

Farhat D, Lincet H. Lipoic acid a multi-level molecular inhibitor of tumorigenesis. Biochim Biophys Acta Rev Cancer. 2020 Jan;1873(1):188317. doi: 10.1016/j.bbcan.2019.188317.

Farkas E. Szupportív kezelés fermentált búzacsíra-kivonattal colorectalis carcinomában Fermented wheat germ extract in the supportive therapy of colorectal cancer. Orv Hetil. 2005 Sep 11;146(37):1925-31.

Farvid Maryam S, Chen Wendy Y, Michels Karin B, Cho Eunyoung, Willett Walter C, Eliassen A Heather et al. Fruit and vegetable consumption in adolescence and early adulthood and risk of breast cancer: population based cohort study BMJ 2016; 353 :i2343

Fasano A, Shea-Donohue T. Mechanisms of disease: the role of intestinal barrier function in the pathogenesis of gastrointestinal autoimmune diseases. Nat Clin Pract Gastroenterol Hepatol. 2005 Sep;2(9):416-22.

Fawell J, Nieuwenhuijsen MJ. Contaminants in drinking water. Br Med Bull. 2003;68:199-208.

Fecher LA, Cummings SD, Keefe MJ, Alani RM. Toward a molecular classification of melanoma. J Clin Oncol. 2007 Apr 20;25(12):1606-20.

Fecka I. Qualitative and quantitative determination of hydrolysable tannins and other polyphenols in herbal products from meadowsweet and dog rose. Phytochem Anal. 2009 May;20(3):177-90.

Federal Communications Commission.. Evaluating Compliance with FCC Guidelines for Human Exposure to Radio Frequency Electromagnetic Fields. Washington, DC: Supplement C to OET Bulletin 65 (01), 1997.

Fehring RJ, Schneider M, Raviele K. Variability in the phases of the menstrual cycle. J Obstet Gynecol Neonatal Nurs. 2006 May-Jun;35(3):376-84.

Feki-Tounsi M, Hamza-Chaffai A. Cadmium as a possible cause of bladder cancer: a review of accumulated evidence. Environ Sci Pollut Res Int. 2014;21(18):10561-10573. doi:10.1007/s11356-014-2970-0

Felley CP, Corthésy-Theulaz I, Rivero JL, Sipponen P, Kaufmann M, Bauerfeind P, Wiesel PH, Brassart D, Pfeifer A, Blum AL, Michetti P. Favourable effect of an acidified milk (LC-1) on Helicobacter pylori gastritis in man. Eur J Gastroenterol Hepatol. 2001 Jan;13(1):25-9.

Felton JS, Fultz E, Dolbeare FA, Knize MG. Effect of microwave pretreatment on heterocyclic aromatic amine mutagens/carcinogens in fried beef patties. Food Chem Toxicol. 1994 Oct;32(10):897-903.

Feng B, Zhu Y, Sun C, Su Z, Tang L, Li C, Zheng G. Basil polysaccharide inhibits hypoxia-induced hepatocellular carcinoma metastasis and progression through suppression of HIF-1α-mediated epithelial-mesenchymal transition. Int J Biol Macromol. 2019 Sep 15;137:32-44. doi: 10.1016/j.ijbiomac.2019.06.189. Epub 2019 Jun 25.

Ferencík M, Ebringer L, Mikes Z, Jahnová A, Ciznár I. Successful modification of human intestinal microflora with oral administration of lactic acid bacteria. Bratisl Lek Listy. 1999 May;100(5):238-45.

Ferguson BJ. Categorization of eosinophilic chronic rhinosinusitis. Curr Opin Otolaryngol Head Neck Surg. 2004 Jun;12(3):237-42.

Fernández-Pérez F, Belchí-Navarro S, Almagro L, Bru R, Pedreño MA, Gómez-Ros LV. Cytotoxic Effect of Natural trans-Resveratrol Obtained from Elicited Vitis vinifera Cell Cultures on Three Cancer Cell Lines. Plant Foods Hum Nutr. 2012 Nov 17.

Fernández-Ponce MT, López-Biedma A, Sánchez-Quesada C, Casas L, Mantell C, Gaforio JJ, Martínez de la Ossa EJ. Selective antitumoural action of pressurized mango leaf extracts against invasive breast cancer. Food Funct. 2017 Oct 18;8(10):3610-3620. doi: 10.1039/c7fo00877e.

Ferrari M, Benini L, Brotto E, Locatelli F, De Iorio F, Bonella F, Tacchella N, Corradini G, Lo Cascio V, Vantini I. Omeprazole reduces the response to capsaicin but not to methacholine in asthmatic patients with proximal reflux. Scand J Gastroenterol. 2007 Mar;42(3):299-307.

Ferrier L, Berard F, Debrauwer L, Chabo C, Langella P, Bueno L, Fioramonti J. Impairment of the intestinal barrier by ethanol involves enteric microflora and mast cell activation in rodents. Am J Pathol. 2006 Apr;168(4):1148-54.

Ferrier L, Berard F, Debrauwer L, Chabo C, Langella P, Bueno L, Fioramonti J. Impairment of the intestinal barrier by ethanol involves enteric microflora and mast cell activation in rodents. Am J Pathol. 2006 Apr;168(4):1148-54.

Fews AP, Henshaw DL, Keitch PA, Close JJ, Wilding RJ. Increased exposure to pollutant aerosols under high voltage power lines. Int J Radiat Biol. 1999 Dec;75(12):1505-21.

Field RW, Krewski D, Lubin JH, Zielinski JM, Alavanja M, Catalan VS, Klotz JB, Letourneau EG, Lynch CF, Lyon JL, Sandler DP, Schoenberg JB, Steck DJ, Stolwijk JA, Weinberg C, Wilcox HB. An overview of the North American residential radon and lung cancer case-control studies. J Toxicol Environ Health A. 2006 Apr;69(7):599-631.

Field T, Henteleff T, Hernandez-Reif M, Martinez E, Mavunda K, Kuhn C, Schanberg S. Children with asthma have improved pulmonary functions after massage therapy. J Pediatr. 1998 May;132(5):854-8.

Firmesse O, Alvaro E, Mogenet A, Bresson JL, Lemée R, Le Ruyet P, Bonhomme C, Lambert D, Andrieux C, Doré J, Corthier G, Furet JP, Rigottier-Gois L. Fate and effects of Camembert cheese microorganisms in the human colonic microbiota of healthy volunteers after regular Camembert consumption. Int J Food Microbiol. 2008 Jul 15;125(2):176-81.

Fischer JL, Mihelc EM, Pollok KE, Smith ML. Chemotherapeutic selectivity conferred by selenium: a role for p53-dependent DNA repair. Mol Cancer Ther. 2007 Jan;6(1):355-61.

Fjeld T, Veiersted B, Sandvik L, Riise G, Levy F. The Effect of Indoor Foliage Plants on Health and Discomfort Symptoms among Office Workers. Ind Built Environ. 1998 July;7(4): 204-209.

Flandrin, J, Montanari M. (eds.). Food: A Culinary History from Antiquity to the Present. New York: Penguin Books, 1999.

Foer J, Siffre M. Caveman: An Interview with Michel Siffre. Cabinet. 2008 Summer (30).

Fogarty MC, Hughes CM, Burke G, Brown JC, Davison GW. Acute and chronic watercress supplementation attenuates exercise-induced peripheral mononuclear cell DNA damage and lipid peroxidation. Br J Nutr. 2012 Apr 5:1-9.

Foliaki S, Annesi-Maesano I, Tuuau-Potoi N, Waqatakirewa L, Cheng S, Douwes J, Pearce N. Risk factors for symptoms of childhood asthma, allergic rhinoconjunctivitis and eczema in the Pacific: an ISAAC Phase III study. Int J Tuberc Lung Dis. 2008 Jul;12(7):799-806.

Forbes EE, Groschwitz K, Abonia JP, Brandt EB, Cohen E, Blanchard C, Ahrens R, Seidu L, McKenzie A, Strait R, Finkelman FD, Foster PS, Matthaei KI, Rothenberg ME, Hogan SP. IL-9- and mast cell-mediated intestinal permeability predisposes to oral antigen hypersensitivity. J Exp Med. 2008 Apr 14;205(4):897-913.

Forestier C, Guelon D, Cluytens V, Gillart T, Sirot J, De Champs C. Oral probiotic and prevention of Pseudomonas aeruginosa infections: a randomized, double-blind, placebo-controlled pilot study in intensive care unit patients. Crit Care. 2008;12(3):R69.

Forget-Dubois N, Boivin M, Dionne G, Pierce T, Tremblay RE, Pérusse D. A longitudinal twin study of the genetic and environmental etiology of maternal hostile-reactive behavior during infancy and toddlerhood. Infant Behav Dev. 2007

Foster S, Hobbs C. Medicinal Plants and Herbs. Boston: Houghton Mifflin, 2002.

Fox RD, Algoculture. Doctorate Disseration, 1983 Jul.

Fraga CG. Relevance, essentiality and toxicity of trace elements in human health. Mol Aspects Med. 2005 Aug-Oct;26(4-5):235-44.

Francavilla R, Lionetti E, Castellaneta SP, Magistà AM, Maurogiovanni G, Bucci N, De Canio A, Indrio F, Cavallo L, Ierardi E, Miniello VL. Inhibition of Helicobacter pylori infection in humans by Lactobacillus reuteri ATCC 55730 and effect on eradication therapy: a pilot study. Helicobacter. 2008 Apr;13(2):127-34.

Francis H, Fletcher G, Anthony C, Pickering C, Oldham L, Hadley E, Custovic A, Niven R. Clinical effects of air filters in homes of asthmatic adults sensitized and exposed to pet allergens. Clin Exp Allergy. 2003 Jan;33(1):101-5.

Frank PI, Morris JA, Hazell ML, Linehan MF, Frank TL. Long term prognosis in preschool children with wheeze: longitudinal postal questionnaire study 1993-2004. BMJ. 2008 Jun 21;336(7658):1423-6. 2008 Jun 16.

Frawley D, Lad V. The Yoga of Herbs. Sante Fe: Lotus Press, 1986.

Frazier AL, Rosenberg SM. Preadolescent and adolescent risk for benign breast disease. J Adolesc Health. 2013 May;52(5 Suppl):S36-40. doi: 10.1016/j.jadohealth.2013.01.007.

Freedman BJ. A dietary free from additives in the management of allergic disease. Clin Allergy. 1977 Sep;7(5):417-21.

Freeman HL, Stansfield SA. Psychosocial effects of urban environments, noise, and crowding. In Lundberg, A. (ed) Environment and Mental Health. London: Lawrence Erlbaum. 1998:147-173.

Freeman W. The Physiology of Perception. Sci. Am. 1991 Feb.

Frenkel M. Is There a Role for Homeopathy in Cancer Care? Questions and Challenges. Curr Oncol Rep. 2015 Sep;17(9):43. doi: 10.1007/s11912-015-0467-8.

Frey A. Electromagnetic field interactions with biological systems. FASEB Jnl. 1993;7:272-28.

Frias J, Song YS, Martínez-Villaluenga C, González de Mejia E, Vidal-Valverde C. Immunoreactivity and amino acid content of fermented soybean products. J Agric Food Chem. 2008 Jan 9;56(1):99-105.

Friedman LS, Harvard Health Publ. Ed. Controlling GERD and Chronic Heartburn. Boston: Harvard Health, 2008.

Friend BA, Shahani KM, Long CA, Vaughn LA. The effect of processing and storage on key enzymes, B vitamins, and lipids of mature human milk. Evaluation of fresh samples and effects of freezing and frozen storage. Pediatr Res. 1983 Jan;17(1):61-4.

Friend BA, Shahani KM. Characterization and evaluation of Aspergillus oryzae lactase coupled to a regenerable support. Biotechnol Bioeng. 1982 Feb;24(2):329-45.

Fritz H, Flower G, Weeks L, Cooley K, Callachan M, McGowan J, Skidmore B, Kirchner L, Seely D. Intravenous Vitamin C and Cancer: A Systematic Review. Integr Cancer Ther. 2014 Jul;13(4):280-300. doi: 10.1177/1534735414534463.

Frumkin H. Beyond toxicity: human health and the natural environment. Am J Prev Med. 2001;20(3):234-40.

Fu G, Zhong Y, Li C, Li Y, Lin X, Liao B, Tsang EW, Wu K, Huang S. Epigenetic regulation of peanut allergen gene Ara h 3 in developing embryos. Planta. 2010 Apr;231(5):1049-60.

Fu JX. Measurement of MEFV in 66 cases of asthma in the convalescent stage and after treatment with Chinese herbs. Zhong Xi Yi Jie He Za Zhi. 1989 Nov;9(11):658-9, 644.

Fu XH. Observation on therapeutic effect of acupuncture on early peripheral facial paralysis. Zhongguo Zhen Jiu. 2007 Jul;27(7):494-6.

Fuhrman BJ, Pfeiffer RM, Wu AH, Xu X, Keefer LK, Veenstra TD, Ziegler RG. Green tea intake is associated with urinary estrogen profiles in Japanese-American women. Nutr J. 2013 Feb 15;12(1):25.

Fuiano N, Fusilli S, Passalacqua G, Incorvaia C. Allergen-specific immunoglobulin E in the skin and nasal mucosa of symptomatic and asymptomatic children sensitized to aeroallergens. J Investig Allergol Clin Immunol. 2010;20(5):425-30.

Fujii T, Ohtsuka Y, Lee T, Kudo T, Shoji H, Sato H, Nagata S, Shimizu T, Yamashiro Y. Bifidobacterium breve enhances transforming growth factor beta1 signaling by regulating Smad7 expression in preterm in-fants. J Pediatr Gastroenterol Nutr. 2006 Jul;43(1):83-8.

Fujii T, Ohtsuka Y, Lee T, Kudo T, Shoji H, Sato H, Nagata S, Shimizu T, Yamashiro Y. Bifidobacterium breve enhances transforming growth factor beta1 signaling by regulating Smad7 expression in preterm infants. J Pediatr Gastroenterol Nutr. 2006 Jul;43(1):83-8.

Fujimiya, Yoshiaki; Suzuki, Youichi; Oshiman, Ko-Ichi; Kobori, Hidekazu; Moriguchi, Koichi; Nakashima, Hisako; Matumoto, Yonezo; Takahara, Shogo; Ebina, Takusaburo; Katakura, Ryuichi. 1998. Selective tumoricidal effect of soluble proteoglucan extracted from the basidiomycete, Agaricus blazei Murill, mediated via natural killer cell activation and apoptosis. Cancer Immunology Immunotherapy, 46(3), 147-159.

Fujimiya, Yoshiaki; Yamamoto, Hajimu; Noji, Masahide; Suzuki, Ikukatsu. 2000. Peroral effect on tumor progression of soluble b-(1,6)-glucans prepared by acid treatment from Agaricus blazei Murr. (Agaricaceae, higher Basidiomycetes). International Journal of Medicinal Mushrooms, 2(1), 43-49.

Fujimori S, Gudis K, Mitsui K, Seo T, Yonezawa M, Tanaka S, Tatsuguchi A, Sakamoto C. A randomized controlled trial on the efficacy of synbiotic versus probiotic or prebiotic treatment to improve the quality of life in patients with ulcerative colitis. Nutrition. 2009 May;25(5):520-5.

Fujimoto S, Furue H, Kimura T, Kondo T, Orita K, Taguchi T, Yoshida K, Ogawa N. (1991). Clinical outcome of postoperative adjuvant immunochemotherapy with sizofiran for patients with resectable gastric cancer: a randomised controlled study. European journal of cancer, 27(9), 1114-8.

Fulgoni VL 3rd. Current protein intake in America: analysis of the National Health and Nutrition Examination Survey, 2003-2004. Am J Clin Nutr. 2008 May;87(5):1554S-1557S.

Fung TT, van Dam RM, Hankinson SE, Stampfer M, Willett WC, Hu FB. Low-carbohydrate diets and mortality: two cohort studies. Ann Intern Med. 2010 Sep 7;153(5):289-98. Protein: Moving Closer to Center Stage.

Furrie E, Macfarlane S, Kennedy A, Cummings JH, Walsh SV, O'neil DA, Macfarlane GT. Synbiotic therapy (Bifidobacterium longum/Synergy 1) initiates resolution of inflammation in patients with active ulcerative colitis: a randomised controlled pilot trial. Gut. 2005 Feb;54(2):242-9.

Fuster JM. Prefrontal neurons in networks of executive memory. Brain Res Bull. 2000 Jul 15;52(5):331-6.

Gabory A, Attig L, Junien C. Sexual dimorphism in environmental epigenetic programming. Mol Cell Endocrinol. 2009 May 25;304(1-2):8-18. 2009 Mar 9.

Gabriel S, Schaffner S, Nguyen H, Moore J, Roy J. The structure of haplotype blocks in the human genome. Science. 2002;296:2225-2229.

Gaddy JA, Radin JN, Loh JT, Zhang F, Washington MK, Peek RM Jr, Algood HM, Cover TL. High dietary salt intake exacerbates Helicobacter pylori-induced gastric carcinogenesis. Infect Immun. 2013 Apr 8.

Gandhi T, Weingart S, Borus J, Seger A, Peterson J, Burdick E, Seger D, Shu K, Federico F, Leape L, Bates D. Adverse drug events in ambulatory care. N Engl J Med. 2003 Apr 17;348(16):1556-64.

Gange R. UVA sunbeds - are there longterm hazards. In Cronley-Dillon J, Rosen E, Marshall J (Eds.):Hazards of Light, Myths and Realities. Oxford, U.K.: Pergamon Press, 1986.

Gao X, Wang W, Wei S, Li W. Review of pharmacological effects of Glycyrrhiza radix and its bioactive compounds. Zhongguo Zhong Yao Za Zhi. 2009 Nov;34(21):2695-700.

Gao XJ, Liu JW, Zhang QG, Zhang JJ, Xu HT, Liu HJ. Nobiletin inhibited hypoxia-induced epithelial-mesenchymal transition of lung cancer cells by inactivating of Notch-1 signaling and switching on miR-200b. Pharmazie. 2015 Apr;70(4):256-62.

Gaón D, Doweck Y, Gómez Zavaglia A, Ruiz Holgado A, Oliver G. Lactose digestion by milk fermented with Lactobacillus acidophilus and Lactobacillus casei of human origin. Medicina (B Aires). 1995;55(3):237-42.

Gaón D, García H, Winter L, Rodríguez N, Quintás R, González SN, Oliver G. Effect of Lactobacillus strains and Saccharomyces boulardii on persistent diarrhea in children. Medicina (B Aires). 2003;63(4):293-8.

Gaón D, Garmendia C, Murrielo NO, de Cucco Games A, Cerchio A, Quintas R, González SN, Oliver G. Effect of Lactobacillus strains (L. casei and L. Acidophilus Strains cerela) on bacterial overgrowth-related chronic diarrhea. Medicina. 2002;62(2):159-63.

Garaczi E, Boros-Gyevi M, Bella Z, Kemény L, Koreck A. Intranasal phototherapy is more effective than fexofenadine hydrochloride in the treatment of seasonal allergic rhinitis: results of a pilot study. Photochem Photobiol. 2011 Mar-Apr;87(2):474-7.

Garami M, Schuler D, Babosa M, Borgulya G, Hauser P, Müller J, Paksy A, Szabó E, Hidvégi M, Fekete G. Fermented wheat germ extract reduces chemotherapy-induced febrile neutropenia in pediatric cancer patients. J Pediatr Hematol Oncol. 2004 Oct;26(10):631-5.

García AM, Sisternas A, Hoyos SP. Occupational exposure to extremely low frequency electric and magnetic fields and Alzheimer disease: a meta-analysis. Int J Epidemiol. 2008 Apr;37(2):329-40.

Garcia Gomez LJ, Sanchez-Muniz FJ. Review: cardiovascular effect of garlic (Allium sativum). Arch Latinoam Nutr. 2000 Sep;50(3):219-29.

Garcia Vilela E, De Lourdes De Abreu Ferrari M, Oswaldo Da Gama Torres H, Guerra Pinto A, Carolina Carneiro Aguirre A, Paiva Martins F, Marcos Andrade Goulart E, Sales Da Cunha A. Influence of Saccharomyces boulardii on the intestinal permeability of patients with Crohn's disease in remission. Scand J Gastroenterol. 2008;43(7):842-8.

Garcia-Lazaro JA, Ahmed B, Schnupp JW. Tuning to natural stimulus dynamics in primary auditory cortex. Curr Biol. 2006 Feb 7;16(3):264-71.

Garcia-Lazaro JA, Ahmed B, Schnupp JW. Tuning to natural stimulus dynamics in primary auditory cortex. Curr Biol. 2006 Feb 7;16(3):264-71.

Garcia-Marcos L, Canflanca IM, Garrido JB, Varela AL, Garcia-Hernandez G, Guillen Grima F, Gonzalez-Diaz C, Carvajal-Urueña I, Arnedo-Pena A, Busquets-Monge RM, Morales Suarez-Varela M, Blanco-Quiros A. Relationship of asthma and rhinoconjunctivitis with obesity, exercise and Mediterranean diet in Spanish schoolchildren. Thorax. 2007 Jun;62(6):503-8.

García-Rivera D, Delgado R, Bougarne N, Haegeman G, Berghe WV. Gallic acid indanone and mangiferin xanthone are strong determinants of immunosuppressive anti-tumour effects of Mangifera indica L. bark in MDA-MB231 breast cancer cells. Cancer Lett. 2011 Jun 1;305(1):21-31.

Garcia-Saenz A, Sánchez de Miguel A, Espinosa A, Valentin A, Aragonés N, Llorca J, Amiano P, Martín Sánchez V, Guevara M, Capelo R, Tardón A, Peiró-Perez R, Jiménez-Moleón JJ, Roca-Barceló A, Pérez-Gómez B, Dierssen-Sotos T, Fernández-Villa T, Moreno-Iribas C, Moreno V, García-Pérez J, Castaño-Vinyals G, Pollán M, Aubé M, Kogevinas M. Evaluating the Association between Artificial Light Exposure and Breast and Prostate Cancer Risk in Spain (MCC-Spain Study). Environ Health Perspect. 2018 Apr 23;126(4):047011. doi: 10.1289/EHP1837.

Gardiner PA, Eakin EG, Healy GN, Owen N. Feasibility of reducing older adults' sedentary time. Am J Prev Med. 2011 Aug;41(2):174-7. PubMed PMID: 21767725.

Gardiner PA, Healy GN, Eakin EG, Clark BK, Dunstan DW, Shaw JE, Zimmet PZ, Owen N. Associations between television viewing and sitting time with metabolic syndrome in older men and women: the Australian Diabetes, Obesity and Lifestyle study. J Am Geriatr Soc. 2011 May;59(5):788-96.

Gardner CD, Fortmann SP, Krauss RM. Association of small low-density lipoprotein particles with the incidence of coronary artery disease in men and women. JAMA. 1996 Sep 18;276(11):875-81.

Gardner ML. Gastrointestinal absorption of intact proteins. Annu Rev Nutr. 1988;8:329-50.

Garland CF, Cuomo RE, Gorham ED, Zeng K, Mohr SB. Cloud cover-adjusted ultraviolet B irradiance and pancreatic cancer incidence in 172 countries. J Steroid Biochem Mol Biol. 2015 Apr 9. pii: S0960-0760(15)00101-6. doi: 10.1016/j.jsbmb.2015.04.004.

Garland CF, Gorham ED, Mohr SB, Grant WB, Giovannucci EL, Lipkin M, Newmark H, Holick MF, Garland FC. Vitamin D and prevention of breast cancer: pooled analysis. J Steroid Biochem Mol Biol. 2007 Mar;103(3-5):708-11.

Gary WK, Fanny WS, David SC. Factors associated with difference in prevalence of asthma in children from three cities in China: multicentre epidemiological survey. BMJ. 2004;329:1-4.

Garzi A, Messina M, Frati F, Carfagna L, Zagordo L, Belcastro M, Parmiani S, Sensi L, Marcucci F. An extensively hydrolysed cow's milk formula improves clinical symptoms of gastroesophageal reflux and reduces the gastric emptying time in infants. Allergol Immunopathol (Madr). 2002 Jan-Feb;30(1):36-41.

Gau SS, Soong WT, Merikangas KR. Correlates of sleep-wake patterns among children and young adolescents in Taiwan. Sleep. 2004 May 1;27(3):512-9.

Gauger J.R. Household appliance magnetic field survey. IEEE PAS-104, No.9:2436-2445, 1985.

Gawrońska A, Dziechciarz P, Horvath A, Szajewska H. A randomized double-blind placebo-controlled trial of Lactobacillus GG for abdominal pain disorders in children. Aliment Pharmacol Ther. 2007 Jan 15;25(2):177-84.

Gazdik F, Kadrabova J, Gazdikova K. Decreased consumption of corticosteroids after selenium supplementation in corticoid-dependent asthmatics. Bratisl Lek Listy. 2002;103(1):22-5.

Geha RS, Beiser A, Ren C, Patterson R, Greenberger PA, Grammer LC, Ditto AM, Harris KE, Shaughnessy MA, Yarnold PR, Corren J, Saxon A. Multicenter, double-blind, placebo-controlled, multiple-challenge evaluation of reported reactions to monosodium glutamate. J Allergy Clin Immunol. 2000 Nov;106(5):973-80.

Geller A, Shrestha R, Yan J. Yeast-Derived β-Glucan in Cancer: Novel Uses of a Traditional Therapeutic. Int J Mol Sci. 2019 Jul 24;20(15):3618. doi: 10.3390/ijms20153618.

Geller SE, Studee L. Botanical and dietary supplements for mood and anxiety in menopausal women. Menopause. 2007 May-Jun;14(3 Pt 1):541-9.

Gerber R. Vibrational Healing. Sante Fe: Bear, 1988.

Gerhauser C. Epigenetic impact of dietary isothiocyanates in cancer chemoprevention. Curr Opin Clin Nutr Metab Care. 2013 Jul;16(4):405-10. doi: 10.1097/MCO.0b013e328362014e.

Gesler WM. Therapeutic landscapes: medical issues in light of the new cultural geography. Soc Sci Med. 1992 Apr;34(7):735-46.

Ghadioungui P. (transl.) The Ebers Papyrus. Academy of Scientific Research. Cairo, 1987.

Ghalaut VS, Sangwan L, Dahiya K, Ghalaut PS, Dhankhar R, Saharan R. Effect of imatinib therapy with and without turmeric powder on nitric oxide levels in chronic myeloid leukemia. J Oncol Pharm Pract. 2012 Jun;18(2):186-90. doi: 10.1177/1078155211416530. Biswas J, Sinha D, Mukherjee S, Roy S, Siddiqi M, Roy M. Curcumin protects DNA damage in a chronically arsenic-exposed population of West Bengal. Hum Exp Toxicol. 2010 Jun;29(6):513-24. doi: 10.1177/0960327109359020.

Gibbons E. Stalking the Healthful Herbs. New York: David McKay, 1966.

Gibson RA. Docosa-hexaenoic acid (DHA) accumulation is regulated by the polyunsaturated fat content of the diet: Is it synthesis or is it incorporation? Asia Pac J Clin Nutr. 2004;13(Suppl):S78.

Gilbert CR, Arum SM, Smith CM. Vitamin D deficiency and chronic lung disease. Can Respir J. 2009 May-Jun;16(3):75-80.

Gill HS, Rutherfurd KJ, Cross ML, Gopal PK. Enhancement of immunity in the elderly by dietary supplementation with the probiotic Bifidobacterium lactis HN019. Am J Clin Nutr. 2001 Dec;74(6):833-9.

Gill HS, Rutherfurd KJ, Cross ML. Dietary probiotic supplementation enhances natural killer cell activity in the elderly: an investigation of age-related immunological changes. J Clin Immunol. 2001 Jul;21(4):264-71.

Ginde AA, Mansbach JM, Camargo CA Jr. Association between serum 25-hydroxyvitamin D level and upper respiratory tract infection in the Third National Health and Nutrition Examination Survey. Arch Intern Med. 2009 Feb 23;169(4):384-90.

Gionchetti P, Rizzello F, Venturi A, Brigidi P, Matteuzzi D, Bazzocchi G, Poggioli G, Miglioli M, Campieri M. Oral bacteriotherapy as maintenance treatment in patients with chronic pouchitis: a double-blind, placebo-controlled trial. Gastroenterology. 2000 Aug;119(2):305-9.

Giovannucci E. The epidemiology of vitamin D and cancer incidence and mortality: Cancer Causes Control. 2005 Mar;16(2):83-95.

Gisler GC, Diaz J, Duran N. Observations on Blood Plasma Chemiluminescence in Normal Subjects and Cancer Patients. Arq Biol Tecnol. 1983;26(3):345-352.

Gittleman AL. Guess What Came to Dinner. New York: Avery, 2001.

Giuseppina Mandalari, Carlo Bisignano, Santa Cirmi, and Michele Navarra. Effectiveness of Citrus Fruits on Helicobacter pylori. Evidence-Based Complementary and Alternative Medicine, vol. 2017, Article ID 8379262, 8 pages, 2017. doi:10.1155/2017/8379262

Glavas-Dodov M, Steffansen B, Crcarevska MS, Geskovski N, Dimchevska S, Kuzmanovska S, Goracinova K. Wheat germ agglutinin-functionalised crosslinked polyelectrolyte microparticles for local colon delivery of 5-FU: in vitro efficacy and in vivo gastrointestinal distribution. J Microencapsul. 2013;30(7):643-56. doi: 10.3109/02652048.2013.770099.

Glinsky VV, Raz A. Modified citrus pectin anti-metastatic properties: one bullet, multiple targets. Carbohydr Res. 2009 Sep 28;344(14):1788-91. doi:10.1016/j.carres.2008.08.038.

Glück U, Gebbers J. Ingested probiotics reduce nasal colonization with pathogenic bacteria (Staphylococcus aureus, Streptococcus pneumoniae, and b-hemolytic streptococci. Am J. Clin. Nutr. 2003;77:517-520.

Goedsche K, Förster M, Kroegel C, Uhlemann C. Repeated cold water stimulations (hydrotherapy according to Kneipp) in patients with COPD. Forsch Komplementmed. 2007 Jun;14(3):158-66.

Goel V, Dolan RJ. The functional anatomy of humor: segregating cognitive and affective components. Nat Neurosci. 2001;4:237-8.

Goheen SC, Gaither K, Anantatmula SM, Mong GM, Sasser LB, Lessor D. Corona discharge influences ozone concentrations near rats. Bioelectromagnetics. 2004 Feb;25(2):107-13.

Gohil K, Packer L. Bioflavonoid-Rich Botanical Extracts Show Antioxidant and Gene Regulatory Activity. Ann N Y Acad Sci. 2002;957:70-7.

Goldin BR, Adlercreutz H, Dwyer JT, Swenson L, Warram JH, Gorbach SL. Effect of diet on excretion of estrogens in pre- and postmenopausal women. Cancer Res. 1981 Sep;41(9 Pt 2):3771-3.

Goldin BR, Adlercreutz H, Gorbach SL, Warram JH, Dwyer JT, Swenson L, Woods MN. Estrogen excretion patterns and plasma levels in vegetarian and omnivorous women. N Engl J Med. 1982 Dec 16;307(25):1542-7.

Goldin BR, Adlercreutz H, Gorbach SL, Warram JH, Dwyer JT, Swenson L, Woods MN. Estrogen excretion patterns and plasma levels in vegetarian and omnivorous women. N Engl J Med. 1982 Dec 16;307(25):1542-7.

Goldin BR, Swenson L, Dwyer J, Sexton M, Gorbach SL. Effect of diet and Lactobacillus acidophilus supplements on human fecal bacterial enzymes. J Natl Cancer Inst. 1980 Feb;64(2):255-61.

Goldstein JL, Aisenberg J, Zakko SF, Berger MF, Dodge WE. Endoscopic ulcer rates in healthy subjects associated with use of aspirin (81 mg q.d.) alone or coadministered with celecoxib or naproxen: a randomized, 1-week trial. Dig Dis Sci. 2008 Mar;53(3):647-56.

Goldstein LS, Dewhirst MW, Repacholi M, Kheifets L. Summary, conclusions and recommendations: adverse temperature levels in the human body. Int J Hyperthermia. 2003 May-Jun;19(3):373-84.

Goldstein N, Arshavskaya TV. Is atmospheric superoxide vitally necessary? Accelerated death of animals in a quasi-neutral electric atmosphere. Z Naturforsch. 1997. May-Jun;52(5-6):396-404.

Goldstein N, Arshavskaya TV. Is atmospheric superoxide vitally necessary? Accelerated death of animals in a quasi-neutral electric atmosphere. Z Naturforsch. 1997. May-Jun;52(5-6):396-404.

Golub E. The Limits of Medicine. New York: Times Books, 1994.

Gomes A, Fernandes E, Lima JL. Fluorescence probes used for detection of reactive oxygen species. J Biochem Biophys Methods. 2005 Dec 31;65(2-3):45-80.

Gomez-Abellan P, Hernandez-Morante JJ, Lujan JA, Madrid JA, Garaulet M. Clock genes are implicated in the human metabolic syndrome. Int J Obes. 2007 Jul 24.

Gong X, Smith JR, Swanson HM, Rubin LP. Carotenoid Lutein Selectively Inhibits Breast cancer Cell Growth and Potentiates the Effect of Chemotherapeutic Agents through ROS-Mediated Mechanisms. Molecules. 2018;23(4):905. Published 2018 Apr 14. doi:10.3390/molecules23040905

Gonzales M, Malcoe LH, Myers OB, Espinoza J. Risk factors for asthma and cough among Hispanic children in the southwestern United States of America, 2003-2004. Rev Panam Salud Publica. 2007 May;21(5):274-81.

González Alvarez R, Arruzazabala ML. Current views of the mechanism of action of prophylactic antiallergic drugs. Allergol Immunopathol (Madr). 1981 Nov-Dec;9(6):501-8.

Gonzalez CA, Riboli E. Diet and cancer prevention: Contributions from the European Prospective Investigation into Cancer and Nutrition (EPIC) study. Eur J Cancer. 2010 Sep;46(14):2555-62.

González CA, Salas-Salvadó J. The potential of nuts in the prevention of cancer. Br J Nutr. 2006 Nov;96 Suppl 2:S87-94. Review. Erratum in: Br J Nutr. 2008 Feb;99(2):447-8.

González J, Fernández M, García Fragoso L. Exclusive breastfeeding reduces asthma in a group of children from the Caguas municipality of Puerto Rico. Bol Asoc Med P R. 2010 Jan-Mar;102(1):10-2.

González Morales JE, Leal de Hernández L, González Spencer D. Asthma associated with gastroesophageal reflux. Rev Alerg Mex. 1998 Jan-Feb;45(1):16-21.

González-Sánchez R, Trujillo X, Trujillo-Hernández B, Vásquez C, Huerta M, Elizalde A. Forskolin versus sodium cromoglycate for prevention of asthma attacks: a single-blinded clinical trial. J Int Med Res. 2006 Mar-Apr;34(2):200-7.

Goossens D, Jonkers D, Russel M, Stobberingh E, Van Den Bogaard A, StockbrUgger R. The effect of Lactobacillus plantarum 299v on the bacterial composition and metabolic activity in faeces of healthy volunteers: a placebo-controlled study on the onset and duration of effects. Aliment Pharmacol Ther. 2003 Sep 1;18(5):495-505.

Goossens DA, Jonkers DM, Russel MG, Stobberingh EE, Stockbrügger RW. The effect of a probiotic drink with Lactobacillus plantarum 299v on the bacterial composition and mucosal biopsies of rectum and ascending colon. Aliment Pharmacol Ther. 2006 Jan 15;23(2):255-63.

Gordon BR. Patch testing for allergies. Curr Opin Otolaryngol Head Neck Surg. 2010 Jun;18(3):191-4.

Gore KV, Rao AK, Guruswamy MN. Physiological studies with Tylophora asthmatica in bronchial asthma. Indian J Med Res. 1980 Jan;71:144-8.

Gore RD, Palaskar SJ, Bartake AR. Wheatgrass: Green Blood can Help to Fight Cancer. J Clin Diagn Res. 2017 Jun;11(6):ZC40-ZC42. doi: 10.7860/JCDR/2017/26316.10057.

Goren AI, Hellmann S. Changes prevalence of asthma among schoolchildren in Israel. Eur Respir J. 1997;10:2279-2284.

Gorham ED, Mohr SB, Garland CF, Chaplin G, Garland FC. Do sunscreens increase risk of melanoma in populations residing at higher latitudes? Ann Epidemiol. 2007 Dec;17(12):956-63.

Gostner JM, Zeisler J, Alam MT, Gruber P, Fuchs D, Becker K, Neubert K, Kleinhappl M, Martini S, Überall F. Cellular reactions to long-term volatile organic compound (VOC) exposures. Sci Rep. 2016 Dec 1;6:37842. doi: 10.1038/srep37842.

Gotteland M, Poliak L, Cruchet S, Brunser O. Effect of regular ingestion of Saccharomyces boulardii plus inulin or Lactobacillus acidophilus LB in children colonized by Helicobacter pylori. Acta Paediatr. 2005 Dec;94(12):1747-51.

Govindan S, Viswanathan S, Vijayasekaran V, Alagappan R. A pilot study on the clinical efficacy of Solanum xanthocarpum and Solanum trilobatum in bronchial asthma. J Ethnopharmacol. 1999 Aug;66(2):205-10.

Govindan S, Viswanathan S, Vijayasekaran V, Alagappan R. Further studies on the clinical efficacy of Solanum xanthocarpum and Solanum trilobatum in bronchial asthma. Phytother Res. 2004 Oct;18(10):805-9.

Grad B, Dean E. Independent confirmation of infrared healer effects. In: White R, Broughton R (Eds.): Research in parapsychology 1983. Metuchen, NJ: Scarecrow Press, 1984:81-83.

Graham C, Sastre A, Cook MR, Kavet R, Gerkovich MM, Riffle DW. Exposure to strong ELF magnetic fields does not alter cardiac autonomic control mechanisms. Bioelectromagnetics. 2000 Sep;21(6):413-21.

Gramaglia C, Gambaro E, Vecchi C, Licandro D, Raina G, Pisani C, Burgio V, Farruggio S, Rolla R, Deantonio L, Grossini E, Krengli M, Zeppegno P. Outcomes of music therapy interventions in cancer patients-A review of the literature. Crit Rev Oncol Hematol. 2019 Jun;138:241-254. doi: 10.1016/j.critrevonc.2019.04.004.

Grant WB, Garland CF. The association of solar ultraviolet B (UVB) with reducing risk of cancer: multifactorial ecologic analysis of geographic variation in age-adjusted cancer mortality rates. Anticancer Res. 2006 Jul-Aug;26(4A):2687-99.

Grant WB, Holick MF. Benefits and requirements of vitamin D for optimal health: a review. Altern Med Rev. 2005 Jun;10(2):94-111.

Grant WB. An estimate of premature cancer mortality in the U.S. due to inadequate doses of solar ultraviolet-B radiation. Cancer. 2002 Mar 15;94(6):1867-75.

Grant WB. Hypothesis—ultraviolet-B irradiance and vitamin D reduce the risk of viral infections and thus their sequelae, including autoimmune diseases and some cancers. Photochem Photobiol. 2008 Mar-Apr;84(2):356-65. 2008 Jan 7.

Grant WB. Solar ultraviolet irradiance and cancer incidence and mortality. Adv Exp Med Biol. 2008;624:16-30.

Grasmuller S, Irnich D. Acupuncture in pain therapy. MMW Fortschr Med. 2007 Jun 21;149(25-26):37-9.

Grasso F, Grillo C, Musumeci F, Triglia A, Rodolico G, Cammisuli F, Rinzivillo C, Fragati G, Santuccio A, Rodolico M. Photon emission from normal and tumour human tissues. Experientia. 1992;48:10-13.

Grasso F, Grillo C, Musumeci F, Triglia A, Rodolico G, Cammisuli F, Rinzivillo C, Fragati G, Santuccio A, Rodolico M. Photon emission from normal and tumour human tissues. Experientia. 1992;48:10-13.

Grasso F, Musumeci F, Triglia A, Rodolico G, Cammisuli F, Rinzivillo C, Fragati G, Santuccio A, Rodolico M. In Stanley P, Kricka L (ed). Ultraweak Luminescence from Cancer Tissues. In Bioluminescence and Chemilu-minescence - Current Status. New York: J Wiley & Sons. 1991:277-280.

Grasso F, Musumeci F, Triglia A. Yanbastiev M. Borisova, S. Self-irradiation effect on yeast cells. Photochemis-try and Photobiology. 1991;54(1):147-149.

Gray H. Anatomy, Descriptive and Surgical. 15th Edition. New York: Random House, 1977.

Gray-Davison F. Ayurvedic Healing. New York: Keats, 2002.

Greskevitch M, Kullman G, Bang KM, Mazurek JM. Respiratory disease in agricultural workers: mortality and morbidity statistics. J Agromedicine. 2007;12(3):5-10.

Griffith HW. Healing Herbs: The Essential Guide. Tucson: Fisher Books, 2000.

Grimm T, Chovanová Z, Muchová J, Sumegová K, Liptáková A, Duracková Z, Högger P. Inhibition of NF-kappaB activation and MMP-9 secretion by plasma of human volunteers after ingestion of maritime pine bark extract (Pycnogenol). J Inflamm (Lond). 2006 Jan 27;3:1.

Grimm T, Schäfer A, Högger P. Antioxidant activity and inhibition of matrix metalloproteinases by metabolites of maritime pine bark extract (pycnogenol). Free Radic Biol Med. 2004 Mar 15;36(6):811-22.

Grimm T, Skrabala R, Chovanová Z, Muchová J, Sumegová K, Liptáková A, Duracková Z, Högger P. Single and multiple dose pharmacokinetics of maritime pine bark extract (pycnogenol) after oral administration to healthy volunteers. BMC Clin Pharmacol. 2006 Aug 3;6:4.

Grissom C. Magnetic field effects in biology: A survey of possible mechanisms with emphasis on radical pair recombination. Chem. Rev. 1995;95:3-24.

Grobstein P. Directed movement in the frog: motor choice, spatial representation, free will? Neurobiology of motor programme selection. Pergamon Press, 1992.

Gronfier C, Wright KP Jr, Kronauer RE, Czeisler CA. Entrainment of the human circadian pacemaker to longer-than-24-h days. Proc Natl Acad Sci U S A. 2007 May 22;104(21):9081-6.

Gropper SS, Smith JL, Groff JL. Advanced nutrition and human metabolism. Belmonth, CA: Wadsworth Publ, 2008.

Groppo FC, Ramacciato JC, Simões RP, Flório FM, Sartoratto A. Antimicrobial activity of garlic, tea tree oil, and chlorhexidine against oral microorganisms. Int Dent J. 2002 Dec;52(6):433-7.

Groschwitz KR, Ahrens R, Osterfeld H, Gurish MF, Han X, Abrink M, Finkelman FD, Pejler G, Hogan SP. Mast cells regulate homeostatic intestinal epithelial migration and barrier function by a chymase/Mcpt4-dependent mechanism. Proc Natl Acad Sci U S A. 2009 Dec 29;106(52):22381-6.

Grosser BI, Monti-Bloch L, Jennings-White C, Berliner DL. Behavioral and electrophysiological effects of androstadienone, a human pheromone. Psychoneuroendocrinology. 2000 Apr;25(3):289-99.

Grzanna R, Lindmark L, Frondoza CG. Ginger—an herbal medicinal product with broad anti-inflammatory actions. J Med Food. 2005 Summer;8(2):125-32.

Gu SX, Zhang AL, Coyle ME, Chen D, Xue CC. Chinese herbal medicine for atopic eczema: an overview of clinical evidence. J Dermatolog Treat. 2016 Aug 18:1-5.

Guager, James, Household Appliance Magnetic Field Data, provided by T.Dan Bracken, Inc., Lockheed Martin Energy Systems, Inc., and IIT Research Institute. 1997 June 24.

Guajardo-Flores D, Serna-Saldívar SO, Gutiérrez-Uribe JA. Evaluation of the antioxidant and antiproliferative activities of extracted saponins and flavonols from germinated black beans (Phaseolus vulgaris L.). Food Chem. 2013 Nov 15;141(2):1497-503.

REFERENCES AND BIBLIOGRAPHY

Guandalini S. The influence of gluten: weaning recommendations for healthy children and children at risk for celiac disease. Nestle Nutr Workshop Ser Pediatr Program. 2007;60:139-51; discussion 151-5.

Guarino A, Canani RB, Spagnuolo MI, Albano F, Di Benedetto L. Oral bacterial therapy reduces the duration of symptoms and of viral excretion in children with mild diarrhea. J Pediatr Gastroenterol Nutr. 1997 Nov;25(5):516-9.

Guerin M, Huntley ME, Olaizola M. Haematococcus astaxanthin: applications for human health and nutrition. Trends Biotechnol. 2003 May;21(5):210-6.

Guerin-Danan C, Chabanet C, Pedone C, Popot F, Vaissade P, Bouley C, Szylit O, Andrieux C. Milk fermented with yogurt cultures and Lactobacillus casei compared with yogurt and gelled milk: influence on intestinal microflora in healthy infants. Am J Clin Nutr. 1998 Jan;67(1):111-7.

Guess BW, Scholz MC, Strum SB, Lam RY, Johnson HJ, Jennrich RI. Modified citrus pectin (MCP) increases the prostate-specific antigen doubling time in men with prostate cancer: a phase II pilot study. Prostate Cancer Prostatic Dis. 2003;6(4):301-4.

Guidelines for Limiting Exposure to Time-Varying Electric, Magnetic, and Electromagnetic Fields (up to 300 GHz). Munich, Germany: Internl. Comm. Non-Ionizing Radiation Protection (ICNIRP). 1998.

Guinot P, Brambilla C, Duchier J, Braquet P, Bonvoisin B, Cournot A. Effect of BN 52063, a specific PAF-acether antagonist, on bronchial provocation test to allergens in asthmatic patients. A preliminary study. Prostaglandins. 1987 Nov;34(5):723-31.

Gundermann KJ, Müller J. Phytodolor—effects and efficacy of a herbal medicine. Wien Med Wochenschr. 2007;157(13-14):343-7.

Guo J, Wei W, Zhan L. Red and processed meat intake and risk of breast cancer: a meta-analysis of prospective studies. Breast cancer Res Treat. 2015 May;151(1):191-8. doi: 10.1007/s10549-015-3380-9.

Guo J. Chronic fatigue syndrome treated by acupuncture and moxibustion in combination with psychological approaches in 310 cases. J Tradit Chin Med. 2007 Jun;27(2):92-5.

Gupta A, Rash GS, Somia NN, Wachowiak MP, Jones J, Desoky A. The motion path of the digits. J Hand Surg. 1998; 23A:1038-1042.

Gupta I, Gupta V, Parihar A, Gupta S, Lüdtke R, Safayhi H, Ammon HP. Effects of Boswellia serrata gum resin in patients with bronchial asthma: results of a double-blind, placebo-controlled, 6-week clinical study. Eur J Med Res. 1998 Nov 17;3(11):511-4.

Gupta YK, Gupta M, Kohli K. Neuroprotective role of melatonin in oxidative stress vulnerable brain. Indian J Physiol Pharmacol. 2003 Oct;47(4):373-86.

Guslandi M, Giollo P, Testoni PA. A pilot trial of Saccharomyces boulardii in ulcerative colitis. Eur J Gastroenterol Hepatol. 2003 Jun;15(6):697-8.

Guslandi M, Mezzi G, Sorghi M, Testoni PA. Saccharomyces boulardii in maintenance treatment of Crohn's disease. Dig Dis Sci. 2000 Jul;45(7):1462-4.

Gutierrez RM, Gonzalez AM, Hoyo-Vadillo C. Alkaloids from Piper: A Review of its Phytochemistry and Pharmacology. Mini Rev Med Chem. 2012 Dec 31.

Gutmanis J. Hawaiian Herbal Medicine. Waipahu, HI: Island Heritage, 2001.

Guyonnet D, Woodcock A, Stefani B, Trevisan C, Hall C. Fermented milk containing Bifidobacterium lactis DN-173 010 improved self-reported digestive comfort amongst a general population of adults. A randomized, open-label, controlled, pilot study. J Dig Dis. 2009 Feb;10(1):61-70.

Gweon EJ, Kim SJ. Resveratrol induces MMP-9 and cell migration via the p38 kinase and PI-3K pathways in HT1080 human fibrosarcoma cells. Oncol Rep. 2013 Feb;29(2):826-34.

Haarala C, Bergman M, Laine M, Revonsuo A, Koivisto M, Hamalainen H. Electromagnetic field emitted by 902 MHz mobile phones shows no effects on children's cognitive function. Bioelectromagnetics. 2005;Suppl 7:S144-50.

Haarala C, Bergman M, Laine M, Revonsuo A, Koivisto M, Hamalainen H. Electromagnetic field emitted by 902 MHz mobile phones shows no effects on children's cognitive function. Bioelectromagnetics. 2005;Suppl 7:S144-50.

Haarman M, Knol J. Quantitative real-time PCR assays to identify and quantify fecal Bifidobacterium species in infants receiving a prebiotic infant formula. Appl Environ Microbiol. 2005 May;71(5):2318-24.

Haas M, Cooperstein R, Peterson D. Disentangling manual muscle testing and Applied Kinesiology: critique and reinterpretation of a literature review. Chiropr Osteopat. 2007 Aug 23;15:11.

Hadji L, Arnoux B, Benveniste J. Effect of dilute histamine on coronary flow of guinea-pig isolated heart. Inhibition by a magnetic field. FASEB Jnl. 1991;5: A1583.

Haggag EG, Abou-Moustafa MA, Boucher W, Theoharides TC. The effect of a herbal water-extract on histamine release from mast cells and on allergic asthma. J Herb Pharmacother. 2003;3(4):41-54.

Hagger-Johnson G, Gow AJ, Burley V, Greenwood D, Cade JE. Sitting Time, Fidgeting, and All-Cause Mortality in the UK Women's Cohort Study. Am J Prev Med. 2015 Sep 4. pii: S0749-3797(15)00345-1. doi: 10.1016/j.amepre.2015.06.025.

Hagins WA, Penn RD, Yoshikami S. Dark current and photocurrent in retinal rods. Biophys J. 1970 May;10(5):380-412.

Hagins WA, Yoshikami S. Proceedings: A role for Ca2+ in excitation of retinal rods and cones. Exp Eye Res. 1974 Mar;18(3):299-305.

Haines JL, Ter-Minassian M, Bazyk A, Gusella JF, Kim DJ, Terwedow H, Pericak-Vance MA, Rimmler JB, Haynes CS, Roses AD, Lee A, Shaner B, Menold M, Seboun E, Fitoussi RP, Gartioux C, Reyes C, Ribierre F, Gyapay G, Weissenbach J, Hauser SL, Goodkin DE, Lincoln R, Usuku K, Oksenberg JR, *et al*. A complete genomic screen for multiple sclerosis underscores a role for the major histocompatability complex. The Multiple Sclerosis Genetics Group. Nat Genet. 1996 Aug;13(4):469-71..

Halász A, Cserháti E. The prognosis of bronchial asthma in childhood in Hungary: a long-term follow-up. J Asthma. 2002 Dec;39(8):693-9.

Hallén A, Jarstrand C, Påhlson C. Treatment of bacterial vaginosis with lactobacilli. Sex Transm Dis. 1992 May-Jun;19(3):146-8.

Halliday GM, Agar NS, Barnetson RS, Ananthaswamy HN, Jones AM. UV-A fingerprint mutations in human skin cancer. Photochem Photobiol. 2005 Jan-Feb;81(1):3-8.

Halpern GM, Miller AH. Medicinal Mushrooms: Ancient Remedies for Modern Ailments. New York: M. Evans, 2002.

Halpern S. Tuning the Human Instrument. Palo Alto, CA: Spectrum Research Institute, 1978.

Hamaguchi R, Okamoto T, Sato M, Hasegawa M, Wada H. Effects of an Alkaline Diet on EGFR-TKI Therapy in EGFR Mutation-positive NSCLC. Anticancer Res. 2017 Sep;37(9):5141-5145. doi: 10.21873/anticanres.11934.

Hamano J, *et al*. A multicenter cohort study on the survival time of cancer patients dying at home or in hospital: Does place matter? CANCER; March 28, 2016 (DOI: 10.1002/cncr.29844)

Hamasaki Y, Kobayashi I, Hayasaki R, Zaitu M, Muro E, Yamamoto S, Ichimaru T, Miyazaki S. The Chinese herbal medicine, shinpi-to, inhibits IgE-mediated leukotriene synthesis in rat basophilic leukemia-2H3 cells. J Ethnopharmacol. 1997 Apr;56(2):123-31.

Hamel P. Through Music to the Self: How to Appreciate and Experience Music. Boulder: Shambala, 1979.

Hameroff SR, Penrose R. Conscious events as orchestrated spacetime selections. J Consc Studies. 1996;3(1):36-53.

Hameroff SR, Penrose R. Orchestrated reduction of quantum coherence in brain microtubules: A model for consciousness. In: Hameroff SN, Kaszniak A, Scott AC (eds.): Toward a Science of Consciousness - The First Tucson Discussions and Debates. Cambridge: MIT Press, 1996.

Hameroff SR, Smith, S, Watt.R. Nonlinear electrodynamics in cytoskeletal protein lattices. In: Adey W, Lawrence A (eds.), Nonlinear Electrodynamics in Biological Systems. 1984:567-583.

Hameroff SR, Watt, R. Information processing in microtubules. J Theor Biology. 1982;98:549-561.

Hameroff SR. Coherence in the cytoskeleton: Implications for biological information processing. In: Fröhlich H. (ed.): Biological Coherence and Response to External Stimuli. Springer, Berlin-New York 1988, pp.242-264.

Hamilton-Miller JM. Probiotics and prebiotics in the elderly. London: Department of Medical Microbiology, Royal Free and University College Medical School, 2004.

Hammermeister J, Brock B, Winterstein D, Page R. Life without TV? cultivation theory and psychosocial health characteristics of television-free individuals and their television-viewing counterparts. Health Commun. 2005;17(3):253-64.

Hammitt WE. The relation between being away and privacy in urban forest recreation environments. Environment and Behaviour. 2000;32 (4):521-540.

Hammond BG, Mayhew DA, Kier LD, Mast RW, Sander WJ. Safety assessment of DHA-rich microalgae from Schizochytrium sp. Regul Toxicol Pharmacol. 2002 Apr;35(2 Pt 1):255-65.

Han ER, Choi IS, Kim HK, Kang YW, Park JG, Lim JR, Choi JH. Inhaled corticosteroid-related tooth problems in asthmatics. J Asthma. 2009 Mar;46(2):160-4.

Han RT, Back SK, Lee H, Lee J, Kim HY, Kim HJ, Na HS. Formaldehyde-Induced Aggravation of Pruritus and Dermatitis Is Associated with the Elevated Expression of Th1 Cytokines in a Rat Model of Atopic Dermatitis. PLoS One. 2016 Dec 22;11(12):e0168466. doi: 10.1371/journal.pone.0168466.

Han SN, Leka LS, Lichtenstein AH, Ausman LM, Meydani SN. Effect of a therapeutic lifestyle change diet on immune functions of moderately hypercholesterolemic humans. J Lipid Res. 2003 Dec;44(12):2304-10.

Hancox RJ, Milne BJ, Poulton R. Association of television viewing during childhood with poor educational achievement. Arch Pediatr Adolesc Med. 2005 Jul;159(7):614-8.

Handwerk B. Are Earthquakes Encouraged by High Tides? National Geographic News. 2004 Oct 22.

Handwerk B. Lobsters Navigate by Magnetism, Study Says. Natl Geogr News. 2003 Jan 6.

Hanifin JP, Stewart KT, Smith P, Tanner R, Rollag M, Brainard GC. High-intensity red light suppresses melatonin. Chronobiol Int. 2006;23(1-2):251-68.

Hanifin JP, Stewart KT, Smith P, Tanner R, Rollag M, Brainard GC. High-intensity red light suppresses melatonin. Chronobiol Int. 2006;23(1-2):251-68.

Hardell E, Kärrman A, van Bavel B, Bao J, Carlberg M, Hardell L. Case-control study on perfluorinated alkyl acids (PFAAs) and the risk of prostate cancer. Environ Int. 2014;63:35-39. doi:10.1016/j.envint.2013.10.005

Hardell L, Carlberg M. Mobile phone and cordless phone use and the risk for glioma – Analysis of pooled case-control studies in Sweden, 1997-2003 and 2007-2009. Pathophysiology. 2015 Mar;22(1):1-13. doi: 10.1016/j.pathophys.2014.10.001.

Hardell L, Carlberg M. Using the Hill viewpoints from 1965 for evaluating strengths of evidence of the risk for brain tumors associated with use of mobile and cordless phones. Rev Environ Health. 2013;28(2-3):97-106. doi: 10.1515/reveh-2013-0006.

Hardin P. Transcription regulation within the circadian clock: the E-box and beyond. J Biol Rhythms. 2004 Oct;19(5):348-60.

Hardin P. Transcription regulation within the circadian clock: the E-box and beyond. J Biol Rhythms. 2004 Oct;19(5):348-60.

Hardman WE, Primerano DA, Legenza MT, Morgan J, Fan J, Denvir J. Dietary walnut altered gene expressions related to tumor growth, survival, and metastasis in breast cancer patients: a pilot clinical trial. Nutr Res. 2019 Mar 10. pii: S0271-5317(18)31190-4. doi: 10.1016/j.nutres.2019.03.004.

Hardman WE. Walnuts have potential for cancer prevention and treatment in mice. J Nutr. 2014 Apr;144(4 Suppl):555S-560S. doi: 10.3945/jn.113.188466.

Harkins T, Grissom C. Magnetic Field Effects on B12 Ethanolamine Ammonia Lyase: Evidence for a Radical Mechanism. Science. 1994;263:958-960.

Harkins T, Grissom C. The Magnetic Field Dependent Step in B12 Ethanolamine Ammonia Lyase is Radical-Pair Recombination. J. Am. Chem. Soc. 1995;117:566-567.

Harland JD, Liburdy RP. Environmental magnetic fields inhibit the antiproliferative action of tamoxifen and melatonin in a human breast cancer cell line. Bioelectromagnetics. 1997;18(8):555-62.

Harrington JJ, Lee-Chiong T Jr. Sleep and older patients. Clin Chest Med. 2007 Dec;28(4):673-84, v.

Harris LA, Chang L. Irritable bowel syndrome: new and emerging therapies. Curr Opin Gastroenterol. 2006 Mar;22(2):128-35.

Harris RB, Foote JA, Hakim IA, Bronson DL, Alberts DS. Fatty acid composition of red blood cell membranes and risk of squamous cell carcinoma of the skin. Cancer Epidemiol Biomarkers Prev. 2005 Apr;14(4):906-12.

Harvald B, Hauge M: Hereditary factors elucidated by twin studies. In Genetics and the Epidemiology of Chronic Disease. Edited by Neel JV, Shaw MV, Schull WJ. Washington, DC: Dept Health, Education and Welfare, 1965:64-76.

Harvey HP, Solomon HJ. Acute anaphylactic shock due to para-aminosalicylic acid. Am Rev Tuberc. 1958 Mar;77(3):492-5.

Hassan AM. Selenium status in patients with aspirin-induced asthma. Ann Clin Biochem. 2008 Sep;45(Pt 5):508-12.

Hassan ZK, Elamin MH, Daghestani MH, Omer SA, Al-Olayan EM, Elobeid MA, Virk, Mohammed OB. Oleuropein Induces Anti-metastatic Effects in Breast cancer. Asian Pac J Cancer Prev. 2012;13(9):4555-9.

Hata K, Ishikawa K, Hori K, Konishi T. Differentiation-inducing activity of lupeol, a lupane-type triterpene from Chinese dandelion root (Hokouei-kon), on a mouse melanoma cell line. Biol Pharm Bull. 2000 Aug;23(8):962-7.

Hata Y, Yamamoto M, Ohni M, Nakajima K, Nakamura Y, Takano T. A placebo-controlled study of the effect of sour milk on blood pressure in hypertensive subjects. Am J Clin Nutr. 1996 Nov;64(5):767-71.

Hatae M, Noda K, Yajima A, Sato S, Terashima Y, Ochiai K, Sasaki H, Mizutani K, Honjo H, Yamamoto T, Ozaki M, Yamamoto K, Hasegawa K, Nishimura R, Kudo T, Kobashi Y, Yakushiji M, Sugiyama T, Hasuo Y, Onishi Y. (1998). Effect of 5'-DFUR used concurrently in radiotherapy and immunotherapy uterine cervical cancer--pilot study. Study of 5'-DFUR for Uterine Cervical Cancer. Gan to kagaku ryoho, 25(5), 705-11.

Hatakka K, Holma R, El-Nezami H, Suomalainen T, Kuisma M, Saxelin M, Poussa T, Mykkänen H, Korpela R. The influence of Lactobacillus rhamnosus LC705 together with Propionibacterium freudenreichii ssp. shermanii JS on potentially carcinogenic bacterial activity in human colon. Int J Food Microbiol. 2008 Dec 10;128(2):406-10.

Hattori K, Sasai M, Yamamoto A, Taniuchi S, Kojima T, Kobayashi Y, Iwamoto H, Yaeshima T, Hayasawa H. Intestinal flora of infants with cow milk hypersensitivity fed on casein-hydrolyzed formula supplemented raffinose. Arerugi. 2000 Dec;49(12):1146-55.

Hattori K, Yamamoto A, Sasai M, Taniuchi S, Kojima T, Kobayashi Y, Iwamoto H, Namba K, Yaeshima T. Effects of administration of bifidobacteria on fecal microflora and clinical symptoms in infants with atopic dermatitis. Arerugi. 2003 Jan;52(1):20-30.

Hayashi K, Narutaki K, Nagaoka Y, Hayashi T, Uesato S. Therapeutic effect of arctiin and arctigenin in immunocompetent and immunocompromised mice infected with influenza A virus. Biol Pharm Bull. 2010;33(7):1199-205.

Haye-Legrand I, Norel X, Labat C, Benveniste J, Brink C. Antigenic contraction of guinea pig tracheal preparations passively sensitized with monoclonal IgE: pharmacological modulation. Int Arch Allergy Appl Immunol. 1988;87(4):342-8.

Hayes AJ, Markovic B. Toxicity of Australian essential oil Backhousia citriodora (Lemon myrtle). Part 1. Antimicrobial activity and in vitro cytotoxicity. Food Chem Toxicol. 2002 Apr;40(4):535-43. doi: 10.1016/s0278-6915(01)00103-x. PMID: 11893412.

He M, Antoine JM, Yang Y, Yang J, Men J, Han H. Influence of live flora on lactose digestion in male adult lactose-malabsorbers after dairy products intake. Wei Sheng Yan Jiu. 2004 Sep;33(5):603-5.

He T, Priebe MG, Zhong Y, Huang C, Harmsen HJ, Raangs GC, Antoine JM, Welling GW, Vonk RJ. Effects of yogurt and bifidobacteria supplementation on the colonic microbiota in lactose-intolerant subjects. J Appl Microbiol. 2008 Feb;104(2):595-604.

Heaney LG, Brightling CE, Menzies-Gow A, Stevenson M, Niven RM; British Thoracic Society Difficult Asthma Network. Refractory asthma in the UK: cross-sectional findings from a UK multicentre registry. Thorax. 2010 Sep;65(9):787-94.

Heaney RP, Dowell MS. Absorbability of the calcium in a high-calcium mineral water. Osteoporos Int. 1994 Nov;4(6):323-4.

Heaney RP, Recker RR, Grote J, Horst RL, Armas LA. Vitamin D(3) is more potent than vitamin D(2) in humans. J Clin Endocrinol Metab. 2011 Mar;96(3):E447-52. doi: 10.1210/jc.2010-2230.

Heap GA, van Heel DA. Genetics and pathogenesis of coeliac disease. Semin Immunol. May 13 2009.

Heckman JD, Ingram AJ, Loyd RD, Luck JV Jr, Mayer PW. Nonunion treatment with pulsed electromagnetic fields. Clin Orthop Relat Res. 1981 Nov-Dec;(161):58-66.

Hedendahl L, Carlberg M, Hardell L. Electromagnetic hypersensitivity–an increasing challenge to the medical profession. Rev Environ Health. 2015;30(4):209-15. doi: 10.1515/reveh-2015-0012.

Heerwagen JH. The psychological aspects of windows and window design'. In Selby, R. I., Anthony, K. H., Choi, J. and Orland, B. (eds) Proceedings of 21st Annual Conference of the Environmental Design Research Asso-ciation. Champaign-Urbana, Illinois, 1990 April:6-9.

Heerwagen JH. The psychological aspects of windows and window design'. In Selby, R. I., Anthony, K. H., Choi, J. and Orland, B. (eds) Proceedings of 21st Annual Conference of the Environmental Design Research Asso-ciation. Champaign-Urbana, Illinois, 1990 April:6-9.

Heine RG, Nethercote M, Rosenbaum J, Allen KJ. Emerging management concepts for eosinophilic esophagitis in children. J Gastroenterol Hepatol. 2011 May 4.

Heinrich H. Assessment of non-sinusoidal, pulsed, or intermittent exposure to low frequency electric and magnetic fields. Health Phys. 2007 Jun;92(6):541-6.

Heinrich U, Gärtner C, Wiebusch M, Eichler O, Sies H, Tronnier H, Stahl W. Supplementation with beta-carotene or a similar amount of mixed carotenoids protects humans from UV-induced erythema. J Nutr. 2003 Jan;133(1):98-101.

Helms JA, Farnham PJ, Segal E, Chang HY. Functional demarcation of active and silent chromatin domains in human HOX loci by noncoding RNAs. Cell. 2007 Jun 29;129(7):1311-23.

Hendel B, Ferreira P. Water & Salt: The Essence of Life. Gaithersburg: Natural Resources, 2003.

Henderson SI, Bangay MJ. Survey of RF exposure levels from mobile telephone base stations in Australia. Bioelectromag. 2006 Jan;27(1):73-6.

Henshaw DL, Ross AN, Fews AP, Preece AW. Enhanced deposition of radon daughter nuclei in the vicinity of power frequency electromagnetic fields. Int J Radiat Biol. 1996 Jan;69(1):25-38.

Herbert V. Vitamin B12: Plant sources, requirements, and assay. Am J Clin Nutr. 1988;48:852-858.

Herman PM, Drost LM. Evaluating the clinical relevance of food sensitivity tests: a single subject experiment. Altern Med Rev. 2004 Jun;9(2):198-207.

Herzog AM, Black KA, Fountaine DJ, Knotts TR. Reflection and attentional recovery as two distinctive benefits of restorative environments. J Environ Psychol. 1997;17:165-70.

Hess AF. Rickets. London: Henry Kimpton, 1930.

Hess-Kosa K. Indoor Air Quality: Sampling Methodologies. Boca Rataon: CRC Press, 2002.

Heyers D, Manns M, Luksch H, Gu¨ ntu¨ rku¨n O, Mouritsen H. A Visual Pathway Links Brain Structures Active during Magnetic Compass Orientation in Migratory Birds. PLoS One. 2007;2(9):e937. 2007.

Hickson M, D'Souza AL, Muthu N, Rogers TR, Want S, Rajkumar C, Bulpitt CJ. Use of probiotic Lactobacillus preparation to prevent diarrhoea associated with antibiotics: randomised double blind placebo controlled trial. BMJ. 2007 Jul 14;335(7610):80.

Hietanen M, Hamalainen AM, Husman T. Hypersensitivity symptoms associated with exposure to cellular telephones: no causal link. Bioelectromagnetics. 2002 May;23(4):264-70.

Higgins CL, Palmer AM, Cahill JL, Nixon RL. Occupational skin disease among Australian healthcare workers: a retrospective analysis from an occupational dermatology clinic, 1993-2014. Contact Dermatitis. 2016 Oct;75(4):213-22. doi: 10.1111/cod.12616.

Hijazi Z, Molla AM, Al-Habashi H, Muawad WM, Molla AM, Sharma PN. Intestinal permeability is increased in bronchial asthma. Arch Dis Child. 2004 Mar;89(3):227-9.

Hill J, Micklewright A, Lewis S, Britton J. Investigation of the effect of short-term change in dietary magnesium intake in asthma. Eur Respir J. 1997 Oct;10(10):2225-9.

Hillecke T, Nickel A, Bolay HV. Scientific perspectives on music therapy. Ann N Y Acad Sci. 2005 Dec;1060:271-82.

Hilton E, Isenberg HD, Alperstein P, France K, Borenstein MT. Ingestion of yogurt containing Lactobacillus acidophilus as prophylaxis for Candidal vaginitis. Ann Intern Med. 1992 Mar 1;116(5):353-7.

Hirayama J, Sahar S, Grimaldi B, Tamaru T, Takamatsu K, Nakahata Y, Sassone-Corsi P. CLOCK-mediated acetylation of BMAL1 controls circadian function. Nature 450, 1086-1090 (13 December 2007)

Hirose Y, Murosaki S, Yamamoto Y, Yoshikai Y, Tsuru T. Daily intake of heat-killed Lactobacillus plantarum L-137 augments acquired immunity in healthy adults. J Nutr. 2006 Dec;136(12):3069-73.

Hjollund NH, Bonde JP, Skotte J. Semen analysis of personnel operating military radar equipment. Reprod Toxicol. 1997 Nov-Dec;11(6):897.

Hlivak P, Jahnova E, Odraska J, Ferencik M, Ebringer L, Mikes Z. Long-term (56-week) oral administration of probiotic Enterococcus faecium M-74 decreases the expression of sICAM-1 and monocyte CD54, and increases that of lymphocyte CD49d in humans. Bratisl Lek Listy. 2005;106(4-5):175-81.

Hlivak P, Odraska J, Ferencik M, Ebringer L, Jahnova E, Mikes Z. One-year application of probiotic strain Enterococcus faecium M-74 decreases serum cholesterol levels. Bratisl Lek Listy. 2005;106(2):67-72.

Ho MW. Assessing Food Quality by Its After-Glow. Inst. Sci in Society. Press release. 2004 May 1.

Hobbs C. Kombucha Manchurian Tea Mushroom: The Essential Guide. Santa Cruz, CA: Botanica Press, 1995.

Hobbs C. Medicinal Mushrooms. Summertown, TN: Botanica Press, 2003.

Hobbs C. Stress & Natural Healing. Loveland, CO: Interweave Press, 1997.

Hoff S, Seiler H, Heinrich J, Kompauer I, Nieters A, Becker N, Nagel G, Gedrich K, Karg G, Wolfram G, Linseisen J. Allergic sensitisation and allergic rhinitis are associated with n-3 polyunsaturated fatty acids in the diet and in red blood cell membranes. Eur J Clin Nutr. 2005 Sep;59(9):1071-80.

Hoffmann D. Holistic Herbal. London: Thorsons, 2002.

Hofmann D, Hecker M, Völp A. Efficacy of dry extract of ivy leaves in children with bronchial asthma-a review of randomized controlled trials. Phytomedicine. 2003 Mar;10(2-3):213-20.

Holick MF. Photobiology of vitamin D. In: Feldman D, Pike JW, Glorieux FH, eds. Vitamin D, Second Edition, Volume I. Burlington, MA: Elsevier, 2005.

Holick MF. Sunlight and vitamin D for bone health and prevention of autoimmune diseases, cancers, and cardiovascular disease. Am J Clin Nutr. 2004 Dec;80(6 Suppl):1678S-88S.

Holick MF. The vitamin D deficiency pandemic and consequences for nonskeletal health: mechanisms of action. Mol Aspects Med. 2008 Dec;29(6):361-8

Holick MF. Vitamin D status: measurement, interpretation, and clinical application. Ann Epidemiol. 2009 Feb;19(2):73-8.

Holick MF. Vitamin D. In: Shils ME, Shike M, Ross AC, Caballero B, Cousins RJ, eds. Modern Nutrition in Health and Disease, 10th ed. Philadelphia: Lippincott Williams & Wilkins, 2006.

Holick MF. Vitamin D: importance in the prevention of cancers, type 1 diabetes, heart disease, and osteoporosis. Am J Clin Nutr. 2004 Mar;79(3):362-71.

Holladay, S.D. Prenatal Immunotoxicant Exposure and Postnatal Autoimmune Disease. Environ Health Perspect. 1999; 107(suppl 5):687-691.

Hollfoth K. Effect of color therapy on health and wellbeing: colors are more than just physics. Pflege.Z 2000;53(2):111-112.

Hollwich F, Dieckhues B, Schrameyer B. The effect of natural and artificial light via the eye on the hormonal and metabolic balance of man. Klin Monbl Augenheilkd. 1977 Jul;171(1):98-104.

Hollwich F, Dieckhues B. Effect of light on the eye on metabolism and hormones. Klin Monbl Augenheilkd. 1989 Nov;195(5):284-90.

Hollwich F. Hartmann C. Influence of light through the eyes on metabolism and hormones. Ophtalmologie. 1990;4(4):385-9.

Hollwich F. The influence of ocular light perception on metabolism in man and in animal. NY: Springer-Verlag, 1979.

Holly EA, Aston DA, Ahn DK, Smith AH. Intraocular melanoma linked to occupations and chemical exposures. Epidemiology. 1996 Jan;7(1):55-61.

Holman CD, Armstrong BK, Heenan PJ. Relationship of cutaneous malignant melanoma to individual sunlight-exposure habits. J Natl Cancer Inst. 1986 Mar;76(3):403-14.

Holmquist G. Susumo Ohno left us January 13, 2000, at the age of 71. Cytogenet and Cell Genet. 2000;88:171-172.

Holt GA. Food & Drug Interactions. Chicago: Precept Press, 1998, 83.

Homma M, Oka K, Niitsuma T, Itoh H. A novel 11 beta-hydroxysteroid dehydrogenase inhibitor contained in saiboku-to, a herbal remedy for steroid-dependent bronchial asthma. J Pharm Pharmacol. 1994 Apr;46(4):305-9.

Honeyman MK. Vegetation and stress: a comparison study of varying amounts of vegetation in countryside and urban scenes. In Relf, D. (ed) The Role of Horticulture in Human Well-Being and Social Development: A National Symposium. Portland: Timber Press. 1992:143-145.

Hönscheid A, Rink L, Haase H. T-lymphocytes: a target for stimulatory and inhibitory effects of zinc ions. Endocr Metab Immune Disord Drug Targets. 2009 Jun;9(2):132-44.

Hood W, Nicholas J, Butler G, Lackland D, Hoel D, Mohr L. Magnetic field exposure of commercial airline pilots. Annals of Epidemiology 2000 Oct 1;10(7):479.

Hooper R, Calvert J, Thompson RL, Deetlefs ME, Burney P. Urban/rural differences in diet and atopy in South Africa. Allergy. 2008 Apr;63(4):425-31.

Hope BE, Massey DG, Fournier-Massey G. Hawaiian materia medica for asthma. Hawaii Med J. 1993 Jun;52(6):160-6.

Horak E, Morass B, Ulmer H. Association between environmental tobacco smoke exposure and wheezing disorders in Austrian preschool children. Swiss Med Wkly. 2007 Nov 3;137(43-44):608-13.

Horne JA, Donlon J, Arendt J. Green light attenuates melatonin output and sleepiness during sleep deprivation. Sleep. 1991 Jun;14(3):233-40.

Horrobin DF. Effects of evening primrose oil in rheumatoid arthritis. Ann Rheum Dis. 1989 Nov;48(11):965-6.

Hoskin M.(ed.). The Cambridge Illustrated History of Astronomy. Cambridge: Cambridge Press, 1997.

Hospers IC, de Vries-Vrolijk K, Brand PL. Double-blind, placebo-controlled cow's milk challenge in children with alleged cow's milk allergies, performed in a general hospital: diagnosis rejected in two-thirds of the children. Ned Tijdschr Geneeskd. 2006 Jun 10;150(23):1292-7.

Hossein G, Halvaei S, Heidarian Y, Dehghani-Ghobadi Z, Hassani M, Hosseini H, Naderi N, Sheikh Hassani S. Pectasol-C Modified Citrus Pectin targets Galectin-3-induced STAT3 activation and synergize paclitaxel cytotoxic effect on ovarian cancer spheroids. Cancer Med. 2019 Jun 13. doi: 10.1002/cam4.2334.

Hosseini S, Pishnamazi S, Sadrzadeh SM, Farid F, Farid R, Watson RR. Pycnogenol((R)) in the Management of Asthma. J Med Food. 2001 Winter;4(4):201-209.

Hostettler S. Hops extract studied to prevent breast cancer. UIC News Center. July 11, 2016.

Hota B, Ellenbogen C, Hayden MK, Aroutcheva A, Rice TW, Weinstein RA. Community-associated methicillin-resistant Staphylococcus aureus skin and soft tissue infections at a public hospital: do public housing and incarceration amplify transmission? Arch Intern Med. 2007 May 28;167(10):1026-33.

Houssen ME, Ragab A, Mesbah A, El-Samanoudy AZ, Othman G, Moustafa AF, Badria FA. Natural anti-inflammatory products and leukotriene inhibitors as complementary therapy for bronchial asthma. Clin Biochem. 2010 Jul;43(10-11):887-90.

Hoyle F. Evolution from Space. Londong: JM Dent, 1981.

Hoyme UB, Saling E. Efficient prematurity prevention is possible by pH-self measurement and immediate therapy of threatening ascending infection. Eur J Obstet Gynecol Reprod Biol. 2004 Aug 10;115(2):148-53.

Hoyos AB. Reduced incidence of necrotizing enterocolitis associated with enteral administration of Lactobacillus acidophilus and Bifidobacterium infantis to neonates in an intensive care unit. Int J Infect Dis. 1999 Summer;3(4):197-202.

Hsiao PC, Lee WJ, Yang SF, Tan P, Chen HY, Lee LM, Chang JL, Lai GM, Chow JM, Chien MH. Nobiletin suppresses the proliferation and induces apoptosis involving MAPKs and caspase-8/-9/-3 signals in human acute myeloid leukemia cells. Tumour Biol. 2014 Dec;35(12):11903-11. doi: 10.1007/s13277-014-2457-0.

Hsieh CH, Lin CY, Hsu CL, Fan KH, Huang SF, Liao CT, Lee LY, Ng SK, Yen TC, Chang JT, Lin JR, Wang HM. Incorporation of Astragalus polysaccharides injection during concurrent chemoradiotherapy in advanced pharyngeal or laryngeal squamous cell carcinoma: preliminary experience of a phase II double-blind, randomized trial. J Cancer Res Clin Oncol. 2020 Jan;146(1):33-41. doi: 10.1007/s00432-019-03033-8.

Hsu HH, Leung WH, Hu GC. Treatment of irritable bowel syndrome with colonic irrigation system: a pilot study. Tech Coloproctol. 2016 Aug;20(8):551-7. doi: 10.1007/s10151-016-1491-x. Mishori R. The Journal of Family Practice, August 2011; vol 60: pp 454-457.

Hsu WH, Pan TM. Monascus purpureus-fermented products and oral cancer: a review. Appl Microbiol Biotechnol. 2012 Mar;93(5):1831-42. doi: 10.1007/s00253-012-3891-9.

Hu C, Kitts DD. Antioxidant, prooxidant, and cytotoxic activities of solvent-fractionated dandelion (Taraxacum officinale) flower extracts in vitro. J Agric Food Chem. 2003 Jan 1;51(1):301-10.

Hu C, Kitts DD. Dandelion (Taraxacum officinale) flower extract suppresses both reactive oxygen species and nitric oxide and prevents lipid oxidation in vitro. Phytomedicine. 2005 Aug;12(8):588-97.

Hu C, Kitts DD. Luteolin and luteolin-7-O-glucoside from dandelion flower suppress iNOS and COX-2 in RAW264.7 cells. Mol Cell Biochem. 2004 Oct;265(1-2):107-13.

Hu FB, Willett WC. Optimal diets for prevention of coronary heart disease. JAMA. 2002 Nov 27;288(20):2569-78.

Hu X, Wu B, Wang P. Displaying of meridian courses travelling over human body surface under natural conditions. Zhen Ci Yan Jiu. 1993;18(2):83-9.

Hu Z, Yang A, Fan H, Wang Y, Zhao Y, Zha X, Zhang H, Tu P. Huaier aqueous extract sensitizes cells to rapamycin and cisplatin through activating mTOR signaling. J Ethnopharmacol. 2016 Jun 20;186:143-150. doi: 10.1016/j.jep.2016.03.069.

Hu Z, Yang A, Su G, Zhao Y, Wang Y, Chai X, Tu P. Huaier restrains proliferative and invasive potential of human hepatoma SKHEP-1 cells partially through decreased Lamin B1 and elevated NOV. Sci Rep. 2016 Aug 9;6:31298. doi: 10.1038/srep31298.

Huang D, Ou B, Prior RL. The chemistry behind antioxidant capacity assays. J Agric Food Chem. 2005 Mar 23;53(6):1841-56.

Huang H, Sjodin A, Chen Y, Ni X, Ma S, Yu H, Ward MH, Udelsman R, Rusiecki J, Zhang Y. Polybrominated Diphenyl Ethers, Polybrominated Biphenyls, and Risk of Papillary Thyroid Cancer: A Nested Case-Control Study. Am J Epidemiol. 2020 Feb 28;189(2):120-132. doi: 10.1093/aje/kwz229. PMID: 31742588; PMCID: PMC7156139.

Huang HB, Pan WH, Chang JW, Chiang HC, Guo YL, Jaakkola JJ, Huang PC. Does exposure to phthalates influence thyroid function and growth hormone homeostasis? The Taiwan Environmental Survey for Toxicants (TEST) 2013. Environ Res. 2017 Feb;153:63-72. doi: 10.1016/j.envres.2016.11.014.

Huang JP, Zhang M, Holman CD, Xie X. Dietary carotenoids and risk of breast cancer in Chinese women. Asia Pac J Clin Nutr. 2007;16 Suppl 1:437-42.

Huang M, Wang W, Wei S. Investigation on medicinal plant resources of Glycyrrhiza uralensis in China and chemical assessment of its underground part. Zhongguo Zhong Yao Za Zhi. 2010 Apr;35(8):947-52.

Huang XE, Hirose K, Wakai K, Matsuo K, Ito H, Xiang J, et al. Comparison of lifestyle risk factors by family history for gastric, breast, lung and colorectal cancer. Asian Pac J Cancer Prev. 2004;5:419-427.

Hubbard HF, Coleman BK, Sarwar G, Corsi RL. Effects of an ozone-generating air purifier on indoor secondary particles in three residential dwellings. Indoor Air. 2005 Dec;15(6):432-44. doi: 10.1111/j.1600-0668.2005.00388.x. PMID: 16268833.

Hudthagosol C, Haddad E, Jongsuwat R. Antioxidant activity comparison of walnuts and fatty fish. J Med Assoc Thai. 2012 Jun;95 Suppl 6:S179-88.

Huesmann LR, Moise-Titus J, Podolski CL, Eron LD. Longitudinal relations between children's exposure to TV violence and their aggressive and violent behavior in young adulthood: 1977-1992. Dev Psychol. 2003 Mar;39(2):201-21.

Huesmann LR, Moise-Titus J, Podolski CL, Eron LD. Longitudinal relations between children's exposure to TV violence and their aggressive and violent behavior in young adulthood: 1977-1992. Dev Psychol. 2003 Mar;39(2):201-21.

Huffman C. Archytas of Tarentum: Pythagorean, philosopher and Mathematician King. Cambridge: Cambridge University Press, 2005.

Hughes MF, Beck BD, Chen Y, Lewis AS, Thomas DJ. Arsenic Exposure and Toxicology: A Historical Perspective. Toxicol Sci. 2011 Jul 12.

Hun L. Bacillus coagulans significantly improved abdominal pain and bloating in patients with IBS. Postgrad Med. 2009 Mar;121(2):119-24.

Hunt T, Madigan S, Williams MT, Olds TS. Use of time in people with chronic obstructive pulmonary disease–a systematic review. Int J Chron Obstruct Pulmon Dis. 2014 Dec 12;9:1377-88. doi: 10.2147/COPD.S74298.

Hunt V. Infinite Mind: Science of the Human Vibrations of Consciousness. Malibu: Malibu Publ. 2000.

Huntley A, Ernst E: Herbal medicines for asthma: a systematic review. Thorax. 2000, 55:925-929.

Hur W, Kim SW, Lee YK, Choi JE, Hong SW, Song MJ, Bae SH, Park T, Um SJ, Yoon

Hur YM, Rushton JP. Genetic and environmental contributions to prosocial behaviour in 2- to 9-year-old South Korean twins. Biol Lett. 2007 Dec 22;3(6):664-6.

Hur YM, Rushton JP. Genetic and environmental contributions to prosocial behaviour in 2- to 9-year-old South Korean twins. Biol Lett. 2007 Aug 28.

Husby S. Dietary antigens: uptake and humoral immunity in man. APMIS Suppl. 1988;1:1-40.

Hyndman SJ, Vickers LM, Htut T, Maunder JW, Peock A, Higenbottam TW. A randomized trial of dehumidification in the control of house dust mite. Clin Exp Allergy. 2000 Aug;30(8):1172-80.

Ibrahim AR, Kawamoto S, Nishimura M, Pak S, Aki T, Diaz-Perales A, Salcedo G, Asturias JA, Hayashi T, Ono K. A new lipid transfer protein homolog identified as an IgE-binding antigen from Japanese cedar pollen. Biosci Biotechnol Biochem. 2010;74(3):504-9.

Idorn M, Thor Straten P. Exercise and cancer: from "healthy" to "therapeutic"? Cancer Immunol Immunother. 2017 May;66(5):667-671. doi: 10.1007/s00262-017-1985-z.

Igarashi T, Izumi H, Uchiumi T, Nishio K, Arao T, Tanabe M, Uramoto H, Sugio K, Yasumoto K, Sasaguri Y, Wang KY, Otsuji Y, Kohno K. Clock and ATF4 transcription system regulates drug resistance in human cancer cell lines. Oncogene. 2007 Jul 19;26(33):4749-60.

Ikeda M, Toyoshima R, Inoue Y, Yamada N, Mishima K, Nomura M, Ozaki N, Okawa M, Takahashi K, Yamauchi T. Mutation screening of the human Clock gene in circadian rhythm sleep disorders. Psychia-try Res. 2002 Mar 15;109(2):121-8.

Ikeda M, Toyoshima R, Inoue Y, Yamada N, Mishima K, Nomura M, Ozaki N, Okawa M, Takahashi K, Yamauchi T. Mutation screening of the human Clock gene in circadian rhythm sleep disorders. Psychia-try Res. 2002 Mar 15;109(2):121-8.

Imase K, Tanaka A, Tokunaga K, Sugano H, Ishida H, Takahashi S. Lactobacillus reuteri tablets suppress Helicobacter pylori infection—a double-blind randomised placebo-controlled cross-over clinical study. Kansenshogaku Zasshi. 2007 Jul;81(4):387-93.

Inbar O, Dotan R, Dlin RA, Neuman I, Bar-Or O. Breathing dry or humid air and exercise-induced asthma during swimming. Eur J Appl Physiol Occup Physiol. 1980;44(1):43-50.

Indrio F, Ladisa G, Mautone A, Montagna O. Effect of a fermented formula on thymus size and stool pH in healthy term infants. Pediatr Res. 2007 Jul;62(1):98-100.

Indrio F, Riezzo G, Raimondi F, Bisceglia M, Cavallo L, Francavilla R. The effects of probiotics on feeding tolerance, bowel habits, and gastrointestinal motility in preterm newborns. J Pediatr. 2008 Jun;152(6):801-6.

Innis SM, Hansen JW. Plasma fatty acid responses, metabolic effects, and safety of microalgal and fungal oils rich in arachidonic and docosahexaenoic acids in healthy adults. Am J Clin Nutr. 1996 Aug;64(2):159-67.

Inoue-Choi M, Sinha R, Gierach GL, Ward MH. Red and processed meat, nitrite, and heme iron intakes and postmenopausal breast cancer risk in the NIH-AARP Diet and Health Study. Int J Cancer. 2015 Oct 27. doi: 10.1002/ijc.29901.

International Agency for Research on Cancer. IARC Monographs evaluate consumption of red meat and processed meat. 26 Oct. 2015.

Ionescu JG. New insights in the pathogenesis of atopic disease. J Med Life. 2009 Apr-Jun;2(2):146-54.

Iovieno A, Lambiase A, Sacchetti M, Stampachiacchiere B, Micera A, Bonini S. Preliminary evidence of the efficacy of probiotic eye-drop treatment in patients with vernal keratoconjunctivitis. Graefes Arch Clin Exp Ophthalmol. 2008 Mar;246(3):435-41.

Irving GR, Iwuji CO, Morgan B, Berry DP, Steward WP, Thomas A, Brown K, Howells LM. Combining curcumin with standard care FOLFOX chemotherapy in patients with inoperable colorectal cancer (CUFOX): study protocol for a randomised control trial. Trials. 2015 Mar 24;16:110. doi: 10.1186/s13063-015-0641-1.

Ishikawa H, Akedo I, Otani T, Suzuki T, Nakamura T, Takeyama I, Ishiguro S, Miyaoka E, Sobue T, Kakizoe T. Randomized trial of dietary fiber and Lactobacillus casei administration for prevention of colorectal tumors. Int J Cancer. 2005 Sep 20;116(5):762-7.

Ishtiaq M, Hanif W, Khan MA, Ashraf M, Butt AM. An ethnomedicinal survey and documentation of important medicinal folklore food phytonims of flora of Samahni valley, (Azad Kashmir) Pakistan. Pak J Biol Sci. 2007 Jul 1;10(13):2241-56.

Isolauri E, Joensuu J, Suomalainen H, Luomala M, Vesikari T. Improved immunogenicity of oral D x RRV reassortant rotavirus vaccine by Lactobacillus casei GG. Vaccine. 1995 Feb;13(3):310-2.

Isolauri E, Juntunen M, Rautanen T, Sillanaukee P, Koivula T. A human Lactobacillus strain (Lactobacillus casei sp strain GG) promotes recovery from acute diarrhea in children. Pediatrics. 1991 Jul;88(1):90-7.

Isolauri E, Kaila M, Mykkänen H, Ling WH, Salminen S. Oral bacteriotherapy for viral gastroenteritis. Dig Dis Sci. 1994 Dec;39(12):2595-600.

Ito, Hitoshi; Shimura, Keishiro; Itoh, Hiroko; Kawade, Mitsuo. 1997. Antitumor effects of a new polysaccharide-protein complex (ATOM) prepared from Agaricus blazei (Iwade strain 101) \"Himematsutake\" and its mechanisms in tumor-bearing mice. Anticancer Research, 17(1A), 277-284.

Itokawa Y. Magnesium intake and cardiovascular disease. Clin Calcium. 2005 Feb;15(2):154-9.

Ivanovic-Zuvic F, de la Vega R, Ivanovic-Zuvic N, Renteria P. Affective disorders and solar activity. Actas Esp Psiquiatr. 2005 Jan-Feb;33(1):7-12.

Ivry GB, Ogle CA, Shim EK. Role of sun exposure in melanoma. Dermatol Surg. 2006 Apr;32(4):481-92.

Iwase T, Kajimura N, Uchiyama M, Ebisawa T, Yoshimura K, Kamei Y, Shibui K, Kim K, Kudo Y, Katoh M, Watanabe T, Nakajima T, Ozeki Y, Sugishita M, Hori T, Ikeda M, Toyoshima R, Inoue Y, Yamada

N, Mishima K, Nomura M, Ozaki N, Okawa M, Takahashi K, Yamauchi T. Mutation screening of the human Clock gene in circadian rhythm sleep disorders. Psychiatry Res. 2002 Mar 15;109(2):121-8.

Izbicki G, Chavko R, Banauch GI, Weiden MD, Berger KI, Aldrich TK, Hall C, Kelly KJ, Prezant DJ. World trade center "sarcoid-like" granulomatous pulmonary disease in New York City fire department rescue workers. Chest. 2007 May;131(5):1414-23.

Izquierdo JL, Martín A, de Lucas P, Rodríguez-González-Moro JM, Almonacid C, Paravisini A. Misdiagnosis of patients receiving inhaled therapies in primary care. Int J Chron Obstruct Pulmon Dis. 2010 Aug 9;5:241-9.

Jaber R. Respiratory and allergic diseases: from upper respiratory tract infections to asthma. Prim Care. 2002 Jun;29(2):231-61.

Jacobs DE, Wilson J, Dixon SL, Smith J, Evens A. The relationship of housing and population health: a 30-year retrospective analysis. Environ Health Perspect. 2009 Apr;117(4):597-604. 2008 Dec 16.

Jacobsen CN, Rosenfeldt Nielsen V, Hayford AE, Møller PL, Michaelsen KF, Paerregaard A, Sandström B, Tvede M, Jakobsen M. Screening of probiotic activities of forty-seven strains of Lactobacillus spp. by in vitro techniques and evaluation of the colonization ability of five selected strains in humans. Appl Environ Microbiol. 1999 Nov;65(11):4949-56.

Jäger T, Scherr C, Shah D, Majewsky V, Wolf U, Betti L, Baumgartner S. The use of plant-based bioassays in homeopathic basic research. Homeopathy. 2015 Oct;104(4):277-82. doi: 10.1016/j.homp.2015.06.009.

Jagetia GC, Aggarwal BB. "Spicing up" of the immune system by curcumin. J Clin Immunol. 2007 Jan;27(1):19-35.

Jagetia GC, Nayak V, Vidyasagar MS. Evaluation of the antineoplastic activity of guduchi (Tinospora cordifolia) in cultured HeLa cells. Cancer Lett. 1998 May 15;127(1-2):71-82.

Jagetia GC, Rao SK. Evaluation of Cytotoxic Effects of Dichloromethane Extract of Guduchi (Tinospora cordifolia Miers ex Hook F & THOMS) on Cultured HeLa Cells. Evid Based Complement Alternat Med. 2006 Jun;3(2):267-72.

Jahanbani R, Ghaffari SM, Salami M, Vahdati K, Sepehri H, Sarvestani NN, Sheibani N, Moosavi-Movahedi AA. Antioxidant and Anticancer Activities of Walnut (Juglans regia L.) Protein Hydrolysates Using Different Proteases. Plant Foods Hum Nutr. 2016 Dec;71(4):402-409.

Jahnova E, Horvathova M, Gazdik F, Weissova S. Effects of selenium supplementation on expression of adhesion molecules in corticoid-dependent asthmatics. Bratisl Lek Listy. 2002;103(1):12-6.

Jain PK, McNaught CE, Anderson AD, MacFie J, Mitchell CJ. Influence of synbiotic containing Lactobacillus acidophilus La5, Bifidobacterium lactis Bb 12, Streptococcus thermophilus, Lactobacillus bulgaricus and oligofructose on gut barrier function and sepsis in critically ill patients: a randomised controlled trial. Clin Nutr. 2004 Aug;23(4):467-75.

Jaiswal M, Prajapati PK, Patgiri BJ Ravishankar B. A Comparative Pharmaco - Clinical Study on Anti-Asthmatic Effect of Shirishaishta Prepared by Bark, Sapwood and Heartwood of Albizia Lebbeck. J Res Ayurv. 2006;27(3):67-74.

Jaiswal M, Prajapati PK, Patgiri BJ, Ravishankar B. Clinical Study on Anti-Asthmatic Effect of Shirishaishta Prepared by Bark, Sapwood and Heartwood of Albizia Lebbeck. Pharmaco. 2006 27(3): 67-74

Jakab F, Mayer A, Hoffmann A, Hidvégi M. First clinical data of a natural immunomodulator in colorectal cancer. Hepatogastroenterology. 2000 Mar-Apr;47(32):393-5.

James MI, Iwuji C, Irving G, Karmokar A, Higgins JA, Griffin-Teal N, Thomas A, Greaves P, Cai H, Patel SR, Morgan B, Dennison A, Metcalfe M, Garcea G, Lloyd DM, Berry DP, Steward WP, Howells LM, Brown K. Curcumin inhibits cancer stem cell phenotypes in ex vivo models of colorectal liver metastases, and is clinically safe and tolerable in combination with FOLFOX chemotherapy. Cancer Lett. 2015 Aug 10;364(2):135-41. doi: 10.1016/j.canlet.2015.05.005.

Janelle KC, Barr SI. Nutrient intakes and eating behavior scores of vegetarian and nonvegetarian women. J Am Diet Assoc. 1995 Feb;95(2):180-6, 189, quiz 187-8.

Janfaza S, Khorsand B, Nikkhah M, Zahiri J. Digging deeper into volatile organic compounds associated with cancer. Biol Methods Protoc. 2019 Nov 27;4(1):bpz014. doi: 10.1093/biomethods/bpz014. PMID: 32161807; PMCID: PMC6994028.

Jang E, Kim SY, Lee NR, Yi CM, Hong DR, Lee WS, Kim JH, Lee KT, Kim BJ, Lee JH, Inn KS. Evaluation of antitumor activity of Artemisia capillaris extract against hepatocellular carcinoma through the inhibition of IL-6/STAT3 signaling axis. Oncol Rep. 2017 Jan;37(1):526-532. doi: 10.3892/or.2016.5283.

Jang YG, Hwang KA, Choi KC. Rosmarinic Acid, a Component of Rosemary Tea, Induced the Cell Cycle Arrest and Apoptosis through Modulation of HDAC2 Expression in Prostate Cancer Cell Lines. Nutrients. 2018 Nov 16;10(11):1784. doi: 10.3390/nu10111784.

Janson C, Anto J, Burney P, Chinn S, de Marco R, Heinrich J, Jarvis D, Kuenzli N, Leynaert B, Luczynska C, Neukirch F, Svanes C, Sunyer J, Wjst M; European Community Respiratory Health Survey II. The European Community Respiratory Health Survey: what are the main results so far? European Community Respiratory Health Survey II. Eur Respir J. 2001 Sep;18(3):598-611.

Janssen S, Solomon G, Schettler T. Chemical Contaminants and Human Disease: The Collaborative on Health and the Environment. 2006. http://www.healthandenvironment.org. Accessed: 2007 Jul.

Jarocka-Cyrta E, Baniukiewicz A, Wasilewska J, Pawlak J, Kaczmarski M. Focal villous atrophy of the duodenum in children who have outgrown cow's milk allergy. Chromoendoscopy and magnification endoscopy evaluation. Med Wieku Rozwoj. 2007 Apr-Jun;11(2 Pt 1):123-7.

Jarvius M, Fryknäs M, D'Arcy P, Sun C, Rickardson L, Gullbo J, Haglund C, Nygren P, Linder S, Larsson R. Piperlongumine induces inhibition of the ubiquitin-proteasome system in cancer cells. Biochem Biophys Res Commun. 2013 Jan 11. doi:pii: S0006-291X(13)00053-3.

Jauhiainen T, Vapaatalo H, Poussa T, Kyrönpalo S, Rasmussen M, Korpela R. Lactobacillus helveticus fermented milk lowers blood pressure in hypertensive subjects in 24-h ambulatory blood pressure measurement. Am J Hypertens. 2005 Dec;18(12 Pt 1):1600-5.

Jayaprakasam B, Doddaga S, Wang R, Holmes D, Goldfarb J, Li XM. Licorice flavonoids inhibit eotaxin-1 secretion by human fetal lung fibroblasts in vitro. J Agric Food Chem. 2009 Feb 11;57(3):820-5.

Jenab M, Bueno-de-Mesquita HB, Ferrari P, van Duijnhoven FJ, Norat T, Pischon T, Jansen EH, Slimani N, Byrnes G, Rinaldi S, Tjønneland A, Olsen A, Overvad K, Boutron-Ruault MC, Clavel-Chapelon F, Morois S, Kaaks R, Linseisen J, Boeing H, Bergmann MM, Trichopoulou A, Misirli G, Trichopoulos D, Berrino F, Vineis P, Panico S, Palli D, Tumino R, Ros MM, van Gils CH, Peeters PH, Brustad M, Lund E, Tormo MJ, Ardanaz E, Rodríguez L, Sánchez MJ, Dorronsoro M, Gonzalez CA, Hallmans G, Palmqvist R, Roddam A, Key TJ, Khaw KT, Autier P, Hainaut P, Riboli E. Association between pre-diagnostic circulating vitamin D concentration and risk of colorectal cancer in European populations: a nested case-control study. BMJ. 2010 Jan 21;340:b5500. doi: 10.1136/bmj.b5500.

Jenab M, Ferrari P, Slimani N, Norat T, Casagrande C, Overad K, Olsen A, Stripp C, Tjønneland A, Boutron-Ruault MC, Clavel-Chapelon F, Kesse E, Nieters A, Bergmann M, Boeing H, Naska A, Trichopoulou A, Palli D, Krogh V, Celentano E, Tumino R, Sacerdote C, Bueno-de-Mesquita HB, Ocké MC, Peeters PH, Engeset D, Quirós JR, González CA, Martínez C, Chirlaque MD, Ardanaz E, Dorronsoro M, Wallström P, Palmqvist R, Van Guelpen B, Bingham S, San Joaquin MA, Saracci R, Kaaks R, Riboli E. Association of nut and seed intake with colorectal cancer risk in the European Prospective Investigation into Cancer and Nutrition. Cancer Epidemiol Biomarkers Prev. 2004 Oct;13(10):1595-603.

Jennings S, Prescott SL. Early dietary exposures and feeding practices: role in pathogenesis and prevention of allergic disease? Postgrad Med J. 2010 Feb;86(1012):94-9.

Jensen B. Foods that Heal. Garden City Park, NY: Avery Publ, 1988, 1993.

Jensen B. Nature Has a Remedy. Los Angeles: Keats, 2001.

Jensen HK. The molecular genetic basis and diagnosis of familial hypercholesterolemia in Denmark. Dan Med Bull. 2002 Nov;49(4):318-45.

Jensen MB, López-de-Dicastillo Bergamo CA, Payet RM, Liu X, Konczak I. Influence of copigment derived from Tasmannia pepper leaf on Davidson's plum anthocyanins. J Food Sci. 2011 Apr;76(3):C447-53.

Jeon HJ, Kang HJ, Jung HJ, Kang YS, Lim CJ, Kim YM, Park EH. Anti-inflammatory activity of Taraxacum officinale. J Ethnopharmacol. 2008 Jan 4;115(1):82-8.

Jeong SC, Koyyalamudi SR, Jeong YT, Song CH, Pang G. Macrophage immunomodulating and antitumor activities of polysaccharides isolated from Agaricus bisporus white button mushrooms. J Med Food. 2012 Jan;15(1):58-65. doi: 10.1089/jmf.2011.1704.

Jernelöv S, Höglund CO, Axelsson J, Axén J, Grönneberg R, Grunewald J, Stierna P, Lekander M. Effects of examination stress on psychological responses, sleep and allergic symptoms in atopic and non-atopic students. Int J Behav Med. 2009;16(4):305-10.

Ji X, Pan C, Li X, Gao Y, Xia L, Quan X, Lv J, Wang R. Trametes robiniophila may induce apoptosis and inhibit MMPs expression in the human gastric carcinoma cell line MKN-45. Oncol Lett. 2017 Feb;13(2):841-846. doi: 10.3892/ol.2016.5517.

Ji Y, Liu YB, Zheng LY, Zhang XQ. Survey of studies on tissue structures and biological characteristics of channel lines. Zhongguo Zhen Jiu. 2007 Jun;27(6):427-32.

Jiang R, Manson JE, Stampfer MJ, Liu S, Willett WC, Hu FB. Nut and peanut butter consumption and risk of type 2 diabetes in women. JAMA. 2002 Nov 27;288(20):2554-60.

Jiang T, Mustapha A, Savaiano DA. Improvement of lactose digestion in humans by ingestion of unfermented milk containing Bifidobacterium longum. J Dairy Sci. 1996 May;79(5):750-7.

Jiménez E, Fernández L, Maldonado A, Martín R, Olivares M, Xaus J, Rodríguez JM. Oral administration of Lactobacillus strains isolated from breast milk as an alternative for the treatment of infectious mastitis during lactation. Appl Environ Microbiol. 2008 Aug;74(15):4650-5.

Jiménez F, Barbaglia Y, Bucci P, Tedeschi FA, Zalazar FE. Molecular detection and genotypification of Helicobacter pylori in gastric biopsies from symptomatic adult patients in Santa Fe, Argentina. Rev Argent Microbiol. 2013 Jan-Mar;45(1):39-43.

Jin CN, Zhang TS, Ji LX, Tian YF. Survey of studies on mechanisms of acupuncture and moxibustion in decreasing blood pressure. Zhongguo Zhen Jiu. 2007 Jun;27(6):467-70.

Jin H, Leng Q, Li C. Dietary flavonoid for preventing colorectal neoplasms. Cochrane Database Syst Rev. 2012 Aug 15;8:CD009350.

Joghatai M, Barari L, Mousavie Anijdan SH, Elmi MM. The Evaluation of Radio-sensitivity of Mung Bean Proteins Aqueous Extract on MCF-7, Hela and Fibroblast Cell Line. Int J Radiat Biol. 2018 Feb 26:1-29. doi: 10.1080/09553002.2018.1446226.

Johansen C. Electromagnetic fields and health effects—epidemiologic studies of cancer, diseases of the central nervous system and arrhythmia-related heart disease. Scand J Work Env Hlth. 2004;30 Spl 1:1-30.

Johansen C. Rehabilitation of cancer patients - research perspectives. Acta Oncol. 2007;46(4):441-5.

Johansson G, Holmén A, Persson L, Högstedt B, Wassén C, Ottova L, Gustafsson JA. Dietary influence on some proposed risk factors for colon cancer: fecal and urinary mutagenic activity and the activity of some intestinal bacterial enzymes. Cancer Detect Prev. 1997;21(3):258-66.

Johansson G, Holmén A, Persson L, Högstedt R, Wassén C, Ottova L, Gustafsson JA. The effect of a shift from a mixed diet to a lacto-vegetarian diet on human urinary and fecal mutagenic activity. Carcinogenesis. 1992 Feb;13(2):153-7.

Johansson G, Ravald N. Comparison of some salivary variables between vegetarians and omnivores. Eur J Oral Sci. 1995 Apr;103(2 (Pt 1)):95-8.

Johansson GK, Ottova L, Gustafsson JA. Shift from a mixed diet to a lactovegetarian diet: influence on some cancer-associated intestinal bacterial enzyme activities. Nutr Cancer. 1990;14(3-4):239-46. PubMed PMID: 2128119.

Johansson ML, Nobaek S, Berggren A, Nyman M, Björck I, Ahrné S, Jeppsson B, Molin G. Survival of Lactobacillus plantarum DSM 9843 (299v), and effect on the short-chain fatty acid content of faeces after ingestion of a rose-hip drink with fermented oats. Int J Food Microbiol. 1998 Jun 30;42(1-2):29-38.

Johnsen NF, Frederiksen K, Christensen J, Skeie G, Lund E, Landberg R, Johansson I, Nilsson LM, Halkjær J, Olsen A, Overvad K, Tjønneland A. Whole-grain products and whole-grain types are associated with lower all-cause and cause-specific mortality in the Scandinavian HELGA cohort. Br J Nutr. 2015 Aug 28;114(4):608-23. doi: 10.1017/S0007114515001701.

Johnson LM. Gitksan medicinal plants—cultural choice and efficacy. J Ethnobiol Ethnomed. 2006 Jun 21;2:29.

Johnston A. A spatial property of the retino-cortical mapping. Spatial Vision. 1986;1(4):319-331.

Johnston RE. Pheromones, the vomeronasal system, and communication. From hormonal responses to individual recognition. Ann N Y Acad Sci. 1998 Nov 30;855:333-48.

Jones MA, Silman AJ, Whiting S, et al. Occurrence of rheumatoid arthritis is not increased in the first degree relatives of a population based inception cohort of inflammatory polyarthritis. Ann Rheum Dis. 1996;55(2): 89-93.

Jones SE, Versalovic J. Probiotic Lactobacillus reuteri biofilms produce antimicrobial and anti-inflammatory factors. BMC Microbiol. 2009 Feb 11;9:35.

José RJ, Roberts J, Bakerly ND. The effectiveness of a social marketing model on case-finding for COPD in a deprived inner city population. Prim Care Respir J. 2010 Jun;19(2):104-8.

Joseph SP, Borrell LN, Shapiro A. Self-reported lifetime asthma and nativity status in U.S. children and adolescents: results from the National Health and Nutrition Examination Survey 1999-2004. J Health Care Poor Underserved. 2010 May;21(2 Suppl):125-39.

Jovanovic-Ignjatic Z, Rakovic D. A review of current research in microwave resonance therapy: novel opportunities in medical treatment. Acupunct Electrother Res. 1999; 24:105-125.

Jovanovic-Ignjatic Z. Microwave Resonant Therapy: Novel Opportunities in Medical Treatment. Acup. & Electro-Therap. Res., The Int. J. 1999;24(2):105-125.

Judson PL, Al Sawah E, Marchion DC, Xiong Y, Bicaku E, Bou Zgheib N, Chon HS, Stickles XB, Hakam A, Wenham RM, Apte SM, Gonzalez-Bosquet J, Chen DT, Lancaster JM. Characterizing the efficacy of fermented wheat germ extract against ovarian cancer and defining the genomic basis of its activity. Int J Gynecol Cancer. 2012 Jul;22(6):960-7. doi: 10.1097/IGC.0b013e318258509d.

Juergens UR, Dethlefsen U, Steinkamp G, Gillissen A, Repges R, Vetter H. Anti-inflammatory activity of 1.8-cineol (eucalyptol) in bronchial asthma: a double-blind placebo-controlled trial. Respir Med. 2003 Mar;97(3):250-6.

Julkunen-Tiitto R. A chemotaxonomic survey of phenolics in leaves of northern Salicaceae species. Phytochemistry. 1986;25(3):663-667.

Jung HA, Yokozawa T, Kim BW, Jung JH, Choi JS. Selective inhibition of prenylated flavonoids from Sophora flavescens against BACE1 and cholinesterases. Am J Chin Med. 2010;38(2):415-29.

Jurenka JS. Anti-inflammatory properties of curcumin, a major constituent of Curcuma longa: a review of preclinical and clinical research. Altern Med Rev. 2009 Feb;14(2):141-153.

Jurkovicová I, Celec P. Sleep apnea syndrome and its complications. Acta Med Austr. 2004 May;31(2):45-50.

Juvonen R, Bloigu A, Peitso A, Silvennoinen-Kassinen S, Saikku P, Leinonen M, Hassi J, Harju T. Training improves physical fitness and decreases CRP also in asthmatic conscripts. J Asthma. 2008 Apr;45(3):237-42.

Kahhak L, Roche A, Dubray C, Arnoux C, Benveniste J. Decrease of ciliary beat frequency by platelet activating factor: protective effect of ketotifen. Inflamm Res. 1996 May;45(5):234-8.

Kähkönen MP, Hopia AI, Vuorela HJ, Rauha JP, Pihlaja K, Kujala TS, Heinonen M. Antioxidant activity of plant extracts containing phenolic compounds. J Agric Food Chem. 1999 Oct;47(10):3954-62.

Kaila M, Isolauri E, Saxelin M, Arvilommi H, Vesikari T. Viable versus inactivated lactobacillus strain GG in acute rotavirus diarrhoea. Arch Dis Child. 1995 Jan;72(1):51-3.

Kaiser S, Dietrich F, de Resende PE, Verza SG, Moraes RC, Morrone FB, Batastini AM, Ortega GG. Cat's claw oxindole alkaloid isomerization induced by cell incubation and cytotoxic activity against T24 and RT4 human bladder cancer cell lines. Planta Med. 2013 Oct;79(15):1413-20. doi: 10.1055/s-0033-1350742. Epub 2013 Aug 23. PMID: 23975868.

Kajander K, Hatakka K, Poussa T, Färkkilä M, Korpela R. A probiotic mixture alleviates symptoms in irritable bowel syndrome patients: a controlled 6-month intervention. Aliment Pharmacol Ther. 2005 Sep 1;22(5):387-94.

Kajander K, Korpela R. Clinical studies on alleviating the symptoms of irritable bowel syndrome. Asia Pac J Clin Nutr. 2006;15(4):576-80.

Kajander K, Krogius-Kurikka L, Rinttilä T, Karjalainen H, Palva A, Korpela R. Effects of multispecies probiotic supplementation on intestinal microbiota in irritable bowel syndrome. Aliment Pharmacol Ther. 2007 Aug 1;26(3):463-73.

Kajander K, Myllyluoma E, Rajilić-Stojanović M, Kyrönpalo S, Rasmussen M, Järvenpää S, Zoetendal EG, de Vos WM, Vapaatalo H, Korpela R. Clinical trial: multispecies probiotic supplementation alleviates the symptoms of irritable bowel syndrome and stabilizes intestinal microbiota. Aliment Pharmacol Ther. 2008 Jan 1;27(1):48-57.

Kalach N, Benhamou PH, Campeotto F, Dupont Ch. Anemia impairs small intestinal absorption measured by intestinal permeability in children. Eur Ann Allergy Clin Immunol. 2007 Jan;39(1):20-2.

Kaliner M, Shelhamer JH, Borson B, Nadel J, Patow C, Marom Z. Human respiratory mucus. Am Rev Respir Dis. 1986 Sep;134(3):612-21.

Kalsbeek A, Perreau-Lenz S, Buijs RM. A network of (autonomic) clock outputs. Chronobiol Int. 2006;23(1-2):201-15.

Kalsbeek A, Perreau-Lenz S, Buijs RM. A network of (autonomic) clock outputs. Chronobiol Int. 2006;23(1-2):201-15.

Kamide Y. We reside in the sun's atmosphere. Biomed Pharmacother. 2005 Oct;59 Suppl 1:S1-4.

Kamycheva E, Jorde R, Figenschau Y, Haug E. Insulin sensitivity in subjects with secondary hyperparathyroidism and the effect of a low serum 25-hydroxyvitamin D level on insulin sensitivity. J Endocrinol In-vest. 2007 Feb;30(2):126-32.

Kanazawa H, Nagino M, Kamiya S, Komatsu S, Mayumi T, Takagi K, Asahara T, Nomoto K, Tanaka R, Nimura Y. Synbiotics reduce postoperative infectious complications: a randomized controlled trial in biliary cancer patients undergoing hepatectomy. Langenbecks Arch Surg. 2005 Apr;390(2):104-13.

Kandel E, Siegelbaum S, Schwartz J. Synaptic transmission. Principles of Neural Science. New York: Elsevier, 1991.

Kandel E, Siegelbaum S, Schwartz J. Synaptic transmission. Principles of Neural Science. New York: Elsevier, 1991.

Kang HJ, Baik HW, Kim SJ, Lee SG, Ahn HY, Park JS, Park SJ, Jang EJ, Park SW, Choi JY, Sung JH, Lee SM. Cordyceps militaris Enhances Cell-Mediated Immunity in Healthy Korean Men. J Med Food. 2015 Oct;18(10):1164-72. doi: 10.1089/jmf.2014.3350.

Kang SK, Kim JK, Ahn SH, Oh JE, Kim JH, Lim DH, Son BK. Relationship between silent gastroesophageal reflux and food sensitization in infants and young children with recurrent wheezing. J Korean Med Sci. 2010 Mar;25(3):425-8.

Kang Y, Li M, Yan W, Li X, Kang J, Zhang Y. Electroacupuncture alters the expression of genes associated with lipid metabolism and immune reaction in liver of hypercholesterolemia mice. Biotechnol Lett. 2007 Aug 18.

Kankaanpää PE, Yang B, Kallio HP, Isolauri E, Salminen SJ. Influence of probiotic supplemented infant formula on composition of plasma lipids in atopic infants. J Nutr Biochem. 2002 Jun;13(6):364-369.

Kano H, Mogami O, Uchida M. Oral administration of milk fermented with Lactobacillus delbrueckii ssp. bulgaricus OLL1073-R-1 to DBA/1 mice inhibits secretion of proinflammatory cytokines. Cytotechnology. 2002 Nov;40(1-3):67-73.

Kapil A, Sharma S. Immunopotentiating compounds from Tinospora cordifolia. J Ethnopharmacol. 1997 Oct;58(2):89-95.

Kaplan C. Indoor air pollution from unprocessed solid fuels in developing countries. Rev Environ Health. 2010 Jul-Sep;25(3):221-42.

Kaplan M, Mutlu EA, Benson M, Fields JZ, Banan A, Keshavarzian A. Use of herbal preparations in the treatment of oxidant-mediated inflammatory disorders. Complement Ther Med. 2007 Sep;15(3):207-16. 2006 Aug 21.

Kaplan R. The nature of the view from home: psychological benefits. Environ Behav. 2001;33(4):507-42.

Kaplan R. The psychological benefits of nearby nature. In: Relf, D. (ed) The Role of Horticulture in Human Well-Being and Social Development: A National Symposium. Portland: Timber Press. 1992:125-133.

Kaplan R. The psychological benefits of nearby nature. In: Relf, D. (ed) The Role of Horticulture in Human Well-Being and Social Development: A National Symposium. Portland: Timber Press. 1992:125-133.

Kaplan R. Wilderness perception and psychological benefits: an analysis of a continuing program. Leisure Sci. 1984;6(3):271-90.

Kaplan S. The restorative environment: nature and human experience. In: Relf, D. (ed) The Role of Horti-culture in Human Well-Being and Social Development: A National Symposium. Portland: Timber Press. 1992:134-142.

Karami S, Bassig B, Stewart PA, et al. Occupational trichloroethylene exposure and risk of lymphatic and haematopoietic cancers: a meta-analysis. Occup Environ Med. 2013;70(8):591-599. doi:10.1136/oemed-2012-101212

Karis TE, Jhon MS. Flow-induced anisotropy in the susceptibility of a particle suspension. Proc Natl Acad Sci USA. 1986 Jul;83(14):4973-4977.

Karkoulias K, Patouchas D, Alahiotis S, Tsiamita M, Vrodakis K, Spiropoulos K. Specific sensitization in wheat flour and contributing factors in traditional bakers. Eur Rev Med Pharmacol Sci. 2007 May-Jun;11(3):141-8.

Karnstedt J. Ions and Consciousness. Whole Self. 1991 Spring.

Karpin VA, Kostriukova NK, Gudkov AB. Human radiation action of radon and its daughter disintegration products. Gig Sanit. 2005 Jul-Aug;(4):13-7.

Karpińska J, Mikołuć B, Motkowski R, Piotrowska-Jastrzebska J. HPLC method for simultaneous determi-nation of retinol, alpha-tocopherol and coenzyme Q10 in human plasma. J Pharm Biomed Anal. 2006 Sep 18;42(2):232-6.

Kashiwada Y, Takanaka K, Tsukada H, Miwa Y, Taga T, Tanaka S, Ikeshiro Y. Sesquiterpene glucosides from anti-leukotriene B4 release fraction of Taraxacum officinale. J Asian Nat Prod Res. 2001;3(3):191-7.

Kathleen K. Harnden, Kimberly L. Blackwell. Increased Fiber Intake Decreases Premenopausal Breast cancer Risk. Pediatrics. 2016 March.

Kato Y, Kawamoto T, Honda KK. Circadian rhythms in cartilage. Clin Calcium. 2006 May;16(5):838-45.

Katz DL, Cushman D, Reynolds J, Njike V, Treu JA, Walker J, Smith E, Katz C. Putting physical activity where it fits in the school day: preliminary results of the ABC (Activity Bursts in the Classroom) for fitness program. Prev Chronic Dis. 2010 Jul;7(4):A82. 2010 Jun 15.

Kawase M, Hashimoto H, Hosoda M, Morita H, Hosono A. Effect of administration of fermented milk containing whey protein concentrate to rats and healthy men on serum lipids and blood pressure. J Dairy Sci. 2000 Feb;83(2):255-63.

Kazaks AG, Uriu-Adams JY, Albertson TE, Shenoy SF, Stern JS. Effect of oral magnesium supplementation on measures of airway resistance and subjective assessment of asthma control and quality of life in men and women with mild to moderate asthma: a randomized placebo controlled trial. J Asthma. 2010 Feb;47(1):83-92.

Kazansky DB. MHC restriction and allogeneic immune responses. J Immunotoxicol. 2008 Oct;5(4):369-84.

Kazłowska K, Hsu T, Hou CC, Yang WC, Tsai GJ. Anti-inflammatory properties of phenolic compounds and crude extract from Porphyra dentata. J Ethnopharmacol. 2010 Mar 2;128(1):123-30.

Ke X, Qian D, Zhu L, Hong S. [Analysis on quality of life and personality characteristics of allergic rhinitis]. Lin Chung Er Bi Yan Hou Tou Jing Wai Ke Za Zhi. 2010 Mar;24(5):200-2.

Kecskés G, Belágyi T, Oláh A. Early jejunal nutrition with combined pre- and probiotics in acute pancreati-tis—prospective, randomized, double-blind investigations. Magy Seb. 2003 Feb;56(1):3-8.

Keil J, Stevenson I. Do cases of the reincarnation type show similar features over many years? A study of Turkish cases. J. Sci. Exploration. 1999;13(2) 189-198.

Keita AV, Söderholm JD. The intestinal barrier and its regulation by neuroimmune factors. Neurogastroen-terol Motil. 2010 Jul;22(7):718-33.

Kekkonen RA, Lummela N, Karjalainen H, Latvala S, Tynkkynen S, Jarvenpaa S, Kautiainen H, Julkunen I, Vapaatalo H, Korpela R. Probiotic intervention has strain-specific anti-inflammatory effects in healthy adults. World J Gastroenterol. 2008 Apr 7;14(13):2029-36.

Kekkonen RA, Sysi-Aho M, Seppanen-Laakso T, Julkunen I, Vapaatalo H, Oresic M, Korpela R. Effect of probiotic Lactobacillus rhamnosus GG intervention on global serum lipidomic profiles in healthy adults. World J Gastroenterol. 2008 May 28;14(20):3188-94.

Kekkonen RA, Vasankari TJ, Vuorimaa T, Haahtela T, Julkunen I, Korpela R. The effect of probiotics on respiratory infections and gastrointestinal symptoms during training in marathon runners. Int J Sport Nutr Exerc Metab. 2007 Aug;17(4):352-63.

Kelder P. Ancient Secret of the Fountain of Youth. New York: Doubleday, 1998.

Keller TL, Zocco D, Sundrud MS, Hendrick M, Edenius M, Yum J, Kim YJ, Lee HK, Cortese JF, Wirth DF, Dignam JD, Rao A, Yeo CY, Mazitschek R, Whitman M. Halofuginone and other febrifugine derivatives inhibit prolyl-tRNA synthetase. Nat Chem Biol. 2012 Feb 12;8(3):311-7.

Kelly HW, Van Natta ML, Covar RA, Tonascia J, Green RP, Strunk RC; CAMP Research Group. Effect of long-term corticosteroid use on bone mineral density in children: a prospective longitudinal assessment in the childhood Asthma Management Program (CAMP) study. Pediatrics. 2008 Jul;122(1):e53-61.

Kelly JH Jr, Sabaté J. Nuts and coronary heart disease: an epidemiological perspective. Br J Nutr. 2006 Nov;96 Suppl 2:S61-7.

Kelly TL, Neri DF, Grill JT, Ryman D, Hunt PD, Dijk DJ, Shanahan TL, Czeisler CA. Nonentrained circadian rhythms of melatonin in submariners scheduled to an 18-hour day. J Biol Rhythms. 1999 Jun;14(3):190-6.

Kelly-Pieper K, Patil SP, Busse P, Yang N, Sampson H, Li XM, Wisnivesky JP, Kattan M. Safety and tolerability of an antiasthma herbal Formula (ASHMI) in adult subjects with asthma: a randomized, double-blinded, placebo-controlled, dose-escalation phase I study. J Altern Complement Med. 2009 Jul;15(7):735-43.

Kenia P, Houghton T, Beardsmore C. Does inhaling menthol affect nasal patency or cough? Pediatr Pulmonol. 2008 Jun;43(6):532-7.

Kensler TW, Curphey TJ, Maxiutenko Y, Roebuck BD. Chemoprotection by organosulfur inducers of phase 2 enzymes: dithiolethiones and dithiins. Drug Metabol Drug Interact. 2000;17(1-4):3-22.

Kent ST, McClure LA, Crosson WL, Arnett DK, Wadley VG, Sathiakumar N. Effect of sunlight exposure on cognitive function among depressed and non-depressed participants: a REGARDS cross-sectional study. Environ Health. 2009 Jul 28;8:34.

Keogh JB, Grieger JA, Noakes M, Clifton PM. Flow-Mediated Dilatation Is Impaired by a High-Saturated Fat Diet but Not by a High-Carbohydrate Diet. Arterioscler Thromb Vasc Biol. 2005 Mar:17

Kerckhoffs DA, Brouns F, Hornstra G, Mensink RP. Effects on the human serum lipoprotein profile of beta-glucan, soy protein and isoflavones, plant sterols and stanols, garlic and tocotrienols. J Nutr. 2002 Sep;132(9):2494-505.

Kerkhof M, Postma DS, Brunekreef B, Reijmerink NE, Wijga AH, de Jongste JC, Gehring U, Koppelman GH. Toll-like receptor 2 and 4 genes influence susceptibility to adverse effects of traffic-related air pollution on childhood asthma. Thorax. 2010 Aug;65(8):690-7.

Kerr CC, Rennie CJ, Robinson PA. Physiology-based modeling of cortical auditory evoked potentials. Biol Cybern. 2008 Feb;98(2):171-84.

Key T, Appleby P, Davey G, Allen N, Spencer E, Travis R. Mortality in British vegetarians: review and preliminary results from EPIC-Oxford. Amer. Jour. Clin. Nutr. Suppl. 2003;78(3): 533S-538S.

Khan S. Vitamin D deficiency and secondary hyperparathyroidism among patients with chronic kidney disease. Am J Med Sci. 2007 Apr;333(4):201-7.

Kheifets L, Monroe J, Vergara X, Mezei G, Afifi AA. Occupational electromagnetic fields and leukemia and brain cancer: an update to two meta-analyses. J Occup Environ Med. 2008 Jun;50(6):677-88.

Kiecolt-Glaser JK, Graham JE, Malarkey WB, Porter K, Lemeshow S, Glaser R. Olfactory influences on mood and autonomic, endocrine, and immune function. Psychoneuroendocrinology. 2008 Apr;33(3):328-39.

Kiecolt-Glaser JK, Heffner KL, Glaser R, Malarkey WB, Porter K, Atkinson C, Laskowski B, Lemeshow S, Marshall GD. How stress and anxiety can alter immediate and late phase skin test responses in allergic rhinitis. Psychoneuroendocrinology. 2009 Jun;34(5):670-80.

Kiefte-de Jong JC, Escher JC, Arends LR, Jaddoe VW, Hofman A, Raat H, Moll HA. Infant nutritional factors and functional constipation in childhood: the Generation R study. Am J Gastroenterol. 2010 Apr;105(4):940-5.

Kiessling G, Schneider J, Jahreis G. Long-term consumption of fermented dairy products over 6 months increases HDL cholesterol. Eur J Clin Nutr. 2002 Sep;56(9):843-9.

Kilara A, Shahani KM. The use of immobilized enzymes in the food industry: a review. CRC Crit Rev Food Sci Nutr. 1979 Dec;12(2):161-98.

Kim EJ, Kim GT, Kim BM, Lim EG, Kim SY, Kim YM. Apoptosis-induced effects of extract from Artemisia annua Linné by modulating PTEN/p53/PDK1/Akt/ signal pathways through PTEN/p53-independent manner in HCT116 colon cancer cells. BMC Complement Altern Med. 2017 Apr 28;17(1):236. doi: 10.1186/s12906-017-1702-7.

Kim HM, Shin HY, Lim KH, Ryu ST, Shin TY, Chae HJ, Kim HR, Lyu YS, An NH, Lim KS. Taraxacum officinale inhibits tumor necrosis factor-alpha production from rat astrocytes. Immunopharmacol Immunotoxicol. 2000 Aug;22(3):519-30.

Kim HS, Kim MK, Lee M, Kwon BS, Suh DH, Song YS. Effect of Red Ginseng on Genotoxicity and Health-Related Quality of Life after Adjuvant Chemotherapy in Patients with Epithelial Ovarian cancer: A Randomized, Double Blind, Placebo-Controlled Trial. Nutrients. 2017 Jul 19;9(7):772. doi: 10.3390/nu9070772.

Kim J, Han Y, Ahn JH, Kim SW, Lee SI, Lee KH, Ahn K. Airborne formaldehyde causes skin barrier dysfunction in atopic dermatitis. Br J Dermatol. 2016 Aug;175(2):357-63. doi: 10.1111/bjd.14357.

Kim LS, Waters RF, Burkholder PM. Immunological activity of larch arabinogalactan and Echinacea: a preliminary, randomized, double-blind, placebo-controlled trial. Altern Med Rev. 2002 Apr;7(2):138-49.

Kim MN, Kim N, Lee SH, Park YS, Hwang JH, Kim JW, Jeong SH, Lee DH, Kim JS, Jung HC, Song IS. The effects of probiotics on PPI-triple therapy for Helicobacter pylori eradication. Helicobacter. 2008 Aug;13(4):261-8.

Kim NI, Jo Y, Ahn SB, Son BK, Kim SH, Park YS, Kim SH, Ju JE. A case of eosinophilic esophagitis with food hypersensitivity. J Neurogastroenterol Motil. 2010 Jul;16(3):315-8.

Kim SJ, Jung JY, Kim HW, Park T. Anti-obesity effects of Juniperus chinensis extract are associated with increased AMP-activated protein kinase expression and phosphorylation in the visceral adipose tissue of rats. Biol Pharm Bull. 2008 Jul;31(7):1415-21.

Kim YG, Moon JT, Lee KM, Chon NR, Park H. The effects of probiotics on symptoms of irritable bowel syndrome. Korean J Gastroenterol. 2006 Jun;47(6):413-9.

Kim YH, Kim KS, Han CS, Yang HC, Park SH, Ko KI, Lee SH, Kim KH, Lee NH, Kim JM, Son K. Inhibitory effects of natural plants of Jeju Island on elastase and MMP-1 expression. Int J Cosmet Sci. 2007 Dec;29(6):487-8.

Kimata H. Differential effects of laughter on allergen-specific immunoglobulin and neurotrophin levels in tears. Percept Mot Skills. 2004 Jun;98(3 Pt 1):901-8.

Kimata H. Effect of viewing a humorous vs. nonhumorous film on bronchial responsiveness in patients with bronchial asthma. Physiol Behav. 2004 Jun;81(4):681-4.

Kimata H. Increase in dermcidin-derived peptides in sweat of patients with atopic eczema caused by a humorous video. J Psychosom Res. 2007 Jan;62(1):57-9.

Kimata H. Laughter counteracts enhancement of plasma neurotrophin levels and allergic skin wheal responses by mobile phone-mediated stress. Behav Med. 2004 Winter;29(4):149-52.

Kimata H. Modulation of fecal polyamines by viewing humorous films in patients with atopic dermatitis. Eur J Gastroenterol Hepatol. 2010 Jun;22(6):724-8.

Kimata H. Reduction of allergic responses in atopic infants by mother's laughter. Eur J Clin Invest. 2004 Sep;34(9):645-6.

Kimata H. Viewing a humorous film decreases IgE production by seminal B cells from patients with atopic eczema. J Psychosom Res. 2009 Feb;66(2):173-5.

Kimata H. Viewing humorous film improves nighttime wakening in children with atopic dermatitis. Indian Pediatr. 2007 Apr;44(4):281-5.

Kimata M, Inagaki N, Nagai H. Effects of luteolin and other flavonoids on IgE-mediated allergic reactions. Planta Med. 2000 Feb;66(1):25-9.

Kimata M, Shichijo M, Miura T, Serizawa I, Inagaki N, Nagai H. Effects of luteolin, quercetin and baicalein on immunoglobulin E-mediated mediator release from human cultured mast cells. Clin Exp Allergy. 2000 Apr;30(4):501-8.

Kimmatkar N, Thawani V, Hingorani L, Khiyani R. Efficacy and tolerability of Boswellia serrata extract in treatment of osteoarthritis of knee—a randomized double blind placebo controlled trial. Phytomedicine. 2003 Jan;10(1):3-7.

Kimura Y, Kido T, Takaku T, Sumiyoshi M, Baba K. 1995. Isolation of an anti-angiogenic substance from Agaricus blazei Murill: its antitumor and antimetastatic actions. Cancer Sci., 95(9), 758-64.

Kimura Y, Tojima H, Fukase S, Takeda K. (1994). Clinical evaluation of sizofilan as assistant immunotherapy in treatment of head and neck cancer. Acta oto-laryngologica, Supplementum 511, 192-5.

Kinoshameg SA, Persinger MA. Suppression of experimental allergic encephalomyelitis in rats by 50-nT, 7-Hz amplitude-modulated nocturnal magnetic fields depends on when after inoculation the fields are applied. Neurosci Lett. 2004 Nov 11;370(2-3):166-70.

Kinoshameg SA, Persinger MA. Suppression of experimental allergic encephalomyelitis in rats by 50-nT, 7-Hz amplitude-modulated nocturnal magnetic fields depends on when after inoculation the fields are applied. J Neulet..2004;08:18.

Kinross JM, von Roon AC, Holmes E, Darzi A, Nicholson JK. The human gut microbiome: implications for future health care. Curr Gastroenterol Rep. 2008 Aug;10(4):396-403.

Kippelen P, Larsson J, Anderson SD, Brannan JD, Dahlén B, Dahlén SE. Effect of sodium cromoglycate on mast cell mediators during hyperpnea in athletes. Med Sci Sports Exerc. 2010 Oct;42(10):1853-60.

Kirjavainen PV, Arvola T, Salminen SJ, Isolauri E. Aberrant composition of gut microbiota of allergic infants: a target of bifidobacterial therapy at weaning? Gut. 2002 Jul;51(1):51-5.

Kirjavainen PV, Salminen SJ, Isolauri E. Probiotic bacteria in the management of atopic disease: underscoring the importance of viability. J Pediatr Gastroenterol Nutr. 2003 Feb;36(2):223-7.

Kirlian SD, Kirlian V. Photography and Visual Observation by Means of High-Frequency Currents. J Sci Appl Photogr. 1963;6(6).

Kirpich IA, Solovieva NV, Leikhter SN, Shidakova NA, Lebedeva OV, Sidorov PI, Bazhukova TA, Soloviev AG, Barve SS, McClain CJ, Cave M. Probiotics restore bowel flora and improve liver enzymes in human alcohol-induced liver injury: a pilot study. Alcohol. 2008 Dec;42(8):675-82.

Kisiel W, Barszcz B. Further sesquiterpenoids and phenolics from Taraxacum officinale. Fitoterapia. 2000 Jun;71(3):269-73.

Kisiel W, Michalska K. Sesquiterpenoids and phenolics from Taraxacum hondoense. Fitoterapia. 2005 Sep;76(6):520-4.

Kitajima H, Sumida Y, Tanaka R, Yuki N, Takayama H, Fujimura M. Early administration of Bifidobacterium breve to preterm infants: randomised controlled trial. Arch Dis Child Fetal Neonatal Ed. 1997 Mar;76(2):F101-7.

Kiyose C, et al. Biodiscrimination of alpha-tocopherol stereoisomers in humans after oral administration. Am J Clin Nutr. 1997 Mar; 65 (3):785-9.

Klarin B, Johansson ML, Molin G, Larsson A, Jeppsson B. Adhesion of the probiotic bacterium Lactobacillus plantarum 299v onto the gut mucosa in critically ill patients: a randomised open trial. Crit Care. 2005 Jun;9(3):R285-93.

Klarin B, Molin G, Jeppsson B, Larsson A. Use of the probiotic Lactobacillus plantarum 299 to reduce pathogenic bacteria in the oropharynx of intubated patients: a randomised controlled open pilot study. Crit Care. 2008;12(6):R136.

Kleffmann J. Daytime Sources of Nitrous Acid (HONO) in the Atmospheric Boundary Layer. Chemphyschem. 2007 Apr 10;8(8):1137-1144.

Klein A, Friedrich U, Vogelsang H, Jahreis G. Lactobacillus acidophilus 74-2 and Bifidobacterium animalis subsp lactis DGCC 420 modulate unspecific cellular immune response in healthy adults. Eur J Clin Nutr. 2008 May;62(5):584-93.

Klein E, Smith D, Laxminarayan R. Trends in Hospitalizations and Deaths in the United States Associated with Infections Caused by Staphylococcus aureus and MRSA, 1999-2004. Emerging Infectious Diseases. University of Florida Rel. 2007 Dec 3.

Klein EA, Thompson IM Jr, Tangen CM, et al. Vitamin E and the risk of prostate cancer: the Selenium and Vitamin E Cancer Prevention Trial (SELECT). JAMA. 2011;306(14):1549-1556. doi: 10.1001/jama.2011.1437

Klein R, Armitage R. Rhythms in human performance: 1 1/2-hour oscillations in cognitive style. Science. 1979 Jun 22;204(4399):1326-8.

Klein R, Landau MG. Healing: The Body Betrayed. Minneapolis: DCI:Chronimed, 1992.

Klein U, Kanellis MJ, Drake D. Effects of four anticaries agents on lesion depth progression in an in vitro caries model. Pediatr Dent. 1999 May-Jun;21(3):176-80.

Klein-Galczinsky C. Pharmacological and clinical effectiveness of a fixed phytogenic combination trembling poplar (Populus tremula), true goldenrod (Solidago virgaurea) and ash (Fraxinus excelsior) in mild to moderate rheumatic complaints. Wien Med Wochenschr. 1999;149(8-10):248-53.

Kleitman N. Sleep and Wakefulness. Univ Chicago Press, 1963.

Klima H, Haas O, Roschger P. Photon emission from blood cells and its possible role in immune system regulation. In: Jezowska-Trzebiatowska B. (ed.): Photon Emission from Biological Systems. Singapore: World Sci. 1987:153-169.

Klima H, Haas O, Roschger P. Photon emission from blood cells and its possible role in immune system regulation. In: Jezowska-Trzebiatowska B., et al. (eds.): Photon Emission from Biological Systems. Singapore: World Scientific, 1987:153-169.

Klimant E, Wright H, Rubin D, Seely D, Markman M. Intravenous vitamin C in the supportive care of cancer patients: a review and rational approach. Curr Oncol. 2018 Apr;25(2):139-148. doi: 10.3747/co.25.3790.

Klingberg TD, Budde BB. The survival and persistence in the human gastrointestinal tract of five potential probiotic lactobacilli consumed as freeze-dried cultures or as probiotic sausage. Int J Food Microbiol. 2006 May 25;109(1-2):157-9.

Kloss J. Back to Eden. Twin Oaks, WI: Lotus Press, 1939-1999.

Kniazeva TA, Kuznetsova LN, Otto MP, Nikiforova TI. Efficacy of chromotherapy in patients with hypertension. Vopr Kurortol Fizioter Lech Fiz Kult. 2006 Jan-Feb;(1):11-3.

Knize MG, Salmon CP, Pais P, Felton JS. Food heating and the formation of heterocyclic aromatic amine and polycyclic aromatic hydrocarbon mutagens/carcinogens. Adv Exp Med Biol. 1999;459:179-93.

Knoll N, Weise A, Claussen U, Sendt W, Marian B, Glei M, Pool-Zobel BL. 2-Dodecylcyclobutanone, a radiolytic product of palmitic acid, is genotoxic in primary human colon cells and in cells from pre-neoplastic lesions. Mutat Res. 2006 Feb 22;594(1-2):10-9.

Knutson TW, Bengtsson U, Dannaeus A, Ahlstedt S, Knutson L. Effects of luminal antigen on intestinal albumin and hyaluronan permeability and ion transport in atopic patients. J Allergy Clin Immunol. 1996 Jun;97(6):1225-32.

Kobayashi I, Hamasaki Y, Sato R, Zaitu M, Muro E, Yamamoto S, Ichimaru T, Miyazaki S. Saiboku-To, a herbal extract mixture, selectively inhibits 5-lipoxygenase activity in leukotriene synthesis in rat baso-philic leukemia-1 cells. J Ethnopharmacol. 1995 Aug 11;48(1):33-41.

Kobayashi M, Tsubono Y, Sasazuki S, Sasaki S, Tsugane S. JPHC Study Group. Vegetables, fruit and risk of gastric cancer in Japan: a 10-year follow-up of the JPHC Study Cohort I. Int J Cancer. 2002;102:39–44.

Koch C. Debunking the Digital Brain. Sci. Am. 1997 Feb.

Kodama N, Komuta K, Nanba H. 2002. Can MaitakeMD-fraction aid cancer patients? Altern Med Rev. 7(3):236-9.)

Kodama N, Komuta K, Nanba H. 2003. Effect of Maitake (Grifola frondosa) D-Fraction on the activation of NK cells in cancer patients. Med Food, 2003 Winter; 6-4, 371-7

Kokwaro JO. Medicinal Plants of East Africa. Nairobi: Univ of Neirobi Press, 2009.

Kollaritsch H, Holst H, Grobara P, Wiedermann G. Prevention of traveler's diarrhea with Saccharomyces boulardii. Results of a placebo controlled double-blind study. Fortschr Med. 1993 Mar 30;111(9):152-6.

Kollerstrom N, Staudenmaier G. Evidence for Lunar-Sidereal Rhythms in Crop Yield: A Review. Biolog Agri & Hort. 2001;19:247–259.

Kollerstrom N, Steffert B. Sex difference in response to stress by lunar month: a pilot study of four years' crisis-call frequency. BMC Psychiatry. 2003 Dec 10;3:20.

Kong LF, Guo LH, Zheng XY. Effect of yiqi bushen huoxue herbs in treating children asthma and on levels of nitric oxide, endothelin-1 and serum endothelial cells. Zhongguo Zhong Xi Yi Jie He Za Zhi. 2001 Sep;21(9):667-9.

Kong W, Li C, Qi Q, Shen J, Chang K. Cardamonin induces G2/M arrest and apoptosis via activation of the JNK-FOXO3a pathway in breast cancer cells. Cell Biol Int. 2019 Aug 8. doi: 10.1002/cbin.11217.

Koo HN, Hong SH, Song BK, Kim CH, Yoo YH, Kim HM. Taraxacum officinale induces cytotoxicity through TNF-alpha and IL-1alpha secretion in Hep G2 cells. Life Sci. 2004 Jan 16;74(9):1149-57.

Koop H, Bachem MG. Serum iron, ferritin, and vitamin B12 during prolonged omeprazole therapy. J Clin Gastroenterol. 1992;14:288-92.

Köpcke W, Krutmann J. Protection from sunburn with beta-Carotene – a meta-analysis. Photochem Photobiol. 2008 Mar-Apr;84(2):284-8.

Korkina LG, Pastore S, Dellambra E, De Luca C. New Molecular and Cellular Targets for Chemoprevention and Treatment of Skin Tumours by Plant Polyphenols: A Critical Review. Curr Med Chem. 2012 Dec 3.

Korschunov VM, Smeianov VV, Efimov BA, Tarabrina NP, Ivanov AA, Baranov AE. Therapeutic use of an antibiotic-resistant Bifidobacterium preparation in men exposed to high-dose gamma-irradiation. J Med Microbiol. 1996 Jan;44(1):70-4.

Kostic AD, Gevers D, Pedamallu CS, Michaud M, Duke F, Earl AM, Ojesina AI, Jung J, Bass AJ, Tabernero J, Baselga J, Liu C, Shivdasani RA, Ogino S, Birren BW, Huttenhower C, Garrett WS, Meyerson M. Genomic analysis identifies association of Fusobacterium with colorectal carcinoma. Genome Res. 2011 Oct 18.

Kostyuk VA, Potapovich AI, Lulli D, Stancato A, De Luca C, Pastore S, Korkina L. Modulation of Human Keratinocyte Responses to Solar UV by Plant Polyphenols as a Basis for Chemoprevention of Non-Melanoma Skin Cancers. Curr Med Chem. 2012 Dec 3.

Kotowska M, Albrecht P, Szajewska H. Saccharomyces boulardii in the prevention of antibiotic-associated diarrhoea in children: a randomized double-blind placebo-controlled trial. Aliment Pharmacol Ther. 2005 Mar 1;21(5):583-90.

Kotzampassi K, Giamarellos-Bourboulis EJ, Voudouris A, Kazamias P, Eleftheriadis E. Benefits of a synbiotic formula (Synbiotic 2000Forte) in critically Ill trauma patients: early results of a randomized controlled trial. World J Surg. 2006 Oct;30(10):1848-55.

Kovács T, Mette H, Per B, Kun L, Schmelczer M, Barta J, Jean-Claude D, Nagy J. Relationship between intestinal permeability and antibodies against food antigens in IgA nephropathy. Orv Hetil. 1996 Jan 14;137(2):65-9.

Kowalchik C, Hylton W (eds). Rodale's Illustrated Encyclopedia of Herbs. Emmaus, PA: 1987.

Kowalczyk E, Krzesiński P, Kura M, Niedworok J, Kowalski J, Błaszczyk J. Pharmacological effects of flavonoids from Scutellaria baicalensis. Przegl Lek. 2006;63(2):95-6.

Kowshik J, Nivetha R, Ranjani S, Venkatesan P, Selvamuthukumar S, Veeravarmal V, Nagini S. Astaxanthin inhibits hallmarks of cancer by targeting the PI3K/NF-ᴋB/STAT3 signalling axis in oral squamous cell carcinoma models. IUBMB Life. 2019 Oct;71(10):1595-1610. doi: 10.1002/iub.2104.

Kozlowski LT, Mehta NY, Sweeney CT, Schwartz SS, Vogler GP, Jarvis MJ, West RJ. Filter ventilation and nicotine content of tobacco in cigarettes from Canada, the United Kingdom, and the United States. Tob Control. 1998 Winter;7(4):369-75.

Krasse P, Carlsson B, Dahl C, Paulsson A, Nilsson A, Sinkiewicz G. Decreased gum bleeding and reduced gingivitis by the probiotic Lactobacillus reuteri. Swed Dent J. 2006;30(2):55-60.

Krause R, Buhring M, Hopfenmuller W, Holick MF, Sharma AM. Ultraviolet B and blood pressure. Lancet. 1998 Aug 29;352(9129):709-10.

Kreig M. Black Market Medicine. New York: Bantam, 1968.

Krishna S, Ganapathi S, Ster IC, et al. A Randomised, Double Blind, Placebo-Controlled Pilot Study of Oral Artesunate Therapy for Colorectal Cancer. EBioMedicine. 2014;2(1):82-90. Published 2014 Nov 15. doi:10.1016/j.ebiom.2014.11.010

Krueger AP, Reed EJ. Biological impact of small air ions. Science. 1976 Sep 24;193(4259):1209-13.

Kruger K, Kamilli I, Schattenkirchner M. Blastocystis hominis as a rare arthritogenic pathogen. Z Rheumatol. 1994 Mar-Apr;53(2):83-5.

Krüger P, Kanzer J, Hummel J, Fricker G, Schubert-Zsilavecz M, Abdel-Tawab M. Permeation of Boswellia extract in the Caco-2 model and possible interactions of its constituents KBA and AKBA with OATP1B3 and MRP2. Eur J Pharm Sci. 2009 Feb 15;36(2-3):275-84.

Krzysiek-Maczka G, Targosz A, Ptak-Belowska A, Korbut E, Szczyrk U, Strzalka M, Brzozowski T. Molecular alterations in fibroblasts exposed to Helicobacter pylori: a missing link in bacterial inflammation progressing into gastric carcinogenesis? J Physiol Pharmacol. 2013 Feb;64(1):77-87.

Kubota A, He F, Kawase M, Harata G, Hiramatsu M, Salminen S, Iino H. Lactobacillus strains stabilize intestinal microbiota in Japanese cedar pollinosis patients. Microbiol Immunol. 2009 Apr;53(4):198-205.

Kuchta K, Schmidt M, Nahrstedt A. German Kava Ban Lifted by Court: The Alleged Hepatotoxicity of Kava (Piper methysticum) as a Case of Ill-Defined Herbal Drug Identity, Lacking Quality Control, and Misguided Regulatory Politics. Planta Med. 2015 Dec;81(18):1647-53.

Kuitunen M, Savilahti E, Sarnesto A. Human alpha-lactalbumin and bovine beta-lactoglobulin absorption in infants. Allergy. 1994 May;49(5):354-60.

Küller R, Laike T. The impact of flicker from fluorescent lighting on well-being, performance and physiological arousal. Ergonomics. 1998 Apr;41(4):433-47.

Kumar A, Panghal S, Mallapur SS, Kumar M, Ram V, Singh BK. Antiinflammatory Activity of Piper longum Fruit Oil. Indian J Pharm Sci. 2009 Jul;71(4):454-6.

Kumar A, Saluja AK, Shah UD, Mayavanshi AV. Pharmacological potential of Albizzia lebbeck: A Review. Pharmacog. 2007 Jan-May; 1(1) 171-174.

Kumar S, Sharma VK, Yadav S, Dey S. Antiproliferative and apoptotic effects of black turtle bean extracts on human breast cancer cell line through extrinsic and intrinsic pathway. Chem Cent J. 2017 Jun 20;11(1):56. doi: 10.1186/s13065-017-0281-5.

Kung HC, Hoyert DL, Xu J, Murphy SL. Deaths: Final Data for 2005. National Vital Statistics Reports. 2008;56(10). http://www.cdc.gov/nchs/data/ nvsr/nvsr56/nvsr56_10.pdf. Accessed: 2008 Jun.

Kunzmann AT, Coleman HG, Huang WY, Kitahara CM, Cantwell MM, Berndt SI. Dietary fiber intake and risk of colorectal cancer and incident and recurrent adenoma in the Prostate, Lung, Colorectal, and Ovarian cancer Screening Trial. Am J Clin Nutr. 2015 Oct;102(4):881-90.

Kuo FF, Kuo JJ. Recent Advances in Acupuncture Research, Institute for Advanced Research in Asian Science and Medicine. Garden City, New York. 1979.

Kuribayashi M, Wang J, Fujiwara O, Doi Y, Nabae K, Tamano S, Ogiso T, Asamoto M, Shirai T. Lack of effects of 1439 MHz electromagnetic near field exposure on the blood-brain barrier in immature and young rats. Bioelectromagnetics. 2005 Oct;26(7):578-88.

Kürklü-Gürleyen E, Öğüt-Erişen M, Çakır O, Uysal Ö, Ak G. Quality of life in patients with recurrent aphthous stomatitis treated with a mucoadhesive patch containing citrus essential oil. Patient Prefer Adherence. 2016 May 27;10:967-73. doi: 10.2147/PPA.S106530.

Kurokawa H, Ito H, Matsui H. Monascus purpureus induced apoptosis on gastric cancer cell by scavenging mitochondrial reactive oxygen species. J Clin Biochem Nutr. 2017 Nov;61(3):189-195. doi: 10.3164/jcbn.17-27.

Kurth T, Barr RG, Gaziano JM, Buring JE. Randomised aspirin assignment and risk of adult-onset asthma in the Women's Health Study. Thorax. 2008 Jun;63(6):514-8. 2008 Mar 13.

Kurugöl Z, Koturoğlu G. Effects of Saccharomyces boulardii in children with acute diarrhoea. Acta Paediatr. 2005 Jan;94(1):44-7.

Kuuler R, Ballal S, Laike T Mikellides B, Tonello G. The impact of light and colour on psychological mood: a cross-cultral study of indoor work environments. Ergonomics. 2006 Nov 15;49(14):1496.

Kuvaeva IB. Permeability of the gastronintestinal tract for macromolecules in health and disease. Hum Physiol. 1979 Mar-Apr;4(2):272-83.

Kuz'mina IaS, Vavilova NN. Kinesitherapy of patients with bronchial asthma and excessive body weight at the early stage of rehabilitation treatment. Vopr Kurortol Fizioter Lech Fiz Kult. 2009 Sep-Oct;(5):17-20.

Kuznetsov VF, Iushchuk ND, Iurko LP, Nabokova NIu. Intestinal dysbacteriosis in yersiniosis patients and the possibility of its correction with biopreparations. Ter Arkh. 1994;66(11):17-8.

Kuznetsova TA, Shevchenko NM, Zviagintseva TN, Besednova NN. Biological activity of fucoidans from brown algae and the prospects of their use in medicine]. Antibiot Khimioter. 2004;49(5):24-30.

Kvamme JM, Wilsgaard T, Florholmen J, Jacobsen BK. Body mass index and disease burden in elderly men and women: the Tromsø Study. Eur J Epidemiol. 2010 Mar;25(3):183-93. 2010 Jan 20.

Kwan HY, Fu X, Liu B, Chao X, Chan CL, Cao H, Su T, Tse AK, Fong WF, Yu ZL. Subcutaneous adipocytes promote melanoma cell growth by activating the Akt signaling pathway: role of palmitic acid. J Biol Chem. 2014 Oct 31;289(44):30525-37. doi: 10.1074/jbc.M114.593210.

Kwan ML, Weltzien E, Kushi LH, Castillo A, Slattery ML, Caan BJ. Dietary patterns and breast cancer recurrence and survival among women with early-stage breast cancer. J Clin Oncol. 2009 Feb 20;27(6):919-26. doi:10.1200/JCO.2008.19.4035.

Kyrø C, Skeie G, Loft S, et al. Intake of whole grains from different cereal and food sources and incidence of colorectal cancer in the Scandinavian HELGA cohort. Cancer Causes Control. 2013;24(7):1363-1374. doi:10.1007/s10552-013-0215-z

Kyrø C, Skeie G, Loft S, Landberg R, Christensen J, Lund E, Nilsson LM, Palmqvist R, Tjønneland A, Olsen A. Intake of whole grains from different cereal and food sources and incidence of colorectal cancer in the Scandinavian HELGA cohort. Cancer Causes Control. 2013 Jul;24(7):1363-74. doi: 10.1007/s10552-013-0215-z.

Lad V. Ayurveda: The Science of Self-Healing. Twin Lakes, WI: Lotus Press.

Laden F, Schwartz J, Speizer FE, Dockery DW. Reduction in fine particulate air

Lakhan SE, Vieira KF. Nutritional and herbal supplements for anxiety and anxiety-related disorders: systematic review. Nutr J. 2010 Oct 7;9:42. doi: 10.1186/1475-2891-9-42.

Lakin-Thomas PL. Transcriptional feedback oscillators: maybe, maybe not. J Bio Rhyth. 2006 Apr;21(2):83-92.

Lam F, Jr, Tsuei JJ, Zhao Z. Studies on the bioenergetic measurement of acupuncture points for determination of correct dosage of allopathic or homeopathic medicine in the treatment of diabetes mellitus. Am J Acupunct. 1990;18:127-33.

Lamaison JL, Carnat A, Petitjean-Freytet C. Tannin content and inhibiting activity of elastase in Rosaceae. Ann Pharm Fr. 1990;48(6):335-40.

Lambing K. Biophoton Measurement as a Supplement to the Conventional Consideration of Food Quality. In: Popp F, Li K, Gu Q (eds.). Recent Advances in Biophoton Research. Singapore: World Scientific Publ. 1992:393-413.

Lancranjan I, Maicanescu M, Rafaila E, Klepsch I, Popescu HI. Gonadic function in workmen with long-term exposure to microwaves. Health Phys. 1975;29:381–383.

Landmark K, Reikvam A. Do vitamins C and E protect against the development of carotid stenosis and cardiovascular disease? Tidsskr Nor Laegeforen. 2005 Jan 20;125(2):159-62.

Landrigan CP, Parry GJ, Bones CB, Hackbarth AD, Goldmann DA, Sharek PJ. Temporal trends in rates of patient harm resulting from medical care. N Engl J Med. 2010 Nov 25;363(22):2124-34. doi: 10.1056/NEJMsa1004404. Erratum in: N Engl J Med. 2010 Dec 23;363(26):2573. PubMed PMID: 21105794.

Laney AS, Cragin LA, Blevins LZ, Sumner AD, Cox-Ganser JM, Kreiss K, Moffatt SG, Lohff CJ. Sarcoidosis, asthma, and asthma-like symptoms among occupants of a historically water-damaged office building. Indoor Air. 2009 Feb;19(1):83-90.

Lang CJ, Hansen M, Roscioli E, Jones J, Murgia C, Leigh Ackland M, Zalewski P, Anderson G, Ruffin R. Dietary zinc mediates inflammation and protects against wasting and metabolic derangement caused by sustained cigarette smoke exposure in mice. Biometals. 2011 Feb;24(1):23-39. 2010 Aug 29.

Langhendries JP, Detry J, Van Hees J, Lamboray JM, Darimont J, Mozin MJ, Secretin MC, Senterre J. Effect of a fermented infant formula containing viable bifidobacteria on the fecal flora composition and pH of healthy full-term infants. J Pediatr Gastroenterol Nutr. 1995 Aug;21(2):177-81.

Lappe FM. Diet for a Small Planet. New York: Ballantine, 1971.

Lappe JM, Travers-Gustafson D, Davies KM, Recker RR, Heaney RP. Vitamin D and calcium supplementation reduces cancer risk: results of a randomized trial. Am J Clin Nutr. 2007 Jun;85(6):1586-91.

Lara-Villoslada F, Sierra S, Boza J, Xaus J, Olivares M. Beneficial effects of consumption of a dairy product containing two probiotic strains, Lactobacillus coryniformis CECT5711 and Lactobacillus gasseri CECT5714 in healthy children. Nutr Hosp. 2007 Jul-Aug;22(4):496-502.

Larsen AI, Olsen J, Svane O. Gender-specific reproductive outcome and exposure to high-frequency electromagnetic radiation among physiotherapists. Scand J Work Environ Health. 1991;17:324–329.

Larsen AI, Skotte J. Can exposure to electromagnetic radiation in diathermy operators be estimated from interview data? A pilot study. Am J Ind Med 1991;19:51–57.

Larsen AI. Congenital malformations and exposure to high-frequency electromagnetic radiation among Danish physiotherapists. Scand J Work Environ Health. 1991;17:318–323.

Larsson SC, Wolk A. Red and processed meat consumption and pancreatic cancer: meta-analysis of prospective studies. Br J Cancer. 2012 Jan 12.

Latour E. Functional electrostimulation and its using in neurorehabilitation. Ortop Traumatol Rehabil. 2006 Dec 29;8(6):593-601.

Lau BH, Riesen SK, Truong KP, Lau EW, Rohdewald P, Barreta RA. Pycnogenol as an adjunct in the management of childhood asthma. J Asthma. 2004;41(8):825-32.

Laubereau B, Filipiak-Pittroff B, von Berg A, Grübl A, Reinhardt D, Wichmann HE, Koletzko S; GINI Study Group. Caesarean section and gastrointestinal symptoms, atopic dermatitis, and sensitisation during the first year of life. Arch Dis Child. 2004 Nov;89(11):993-7.

Laura AG, Armas, B, Heaney H, Heaney R. Vitamin D2 Is Much Less Effective than Vitamin D3 in Humans. J Clin Endocr & Metab. 2004;89(11):5387-5391.

Laurière M, Pecquet C, Bouchez-Mahiout I, Snégaroff J, Bayrou O, Raison-Peyron N, Vigan M. Hydrolysed wheat proteins present in cosmetics can induce immediate hypersensitivities. Contact Dermatitis. 2006 May;54(5):283-9.

LaValle JB. The Cox-2 Connection. Rochester, VT: Healing Arts, 2001.

Laverty WH, Kelly IW. Cyclical calendar and lunar patterns in automobile property accidents and injury accidents. Percept Mot Skills. 1998 Feb;86(1):299-302.

Lazarou J, Pomeranz BH, Corey PN. Incidence of adverse drug reactions in hospitalized patients: a meta-analysis of prospective studies. JAMA. 1998 Apr.

Le Bon AM, Siess MH. Organosulfur compounds from Allium and the chemoprevention of cancer. Drug Metabol Drug Interact. 2000;17(1-4):51-79.

Leal AL, Eslava-Schmalbach J, Alvarez C, Buitrago G, Méndez M; Grupo para el Control de la Resistencia Bacteriana en Bogotá. Endemic tendencies and bacterial resistance markers in third-level hospitals in Bogotá, Colombia. Rev Salud Publica (Bogota). 2006 May;8 Suppl 1:59-70.

Lean G. US study links more than 200 diseases to pollution. London Independent. 2004 Nov 14.

Leander M, Cronqvist A, Janson C, Uddenfeldt M, Rask-Andersen A. Health-related quality of life predicts onset of asthma in a longitudinal population study. Respir Med. 2009 Feb;103(2):194-200.

Lecheler J, Pfannebecker B, Nguyen DT, Petzold U, Munzel U, Kremer HJ, Maus J. Prevention of exercise-induced asthma by a fixed combination of disodium cromoglycate plus reproterol compared with montelukast in young patients. Arzneimittelforschung. 2008;58(6):303-9.

Leder D. Spooky actions at a distance: physics, psi, and distant healing. J Altern Complement Med. 2005 Oct;11(5):923-30.

Lee E, Haa K, Yook JM, Jin MH, Seo CS, Son KH, Kim HP, Bae KH, Kang SS, Son JK, Chang HW. Anti-asthmatic activity of an ethanol extract from Saururus chinensis. Biol Pharm Bull. 2006 Feb;29(2):211-5.

Lee H, Kim JS, Kim E. Fucoidan from seaweed Fucus vesiculosus inhibits lung cancer cell via PI3K-Akt-mTOR pathways. PLoS One. 2012;7(11):e50624.

Lee JY, Kim CJ. Determination of allergenic egg proteins in food by protein-, mass spectrometry-, and DNA-based methods. J AOAC Int. 2010 Mar-Apr;93(2):462-77.

Lee KH, Yeh MH, Kao ST, Hung CM, Chen BC, Liu CJ, Yeh CC. Xia-bai-san inhibits lipopolysaccharide-induced activation of intercellular adhesion molecule-1 and nuclear factor-kappa B in human lung cells. J Ethnopharmacol. 2009 Jul 30;124(3):530-8.

Lee KR, Kozukue N, Han JS, Park JH, Chang EY, Baek EJ, Chang JS, Friedman M. Glycoalkaloids and metabolites inhibit the growth of human colon (HT29) and liver (HepG2) cancer cells. J Agric Food Chem. 2004 May 19;52(10):2832-9.

Lee MC, Lin LH, Hung KL, Wu HY. Oral bacterial therapy promotes recovery from acute diarrhea in children. Acta Paediatr Taiwan. 2001 Sep-Oct;42(5):301-5.

Lee SJ, Cho SJ, Park EA. Effects of probiotics on enteric flora and feeding tolerance in preterm infants. Neonatology. 2007;91(3):174-9.

Lee SJ, Shim YH, Cho SJ, Lee JW. Probiotics prophylaxis in children with persistent primary vesicoureteral reflux. Pediatr Nephrol. 2007 Sep;22(9):1315-20.

Lee TH, Hsueh PR, Yeh WC, Wang HP, Wang TH, Lin JT. Low frequency of bacteremia after endoscopic mucosal resection. Gastrointest Endosc. 2000 Aug;52(2):223-5.

Lee W, Kim KY, Yu SN, Kim SH, Chun SS, Ji JH, Yu HS, Ahn SC. Pipernonaline from Piper longum Linn. induces ROS-mediated apoptosis in human prostate cancer PC-3 cells. Biochem Biophys Res Commun. 2013 Jan 4;430(1):406-12.

Lee YJ, Lee YJ, Im JH, Won SY, Kim YB, Cho MK, Nam HS, Choi YJ, Lee SH. Synergistic anti-cancer effects of resveratrol and chemotherapeutic agent clofarabine against human malignant mesothelioma MSTO-211H cells. Food Chem Toxicol. 2012 Nov 9;52C:61-68.

Lee YM, Han SI, Song BC, Yeum KJ. Bioactives in Commonly Consumed Cereal Grains: Implications for Oxidative Stress and Inflammation. J Med Food. 2015 Nov;18(11):1179-86. doi: 10.1089/jmf.2014.3394.

Lee YS, Kim SH, Jung SH, Kim JK, Pan CH, Lim SS. Aldose reductase inhibitory compounds from Glycyrrhiza uralensis. Biol Pharm Bull. 2010;33(5):917-21.

Lefort J, Sedivy P, Desquand S, Randon J, Coeffier E, Maridonneau-Parini I, Floch A, Benveniste J, Vargaftig BB. Pharmacological profile of 48740 R.P., a PAF-acether antagonist. Eur J Pharmacol. 1988 Jun 10;150(3):257-68.

Léger D, Annesi-Maesano I, Carat F, Rugina M, Chanal I, Pribil C, El Hasnaoui A, Bousquet J. Allergic rhinitis and its consequences on quality of sleep: An unexplored area. Arch Intern Med. 2006 Sep 18;166(16):1744-8.

Lehmann B. The vitamin D3 pathway in human skin and its role for regulation of biological processes. Photochem Photobiol. 2005 Nov-Dec;81(6):1246-51.

Leitzmann C. Vegetarian diets: what are the advantages? Forum Nutr. 2005;(57):147-56.

Lempereur M, Majewska C, Brunquers A, Wongpramud S, Valet B, Janssens P, Dillemans M, Van Nedervelde L, Gallo D. Tetrahydro-iso-alpha Acids Antagonize Estrogen Receptor Alpha Activity in MCF-7 Breast cancer Cells. Int J Endocrinol. 2016;2016:9747863. doi: 10.1155/2016/9747863.

Lenn NJ, Beebe B, Moore RY (1977) Postnatal development of the suprachiasmatic nucleus of the rat. Cell Tissue Res. 178:463-475.

Léonard R, Wopfner N, Pabst M, Stadlmann J, Petersen BO, Duus JØ, Himly M, Radauer C, Gadermaier G, Razzazi-Fazeli E, Ferreira F, Altmann F. A new allergen from ragweed (Ambrosia artemisiifolia) with homology to art v 1 from mugwort. J Biol Chem. 2010 Aug 27;285(35):27192-200.

Lerman RH, Minich DM, Darland G, Lamb JJ, Chang JL, Hsi A, Bland JS, Tripp ML. Subjects with elevated LDL cholesterol and metabolic syndrome benefit from supplementation with soy protein, phytosterols, hops rho iso-alpha acids, and Acacia nilotica proanthocyanidins. J Clin Lipidol. 2010 Jan-Feb;4(1):59-68.

Lerman-Garber I, Ichazo-Cerro S, Zamora-González J, Cardoso-Saldaña G, Posadas-Romero C. Effect of a high-monounsaturated fat diet enriched with avocado in NIDDM patients. Diabetes Care. 1994 Apr;17(4):311-5.

Leroux E, Ducros A. Cluster headache. Orphanet J Rare Dis. 2008 Jul 23;3:20.

Lesinski GB, Reville PK, Mace TA, Young GS, Ahn-Jarvis J, Thomas-Ahner J, Vodovotz Y, Ameen Z, Grainger E, Riedl K, Schwartz S, Clinton SK. Consumption of Soy Isoflavone in Men with Prostate Cancer Is Associated with Reduced Proinflammatory Cytokines and Immunosuppressive Cells. Cancer Prev Res (Phila). 2015 Nov;8(11):1036-44. doi: 10.1158/1940-6207.CAPR-14-0464.

Leu YL, Shi LS, Damu AG. Chemical constituents of Taraxacum formosanum. Chem Pharm Bull. 2003 May;51(5):599-601.

Leu YL, Wang YL, Huang SC, Shi LS. Chemical constituents from roots of Taraxacum formosanum. Chem Pharm Bull. 2005 Jul;53(7):853-5.

Leung DY, Shanahan WR Jr, Li XM, Sampson HA. New approaches for the treatment of anaphylaxis. Novartis Found Symp. 2004;257:248-60; discussion 260-4, 276-85.

Levinson D. Adverse Events in Hospitals: National Incidence Among Medicare Beneficiaries. Dept of Health and Human Services. Nov. 2010. OEI-06-09-00090.

Lewerin C, Jacobsson S, Lindstedt G, Nilsson-Ehle H. Serum biomarkers for atrophic gastritis and antibodies against Helicobacter pylori in the elderly: Implications for vitamin B12, folic acid and iron status and response to oral vitamin therapy. Scand J Gastroenterol. 2008;43(9):1050-6.

Lewis WH, Elvin-Lewis MPF. Medical Botany: Plants Affecting Man's Health. New York: Wiley, 1977.

Lewontin R. The Genetic Basis of Evolutionary Change. New York: Columbia Univ Press, 1974.

Leyel CF. Culpeper's English Physician & Complete Herbal. Hollywood, CA: Wilshire, 1971.

Leynadier F. Mast cells and basophils in asthma. Ann Biol Clin (Paris). 1989;47(6):351-6.

Li DK, Odouli R, Wi S, Janevic T, Golditch I, Bracken TD, Senior R, Rankin R, Iriye R. A population-based prospective cohort study of personal exposure to magnetic fields during pregnancy and the risk of miscarriage. Epidemiology. 2002 Jan;13(1):9-20.

Li J, Malakhova M, Mottamal M, Reddy K, Kurinov I, Carper A, Langfald A, Oi N, Kim MO, Zhu F, Sosa CP, Zhou K, Bode AM, Dong Z. Norathyriol suppresses skin cancers induced by solar ultraviolet radiation by targeting ERK kinases. Cancer Res. 2012 Jan 1;72(1):260-70

Li KH. Bioluminescence and stimulated coherent radiation. Laser und Elektrooptik 3. 1981:32-35.

Li MH, Zhang HL, Yang BY. Effects of ginkgo leaf concentrated oral liquor in treating asthma. Zhongguo Zhong Xi Yi Jie He Za Zhi. 1997 Apr;17(4):216-8. 5.

Li N, Wang DL, Wang CW, Wu B. Discussion on randomized controlled trials about clinical researches of acupuncture and moxibustion medicine. Zhongguo Zhen Jiu. 2007 Jul;27(7):529-32.

Li Q, Gandhi OP. Calculation of magnetic field-induced current densities for humans from EAS countertop activation/deactivation devices that use ferromagnetic cores. Phys Med Biol. 2005 Jan 21;50(2):373-85.

Li Q, Li XL, Yang X, Bao JM, Shen XH. Effects of antiallergic herbal agents on cystic fibrosis transmembrane conductance regulator in nasal mucosal epithelia of allergic rhinitis rabbits. Chin Med J (Engl). 2009 Dec 20;122(24):3020-4.

Li S, Li W, Wang Y, Asada Y, Koike K. Prenylflavonoids from Glycyrrhiza uralensis and their protein tyrosine phosphatase-1B inhibitory activities. Bioorg Med Chem Lett. 2010 Sep 15;20(18):5398-401.

Li WQ, Zhang JY, Ma JL, Li ZX, Zhang L, Zhang Y, Guo Y, Zhou T, Li JY, Shen L, Liu WD, Han ZX, Blot WJ, Gail MH, Pan KF, You WC. Effects of Helicobacter pylori treatment and vitamin and garlic supplementation on gastric cancer incidence and mortality: follow-up of a randomized intervention trial. BMJ. 2019 Sep 11;366:l5016. doi: 10.1136/bmj.l5016. PMID: 31511230; PMCID: PMC6737461.

Li X, Qu L, Dong Y, Han L, Liu E, Fang S, Zhang Y, Wang T. A review of recent research progress on the astragalus genus. Molecules. 2014 Nov 17;19(11):18850-80. doi: 10.3390/molecules191118850. PMID: 25407722; PMCID: PMC6270929.

Li X, Yang G, Li X, Zhang Y, Yang J, Chang J, Sun X, Zhou X, Guo Y, Xu Y, Liu J, Bensoussan A. Traditional chinese medicine in cancer care: a review of controlled clinical studies published in chinese. PLoS One. 2013;8(4):e60338.

Li XZ, Ramzan I. Role of ethanol in kava hepatotoxicity. Phytother Res. 2010 Apr;24(4):475-80. doi: 10.1002/ptr.3046.

Li Y, Fletcher T, Mucs D, et al. Half-lives of PFOS, PFHxS and PFOA after end of exposure to contaminated drinking water. Occup Environ Med. 2018;75(1):46-51. doi:10.1136/oemed-2017-104651

Li YQ, Yuan W, Zhang SL. Clinical and experimental study of xiao er ke cuan ling oral liquid in the treatment of infantile bronchopneumonia. Zhongguo Zhong Xi Yi Jie He Za Zhi. 1992 Dec;12(12):719-21, 737, 708.

Liao H, Xi P, Chen Q, Yi L, Zhao Y. Clinical study on acupuncture moxibustion, acupuncture plus moxibustion at Weiwanxiashu (EX-B3) for treatment of diabetes. Zhongguo Zhen Jiu. 2007 Jul;27(7):482-4.

Liao W, Lai T, Chen L, Fu J, Sreenivasan ST, Yu Z, Ren J. Synthesis and Characterization of a Walnut Peptides-Zinc Complex and Its Antiproliferative Activity against Human Breast Carcinoma Cells through the Induction of Apoptosis. J Agric Food Chem. 2016 Feb 24;64(7):1509-19. doi: 10.1021/acs.jafc.5b04924.

Lieber AL. Human aggression and the lunar synodic cycle. J Clin Psychiatry. 1978 May;39(5):385-92.

Lied GA, Lillestøl K, Valeur J, Berstad A. Intestinal B cell-activating factor: an indicator of non-IgE-mediated hypersensitivity reactions to food? Aliment Pharmacol Ther. 2010 Jul;32(1):66-73.

Lieske JC, Goldfarb DS, De Simone C, Regnier C. Use of a probiotic to decrease enteric hyperoxaluria. Kidney Int. 2005 Sep;68(3):1244-9.

Lim W, Park S, Bazer FW, Song G. Apigenin Reduces Survival of Choriocarcinoma Cells by Inducing Apoptosis via the PI3K/AKT and ERK1/2 MAPK Pathways. J Cell Physiol. 2016 Dec;231(12):2690-9. doi: 10.1002/jcp.25372.

Lin HC, Hsu CH, Chen HL, Chung MY, Hsu JF, Lien RI, Tsao LY, Chen CH, Su BH. Oral probiotics prevent necrotizing enterocolitis in very low birth weight preterm infants: a multicenter, randomized, controlled trial. Pediatrics. 2008 Oct;122(4):693-700.

Lin HC, Su BH, Chen AC, Lin TW, Tsai CH, Yeh TF, Oh W. Oral probiotics reduce the incidence and severity of necrotizing enterocolitis in very low birth weight infants. Pediatrics. 2005 Jan;115(1):1-4.

Ling WH, Hänninen O. Shifting from a conventional diet to an uncooked vegan diet reversibly alters fecal hydrolytic activities in humans. J Nutr. 1992 Apr;122(4):924-30.

Lininger S, Gaby A, Austin S, Brown D, Wright J, Duncan A. The Natural Pharmacy. New York: Three Rivers, 1999.

Linsalata M, Russo F, Berloco P, Caruso ML, Matteo GD, Cifone MG, Simone CD, Ierardi E, Di Leo A. The influence of Lactobacillus brevis on ornithine decarboxylase activity and polyamine profiles in Helicobacter pylori-infected gastric mucosa. Helicobacter. 2004 Apr;9(2):165-72.

Lipkind M. Can the vitalistic Entelechia principle be a working instrument ? (The theory of the biological field of Alexander G.Gurvich). In: Popp F, Li K, Gu Q (eds.). Recent Advances in Biophoton Research. Sin-gapore: World Sci Publ, 1992:469-494.

Lipkind M. Registration of spontaneous photon emission from virus-infected cell cultures: development of experimental system. Indian J Exp Biol. 2003 May;41(5):457-72.

Lipski E. Digestive Wellness. Los Angeles, CA: Keats, 2000.

Litime M, Aïssa J, Benveniste J. Antigen signaling at high dilution. FASEB Jnl. 1993;7: A602.

Litscher G. Bioengineering assessment of acupuncture, part 5: cerebral near-infrared spectroscopy. Crit Rev Biomed Eng. 2006;34(6):439-.

REFERENCES AND BIBLIOGRAPHY

Liu GM, Cao MJ, Huang YY, Cai QF, Weng WY, Su WJ. Comparative study of in vitro digestibility of major allergen tropomyosin and other food proteins of Chinese mitten crab (Eriocheir sinensis). J Sci Food Agric. 2010 Aug 15;90(10):1614-20.

Liu H, Schmitz JC, Wei J, Cao S, Beumer JH, Strychor S, Cheng L, Liu M, Wang C, Wu N, Zhao X, Zhang Y, Liao J, Chu E, Lin X. Clove extract inhibits tumor growth and promotes cell cycle arrest and apoptosis. Oncol Res. 2014;21(5):247-59. doi: 10.3727/096504014X13946388748910.

Liu J, Li X, Liu J, Ma L, Li X, Fønnebø V. Traditional Chinese medicine in cancer care: a review of case reports published in Chinese literature. Forsch Komplementmed. 2011;18(5):257-63.

Liu J, Zhang J, Shi Y, Grimsgaard S, Alraek T, Fønnebø V. Chinese red yeast rice (Monascus purpureus) for primary hyperlipidemia: a meta-analysis of randomized controlled trials. Chin Med. 2006 Nov 23;1:4.

Liu JY, Hu JH, Zhu QG, Li FQ, Wang J, Sun HJ. Effect of matrine on the expression of substance P receptor and inflammatory cytokines production in human skin keratinocytes and fibroblasts. Int Immunopharmacol. 2007 Jun;7(6):816-23.

Liu L, Fan J, Ai G, Liu J, Luo N, Li C, Cheng Z. Berberine in combination with cisplatin induces necroptosis and apoptosis in ovarian cancer cells. Biol Res. 2019 Jul 18;52(1):37. doi: 10.1186/s40659-019-0243-6.

Liu Q, Chen X, Yang G, Min X, Deng M. Apigenin inhibits cell migration through MAPK pathways in human bladder smooth muscle cells. Biocell. 2011 Dec;35(3):71-9.

Liu T, Valdez R, Yoon PW, Crocker D, Moonesinghe R, Khoury MJ. The association between family history of asthma and the prevalence of asthma among US adults: National Health and Nutrition Examination Survey, 1999-2004. Genet Med. 2009 May;11(5):323-8.

Liu XJ, Cao MA, Li WH, Shen CS, Yan SQ, Yuan CS. Alkaloids from Sophora flavescens Aiton. Fitoterapia. 2010 Sep;81(6):524-7.

Liu Y, Hua W, Li Y, Xian X, Zhao Z, Liu C, Zou J, Li J, Fang X, Zhu Y. Berberine suppresses colon cancer cell proliferation by inhibiting the SCAP/SREBP-1 signaling pathway-mediated lipogenesis. Biochem Pharmacol. 2020 Apr;174:113776. doi: 10.1016/j.bcp.2019.113776.

Livanova L, Levshina I, Nozdracheva L, Elbakidze MG, Airapetiants MG. The protective action of negative air ions in acute stress in rats with different typological behavioral characteristics. Zh Vyssh Nerv Deiat Im I P Pavlova. 1998 May-Jun;48(3):554-7.

Livanova L, Levshina I, Nozdracheva L, Elbakidze MG, Airapetiants MG. The protective action of negative air ions in acute stress in rats with different typological behavioral characteristics. Zh Vyssh Nerv Deiat Im I P Pavlova. 1998 May-Jun;48(3):554-7.

Lloyd D, Murray D. Redox rhythmicity: clocks at the core of temporal coherence.BioEss. 2007;29(5):465-473.

Lloyd D, Murray D. Redox rhythmicity: clocks at the core of temporal coherence.BioEss. 2007;29(5):465-473.

Lloyd JU. American Materia Medica, Therapeutics and Pharmacognosy. Portland, OR: Eclect Med Publ, 1989-1983.

Lloyd Spencer J. Immunization via the anal mucosa and adjacent skin to protect against respiratory virus infections and allergic rhinitis: a hypothesis. Med Hypotheses. 2010 Mar;74(3):542-6.

Lloyd-Still JD, Powers CA, Hoffman DR, Boyd-Trull K, Lester LA, Benisek DC, Arterburn LM. Bioavailability and safety of a high dose of docosahexaenoic acid triacylglycerol of algal origin in cystic fibrosis patients: a randomized, controlled study. Nutrition. 2006 Jan;22(1):36-46.

Locke GR 3rd, Talley NJ, Fett SL, Zinsmeister AR, Melton LJ 3rd. Prevalence and clinical spectrum of gastroesophageal reflux: a population-based study in Olmsted County, Minnesota. Gastroenterology. 1997 May;112(5):1448-56.

Loguercio C, Abbiati R, Rinaldi M, Romano A, Del Vecchio Blanco C, Coltorti M. Long-term effects of Enterococcus faecium SF68 versus lactulose in the treatment of patients with cirrhosis and grade 1-2 hepatic encephalopathy. J Hepatol. 1995 Jul;23(1):39-46.

Loguercio C, Del Vecchio Blanco C, Coltorti M. Enterococcus lactic acid bacteria strain SF68 and lactulose in hepatic encephalopathy: a controlled study. J Int Med Res. 1987 Nov-Dec;15(6):335-43.

Loizzo MR, Saab AM, Tundis R, Statti GA, Menichini F, Lampronti I, Gambari R, Cinatl J, Doerr HW. Phytochemical analysis and in vitro antiviral activities of the essential oils of seven Lebanon species. Chem Biodivers. 2008 Mar;5(3):461-70.

Lomax AR, Calder PC. Probiotics, immune function, infection and inflammation: a review of the evidence from studies conducted in humans. Curr Pharm Des. 2009;15(13):1428-518.

Looi CY, Arya A, Cheah FK, Muharram B, Leong KH, Mohamad K, Wong WF, Rai N, Mustafa MR. Induction of Apoptosis in Human Breast cancer Cells Centratherum anthelminticum (L.) Seeds. PLoS One. 2013;8(2):e56643. doi: 10.1371/journal.pone.0056643.

Lopes EA, Fanelli-Galvani A, Prisco CC, Gonçalves RC, Jacob CM, Cabral AL, Martins MA, Carvalho CR. Assessment of muscle shortening and static posture in children with persistent asthma. Eur J Pediatr. 2007 Jul;166(7):715-21.

371

NATURAL CANCER SCIENCE

López A, El-Naggar T, Dueñas M, Ortega T, Estrella I, Hernández T, Gómez-Serranillos MP, Palomino OM, Carretero ME. Effect of cooking and germination on phenolic composition and biological properties of dark beans (Phaseolus vulgaris L.). Food Chem. 2013 May 1;138(1):547-55.

López N, de Barros-Mazón S, Vilela MM, Silva CM, Ribeiro JD. Genetic and environmental influences on atopic immune response in early life. J Investig Allergol Clin Immunol. 1999 Nov-Dec;9(6):392-8.

Lopez-Garcia E, Schulze MB, Meigs JB, Manson JE, Rifai N, Stampfer MJ, Willett WC, Hu FB. Consumption of trans fatty acids is related to plasma biomarkers of inflammation and endothelial dysfunction. J Nutr. 2005 Mar;135(3):562-6.

Lorea Baroja M, Kirjavainen PV, Hekmat S, Reid G. Anti-inflammatory effects of probiotic yogurt in inflammatory bowel disease patients. Clin Exp Immunol. 2007 Sep;149(3):470-9.

Lorenz I, Schneider EM, Stolz P, Brack A, Strube J. Sensitive flow cytometric method to test basophil activation influenced by homeopathic histamine dilutions. Forsch Komplementarmed Klass Naturheilkd. 2003 Dec;10(6):316-24.

Lorenzoni DC, Pinheiro LP, Nascimento HS, Menegardo CS, Silva RG, Bautz WG, Henriques JF, Almeida-Coburn KL, da Gama-de-Souza LN. Could formaldehyde induce mutagenic and cytotoxic effects in buccal epithelial cells during anatomy classes? Med Oral Patol Oral Cir Bucal. 2017 Jan 1;22(1):e58-e63.

Lou J, Wang Y, Wang X, Jiang Y. Uncoupling protein 2 regulates palmitic acid-induced hepatoma cell autophagy. Biomed Res Int. 2014;2014:810401. doi: 10.1155/2014/810401.

Loughnan ME, Nicholls N, Tapper NJ. Demographic, seasonal, and spatial differences in acute myocardial infarction admissions to hospital in Melbourne Australia. Int J Health Geogr. 2008 Jul 30;7:42.

Lovejoy S, Pecknold S, Schertzer D. Stratified multifractal magnetization and surface geomagnetic fields-I. Spectral analysis and modeling. Geophysical Journal International. 2001 145(1):112-126.

Lovelock, J. Gaia: A New Look at Life on Earth. Oxford: Oxford Press, 1979.

Lovely RH. Recent studies in the behavioral toxicology of ELF electric and magnetic fields. Prog Clin Biol Res. 1988;257:327-47.

Loving RT, Kripke DF, Knickerbocker NC, Grandner MA. Bright green light treatment of depression for older adults. BMC Psychiatry. 2005 Nov 9;5:42.

Lu C, Sun H, Huang J, Yin S, Hou W, Zhang J, Wang Y, Xu Y, Xu H. Long-Term Sleep Duration as a Risk Factor for Breast cancer: Evidence from a Systematic Review and Dose-Response Meta-Analysis. Biomed Res Int. 2017;2017:4845059. doi: 10.1155/2017/4845059.

Lu J, Cui Y, Shi R. A Practical English-Chinese Library of Traditional Chinese Medicine: Chinese Acupuncture and Moxibustion. Shanghai: Publishing House of the Shanghai College of Traditional Chinese Medicine, 1988.

Lu J, Wang CM, Xu ST, Song LL, Zhao XM, Wang QY, Sheng GY. Role of helicobacter pylori infection in the pathogenesis and clinical outcome of childhood acute idiopathic thrombocytopenic purpura. Zhonghua Xue Ye Xue Za Zhi. 2013 Jan;34(1):41-4.

Lu MK, Shih YW, Chang Chien TT, Fang LH, Huang HC, Chen PS. α-Solanine inhibits human melanoma cell migration and invasion by reducing matrix metalloproteinase-2/9 activities. Biol Pharm Bull. 2010;33(10):1685-91.

Lu Z, Zhou R, Kong Y, Wang J, Xia W, Guo J, Liu J, Sun H, Liu K, Yang J, Mi M, Xu H. S-equol, a Secondary Metabolite of Natural Anticancer Isoflavone Daidzein, Inhibits Prostate Cancer Growth In Vitro and In Vivo, Though Activating the Akt/FOXO3a Pathway. Curr Cancer Drug Targets. 2015 Dec 6.

Lucas A, Brooke OG, Cole TJ, Morley R, Bamford MF. Food and drug reactions, wheezing, and eczema in preterm infants. Arch Dis Child. 1990 Apr;65(4):411-5. 8; .

Lucendo AJ, Lucendo B. An update on the immunopathogenesis of eosinophilic esophagitis. Expert Rev Gastroenterol Hepatol. 2010 Apr;4(2):141-8.

Luna Vital DA, González de Mejía E, Dia VP, Loarca-Piña G. Peptides in common bean fractions inhibit human colorectal cancer cells. Food Chem. 2014 Aug 15;157:347-55. doi: 10.1016/j.foodchem.2014.02.050.

Lunardi AC, Marques da Silva CC, Rodrigues Mendes FA, Marques AP, Stelmach R, Fernandes Carvalho CR. Musculoskeletal dysfunction and pain in adults with asthma. J Asthma. 2011 Feb;48(1):105-10.

Luo J, Margolis KL, Wactawski-Wende J, Horn K, Messina C, Stefanick ML, Tindle HA, Tong E, Rohan TE. Association of active and passive smoking with risk of breast cancer among postmenopausal women: a prospective cohort study. BMJ. 2011 Mar 1;342:d1016.

Luu HN, Blot WJ, Xiang YB, Cai H, Hargreaves MK, Li H, Yang G, Signorello L, Gao YT, Zheng W, Shu XO. Prospective evaluation of the association of nut/peanut consumption and mortality. JAMA Intern Med. 2015 May;175(5):755-66. doi: 10.1001/jamainternmed.2014.8347.

Lux S, Scharlau D, Schlörmann W, Birringer M, Glei M. In vitro fermented nuts exhibit chemopreventive effects in HT29 colon cancer cells. Br J Nutr. 2012 Oct;108(7):1177-86.

Lv X, Liu F, Shang Y, Chen SZ. Honokiol exhibits enhanced antitumor effects with chloroquine by inducing cell death and inhibiting autophagy in human non-small cell lung cancer cells. Oncol Rep. 2015 Jun 29. doi: 10.3892/or.2015.4091.

Lv X, Xi L, Han D, Zhang L. Evaluation of the psychological status in seasonal allergic rhinitis patients. ORL J Otorhinolaryngol Relat Spec. 2010;72(2):84-90.

Lv Y, So KF, Wong NK, Xiao J. Anti-cancer activities of S-allylmercaptocysteine from aged garlic. Chin J Nat Med. 2019 Jan;17(1):43-49. doi: 10.1016/S1875-5364(19)30008-1.

Lydic R, Schoene WC, Czeisler CA, Moore-Ede MC. Suprachiasmatic region of the human hypothalamus: homolog to the primate circadian pacemaker? Sleep. 1980;2(3):355-61.

Lykken DT, Tellegen A, DeRubeis R: Volunteer bias in twin research: the rule of two-thirds. Soc Biol 1978, 25(1): 1-9. Phillips DI: Twin studies in medical research: can they tell us whether diseases are genetically determined? Lancet 1993;341(8851): 1008-1009.

Lynch BM, Dunstan DW, Healy GN, Winkler E, Eakin E, Owen N. Objectively measured physical activity and sedentary time of breast cancer survivors, and associations with adiposity: findings from NHANES (2003-2006). Cancer Causes Control. 2010 Feb;21(2):283-8.

Lynch BM, Friedenreich CM, Winkler EA, Healy GN, Vallance JK, Eakin EG, Owen N. Associations of objectively assessed physical activity and sedentary time with biomarkers of breast cancer risk in postmenopausal women: findings from NHANES (2003-2006). Breast cancer Res Treat. 2011 Nov;130(1):183-94.

Lynch M, Walsh B. Genetics and Analysis of Quantitative Traits. Sunderland, MA: Sinauer, 1998

Lythcott GI. Anaphylaxis to viomycin. Am Rev Tuberc. 1957 Jan;75(1):135-8.

Lythgoe JN. Visual pigments and environmental light. Vision Res. 1984;24(11):1539-50.

Lytle CD, Sagripanti JL. Predicted inactivation of viruses of relevance to biodefense by solar radiation. J Virol. 2005 Nov;79(22):14244-52.

Ma MW, Gao XS, Yu HL, Qi X, Sun SQ, Wang D. Cordyceps sinensis Promotes the Growth of Prostate Cancer Cells. Nutr Cancer. 2018 Oct;70(7):1166-1172. doi: 10.1080/01635581.2018.1504091.

Ma X, Jin S, Zhang Y, Wan L, Zhao Y, Zhou L. Inhibitory effects of nobiletin on hepatocellular carcinoma in vitro and in vivo. Phytother Res. 2014 Apr;28(4):560-7. doi: 10.1002/ptr.5024. Epub 2013 Jul 1,

Ma XP, Muzhapaer D. Efficacy of sublingual immunotherapy in children with dust mite allergic asthma. Zhongguo Dang Dai Er Ke Za Zhi. 2010 May;12(5):344-7.

Maas J, Jayson, J. K.. & Kleiber, D. A. Effects of spectral differences in illumination on fatigue. J Appl Psychol. 1974;59:524-526.

Maas J, Jayson, J. K.. & Kleiber, D. A. Effects of spectral differences in illumination on fatigue. J Appl Psychol. 1974;59:524-526.

Mabey R, ed. The New Age Herbalist. New York: Simon & Schuster, 1941.

Maccabee PJ, Amassian VE, Cracco RQ, Cracco JB, Eberle L, Rudell A. Stimulation of the human nervous system using the magnetic coil. J Clin Neurophysiol. 1991 Jan;8(1):38-55.

MacEwen BT, MacDonald DJ, Burr JF. A systematic review of standing and treadmill desks in the workplace. Prev Med. 2015 Jan;70:50-8. doi: 10.1016/j.ypmed.2014.11.011.

Maciorkowska E, Kaczmarski M, Andrzej K. Endoscopic evaluation of upper gastrointestinal tract mucosa in children with food hypersensitivity. Med Wieku Rozwoj. 2000 Jan-Mar;4(1):37-48.

Macke S, Jerz G, Empl MT, Steinberg P, Winterhalter P. Activity-guided isolation of resveratrol oligomers from a grapevine-shoot extract using countercurrent chromatography. J Agric Food Chem. 2012 Dec 5;60(48):11919-27.

Mackerras D, Cunningham J, Hunt A, Brent P. Re: "effect of supplemental folic acid in pregnancy on childhood asthma: a prospective birth cohort study". Am J Epidemiol. 2010 Mar 15;171(6):746-7; author reply 747. 2010 Feb 9.

Madden JA, Plummer SF, Tang J, Garaiova I, Plummer NT, Herbison M, Hunter JO, Shimada T, Cheng L, Shirakawa T. Effect of probiotics on preventing disruption of the intestinal microflora following antibiotic therapy: a double-blind, placebo-controlled pilot study. Int Immunopharmacol. 2005 Jun;5(6):1091-7.

Maes HH, Silberg JL, Neale MC, Eaves LJ. Genetic and cultural transmission of antisocial behavior: an extended twin parent model. Twin Res Hum Genet. 2007 Feb;10(1):136-50.

Magnusson A, Stefansson JG. Prevalence of seasonal affective disorder in Iceland. Arch Gen Psychiatry. 1993 Dec;50(12):941-6.

Mah KW, Chin VI, Wong WS, Lay C, Tannock GW, Shek LP, Aw MM, Chua KY, Wong HB, Panchalingham A, Lee BW. Effect of a milk formula containing probiotics on the fecal microbiota of asian infants at risk of atopic diseases. Pediatr Res. 2007 Dec;62(6):674-9.

Maier R, Greter SE, Maier N. Effects of pulsed electromagnetic fields on cognitive processes - a pilot study on pulsed field interference with cognitive regeneration. Acta Neurol Scand. 2004 Jul;110(1):46-52.

Maier S, Heitzler T, Asmus K, Brötz E, Hardter U, Hesselbach K, Paululat T, Bechthold A. Functional characterization of different ORFs including luciferase-like monooxygenase genes from the mensacarcin gene cluster. Chembiochem. 2015 May 26;16(8):1175-82. doi: 10.1002/cbic.201500048.

Maier T, Korting HC. Sunscreens - which and what for? Skin Pharmacol Physiol. 2005 Nov-Dec;18(6):253-62.

Mainardi T, Kapoor S, Bielory L. Complementary and alternative medicine: herbs, phytochemicals and vitamins and their immunologic effects. J Allergy Clin Immunol. 2009 Feb;123(2):283-94; quiz 295-6.

Majamaa H, Isolauri E, Saxelin M, Vesikari T. Lactic acid bacteria in the treatment of acute rotavirus gastroenteritis. J Pediatr Gastroenterol Nutr. 1995 Apr;20(3):333-8.

Makomaski Illing EM, Kaiserman MJ. Mortality attributable to tobacco use in Canada and its regions, 1998. Can J Public Health. 2004;95(1):38-44.

Makrides M, Neumann M, Gibson R. Effect of maternal docosahexaenoic acid (DHA) supplementation on breast milk composition. Europ Jrnl of Clin Nutr. 1996;50:352-357.

Maliakal PP, Wanwimolruk S. Effect of herbal teas on hepatic drug metabolizing enzymes in rats. J Pharm Pharmacol. 2001 Oct;53(10):1323-9.

Mälkönen T, Alanko K, Jolanki R, Luukkonen R, Aalto-Korte K, Lauerma A, Susitaival P. Long-term follow-up study of occupational hand eczema. Br J Dermatol. 2010 Aug 13.

Mallol J, Solé D, Baeza-Bacab M, Aguirre-Camposano V, Soto-Quiros M, Baena-Cagnani C; Latin American ISAAC Group. Regional variation in asthma symptom prevalence in Latin American children. J Asthma. 2010 Aug;47(6):644-50.

Mancini A, Imperlini E, Nigro E, Montagnese C, Daniele A, Orrù S, Buono P. Biological and Nutritional Properties of Palm Oil and Palmitic Acid: Effects on Health. Molecules. 2015 Sep 18;20(9):17339-61. doi: 10.3390/molecules200917339.

Mancini FR, Cano-Sancho G, Gambaretti J, et al. Perfluorinated alkylated substances serum concentration and breast cancer risk: Evidence from a nested case-control study in the French E3N cohort. Int J Cancer. 2020;146(4):917-928. doi:10.1002/ijc.32357

Maneechotesuwan K, Supawita S, Kasetsinsombat K, Wongkajornsilp A, Barnes PJ. Sputum indoleamine-2, 3-dioxygenase activity is increased in asthmatic airways by using inhaled corticosteroids. J Allergy Clin Immunol. 2008 Jan;121(1):43-50.

Manley KJ, Fraenkel MB, Mayall BC, Power DA. Probiotic treatment of vancomycin-resistant enterococci: a randomised controlled trial. Med J Aust. 2007 May 7;186(9):454-7.

Mansour HA, Monk TH, Nimgaonkar VL. Circadian genes and bipolar disorder. Ann Med. 2005;37(3):196-205.

Månsson HL. Fatty acids in bovine milk fat. Food Nutr Res. 2008;52. doi: 10.3402/fnr.v52i0.1821.

Manthey JA, Bendele P. Anti-inflammatory activity of an orange peel polymethoxylated flavone, 3',4',3,5,6,7,8-heptamethoxyflavone, in the rat carrageenan/paw edema and mouse lipopolysaccharide-challenge assays. J Agric Food Chem. 2008 Oct 22;56(20):9399-403.

Manz F. Hydration and disease. J Am Coll Nutr. 2007 Oct;26(5 Suppl):535S-541S.

Manzoni P, Mostert M, Leonessa ML, Priolo C, Farina D, Monetti C, Latino MA, Gomirato G. Oral supplementation with Lactobacillus casei subspecies rhamnosus prevents enteric colonization by Candida species in preterm neonates: a randomized study. Clin Infect Dis. 2006 Jun 15;42(12):1735-42.

Marasanov SB, Matveev II. Correlation between protracted premedication and complication in cancer patients operated on during intense solar activity. Vopr Onkol. 2007;53(1):96-9.

Marcos A, Wärnberg J, Nova E, Gómez S, Alvarez A, Alvarez R, Mateos JA, Cobo JM. The effect of milk fermented by yogurt cultures plus Lactobacillus casei DN-114001 on the immune response of subjects under academic examination stress. Eur J Nutr. 2004 Dec;43(6):381-9.

Marcsek Z, Kocsis Z, Jakab M, Szende B, Tompa A. The efficacy of tamoxifen in estrogen receptor-positive breast cancer cells is enhanced by a medical nutriment. Cancer Biother Radiopharm. 2004 Dec;19(6):746-53. doi: 10.1089/cbr.2004.19.746.

Marcucci F, Duse M, Frati F, Incorvaia C, Marseglia GL, La Rosa M. The future of sublingual immunotherapy. Int J Immunopathol Pharmacol. 2009 Oct-Dec;22(4 Suppl):31-3.

Marengo A, Rosso C, Bugianesi E. Liver Cancer: Connections with Obesity, Fatty Liver, and Cirrhosis. Annu Rev Med. 2016;67:103-17. doi: 10.1146/annurev-med-090514-013832.

Margioris AN. Fatty acids and postprandial inflammation. Curr Opin Clin Nutr Metab Care. 2009 Mar;12(2):129-37.

Marin C, Ramirez R, Delgado-Lista J, Yubero-Serrano EM, Perez-Martinez P, Carracedo J, Garcia-Rios A, Rodriguez F, Gutierrez-Mariscal FM, Gomez P, Perez-Jimenez F, Lopez-Miranda J. Mediterranean diet reduces endothelial damage and improves the regenerative capacity of endothelium. Am J Clin Nutr. 2011 Feb;93(2):267-74.

Marks C. Commissurotomy, Consciousness, and Unity of Mind. Cambridge: MIT Press, 1981.

Marks L. The Unity of the Senses: Interrelations among the Modalities. New York: Academic Press, 1978.

Marteau P, Pochart P, Bouhnik Y, Zidi S, Goderel I, Rambaud JC. Survival of Lactobacillus acidophilus and Bifidobacterium sp. in the small intestine following ingestion in fermented milk. A rational basis for the use of probiotics in man. Gastroenterol Clin Biol. 1992;16(1):25-8.

Marth K, Novatchkova M, Focke-Tejkl M, Jenisch S, Jäger S, Kabelitz D, Valenta R. Tracing antigen signatures in the human IgE repertoire. Mol Immunol. 2010 Aug;47(14):2323-9.

Martin IR, Wickens K, Patchett K, Kent R, Fitzharris P, Siebers R, Lewis S, Crane J, Holbrook N, Town GI, Smith S. Cat allergen levels in public places in New Zealand. N Z Med J. 1998 Sep 25;111(1074):356-8.

Martin LJ, Li Q, Melnichouk O, Greenberg C, Minkin S, Hislop G, Boyd NF. A randomized trial of dietary intervention for breast cancer prevention. Cancer Res. 2011 Jan 1;71(1):123-33.

Martinez M. Docosahexaenoic acid therapy in docosahexaenoic acid-deficient patients with disorders of peroxisomal biogenesis. Versicherungsmedizin. 1996;31 Suppl:145-152

Martinez V, Mariano A, Teresa OR, Lazcano ME, Bye R. Anti-inflammatory active compounds from the n-hexane extract of Euphorbia hirta. Rev Soc Quim Méx. 1999;43:103–5.

Martínez-Augustin O, Boza JJ, Del Pino JI, Lucena J, Martínez-Valverde A, Gil A. Dietary nucleotides might influence the humoral immune response against cow's milk proteins in preterm neonates. Biol Neonate. 1997;71(4):215-23.

Martínez-Gómez D, Guallar-Castillon P, Mota J, Lopez-Garcia E, Rodriguez-Artalejo F. Physical Activity, Sitting Time and Mortality in Older Adults with Diabetes. Int J Sports Med. 2015 Sep 2.

Martins N, Petropoulos S, Ferreira IC. Chemical composition and bioactive compounds of garlic (Allium sativum L.) as affected by pre- and post-harvest conditions: A review. Food Chem. 2016 Nov 15;211:41-50. doi: 10.1016/j.foodchem.2016.05.029.

Martin-Venegas R, Roig-Perez S, Ferrer R, Moreno JJ. Arachidonic acid cascade and epithelial barrier function during Caco-2 cell differentiation. J Lipid Res. 2006 Apr;3.

Marushko IuV. The development of a treatment method for streptococcal tonsillitis in children. Lik Sprava. 2000 Jan-Feb;(1):79-82.

Maryam S. Farvid, A. Heather Eliassen, Eunyoung Cho, Xiaomei Liao, Wendy Y. Chen, Walter C. Willett. Dietary Fiber Intake and Breast Cancer Risk. Pediatrics. 2016 March.

Marzouk MS, Moharram FA, Gamal-Eldeen A, Damlakhy IM. Spectroscopic identification of new ellagitannins and a trigalloyl-glucosylkaempferol from an extract of Euphorbia cotinifolia L. with antitumour and antioxidant activity. Z Naturforsch C. 2012 Mar-Apr;67(3-4):151-62.

Maslowski KM, Mackay CR. Diet, gut microbiota and immune responses. Nat Immunol. 2011 Jan;12(1):5-9.

Massey DG, Chien YK, Fournier-Massey G. Mamane: scientific therapy for asthma? Hawaii Med J. 1994;53:350-1. 363.

Mastorakos G, Pavlatou M. Exercise as a stress model and the interplay between the hypothalamus-pituitary-adrenal and the hypothalamus-pituitary-thyroid axes. Horm Metab Res. 2005 Sep;37(9):577-84.

Masuno T, Kishimoto S, Ogura T, Honma T, Niitani H, Fukuoka M, Ogawa N. A comparative trial of LC9018 plus doxorubicin and doxorubicin alone for the treatment of malignant pleural effusion secondary to lung cancer. Cancer. 1991 Oct 1;68(7):1495-500.

Mater DD, Bretigny L, Firmesse O, Flores MJ, Mogenet A, Bresson JL, Corthier G. Streptococcus thermophilus and Lactobacillus delbrueckii subsp. bulgaricus survive gastrointestinal transit of healthy volunteers consuming yogurt. FEMS Microbiol Lett. 2005 Sep 15;250(2):185-7.

Mathur BN, Shahani KM. Use of total whey constituents for human food. J Dairy Sci. 1979 Jan;62(1):99-105.

Matito C, Agell N, Sanchez-Tena S, Torres JL, Cascante M. Protective effect of structurally diverse grape procyanidin fractions against UV-induced cell damage and death. J Agric Food Chem. 2011 May 11;59(9):4489-95.

Matsumoto M, Benno Y. Anti-inflammatory metabolite production in the gut from the consumption of probiotic yogurt containing Bifidobacterium animalis subsp. lactis LKM512. Biosci Biotechnol Biochem. 2006 Jun;70(6):1287-92.

Matsumoto M, Benno Y. Consumption of Bifidobacterium lactis LKM512 yogurt reduces gut mutagenicity by increasing gut polyamine contents in healthy adult subjects. Mutat Res. 2004 Dec 21;568(2):147-53.

Matsumoto Y, Noguchi E, Imoto Y, Nanatsue K, Takeshita K, Shibasaki M, Arinami T, Fujieda S. Upregulation of IL17RB during natural allergen exposure in patients with seasonal allergic rhinitis. Allergol Int. 2011 Mar;60(1):87-92.

Matsumura Y, Nishigori C, Yagi T, Imamura S, Takebe H. Characterization of p53 gene mutations in basal-cell carcinomas: comparison between sun-exposed and less-exposed skin areas. Int J Cancer. 1996 Mar 15;65(6):778-80.

Matsuzaki T, Saito M, Usuku K, Nose H, Izumo S, Arimura K, Osame M. A prospective uncontrolled trial of fermented milk drink containing viable Lactobacillus casei strain Shirota in the treatment of HTLV-1 associated myelopathy/tropical spastic paraparesis. J Neurol Sci. 2005 Oct 15;237(1-2):75-81.

Matutinovic Z, Galic M. Relative magnetic hearing threshold. Laryngol Rhinol Otol. 1982 Jan;61(1):38-41.

Maurer HR. Bromelain: biochemistry, pharmacology and medical use. Cell Mol Life Sci. 2001 Aug;58(9):1234-45.

Maxwell T, Chun SY, Lee KS, Kim S, Nam KS. The anti-metastatic effects of the phytoestrogen arctigenin on human breast cancer cell lines regardless of the status of ER expression. Int J Oncol. 2017 Feb;50(2):727-735. doi: 10.3892/ijo.2016.3825.

Mayes MD. Epidemiologic studies of environmental agents and systemic autoimmune diseases. Environ Health Perspect. 1999 Oct;107 Suppl 5:743-8.

Mayron L, Ott J, Nations R, Mayron E. Light, radiation and academic behaviour: Initial studies on the effects of full-spectrum lighting and radiation shielding on behaviour and academic performance of school children. Acad Ther. 1974;10, 33-47.

Mayron L. Hyperactivity from fluorescent lighting - fact or fancy: A commentary on the report by O'Leary, Rosenbaum and Hughes. J Abnorm Child Psychol. 1978;6:291-294.

Mazzio EA, Soliman KF. In vitro screening for the tumoricidal properties of international medicinal herbs. Phytother Res. 2009 Mar;23(3):385-98.

McAlindon TE. Nutraceuticals: do they work and when should we use them? Best Pract Res Clin Rheumatol. 2006 Feb;20(1):99-115.

McCarney RW, Lasserson TJ, Linde K, Brinkhaus B. An overview of two Cochrane systematic reviews of complementary treatments for chronic asthma: acupuncture and homeopathy. Respir Med. 2004 Aug;98(8):687-96.

McCarney RW, Linde K, Lasserson TJ. Homeopathy for chronic asthma. Cochrane Database Syst Rev. 2004;(1):CD000353.

McClung CA. Role for the Clock gene in bipolar disorder. Cold Spring Harb Symp Quant Biol. 2007;72:637-44.

McColl SL, Veitch JA. Full-spectrum fluorescent lighting: a review of its effects on physiology and health. Psychol Med. 2001 Aug;31(6):949-64.

McConnaughey E. Sea Vegetables. Happy Camp, CA: Naturegraph, 1985.

McConnel JV, Cornwell PR, Clay M. An apparatus for conditioning Planaria. Am J Psychol. 1960 Dec;73:618-22.

McCulloch M, Jezierski T, Broffman M, Hubbard A, Turner K, Janecki T. Diagnostic accuracy of canine scent detection in early- and late-stage lung and breast cancers. Integr Cancer Ther. 2006 Mar;5(1):30-9.

McDougall J, McDougall M. The McDougal Plan. Clinton, NJ: New Win, 1983.

McGuire BW, Sia LL, Haynes JD, Kisicki JC, Gutierrez ML, Stokstad EL. Absorption kinetics of orally administered leucovorin calcium. NCI Monogr. 1987;(5):47-56.

McGuire BW, Sia LL, Leese PT, Gutierrez ML, Stokstad EL. Pharmacokinetics of leucovorin calcium after intravenous, intramuscular, and oral administration. Clin Pharm. 1988 Jan;7(1):52-8.

McKenzie H, Main J, Pennington CR, Parratt D. Antibody to selected strains of Saccharomyces cerevisiae (baker's and brewer's yeast) and Candida albicans in Crohn's disease. Gut. 1990 May;31(5):536-8.

McLachlan CN. beta-casein A1, ischaemic heart disease mortality, and other illnesses. Med Hypotheses. 2001 Feb;56(2):262-72.

McLay RN, Daylo AA, Hammer PS. No effect of lunar cycle on psychiatric admissions or emergency evaluations. Mil Med. 2006 Dec;171(12):1239-42.

McNally ME, Atkinson SA, Cole DE. Contribution of sulfate and sulfoesters to total sulfur intake in infants fed human milk. J Nutr. 1991 Aug;121(8):1250-4.

McNaught CE, Woodcock NP, Anderson AD, MacFie J. A prospective randomised trial of probiotics in critically ill patients. Clin Nutr. 2005 Apr;24(2):211-9.

McNaught CE, Woodcock NP, MacFie J, Mitchell CJ. A prospective randomised study of the probiotic Lactobacillus plantarum 299V on indices of gut barrier function in elective surgical patients. Gut. 2002 Dec;51(6):827-31.

McQuistan TJ, Simonich MT, Pratt MM, Pereira CB, Hendricks JD, Dashwood RH, Williams DE, Bailey GS. Cancer chemoprevention by dietary chlorophylls: A 12,000-animal dose-dose matrix biomarker and tumor study. Food Chem Toxicol. 2011 Nov 3.

McTaggart L. The Field. New York: Quill, 2003.

Meeker JD, Ferguson KK. Relationship between Urinary Phthalate and Bisphenol A Concentrations and Serum Thyroid Measures in U.S. Adults and Adolescents from NHANES 2007-08. Environ Health Perspect. 2011 Jul 11.

Mehra PN, Puri HS. Studies on Gaduchi satwa. Indian J Pharm. 1969;31:180-2.

Mehta BK, Mehta D, Verma M. Novel steroids from the seeds of Centratherum anthelminticum. Nat Prod Res. 2005 Jul;19(5):435-42.

Meier B, Shao Y, Julkunen-Tiitto R, Bettschart A, Sticher O. A chemotaxonomic survey of phenolic compounds in Swiss willow species. Planta Med. 1992;58:A698.

Meier B, Sticher O, Julkunen-Tiitto R. Pharmaceutical aspects of the use of willows in herbal remedies. Planta Med. 1988;54(6):559-560.

Meinecke FW. Sequelae and rehabilitation of spinal cord injuries. Curr Opin Neurol Neurosurg. 1991 Oct;4(5):714-9.

Meiyanto E, Hermawan A, Anindyajati. Natural products for cancer-targeted therapy: citrus flavonoids as potent chemopreventive agents. Asian Pac J Cancer Prev. 2012;13(2):427-36.

Melcion C, Verroust P, Baud L, Ardaillou N, Morel-Maroger L, Ardaillou R. Protective effect of procyanidolic oligomers on the heterologous phase of glomerulonephritis induced by anti-glomerular basement membrane antibodies. C R Seances Acad Sci III. 1982 Dec 6;295(12):721-6.

Melkonian SC, Daniel CR, Ye Y, Pierzynski JA, Roth JA, Wu X. Glycemic Index, Glycemic Load, and Lung Cancer Risk in Non-Hispanic Whites. Cancer Epidemiol Biomarkers Prev. 2016 Mar;25(3):532-9. doi: 10.1158/1055-9965.EPI-15-0765.

Melzack R, Coderre TJ, Katz J, Vaccarino AL. Central neuroplasticity and pathological pain. Ann N Y Acad Sci. 2001 Mar;933:157-74.

Melzack R, Wall PD. Pain mechanisms: a new theory. Science. 1965 Nov 19;150(699):971-9.

Melzack R. Evolution of the neuromatrix theory of pain. The prithvi raj lecture: presented at the third world congress of world institute of pain, barcelona 2004. Pain Pract. 2005 Jun;5(2):85-94.

Melzack R. Pain—an overview. Acta Anaesthesiol Scand. 1999 Oct;43(9):880-4.

Merchant RE and Andre CA. 2001. A review of recent clinical trials of the nutritional supplement Chlorella pyrenoidosa in the treatment of fibromyalgia, hypertension, and ulcerative colitis. Altern Ther Health Med. May-Jun;7(3):79-91.

Messina M. Insights gained from 20 years of soy research. J Nutr. 2010 Dec;140(12):2289S-2295S. 2010 Oct 27.

Meyer A, Kirsch H, Domergue F, Abbadi A, Sperling P, Bauer J, Cirpus P, Zank TK, Moreau H, Roscoe TJ, Zahringer U, Heinz E. Novel fatty acid elongases and their use for the reconstitution of docosahexaenoic acid biosynthesis. J Lipid Res. 2004 Oct;45(10):1899-909.

Meyer AL, Elmadfa I, Herbacek I, Micksche M. Probiotic, as well as conventional yogurt, can enhance the stimulated production of proinflammatory cytokines. J Hum Nutr Diet. 2007 Dec;20(6):590-8.

Michaelsen KF. Probiotics, breastfeeding and atopic eczema. Acta Derm Venereol Suppl (Stockh). 2005 Nov;(215):21-4.

Michalska K, Kisiel W. Sesquiterpene lactones from Taraxacum obovatum. Planta Med. 2003 Feb;69(2):181-3.

Michetti P, Dorta G, Wiesel PH, Brassart D, Verdu E, Herranz M, Felley C, Porta N, Rouvet M, Blum AL, Corthésy-Theulaz I. Effect of whey-based culture supernatant of Lactobacillus acidophilus (johnsonii) La1 on Helicobacter pylori infection in humans. Digestion. 1999;60(3):203-9.

Michielutti F, Bertini M, Presciuttini B, Andreotti G. Clinical assessment of a new oral bacterial treatment for children with acute diarrhea. Minerva Med. 1996 Nov;87(11):545-50.

Mickleborough TD, Lindley MR, Ray S. Dietary salt, airway inflammation, and diffusion capacity in exercise-induced asthma. Med Sci Sports Exerc. 2005 Jun;37(6):904-14.

Mikoluc B, Motkowski R, Karpinska J, Piotrowska-Jastrzebska J. Plasma levels of vitamins A and E, coenzyme Q10, and anti-ox-LDL antibody titer in children treated with an elimination diet due to food hypersensitivity. Int J Vitam Nutr Res. 2009 Sep;79(5-6):328-36.

Milazzo S, Russell N, Ernst E. Efficacy of homeopathic therapy in cancer treatment. Eur J Cancer. 2006 Feb;42(3):282-9. Epub 2006 Jan 11.

Miles LE, Raynal DM, Wilson MA. Blind man living in normal society has circadian rhythms of 24.9 hours. Science. 1977 Oct 28;198(4315):421-3.

Milgrom P, Ly KA, Roberts MC, Rothen M, Mueller G, Yamaguchi DK. Mutans streptococci dose response to xylitol chewing gum. J Dent Res. 2006 Feb;85(2):177-81.

Millen AE, Tucker MA, Hartge P, Halpern A, Elder DE, Guerry D 4th, Holly EA, Sagebiel RW, Potischman N. Diet and melanoma in a case-control study. Cancer Epidem Biomarkers Prev. 2004 Jun;13(6):1042-51.

Miller AL. The etiologies, pathophysiology, and alternative/complementary treatment of asthma. Altern Med Rev. 2001 Feb;6(1):20-47.

Miller GT. Living in the Environment. Belmont, CA: Wadsworth, 1996.

Miller JD, Morin LP, Schwartz WJ, Moore RY. New insights into the mammalian circadian clock. Sleep. 1996 Oct;19(8):641-67.

Miller K. Cholesterol and In-Hospital Mortality in Elderly Patients. Am Family Phys. 2004 May.

Mindell E, Hopkins V. Prescription Alternatives. New Canaan, CT: Keats, 1998.

Miranda H, Outeiro TF. The sour side of neurodegenerative disorders: the effects of protein glycation. J Pathol. 2010 May;221(1):13-25.

Mirkin V, Berrebi A, Rakhman I, Haran M, Shvidel L. The role of the plant Artemisa in Apoptosis of B Cells in Leukemia. Harefuah. 2017 Feb;156(2):86-88.

Mishkin M, Appenzeller T. The Anatomy of Memory. Sci. Am. 1987 June.

Mitchell AE, Hong YJ, Koh E, Barrett DM, Bryant DE, Denison RF, Kaffka S. Ten-year comparison of the influence of organic and conventional crop management practices on the content of flavonoids in tomatoes. J Agric Food Chem. 2007 Jul 25;55(15):6154-9.

Miyake Y, Sasaki S, Tanaka K, Hirota Y. Dairy food, calcium and vitamin D intake in pregnancy, and wheeze and eczema in infants. Eur Respir J. 2010 Jun;35(6):1228-34. 2009 Oct 19.

Miyazaki K, Mizutani H, Katabuchi H, Fukuma K, Fujisaki S, Okamura H. Activated (HLA-DR+) T-lymphocyte subsets in cervical carcinoma and effects of radiotherapy and immunotherapy with sizofiran on cell-mediated immunity and survival. Gynecol Oncol. 1995 Mar;56(3):412-20.

Mizuno, Masashi; Morimoto, Mikio; Minato, Ken-Ichiro; Tsuchida, Hironobu. 1998. Polysaccharides from Agaricus blazei stimulate lymphocyte T-cell subsets in mice. Bioscience, Biotechnology, and Biochemistry, 62(3), 434-437.

Modern Biology. Austin: Harcourt Brace, 1993.

Moertel CG, Fleming TR, Creagan ET, Rubin J, O'Connell MJ, Ames MM. High-dose vitamin C versus placebo in the treatment of patients with advanced cancer who have had no prior chemotherapy. A randomized double-blind comparison. N Engl J Med. 1985 Jan 17;312(3):137-41. doi: 10.1056/NEJM198501173120301.

Mohamed S, Saka S, EL-Sharkawy SH, Ali AM, Muid S. Antimycotic screening of 58 Malaysian plants against plant pathogens. Pestic Sci. 1996;47:259–64.

Mohammad MA, Molloy A, Scott J, Hussein L. Plasma cobalamin and folate and their metabolic markers methylmalonic acid and total homocysteine among Egyptian children before and after nutritional supplementation with the probiotic bacteria Lactobacillus acidophilus in yoghurt matrix. Int J Food Sci Nutr. 2006 Nov-Dec;57(7-8):470-80.

Mohan R, Koebnick C, Schildt J, Mueller M, Radke M, Blaut M. Effects of Bifidobacterium lactis Bb12 supplementation on body weight, fecal pH, acetate, lactate, calprotectin, and IgA in preterm infants. Pediatr Res. 2008 Oct;64(4):418-22.

Mohan R, Koebnick C, Schildt J, Schmidt S, Mueller M, Possner M, Radke M, Blaut M. Effects of Bifidobacterium lactis Bb12 supplementation on intestinal microbiota of preterm infants: a double-blind, placebo-controlled, randomized study. J Clin Microbiol. 2006 Nov;44(11):4025-31.

Mohr SB, Garland CF, Gorham ED, Grant WB, Garland FC. Is ultraviolet B irradiance inversely associated with incidence rates of endometrial cancer: an ecological study of 107 countries. Prev Med. 2007 Nov;45(5):327-31.

Mohr SB. A brief history of vitamin d and cancer prevention. Ann Epidemiol. 2009 Feb;19(2):79-83.

Mokhtar N, Chan SC. Use of complementary medicine amongst asthmatic patients in primary care. Med J Malaysia. 2006 Mar;61(1):125-7.

Monarca S. Zerbini I, Simonati C, Gelatti U. Drinking water hardness and chronic degenerative diseases. Part II. Cardiovascular diseases. Ann. Ig. 2003;15:41-56.

Monti DA, Mitchell E, Bazzan AJ, Littman S, Zabrecky G, Yeo CJ, Pillai MV, Newberg AB, Deshmukh S, Levine M. Phase I evaluation of intravenous ascorbic acid in combination with gemcitabine and erlotinib in patients with metastatic pancreatic cancer. PLoS One. 2012;7(1):e29794. doi: 10.1371/journal.pone.0029794.

Moon JY, Cho M, Ahn KS, Cho SK. Nobiletin induces apoptosis and potentiates the effects of the anticancer drug 5-fluorouracil in p53-mutated SNU-16 human gastric cancer cells. Nutr Cancer. 2013;65(2):286-95. doi: 10.1080/01635581.2013.756529.

Moore M. The Miracle Food. Huffington Post. Accessed Jan 4, 2017

Moore PS, Chang Y. Why do viruses cause cancer? Highlights of the first century of human tumour virology. Nat Rev Cancer. 2010;10(12):878-889. doi:10.1038/nrc2961

Moore R. Circadian Rhythms: A Clock for the Ages. Science 1999 June 25;284(5423):2102 – 2103.

Moore RY, Speh JC. Serotonin innervation of the primate suprachiasmatic nucleus. Brain Res. 2004 Jun 4;1010(1-2):169-73.

Moore RY, Speh JC. Serotonin innervation of the primate suprachiasmatic nucleus. Brain Res. 2004 Jun 4;1010(1-2):169-73.

Moore RY. Neural control of the pineal gland. Behav Brain Res. 1996;73(1-2):125-30.

Moore RY. Organization and function of a central nervous system circadian oscillator: the suprachiasmatic hypothalamic nucleus. Fed Proc. 1983 Aug;42(11):2783-9.

Moorhead KJ, Morgan HC. Spirulina: Nature's Superfood. Kailua-Kona, HI: Nutrex, 1995.

Moreira A, Delgado L, Haahtela T, Fonseca J, Moreira P, Lopes C, Mota J, Santos P, Rytilä P, Castel-Branco MG. Physical training does not increase allergic inflammation in asthmatic children. Eur Respir J. 2008 Dec;32(6):1570-5.

Moreira P, Moreira A, Padrão P, Delgado L. The role of economic and educational factors in asthma: evidence from the Portuguese health survey. Public Health. 2008 Apr;122(4):434-9. 2007 Oct 17.

Morel AF, Dias GO, Porto C, Simionatto E, Stuker CZ, Dalcol II. Antimicrobial activity of extractives of Solidago microglossa. Fitoterapia. 2006 Sep;77(6):453-5.

Morgan LL, Miller AB, Sasco A, Davis DL. Mobile phone radiation causes brain tumors and should be classified as a probable human carcinogen (2A) (review). Int J Oncol. 2015;46(5):1865-1871. doi:10.3892/ijo.2015.2908

Morick H. Introduction to the Philosophy of Mind: Readings from Descartes to Strawson. Glenview, Ill: Scott Foresman, 1970.

Morimoto K, Takeshita T, Nanno M, Tokudome S, Nakayama K. Modulation of natural killer cell activity by supplementation of fermented milk containing Lactobacillus casei in habitual smokers. Prev Med. 2005 May;40(5):589-94.

Morton C. Velocity Alters Electric Field. www.amasci.com/ freenrg/ morton1.html. Accessed: 2007 July.

Moshe M. Method and apparatus for predicting the occurrence of an earthquake by identifying electromagnetic precursors. US Patent Issued on May 28, 1996. Number 5521508.

Moss M. E. Coli Path Shows Flaws in Ground Beef Inspection. NY Times 2009 Oct 3.

Motoyama H. Acupuncture Meridians. Science & Medicine. 1999 July/August.

Motoyama H. Before Polarization Current and the Acupuncture Meridians. Journal of Holistic Medicine. 1986;8(1&2).

Motoyama H. Deficient/ Excessive Patterns Found in Meridian Functioning in Cases of Liver Disease. Subtle Energy & Energy Medicine. 2000; 11(2).

Motoyama H. Energetic Medicine: new science of healing: An interview with A. Jackson. www.shareintl.org/archives/health-healing/hh_adjenergetic.html. Acc. 2007 Oct.

Motoyama H. Smith, W. Harada T. Pre-Polarization Resistance of the Skin as Determined by the Single Square Voltage Pulse. Psychophysiology. 1984;21(5).

Mourouti N, Kontogianni MD, Papavagelis C, Plytzanopoulou P, Vassilakou T, Psaltopoulou T, Malamos N, Linos A, Panagiotakos DB. Meat consumption and breast cancer: a case-control study in women. Meat Sci. 2015 Feb;100:195-201.

Moussaieff A, Shein NA, Tsenter J, Grigoriadis S, Simeonidou C, Alexandrovich AG, Trembovler V, Ben-Neriah Y, Schmitz ML, Fiebich BL, Munoz E, Mechoulam R, Shohami E. Incensole acetate: a novel neuroprotective agent isolated from Boswellia carterii. J Cereb Blood Flow Metab. 2008 Jul;28(7):1341-52.

Moyle A. Nature Cure for Asthma and Hay Fever. Wellingborough, U.K.: Thorsons, 1978.

Mozafar A. Is there vitamin B12 in plants or not? A plant nutritionist's view. Veg Nutr. 1997;1/2:50-52.

Mozaffarian D, Aro A, Willett WC. Health effects of trans-fatty acids: experimental and observational evidence. Eur J Clin Nutr. 2009 May;63 Suppl 2:S5-21.

Muka T, Kraja B, Ruiter R, Lahousse L, de Keyser CE, Hofman A, Franco OH, Brusselle G, Stricker BH, de Jong JC. Dietary mineral intake and lung cancer risk: the Rotterdam Study. Eur J Nutr. 2016 Apr 12.

Muller H, Lindman AS, Blomfeldt A, Seljeflot I, Pedersen JI. A diet rich in coconut oil reduces diurnal postprandial variations in circulating tissue plasminogen activator antigen and fasting lipoprotein (a) compared with a diet rich in unsaturated fat in humans. J Nutr. 2003 Nov;133(11):3422-7.

Müller S, Pühl S, Vieth M, Stolte M. Analysis of symptoms and endoscopic findings in 117 patients with histological diagnoses of eosinophilic esophagitis. Endoscopy. 2007 Apr;39(4):339-44.

Mullié C, Yazourh A, Thibault H, Odou MF, Singer E, Kalach N, Kremp O, Romond MB. Increased poliovirus-specific intestinal antibody response coincides with promotion of Bifidobacterium longum-infantis and Bifidobacterium breve in infants: a randomized, double-blind, placebo-controlled trial. Pediatr Res. 2004 Nov;56(5):791-5.

Mumby DG, Wood ER, Pinel J. Object-recognition memory is only mildly impaired in rats with lesions of the hippocampus and amygdala. Psychobio. 1992;20: 18-27.

Murata M, Morishige F, Yamaguchi H. Prolongation of survival times of terminal cancer patients by administration of large doses of ascorbate. Int J Vitam Nutr Res Suppl. 1982;23:103-13.

Murata K, Takano F, Fushiya S, Oshima Y. Potentiation by febrifugine of host defense in mice against Plasmodium berghei NK65. Biochem Pharmacol. 1999 Nov 15;58(10):1593-601.

Murchie G. The Seven Mysteries of Life. Boston: Houghton Mifflin Company, 1978.

Murchie G. The Seven Mysteries of Life. Boston: Houghton Mifflin Company, 1978.

Murphy R. Organon Philosophy Workbook. Blacksburg, VA: HANA, 1994.

Murray M and Pizzorno J. Encyclopedia of Natural Medicine. 2nd Edition. Roseville, CA: Prima Publishing, 1998.

Musaev AV, Nasrullaeva SN, Zeïnalov RG. Effects of solar activity on some demographic indices and morbidity in Azerbaijan with reference to A. L. Chizhevsky's theory. Vopr Kurortol Fizioter Lech Fiz Kult. 2007 May-Jun;(3):38-42.

Mustapha A, Jiang T, Savaiano DA. Improvement of lactose digestion by humans following ingestion of unfermented acidophilus milk: influence of bile sensitivity, lactose transport, and acid tolerance of Lactobacillus acidophilus. J Dairy Sci. 1997 Aug;80(8):1537-45.

Muzzarelli L, Force M, Sebold M. Aromatherapy and reducing preprocedural anxiety: A controlled prospective study. Gastroenterol Nurs. 2006 Nov-Dec;29(6):466-71.

Myllyluoma E, Ahonen AM, Korpela R, Vapaatalo H, Kankuri E. Effects of multispecies probiotic combination on helicobacter pylori infection in vitro. Clin Vaccine Immunol. 2008 Sep;15(9):1472-82.

Myneni AA, Chang SC, Niu R, Liu L, Swanson MK, Li J, Su J, Giovino GA, Yu S, Zhang ZF, Mu L. Raw Garlic Consumption and Lung Cancer in a Chinese Population. Cancer Epidemiol Biomarkers Prev. 2016 Apr;25(4):624-33. doi: 10.1158/1055-9965.EPI-15-0760.

Myobatake Y, Takeuchi T, Kuramochi K, Kuriyama I, Ishido T, Hirano K, Sugawara F, Yoshida H, Mizushina Y. Pinophilins A and B, inhibitors of mammalian A-, B-, and Y-family DNA polymerases and human cancer cell proliferation. J Nat Prod. 2012 Feb 24;75(2):135-41.

Myss C. Anatomy of the Spirit. New York: Harmony, 1996.

Naderi-Kalali B, Allameh A, Rasaee MJ, Bach HJ, Behechti A, Doods K, Kettrup A, Schramm KW. Suppressive effects of caraway (Carum carvi) extracts on 2, 3, 7, 8-tetrachloro-dibenzo-p-dioxin-dependent gene expression of cytochrome P450 1A1 in the rat H4IIE cells. Toxicol In Vitro. 2005 Apr;19(3):373-7. doi: 10.1016/j.tiv.2004.11.003.

Nadkarni AK, Nadkarni KM. Indian Materia Medica. (Vols 1 and 2). Bombay: Popular Pradashan, 1908, 1976.

Nagai T, Arai Y, Emori M, Nunome SY, Yabe T, Takeda T, Yamada H. Anti-allergic activity of a Kampo (Japanese herbal) medicine "Sho-seiryu-to (Xiao-Qing-Long-Tang)" on airway inflammation in a mouse model. Int Immunopharmacol. 2004 Oct;4(10-11):1353-65.

Nagata, Jun-ichi; Arakaki, Nana; Kinjo, Kazuhiko; Saito, Morio; Chinen, Isao. 2001. Effects of polysaccharides from Tricholma giganteum and Agaricus blazei on antitumor activity in tumor-bearing mice and NO production from mouse peritoneal macrophage. Nippon Shokuhin Kagaku Kogaku Kaishi, 48(12), 939-942.

Nagel G, Linseisen J. Dietary intake of fatty acids, antioxidants and selected food groups and asthma in adults. Eur J Clin Nutr. 2005 Jan;59(1):8-15.

Nagel G, Weinmayr G, Kleiner A, Garcia-Marcos L, Strachan DP; ISAAC Phase Two Study Group. Effect of diet on asthma and allergic sensitisation in the International Study on Allergies and Asthma in Childhood (ISAAC) Phase Two. Thorax. 2010 Jun;65(6):516-22.

Nagel JM, Brinkoetter M, Magkos F, Liu X, Chamberland JP, Shah S, Zhou J, Blackburn G, Mantzoros CS. Dietary walnuts inhibit colorectal cancer growth in mice by suppressing angiogenesis. Nutrition. 2012 Jan;28(1):67-75. doi: 10.1016/j.nut.2011.03.004.

Naghii MR, Samman S. The role of boron in nutrition and metabolism. Prog Food Nutr Sci. 1993 Oct-Dec;17(4):331-49.

Nair PK, Rodriguez S, Ramachandran R, Alamo A, Melnick SJ, Escalon E, Garcia PI Jr, Wnuk SF, Ramachandran C. Immune stimulating properties of a novel polysaccharide from the medicinal plant Tinospora cordifolia. Int Immunopharmacol. 2004 Dec 15;4(13):1645-59.

Naito S, Koga H, Yamaguchi I, Fujimoto N, Hasui Y, Kuramoto H, Iguchi A, Kinukawa N; Kyushu University Urological Oncology Group. Prevention of recurrence with epirubicin and Lactobacillus casei after transurethral resection of bladder cancer. J Urol. 2008 Feb;179(2):485-90.

Nakamura K, Urayama K, Hoshino Y. Lumbar cerebrospinal fluid pulse wave rising from pulsations of both the spinal cord and the brain in humans. Spinal Cord. 1997 Nov;35(11):735-9.

Nakano T, Oka K, Hanba K, Morita S. (1996). Intratumoral administration of sizofiran activates Langerhans cell and T-cell infiltration in cervical cancer. Clinical immunology and immunopathology, 79(1), 79-86.

Nakatani K, Yau KW. Calcium and light adaptation in retinal rods and cones. Nature. 1988 Jul 7;334(6177): 69-71.

Nakatani K, Yau KW. Calcium and light adaptation in retinal rods and cones. Nature. 1988 Jul 7;334(6177): 69-71.

Nam S, Scuto A, Yang F, Chen W, Park S, Yoo HS, Konig H, Bhatia R, Cheng X, Merz KH, Eisenbrand G, Jove R. Indirubin derivatives induce apoptosis of leukemia cells involving inhibition of Stat5 signaling. Mol Oncol. 2012 Feb 17.

Napoli N, Thompson J, Civitelli R, Villareal R. Effects of dietary calcium compared with calcium supplements on estrogen metabolism and bone mineral density. Am J Clin Nutr. 2007;85(5): 1428-1433.

Napoli, J.E., Brand-Miller, J.C., Conway, P. (2003) Bifidogenic effects of feeding infant formula containing galactooligosaccharides in healthy formula-fed infants. Asia Pac J Clin Nutr. 12(Suppl): S60

Narayanapillai SC, Lin SH, Leitzman P, Upadhyaya P, Baglole CJ, Xing C. Dihydromethysticin (DHM) Blocks Tobacco Carcinogen 4-(Methylnitrosamino)-1-(3-pyridyl)-1-butanone (NNK)-Induced O(6)-Methylguanine in a Manner Independent of the Aryl Hydrocarbon Receptor (AhR) Pathway in C57BL/6 Female Mice. Chem Res Toxicol. 2016 Nov 21;29(11):1828-1834.

Nariya M, Shukla V, Jain S, Ravishankar B. Comparison of enteroprotective efficacy of triphala formulations (Indian Herbal Drug) on methotrexate-induced small intestinal damage in rats. Phytother Res. 2009 Aug;23(8):1092-8.

Naruszewicz M, Daniewski M, Nowicka G, Kozlowska-Wojciechowska M. Trans-unsaturated fatty acids and acrylamide in food as potential atherosclerosis progression factors. Based on own studies. Acta Microbiol Pol. 2003;52 Suppl:75-81.

Naruszewicz M, Johansson ML, Zapolska-Downar D, Bukowska H. Effect of Lactobacillus plantarum 299v on cardiovascular disease risk factors in smokers. Am J Clin Nutr. 2002 Dec;76(6):1249-55.

Narva M, Nevala R, Poussa T, Korpela R. The effect of Lactobacillus helveticus fermented milk on acute changes in calcium metabolism in postmenopausal women. Eur J Nutr. 2004 Apr;43(2):61-8.

Näse L, Hatakka K, Savilahti E, Saxelin M, Pönkä A, Poussa T, Korpela R, Meurman JH. Effect of long-term consumption of a probiotic bacterium, Lactobacillus rhamnosus GG, in milk on dental caries and caries risk in children. Caries Res. 2001 Nov-Dec;35(6):412-20.

Natarajan E, Grissom C. The Origin of Magnetic Field Dependent Recombination in Alkylcobalamin Radical Pairs. Photochem Photobiol. 1996;64: 286-295.

National Cancer Institute. Formaldehyde and Cancer Risk. Accessed Jan. 11, 2017

National Cooperation Group on Childhood Asthma. A nationwide survey in China on prevalence of asthma in urban children. Chin J Pediatr. pp. 123-127.

National Institutes of Health. Iron Fact Sheet. Accessed April 18, 2016

National Toxicology Program. Final Report on Carcinogens Background Document for Formaldehyde. Rep Carcinog Backgr Doc. 2010 Jan;(10-5981):i-512.

Navarro Silvera SA, Rohan TE. Trace elements and cancer risk: a review of the epidemiologic evidence. Cancer Causes Control. 2007 Feb;18(1):7-27.

NDL, BHNRC, ARS, USDA. Oxygen Radical Absorbance Capacity (ORAC) of Selected Foods - 2007. Beltsville, MD: USDA-ARS. 2007.

Negri A, Naponelli V, Rizzi F, Bettuzzi S. Molecular Targets of Epigallocatechin-Gallate (EGCG): A Special Focus on Signal Transduction and Cancer. Nutrients. 2018;10(12):1936. Published 2018 Dec 6. doi:10.3390/nu10121936

Nerín C, Canellas E, Aznar M, Silcock P. Food Addit Contam Part A Chem Anal Control Expo Risk Assess. Analytical methods for the screening of potential volatile migrants from acrylic-base adhesives used in food-contact materials. 2009 Dec;26(12):1592-601.

Nestel PJ. Adulthood - prevention: Cardiovascular disease. Med J Aust. 2002 Jun 3;176(11 Suppl):S118-9.

Nestor PJ, Graham KS, Bozeat S, Simons JS, Hodges JR. Memory consolidation and the hippocampus: further evidence from studies of autobiographical memory in semantic dementia and frontal variant frontotemporal dementia. Neuropsychologia. 2002;40(6):633-54.

New Study Shows Small Serving of Peanuts Reduces Chronic Disease and Death Risk. PR Newswire Press Release. Dec. 7, 2016

New York State. PM2.5 Monitoring. Fine Particulate Matter Monitoring. Accessed May 4, 2016.

Newall CA, Anderson LA, Phillipson JD (eds). Herbal Medicines: A Guide for Health-Care Professionals. London: Pharmaceut Press; 1996.

Newmark T, Schulick P. Beyond Aspirin. Prescott, AZ: Holm, 2000.

Newton PE. The Effect of Sound on Plant Grwoth. JAES. 1971 Mar;19(3): 202-205.

Neyestani TR, Shariatzadeh N, Gharavi A, Kalayi A, Khalaji N. Physiological dose of lycopene suppressed oxidative stress and enhanced serum levels of immunoglobulin M in patients with Type 2 diabetes mellitus: a possible role in the prevention of long-term complications. J Endocrinol Invest. 2007 Nov;30(10):833-8.

Ngai SP, Jones AY, Hui-Chan CW, Ko FW, Hui DS. Effect of Acu-TENS on post-exercise expiratory lung volume in subjects with asthma-A randomized controlled trial. Respir Physiol Neurobiol. 2009 Jul 31;167(3):348-53. 2009 Jun 18.

Ngo SN, Williams DB, Head RJ. Rosemary and cancer prevention: preclinical perspectives. Crit Rev Food Sci Nutr. 2011 Dec;51(10):946-54. doi: 10.1080/10408398.2010.490883. PMID: 21955093.

Nhu-Trang TT, Casabianca H, Grenier-Loustalot MF. Authenticity control of essential oils containing citronellal and citral by chiral and stable-isotope gas-chromatographic analysis. Anal Bioanal Chem. 2006 Dec;386(7-8):2141-52.

Nicastro HL, Ross SA, Milner JA. Garlic and onions: their cancer prevention properties. Cancer Prev Res (Phila). 2015 Mar;8(3):181-9. doi: 10.1158/1940-6207.CAPR-14-0172.

Nicholas JS, Lackland DT, Butler GC, Mohr LC Jr, Dunbar JB, Kaune WT, Grosche B, Hoel DG. Cosmic radiation and magnetic field exposure to airline flight crews. Am J Ind Med. 1998 Dec;34(6):574-80.

Nicholls SJ, Lundman P, Harmer JA, Cutri B, Griffiths KA, Rye KA, Barter PJ, Celermajer DS. Consumption of saturated fat impairs the anti-inflammatory properties of high-density lipoproteins and endothelial function. J Am Coll Cardiol. 2006 Aug 15;48(4):715-20.

Niederau C, Göpfert E. The effect of chelidonium- and turmeric root extract on upper abdominal pain due to functional disorders of the biliary system. Results from a placebo-controlled double-blind study. Med Klin. 1999 Aug 15;94(8):425-30.

381

Niedzielin K, Kordecki H, Birkenfeld B. A controlled, double-blind, randomized study on the efficacy of Lactobacillus plantarum 299V in patients with irritable bowel syndrome. Eur J Gastroenterol Hepatol. 2001 Oct;13(10):1143-7.

Nielsen LR, Mosekilde L. Vitamin D and breast cancer. Ugeskr Laeger. 2007 Apr 2;169(14):1299-302.

Nielsen OH, Jørgensen S, Pedersen K, Justesen T. Microbiological evaluation of jejunal aspirates and faecal samples after oral administration of bifidobacteria and lactic acid bacteria. J Appl Bacteriol. 1994 May;76(5):469-74.

Nielsen RG, Bindslev-Jensen C, Kruse-Andersen S, Husby S. Severe gastroesophageal reflux disease and cow milk hypersensitivity in infants and children: disease association and evaluation of a new challenge procedure. J Pediatr Gastroenterol Nutr. 2004 Oct;39(4):383-91.

Nielsen SE, Young JF, Daneshvar B, Lauridsen ST, Knuthsen P, Sandström B, Dragsted LO. Effect of parsley (Petroselinum crispum) intake on urinary apigenin excretion, blood antioxidant enzymes and biomarkers for oxidative stress in human subjects. Br J Nutr. 1999 Jun;81(6):447-55.

Nievergelt CM, Kripke DF, Remick RA, Sadovnick AD, McElroy SL, Keck PE Jr, Kelsoe JR. Examination of the clock gene Cryptochrome 1 in bipolar disorder: mutational analysis and absence of evidence for linkage or association. Psychiatr Genet. 2005 Mar;15(1):45-52.

Niggli H. Temperature dependence of ultraweak photon emission in fibroblastic differentiation after irradiation with artificial sunlight. Indian J Exp Biol. 2003 May;41:419-423.

Nightingale JA, Rogers DF, Hart LA, Kharitonov SA, Chung KF, Barnes PJ. Effect of inhaled endotoxin on induced sputum in normal, atopic, and atopic asthmatic subjects. Thorax. 1998 Jul;53(7):563-71.

Niimi A, Nguyen LT, Usmani O, Mann B, Chung KF. Reduced pH and chloride levels in exhaled breath condensate of patients with chronic cough. Thorax. 2004 Jul;59(7):608-12.

Nilson KM, Vakil JR, Shahani KM. B-complex vitamin content of cheddar cheese. J Nutr. 1965 Aug;86:362-8.

Ninan TK, Russell G. Respiratory symptoms and atopy in Aberdeen schoolchildren: evidence from two surveys 25 years apart. BMJ. 1992;304:873-875.

Nishigori C, Hattori Y, Toyokuni S. Role of reactive oxygen species in skin carcinogenesis. Antioxid Redox Signal. 2004 Jun;6(3):561-70.

Njoroge GN, Bussmann RW. Traditional management of ear, nose and throat (ENT) diseases in Central Kenya. J Ethnobiol Ethnomed. 2006 Dec 27;2:54.

Nobaek S, Johansson ML, Molin G, Ahrné S, Jeppsson B. Alteration of intestinal microflora is associated with reduction in abdominal bloating and pain in patients with irritable bowel syndrome. Am J Gastroenterol. 2000 May;95(5):1231-8.

Nodake Y, Fukumoto S, Fukasawa M, Sakakibara R, Yamasaki N. Reduction of the immunogenicity of beta-lactoglobulin from cow's milk by conjugation with a dextran derivative. Biosci Biotechnol Biochem. 2010;74(4):721-6.

Nokerbek S, Sakipova Z, Chalupová M, Nejezchlebová M, Hošek J. Cytotoxic, anti-cancer, and anti-microbial effects of different extracts obtained from Artemisia rupestris. Ceska Slov Farm. 2017 Spring;66(1):15-22.

Noone EJ, Roche HM, Nugent AP, Gibney MJ. The effect of dietary supplementation using isomeric blends of conjugated linoleic acid on lipid metabolism in healthy human subjects. Br J Nutr. 2002 Sep;88(3):243-51.

Noorbakhsh R, Mortazavi SA, Sankian M, Shahidi F, Assarehzadegan MA, Varasteh A. Cloning, expression, characterization, and computational approach for cross-reactivity prediction of manganese superoxide dismutase allergen from pistachio nut. Allergol Int. 2010 Sep;59(3):295-304.

Nopchinda S, Varavithya W, Phuapradit P, Sangchai R, Suthutvoravut U, Chantraruksa V, Haschke F. Effect of bifidobacterium Bb12 with or without Streptococcus thermophilus supplemented formula on nutritional status. J Med Assoc Thai. 2002 Nov;85 Suppl 4:S1225-31.

Norat T, Dossus L, Rinaldi S, Overvad K, Grønbaek H, Tjønneland A, Olsen A, Clavel-Chapelon F, Boutron-Ruault MC, Boeing H, Lahmann PH, Linseisen J, Nagel G, Trichopoulou A, Trichopoulos D, Kalapothaki V, Sieri S, Palli D, Panico S, Tumino R, Sacerdote C, Bueno-de-Mesquita HB, Peeters PH, van Gils CH, Agudo A, Amiano P, Ardanoz E, Martinez C, Quirós R, Tormo MJ, Bingham S, Key TJ, Allen NE, Ferrari P, Slimani N, Riboli E, Kaaks R. Diet, serum insulin-like growth factor-I and IGF-binding protein-3 in European women. Eur J Clin Nutr. 2007 Jan;61(1):91-8.

Norlela S, Izham C, Khalid BA. Colonic irrigation-induced hyponatremia. Malays J Pathol. 2004 Dec;26(2):117-8.

Norris R. "Flush-free niacin": Dietary supplement may be "benefit-free." Prev Cardio. 2006 Winter: 64.

North J. The Fontana History of Astronomy and Cosmology. London: Fontana Press, 1994.

Nova E, Toro O, Varela P, López-Vidriero I, Morandé G, Marcos A. Effects of a nutritional intervention with yogurt on lymphocyte subsets and cytokine production capacity in anorexia nervosa patients. Eur J Nutr. 2006 Jun;45(4):225-33.

Novembre E, Dini L, Bernardini R, Resti M, Vierucci A. Unusual reactions to food additives. Pediatr Med Chir. 1992 Jan-Feb;14(1):39-42.

Novick RM, Nelson ML, McKinley MA, Anderson GL, Keenan JJ. The effect of clothing care activities on textile formaldehyde content. J Toxicol Environ Health A. 2013;76(14):883-93. doi: 10.1080/15287394.2013.821439.

NRPB 2003. Health Effects from Radiofrequency Electromagnetic Fields. Report of an Independent Advisory Group on Non-ionising Radiation. Chilton, Didcot, UK:National Radiation Protection Board.

Nwaru BI, Erkkola M, Ahonen S, Kaila M, Haapala AM, Kronberg-Kippilä C, Salmelin R, Veijola R, Ilonen J, Simell O, Knip M, Virtanen SM. Age at the introduction of solid foods during the first year and allergic sensitization at age 5 years. Pediatrics. 2010 Jan;125(1):50-9. 2009 Dec 7.

NYC Health. New York City Trends in Air Pollution and its Health Consequence. May 2013.

O'Connor J., Bensky D. (ed). Shanghai College of Traditional Chinese Medicine: Acupuncture: A Comprehensive Text. Seattle: Eastland Press, 1981.

O'Dwyer JJ. College Physics. Pacific Grove, CA: Brooks/Cole, 1990.

O'Brien SJ, Shannon JE, Gail MH. A molecular approach to the identification and individualization of human and animal cells in culture: isozyme and allozyme genetic signatures. In Vitro. 1980 Feb;16(2):119-35.

Oehme FW (ed.). Toxicity of heavy metals in the environment. Part 1. New York: M.Dekker, 1979.

Ogawa T, Hashikawa S, Asai Y, Sakamoto H, Yasuda K, Makimura Y. A new synbiotic, Lactobacillus casei subsp. casei together with dextran, reduces murine and human allergic reaction. FEMS Immunol Med Microbiol. 2006 Apr;46(3):400-9.

Oh B, Kim BS, Kim JW, Kim JS, Koh SJ, Kim BG, Lee KL, Chun J. Probiotics on Gut Microbiota… Helicobacter pylori Eradication Helicobacter. 2016 Jun;21(3):165-74. doi: 10.1111/hel.12270.

Oh CK, Lücker PW, Wetzelsberger N, Kuhlmann F. The determination of magnesium, calcium, sodium and potassium in assorted foods with special attention to the loss of electrolytes after various forms of food preparations. Mag.-Bull. 1986;8:297-302.

Oh SY, Chung J, Kim MK, Kwon SO, Cho BH. Antioxidant nutrient intakes and corresponding biomarkers associated with the risk of atopic dermatitis in young children. Eur J Clin Nutr. 2010 Mar;64(3):245-52. 2010 Jan 27.

Ohashi Y, Nakai S, Tsukamoto T, Masumori N, Akaza H, Miyanaga N, Kitamura T, Kawabe K, Kotake T, Kuroda M, Naito S, Koga H, Saito Y, Nomata K, Kitagawa M, Aso Y. Habitual intake of lactic acid bacteria and risk reduction of bladder cancer. Urol Int. 2002;68(4):273-80.

Ok IS, Kim SH, Kim BK, Lee JC, Lee YC. Pinellia ternata, Citrus reticulata, and their combinational prescription inhibit eosinophil infiltration and airway hyperresponsiveness by suppressing CCR3+ and Th2 cytokines production in the ovalbumin-induced asthma model. Mediators Inflamm. 2009;2009:413270.

Okamura H. Clock genes in cell clocks: roles, actions, and mysteries. J Biol Rhythms. 2004 Oct;19(5):388-99.

Okamura T, Maehara Y, Sugimachi K. Phase II clinical study of LC9018 on carcinomatous peritonitis of gastric cancer. Subgroup for Carcinomatous Peritonitis, Cooperative, Study Group of LC9018. Gan To Kagaku Ryoho. 1989 Jun;16(6):2257-62.

Okawa T, Niibe H, Arai T, Sekiba K, Noda K, Takeuchi S, Hashimoto S, Ogawa N. Effect of LC9018 combined with radiation therapy on carcinoma of the uterine cervix. A phase III, multicenter, randomized, controlled study. Cancer. 1993 Sep 15;72(6):1949-54.

Okayama Y, Begishvili TB, Church MK. Comparison of mechanisms of IL-3 induced histamine release and IL-3 priming effect on human basophils. Clin Exp Allergy. 1993 Nov;23(11):901-10.

Okuyama Y, Ozasa K, Oki K, Nishino H, Fujimoto S, Watanabe Y. Inverse associations between serum concentrations of zeaxanthin and other carotenoids and colorectal neoplasm in Japanese. Int J Clin Oncol. 2013 Feb 5.

Oláh A, Belágyi T, Issekutz A, Gamal ME, Bengmark S. Randomized clinical trial of specific lactobacillus and fibre supplement to early enteral nutrition in patients with acute pancreatitis. Br J Surg. 2002 Sep;89(9):1103-7.

Ołdak E, Kurzatkowska B, Stasiak-Barmuta A. Natural course of sensitization in children: follow-up study from birth to 6 years of age, I. Evaluation of total serum IgE and specific IgE antibodies with regard to atopic family history. Rocz Akad Med Bialymst. 2000;45:87-95.

Ole D. Rughede, On the Theory and Physics of the Aether. Progress in Physics. 2006; (1).

O'Leary KD, Rosenbaum A, Hughes PC. Fluorescent lighting: a purported source of hyperactive behavior. J Abnorm Child Psychol. 1978 Sep;6(3):285-9.

Oleĭnichenko EV, Mitrokhin SD, Nonikov VE, Minaev VI. Effectiveness of acipole in prevention of enteric dysbacteriosis due to antibacterial therapy. Antibiot Khimioter. 1999;44(1):23-5.

Olivares M, Díaz-Ropero MA, Gómez N, Lara-Villoslada F, Sierra S, Maldonado JA, Martín R, López-Huertas E, Rodríguez JM, Xaus J. Oral administration of two probiotic strains, Lactobacillus gasseri

CECT5714 and Lactobacillus coryniformis CECT5711, enhances the intestinal function of healthy adults. Int J Food Microbiol. 2006 Mar 15;107(2):104-11.

Olivares M, Paz Díaz-Ropero M, Gómez N, Sierra S, Lara-Villoslada F, Martín R, Miguel Rodríguez J, Xaus J. Dietary deprivation of fermented foods causes a fall in innate immune response. Lactic acid bacteria can counteract the immunological effect of this deprivation. J Dairy Res. 2006 Nov;73(4):492-8.

Olney JW. Excitotoxins in foods. Neurotoxicology. 1994;15:535-44.

Olsen LR, Grillo MP, Skonberg C. Constituents in kava extracts potentially involved in hepatotoxicity: a review. Chem Res Toxicol. 2011 Jul 18;24(7):992-1002. doi: 10.1021/tx100412m.

O'Mahony L, McCarthy J, Kelly P, Hurley G, Luo F, Chen K, O'Sullivan GC, Kiely B, Collins JK, Shanahan F, Quigley EM. Lactobacillus and bifidobacterium in irritable bowel syndrome: symptom responses and relationship to cytokine profiles. Gastroenterology. 2005 Mar;128(3):541-51.

Ombra MN, d'Acierno A, Nazzaro F, Riccardi R, Spigno P, Zaccardelli M, Pane C, Maione M, Fratianni F. Phenolic Composition and Antioxidant and Antiproliferative Activities of the Extracts of Twelve Common Bean (Phaseolus vulgaris L.) Endemic Ecotypes of Southern Italy before and after Cooking. Oxid Med Cell Longev. 2016;2016:1398298. doi: 10.1155/2016/1398298.

Onder G, et al. Serum cholesterol levels and in-hospital mortality in the elderly. Am J Med. 2003 Sept;115:265-71.

Ong KW, Hsu A, Tan BK. Chlorogenic acid stimulates glucose transport in skeletal muscle via AMPK activation: a contributor to the beneficial effects of coffee on diabetes. PLoS One. 2012;7(3):e32718.

Onwulata CI, Rao DR, Vankineni P. Relative efficiency of yogurt, sweet acidophilus milk, hydrolyzed-lactose milk, and a commercial lactase tablet in alleviating lactose maldigestion. Am J Clin Nutr. 1989 Jun;49(6):1233-7.

Oosterga M, ten Vaarwerk IA, DeJongste MJ, Staal MJ. Spinal cord stimulation in refractory angina pectoris—clinical results and mechanisms. Z Kardiol. 1997;86 Suppl 1:107-13.

Oozeer R, Leplingard A, Mater DD, Mogenet A, Michelin R, Seksek I, Marteau P, Doré J, Bresson JL, Corthier G. Survival of Lactobacillus casei in the human digestive tract after consumption of fermented milk. Appl Environ Microbiol. 2006 Aug;72(8):5615-7.

Oreskovic NM, Sawicki GS, Kinane TB, Winickoff JP, Perrin JM. Travel patterns to school among children with asthma. Clin Pediatr. 2009 Jul;48(6):632-40. 2009 May 6.

Ortiz LM, Lombardi P, Tillhon M, Scovassi AI. Berberine, an epiphany against cancer. Molecules. 2014 Aug 15;19(8):12349-67. doi: 10.3390/molecules190812349

Ortiz-Andrellucchi A, Sánchez-Villegas A, Rodríguez-Gallego C, Lemes A, Molero T, Soria A, Peña-Quintana L, Santana M, Ramírez O, García J, Cabrera F, Cobo J, Serra-Majem L. Immunomodulatory effects of the intake of fermented milk with Lactobacillus casei DN114001 in lactating mothers and their children. Br J Nutr. 2008 Oct;100(4):834-45.

Osguthorpe JD. Immunotherapy. Curr Opin Otolaryngol Head Neck Surg. 2010 Jun;18(3):206-12.

Osman AM, Bayoumi HM, Al-Harthi SE, Damanhouri ZA, Elshal MF. Modulation of doxorubicin cytotoxicity by resveratrol in a human breast cancer cell line. Cancer Cell Int. 2012 Nov 16;12(1):47.

Ostlund RE Jr. Phytosterols and cholesterol metabolism. Curr Opin Lipidol. 2004 Feb;15(1):37-41.

Ostrander S, Schroeder L, Ostrander N. Super-Learning. New York: Delta, 1979.

Otani S. Memory trace in prefrontal cortex: theory for the cognitive switch. Biol Rev Camb Philos Soc. 2002 Nov;77(4):563-77.

Otsuki N, Dang NH, Kumagai E, Kondo A, Iwata S, Morimoto C. Aqueous extract of Carica papaya leaves exhibits anti-tumor activity and immunomodulatory effects. J Ethnopharmacol. 2010 Feb 17;127(3):760-7.

Ott J. Color and Light: Their Effects on Plants, Animals, and People (Series of seven articles in seven issues). Internl J Biosoc Res. 1985-1991.

Ott J. Health and Light: The Effects of Natural and Artificial Light on Man and Other Living Things. Self published, 1973,

Otto SJ, van Houwelingen AC, Hornstra G. The effect of supplementation with docosahexaenoic and arachidonic acid derived from single cell oils on plasma and erythrocyte fatty acids of pregnant women in the second trimester. Prost Leuk Essent Fatty Acids. 2000 Nov;63(5):323-8.

Ou CC, Tsao SM, Lin MC, Yin MC. Protective action on human LDL against oxidation and glycation by four organosulfur compounds derived from garlic. Lipids. 2003 Mar;38(3):219-24.

Ouellet-Hellstrom R, Stewart WF. Miscarriages among female physical therapists who report using radio- and microwave-frequency electromagnetic radiation. Am J Epidemiol. 1993 Nov 15;138(10):775-86.

Ouwehand AC, Bergsma N, Parhiala R, Lahtinen S, Gueimonde M, Finne-Soveri H, Strandberg T, Pitkälä K, Salminen S. Bifidobacterium microbiota and parameters of immune function in elderly subjects. FEMS Immunol Med Microbiol. 2008 Jun;53(1):18-25.

Ouwehand AC, Tiihonen K, Saarinen M, Putaala H, Rautonen N. Influence of a combination of Lactobacillus acidophilus NCFM and lactitol on healthy elderly: intestinal and immune parameters. Br J Nutr. 2009 Feb;101(3):367-75.

REFERENCES AND BIBLIOGRAPHY

Owczarek K, Hrabec E, Fichna J, Sosnowska D, Koziołkiewicz M, Szymański J, Lewandowska U. Flavanols from Japanese quince (Chaenomeles japonica) fruit suppress expression of cyclooxygenase-2, metallo-proteinase-9, and nuclear factor-kappaB in human colon cancer cells. Acta Biochim Pol. 2017;64(3):567-576. doi: 10.18388/abp.2017_1599.

Ozkan TB, Sahin E, Erdemir G, Budak F. Effect of Saccharomyces boulardii in children with acute gastro-enteritis and its relationship to the immune response. J Int Med Res. 2007 Mar-Apr;35(2):201-12.

Ozone Hole Healing Gradually. Associated Press. 2005 Sept 16, 03:18 pm ET.

Paavonen EJ, Pennonen M, Roine M, Valkonen S, Lahikainen AR. TV exposure associated with sleep disturbances in 5- to 6-year-old children. J Sleep Res. 2006 Jun;15(2):154-61.

Pacione M. Urban environmental quality and human wellbeing-a social geographical perspective. Landscape and Urban Planning 2003;986:1-12.

Padayatty SJ, Sun H, Wang Y, Riordan HD, Hewitt SM, Katz A, Wesley RA, Levine M. Vitamin C pharma-cokinetics: implications for oral and intravenous use. Ann Intern Med. 2004 Apr 6;140(7):533-7. doi: 10.7326/0003-4819-140-7-200404060-00010.

Paineau D, Carcano D, Leyer G, Darquy S, Alyanakian MA, Simoneau G, Bergmann JF, Brassart D, Bornet F, Ouwehand AC. Effects of seven potential probiotic strains on specific immune responses in healthy adults: a double-blind, randomized, controlled trial. FEMS Immunol Med Microbiol. 2008 Jun;53(1):107-13.

Pakhale S, Doucette S, Vandemheen K, Boulet LP, McIvor RA, Fitzgerald JM, Hernandez P, Lemiere C, Sharma S, Field SK, Alvarez GG, Dales RE, Aaron SD. A comparison of obese and nonobese people with asthma: exploring an asthma-obesity interaction. Chest. 2010 Jun;137(6):1316-23. 2010 Feb 12.

Palacios R, Sugawara I. Hydrocortisone abrogates proliferation of T cells in autologous mixed lymphocyte reaction by rendering the interleukin-2 Producer T cells unresponsive to interleukin-1 and unable to synthesize the T-cell growth factor. Scand J Immunol. 1982 Jan;15(1):25-31. 7.

Palacios R. HLA-DR antigens render interleukin-2-producer T lymphocytes sensitive to interleukin-1. Scand J Immunol. 1981 Sep;14(3):321-6.

Palm TA. The geographical distribution and aetiology of rickets. Practitioner. 1890;45:270-90, 321-42.

Palmer JB, Lane D, Mayo D, Schluchter M, Leeming R. Effects of Music Therapy on Anesthesia Require-ments and Anxiety in Women Undergoing Ambulatory Breast Surgery for Cancer Diagnosis and Treatment: A Randomized Controlled Trial. J Clin Oncol. 2015 Oct 1;33(28):3162-8. doi: 10.1200/JCO.2014.59.6049. Epub 2015 Aug 17.

Palumbo A. Gravitational and geomagnetic tidal source of earthquake triggering. Ital Phys. 1989 Nov;12(6).

Pan S, Yuan C, Tagmount A, et al. Parabens and Human Epidermal Growth Factor Receptor Ligand Cross-Talk in Breast cancer Cells. Environ Health Perspect. 2016;124(5):563-569. doi:10.1289/ehp.1409200

Panahi Y, Saadat A, Beiraghdar F, Sahebkar A. Adjuvant therapy with bioavailability-boosted curcuminoids suppresses systemic inflammation and improves quality of life in patients with solid tumors: a random-ized double-blind placebo-controlled trial. Phytother Res. 2014 Oct;28(10):1461-7. doi: 10.1002/ptr.5149.

Panahi Y, Saadat A, Sahebkar A, Hashemian F, Taghikhani M, Abolhasani E. Effect of Ginger on acute and delayed chemotherapy-induced nausea and vomiting: a pilot, randomized, open-label clinical trial. In-tegr Cancer Ther. 2012 Sep;11(3):204-11. doi: 10.1177/1534735411433201.

Pandey PR, Xing F, Sharma S, Watabe M, Pai SK, Iiizumi-Gairani M, Fukuda K, Hirota S, Mo YY, Watabe K. Elevated lipogenesis in epithelial stem-like cell confers survival advantage in ductal carcinoma in situ of breast cancer. Oncogene. 2012 Dec 3.

Panghal S, Mallapur SS, Kumar M, Ram V, Singh BK. Antiinflammatory Activity of Piper longum Fruit Oil. Indian J Pharm Sci. 2009 Jul;71(4):454-6.

Panigrahi P, Parida S, Pradhan L, Mohapatra SS, Misra PR, Johnson JA, Chaudhry R, Taylor S, Hansen NI, Gewolb IH. Long-term colonization of a Lactobacillus plantarum synbiotic preparation in the neonatal gut. J Pediatr Gastroenterol Nutr. 2008 Jul;47(1):45-53.

Papandreou C, Becerra-Tomás N, Bulló M, Martínez-González MÁ, Corella D, Estruch R, Ros E, Arós F, Schroder H, Fitó M, Serra-Majem L, Lapetra J, Fiol M, Ruiz-Canela M, Sorli JV, Salas-Salvadó J. Leg-ume consumption and risk of all-cause, cardiovascular, and cancer mortality in the PREDIMED study. Clin Nutr. 2018 Jan 9. pii: S0261-5614(17)31439-5. doi: 10.1016/j.clnu.2017.12.019.

Pápay ZE, Kósa A, Boldizsár I, Ruszkai A, Balogh E, Klebovich I, Antal I. Pharmaceutical and formulation aspects of Petroselinum crispum extract. Acta Pharm Hung. 2012;82(1):3-14.

Parcell S. Sulfur in human nutrition and applications in medicine. Altern Med Rev. 2002 Feb;7(1):22-44.

Park AE, Fernandez JJ, Schmedders K, Cohen MS. The Fibonacci sequence: relationship to the human hand. J Hand Surg. 2003 Jan;28(1):157-60.

Park BJ, Tsunetsugu Y, Kasetani T, Kagawa T, Miyazaki Y. The physiological effects of Shinrin-yoku (taking in the forest atmosphere or forest bathing): evidence from field experiments in 24 forests across Japan. Environ Health Prev Med. 2010 Jan;15(1):18-26.

Park EJ, Pezzuto JM. Antioxidant Marine Products in Cancer Chemoprevention. Antioxid Redox Signal. 2013 Mar 19.

Park SY, Park GY, Ko WS, Kim Y. Dichroa febrifuga inhibits the production of IL-1beta and IL-6 through blocking NF-kappaB, MAPK and Akt activation in macrophages. J Ethnopharmacol. 2009 Sep 7;125(2):246-51.

Parra D, De Morentin BM, Cobo JM, Mateos A, Martinez JA. Monocyte function in healthy middle-aged people receiving fermented milk containing Lactobacillus casei. J Nutr Health Aging. 2004;8(4):208-11.

Parra MD, Martínez de Morentin BE, Cobo JM, Mateos A, Martínez JA. Daily ingestion of fermented milk containing Lactobacillus casei DN114001 improves innate-defense capacity in healthy middle-aged people. J Physiol Biochem. 2004 Jun;60(2):85-91.

Parrón T, Requena M, Hernández AF, Alarcón R. Environmental exposure to pesticides and cancer risk in multiple human organ systems. Toxicol Lett. 2014;230(2):157-165. doi:10.1016/j.toxlet.2013.11.009

Partonen T, Haukka J, Nevanlinna H, Lönnqvist J. Analysis of the seasonal pattern in suicide. J Affect Disord. 2004 Aug;81(2):133-9.

Partonen T, Haukka J, Nevanlinna H, Lönnqvist J. Analysis of the seasonal pattern in suicide. J Affect Disord. 2004 Aug;81(2):133-9.

Partonen T, Haukka J, Viilo K, Hakko H, Pirkola S, Isometsä E, Lönnqvist J, Särkioja T, Väisänen E, Räsänen P. Cyclic time patterns of death from suicide in N. Finland. J Affect Disrd. 2004 Jan;78(1):11-9.

Partonen T. Magnetoreception attributed to the efficacy of light therapy. Med Hypoth. 1998 Nov;51(5):447-8.

Partridge MR, Dockrell M, Smith NM: The use of complementary medicines by those with asthma. Respir Med 2003, 97:436-438.

Pascual A, Avgustinova A, Mejetta S, Martín M, Castellanos A, Attolini CS, Berenguer A, Prats N, Toll A, Hueto JA, Bescós C, Di Croce L, Benitah SA. Targeting metastasis-initiating cells through the fatty acid receptor CD36. Nature. 2016 Dec 7. doi: 10.1038/nature20791.

Patel AV, Bernstein L, Deka A, Feigelson HS, Campbell PT, Gapstur SM, Colditz GA, Thun MJ. Leisure time spent sitting in relation to total mortality in a prospective cohort of US adults. Am J Epidemiol. 2010 Aug 15;172(4):419-29.

Patel DS, Rafferty GF, Lee S, Hannam S, Greenough A. Work of breathing and volume targeted ventilation in respiratory distress. Arch Dis Child Fetal Neonatal Ed. 2010 Nov;95(6):F443-6.

Patriarca G, Nucera E, Pollastrini E, Roncallo C, De Pasquale T, Lombardo C, Pedone C, Gasbarrini G, Buonomo A, Schiavino D. Oral specific desensitization in food-allergic children. Dig Dis Sci. 2007 Jul;52(7):1662-72.

Patterson DB. Anaphylactic shock from chloromycetin. Northwest Med. 1950 May;49(5):352-3.Agarwal KN, Bhasin SK. Feasibility studies to control acute diarrhoea in children by feeding fermented milk preparations Actimel and Indian Dahi. Eur J Clin Nutr. 2002 Dec;56 Suppl 4:S56-9.

Patwardhan B, Gautam M. Botanical immunodrugs: scope and opportunities. Drug Discov Today. 2005 Apr 1;10(7):495-502.

Paul M, Somkuti GA. Hydrolytic breakdown of lactoferricin by lactic acid bacteria. J Ind Microbiol Biotechnol. 2010 Feb;37(2):173-8. Epub 2009 Nov 19.

Payment P, Franco E, Richardson L, Siemiatyck, J. Gastrointestinal health effects associated with the consumption of drinking water produced by point-of-use domestic reverse-osmosis filtration units. Appl. Environ. Microbiol. 1991;57:945-948.

Peat JK, van den Berg RH, Green WF, Mellis CM, Leeder SR, Woolcock AJ. Changing prevalence of asthma in Australian children. BMJ. 1994;308:1591-1596.

Pedemonte M, Rodríguez-Alvez A, Velluti RA. Electroencephalographic frequencies associated with heart changes in RR interval variability during paradoxical sleep. Auton Neurosci. 2005 Dec 30;123(1-2):82-6.

Pedemonte M, Rodríguez-Alvez A, Velluti RA. Electroencephalographic frequencies associated with heart changes in RR interval variability during paradoxical sleep. Auton Neurosci. 2005 Dec 30;123(1-2):82-6.

Pedone CA, Arnaud CC, Postaire ER, Bouley CF, Reinert P. Multicentric study of the effect of milk fermented by Lactobacillus casei on the incidence of diarrhoea. Int J Clin Pract. 2000 Nov;54(9):568-71.

Pedone CA, Bernabeu AO, Postaire ER, Bouley CF, Reinert P. The effect of supplementation with milk fermented by Lactobacillus casei (strain DN-114 001) on acute diarrhoea in children attending day care centres. Int J Clin Pract. 1999 Apr-May;53(3):179-84.

Pedrosa MC, Golner BB, Goldin BR, Barakat S, Dallal GE, Russell RM. Survival of yogurt-containing organisms and Lactobacillus gasseri (ADH) and their effect on bacterial enzyme activity in the gastrointestinal tract of healthy and hypochlorhydric elderly subjects. Am J Clin Nutr. 1995 Feb;61(2):353-9.

Pehowich DJ, Gomes AV, Barnes JA. Fatty acid composition and possible health effects of coconut constituents. West Indian Med J. 2000 Jun;49(2):128-33.

Peluso I, Yarla NS, Ambra R, Pastore G, Perry G. MAPK signalling pathway in cancers: Olive products as cancer preventive and therapeutic agents. Semin Cancer Biol. 2017 Sep 11. pii: S1044-579X(17)30165-7. doi: 10.1016/j.semcancer.2017.09.002.

Penev PD. Association between sleep and morning testosterone levels in older men. Sleep. 2007 Apr 1;30(4):427-32.

Penn RD, Hagins WA. Kinetics of the photocurrent of retinal rods. Biophys J. 1972 Aug;12(8):1073-94.

Penn RD, Hagins WA. Signal transmission along retinal rods and the origin of the electroretinographic a-wave. Nature. 1969 Jul 12;223(5202):201-4.

Penson RT, Kyriakou H, Zuckerman D, Chabner BA, Lynch TJ Jr. Teams: communication in multidisciplinary care. Oncologist. 2006 May;11(5):520-6.

Peral MC, Martinez MA, Valdez JC. Bacteriotherapy with Lactobacillus plantarum in burns. Int Wound J. 2009 Feb;6(1):73-81.

Perez-Galvez A, Martin HD, Sies H, Stahl W. Incorporation of carotenoids from paprika oleoresin into human chylomicrons. Br J Nutr. 2003 Jun;89(6):787-93.

Pérez-López FR. Vitamin D and its implications for musculoskeletal health in women: an update. Maturitas. 2007 Oct 20;58(2):117-37.

Perez-Pena R. Secrets of the Mummy's Medicine Chest. NY Times. 2005 Sept 10.

Pérez-Sánchez A, Barrajón-Catalán E, Ruiz-Torres V, Agulló-Chazarra L, Herranz-López M, Valdés A, Cifuentes A, Micol V. Rosemary (Rosmarinus officinalis) extract causes ROS-induced necrotic cell death and inhibits tumor growth in vivo. Sci Rep. 2019 Jan 28;9(1):808. doi: 10.1038/s41598-018-37173-7.

Peroxisomes from pepper fruits (Capsicum annuum L.): purification, characterisation and antioxidant activity. J Plant Physiol. 2003 Dec;160(12):1507-16.

Perreau-Lenz S, Kalsbeek A, Van Der Vliet J, Pevet P, Buijs RM. In vivo evidence for a controlled offset of melatonin synthesis at dawn by the suprachiasmatic nucleus in the rat. Neuroscience. 2005;130(3):797-803.

Perrin RN. Lymphatic drainage of the neuraxis in chronic fatigue syndrome: a hypothetical model for the cranial rhythmic impulse. J Am Osteopath Assoc. 2007 Jun;107(6):218-24.

Persinger M.A. Psi phenomena and temporal lobe activity: The geomagnetic factor. In L.A. Henkel & R.E. Berger (Eds.), Research in parapsychology. (121- 156). Metuchen, NJ: Scarecrow Press, 1989.

Persinger M.A., Krippner S. Dream ESP experiments and geomagnetic activity. Journal of the American Society of Psychical Research. 1989;83:101- 106.

Persson R, Orbaek P, Kecklund G, Akerstedt T. Impact of an 84-hour workweek on biomarkers for stress, metabolic processes and diurnal rhythm. Scand J Work Environ Health. 2006 Oct;32(5):349-58.

Pert C. Molecules of Emotion. New York: Scribner, 1997.

Peterson CG, Hansson T, Skott A, Bengtsson U, Ahlstedt S, Magnussons J. Detection of local mast-cell activity in patients with food hypersensitivity. J Investig Allergol Clin Immunol. 2007;17(5):314-20.

Peterson KA, Samuelson WM, Ryujin DT, Young DC, Thomas KL, Hilden K, Fang JC. The role of gastroesophageal reflux in exercise-triggered asthma: a randomized controlled trial. Dig Dis Sci. 2009 Mar;54(3):564-71. 2008 Aug 8.

Petiot JF, Sainte-Laudy J, Benveniste J. Interpretation of results on a human basophil degranulation test. Ann Biol Clin (Paris). 1981;39(6):355-9.

Petlevski R, Hadzija M, Slijepcević M, Juretić D, Petrik J. Glutathione S-transferases and malondialdehyde in the liver of NOD mice on short-term treatment with plant mixture extract P-9801091. Phytother Res. 2003 Apr;17(4):311-4.

Petricevic L, Unger FM, Viernstein H, Kiss H. Randomized, double-blind, placebo-controlled study of oral lactobacilli to improve the vaginal flora of postmenopausal women. Eur J Obstet Gynecol Reprod Biol. 2008 Nov;141(1):54-7.

Petricevic L, Witt A. The role of Lactobacillus casei rhamnosus Lcr35 in restoring the normal vaginal flora after antibiotic treatment of bacterial vaginosis. BJOG. 2008 Oct;115(11):1369-74.

Petrunov B, Marinova S, Markova R, Nenkov P, Nikolaeva S, Nikolova M, Taskov H, Cvetanov J. Cellular and humoral systemic and mucosal immune responses stimulated in volunteers by an oral polybacterial immunomodulator "Dentavax". Int Immunopharmacol. 2006 Jul;6(7):1181-93.

Petti S, Tarsitani G, D'Arca AS. A randomized clinical trial of the effect of yoghurt on the human salivary microflora. Arch Oral Biol. 2001 Aug;46(8):705-12.

Pfundstein B, El Desouky SK, Hull WE, Haubner R, Erben G, Owen RW. Polyphenolic compounds in the fruits of Egyptian medicinal plants (Terminalia bellerica, Terminalia chebula and Terminalia horrida): characterization, quantitation and determination of antioxidant capacities. Phytochemistry. 2010 Jul;71(10):1132-48.

Phuapradit P, Varavithya W, Vathanophas K, Sangchai R, Podhipak A, Suthutvoravut U, Nopchinda S, Chantraruksa V, Haschke F. Reduction of rotavirus infection in children receiving bifidobacteria-supplemented formula. J Med Assoc Thai. 1999 Nov;82 Suppl 1:S43-8.

Physicians' Desk Reference. Montvale, NJ: Thomson, 2003-2008.

Piemontese L, Messia MC, Marconi E, Falasca L, Zivoli R, Gambacorta L, Perrone G, Solfrizzo M. Effect of gaseous ozone treatments on DON, microbial contaminants and technological parameters of wheat and semolina. Food Addit Contam Part A Chem Anal Control Expo Risk Assess. 2018 Apr;35(4):760-771. doi: 10.1080/19440049.2017.1419285. Epub 2018 Jan 19. PMID: 29279049.

Pierce SK, Klinman NR. Antibody-specific immunoregulation. J Exp Med. 1977 Aug 1;146(2):509-19.

Pieterse Z, Jerling JC, Oosthuizen W, Kruger HS, Hanekom SM, Smuts CM, Schutte AE. Substitution of high monounsaturated fatty acid avocado for mixed dietary fats during an energy-restricted diet: effects on weight loss, serum lipids, fibrinogen, and vascular function. Nutrition. 2005 Jan;21(1):67-75

Piggins HD. Human clock genes. Ann Med. 2002;34(5):394-400.

Pike MG, Heddle RJ, Boulton P, Turner MW, Atherton DJ. Increased intestinal permeability in atopic eczema. J Invest Dermatol. 1986 Feb;86(2):101-4.

Piluso LG, Moffatt-Smith C. Disinfection using ultraviolet radiation as an antimicrobial agent: a review and synthesis of mechanisms and concerns. PDA J Pharm Sci Technol. 2006 Jan-Feb;60(1):1-16.

Piluso LG, Moffatt-Smith C. Disinfection using ultraviolet radiation as an antimicrobial agent: a review and synthesis of mechanisms and concerns. PDA J Pharm Sci Technol. 2006 Jan-Feb;60(1):1-16.

Pines JM, Prabhu A, Hilton JA, Hollander JE, Datner EM. The effect of emergency department crowding on length of stay and medication treatment times in discharged patients with acute asthma. Acad Emerg Med. 2010 Aug;17(8):834-9.

Pines M, Nagler A. Halofuginone: a novel antifibrotic therapy. Gen Pharmacol. 1998 Apr;30(4):445-50.

Pinkerton LE, Hein MJ, Stayner LT. Mortality among a cohort of garment workers exposed to formaldehyde: an update. Occup Environ Med. 2004 Mar;61(3):193-200.

Pinner KD, Wales CT, Gristock RA, Vo HT, So N, Jacobs AT. Flavokawains A and B from kava (Piper methysticum) activate heat shock and antioxidant responses and protect against hydrogen peroxide-induced cell death in HepG2 hepatocytes. Pharm Biol. 2016 Sep;54(9):1503-12. doi: 10.3109/13880209.2015.1107104.

Pitkala KH, Strandberg TE, Finne Soveri UH, Ouwehand AC, Poussa T, Salminen S. Fermented cereal with specific bifidobacteria normalizes bowel movements in elderly nursing home residents. A randomized, controlled trial. J Nutr Health Aging. 2007 Jul-Aug;11(4):305-11.

Pittas AG, Harris SS, Stark PC, Dawson-Hughes B. The effects of calcium and vitamin D supplementation on blood glucose and markers of inflammation in nondiabetic adults. Diab Care. 2007 Apr;30(4):980-6.

Pitten FA, Scholler M, Krüger U, Effendy I, Kramer A. Filamentous fungi and yeasts on mattresses covered with different encasings. Eur J Dermatol. 2001 Nov-Dec;11(6):534-7.

Pitt-Rivers R, Trotter WR. The Thyroid Gland. London: Butterworth Publisher, 1954.

Plaut M, Valentine MD. Clinical practice. Allergic rhinitis. N Engl J Med. 2005 Nov 3;353(18):1934-44.

Plaut TE, Jones TB. Dr. Tom Plaut's Asthma guide for people of all ages. Amherst, MA: Pedipress, 1999.

Plaza V, Miguel E, Bellido-Casado J, Lozano MP, Ríos L, Bolíbar I. [Usefulness of the Guidelines of the Spanish Society of Pulmonology and Thoracic Surgery (SEPAR) in identifying the causes of chronic cough]. Arch Bronconeumol. 2006 Feb;42(2):68-73.

Plein K, Hotz J. Therapeutic effects of Saccharomyces boulardii on mild residual symptoms in a stable phase of Crohn's disease with special respect to chronic diarrhea—a pilot study. Z Gastroenterol. 1993 Feb;31(2):129-34.

Plitzko B, Kaweesa EN, Loesgen S. The natural product mensacarcin induces mitochondrial toxicity and apoptosis in melanoma cells. J Biol Chem. 2017 Dec 22;292(51):21102-21116. doi: 10.1074/jbc.M116.774836.

Plohmann B, Bader G, Hiller K, Franz G. Immunomodulatory and antitumoral effects of triterpenoid saponins. Pharmazie. 1997 Dec;52(12):953-7.

Plotnikoff GA, Quigley JM. Prevalence of severe hypovitaminosis D in patients with persistent, nonspecific musculoskeletal pain. Mayo Clin Proc 2003;78: 1463-70.

Pobłocka-Olech L, Krauze-Baranowska M. SPE-HPTLC of procyanidins from the barks of different species and clones of Salix. J Pharm Biomed Anal. 2008 Nov 4;48(3):965-8.

Polito A, Aboab J, Annane D. The hypothalamic pituitary adrenal axis in sepsis. Novartis Found Symp. 2007;280:182-203.

Polk S, Sunyer J, Muñoz-Ortiz L, Barnes M, Torrent M, Figueroa C, Harris J, Vall O, Antó JM, Cullinan P. A prospective study of Fel d1 and Der p1 exposure in infancy and childhood wheezing. Am J Respir Crit Care Med. 2004 Aug 1;170(3):273-8.

Pollastri MP, Whitty A, Merrill JC, Tang X, Ashton TD, Amar S. Identification and characterization of kava-derived compounds mediating TNF-alpha suppression. Chem Biol Drug Des. 2009 Aug;74(2):121-8. doi: 10.1111/j.1747-0285.2009.00838.x.

Pollini F, Capristo C, Boner AL. Upper respiratory tract infections and atopy. Int J Immunopathol Pharmacol. 2010 Jan-Mar;23(1 Suppl):32-7.

Pollo LA, Bosi CF, Leite AS, Rigotto C, Kratz J, Simões CM, Fonseca DE, Coimbra D, Caramori G, Nepel A, Campos FR, Barison A, Biavatti MW. Polyacetylenes from the leaves of Vernonia scorpioides (Asteraceae) and their antiproliferative and antiherpetic activities. Phytochemistry. 2013 Nov;95:375-83. doi: 10.1016/j.phytochem.2013.07.011.

Ponsonby AL, McMichael A, van der Mei I. Ultraviolet radiation and autoimmune disease: insights from epidemiological research. Toxicology. 2002 Dec 27;181-182:71-8.

Pont AR, Charron AR, Brand RM. Active ingredients in sunscreens act as topical penetration enhancers for the herbicide 2,4-dichlorophenoxyacetic acid. Toxicol Appl Pharmacol. 2004 Mar 15;195(3):348-54.

Pool R. Is there an EMF-Cancer connection? Science. 1990;249: 1096-1098.

Popadic D, Savic E, Ramic Z, Djordjevic V, Trajkovic V, Medenica L, Popadic S. Aloe-emodin inhibits proliferation of adult human keratinocytes in vitro. J Cosmet Sci. 2012 Sep-Oct;63(5):297-302.

Popat R, Plesner T, Davies F, Cook G, Cook M, Elliott P, Jacobson E, Gumbleton T, Oakervee H, Cavenagh J. A phase 2 study of SRT501 (resveratrol) with bortezomib for patients with relapsed and or refractory multiple myeloma. Br J Haematol. 2012 Dec 4.

Pope CA 3rd, Burnett RT, Thun MJ, Calle EE, Krewski D, Ito K, Thurston GD. Lung cancer, cardiopulmonary mortality, and long-term exposure to fine particulate air pollution. JAMA. 2002 Mar 6;287(9):1132-41. doi: 10.1001/jama.287.9.1132. PMID: 11879110; PMCID: PMC4037163.

Pope CA 3rd, Coleman N, Pond ZA, Burnett RT. Fine particulate air pollution and human mortality: 25+ years of cohort studies. Environ Res. 2020 Apr;183:108924. doi: 10.1016/j.envres.2019.108924. Epub 2019 Nov 14. PMID: 31831155.

Popp F Chang J. Mechanism of interaction between electromagnetic fields and living organisms. Science in China. 2000 Series C;43(5):507-518.

Popp F, Chang J, Herzog A, Yan Z, Yan Y. Evidence of non-classical (squeezed) light in biological systems. Physics Lett. 2002;293:98-102.

Popp F, Yan Y. Delayed luminescence of biological systems in terms of coherent states. Phys.Lett. 2000;293:91-97.

Popp F. Molecular Aspects of Carcinogenesis. In Deutsch E, Moser K, Rainer H, Stacher A (eds.). Molecular Base of Malignancy. Stuttgart: G.Thieme, 1976:47-55.

Popper KR, Eccles, JC. The Self and Its Brain. London: Routledge, 1983.

Portaluppi F, Hermida RC. Circadian rhythms in cardiac arrhythmias and opportunities for their chronotherapy. Adv Drug Deliv Rev. 2007 Aug 31;59(9-10):940-51.

Postlethwait EM. Scavenger receptors clear the air. J Clin Invest. 2007 Mar;117(3):601-4.

Postma DS. Gender Differences in Asthma Development and Progression. Gender Medicine. 2007;4:S133-146.

Potterton D. (Ed.) Culpeper's Color Herbal. New York: Sterling, 1983.

Poulos LM, Toelle BG, Marks GB. The burden of asthma in children: an Australian perspective. Paediatr Respir Rev. 2005 Mar;6(1):20-7.

Pourzand A, Tajaddini A, Pirouzpanah S, et al. Associations between Dietary Allium Vegetables and Risk of Breast cancer: A Hospital-Based Matched Case-Control Study [published correction appears in J Breast cancer. 2018 Jun;21(2):231]. J Breast cancer. 2016;19(3):292–300. doi:10.4048/jbc.2016.19.3.292

Prasad R, Katiyar SK. Honokiol, an Active Compound of Magnolia Plant, Inhibits Growth, and Progression of Cancers of Different Organs. Adv Exp Med Biol. 2016;928:245-265. doi: 10.1007/978-3-319-41334-1_11.

Prasad S, Tyagi AK. Ginger and its constituents: role in prevention and treatment of gastrointestinal cancer. Gastroenterol Res Pract. 2015;2015:142979. doi: 10.1155/2015/142979.

Prato FS, Frappier JR, Shivers RR, Kavaliers M, Zabel P, Drost D, Lee TY. Magnetic resonance imaging increases the blood-brain barrier permeability to 153-gadolinium diethylenetriaminepentaacetic acid in rats. Brain Res. 1990 Jul 23;523(2):301-4.

Prato FS, Frappier JR, Shivers RR, Kavaliers M, Zabel P, Drost D, Lee TY. Magnetic resonance imaging increases the blood-brain barrier permeability to 153-gadolinium diethylenetriaminepentaacetic acid in rats. Brain Res. 1990 Jul 23;523(2):301-4.

Pregliasco F, Anselmi G, Fonte L, Giussani F, Schieppati S, Soletti L. A new chance of preventing winter diseases by the administration of synbiotic formulations. J Clin Gastroenterol. 2008 Sep;42 Suppl 3 Pt 2:S224-33.

Preisinger E, Quittan M. Thermo- and hydrotherapy. Wien Med Wochenschr. 1994;144(20-21):520-6.

Prescott SL, Wickens K, Westcott L, Jung W, Currie H, Black PN, Stanley TV, Mitchell EA, Fitzharris P, Siebers R, Wu L, Crane J; Probiotic Study Group. Supplementation with Lactobacillus rhamnosus or Bifidobacterium lactis probiotics in pregnancy increases cord blood interferon-gamma and breast milk transforming growth factor-beta and immunoglobin A detection. Clin Exp Allergy. 2008 Oct;38(10):1606-14.

Pribram K. Brain and perception: holonomy and structure in figural processing. Hillsdale, N. J.: Lawrence Erlbaum Assoc., 1991.

Priftis KN, Panagiotakos DB, Anthracopoulos MB, Papadimitriou A, Nicolaidou P. Aims, methods and preliminary findings of the Physical Activity, Nutrition and Allergies in Children Examined in Athens (PANACEA) epidemiological study. BMC Public Health. 2007 Jul 4;7:140.

Prince SA, Gresty KM, Reed JL, Wright E, Tremblay MS, Reid RD. Individual, social and physical environmental correlates of sedentary behaviours in adults: a systematic review protocol. Syst Rev. 2014 Oct 21;3:120. doi: 10.1186/2046-4053-3-120.

Prioult G, Fliss I, Pecquet S. Effect of probiotic bacteria on induction and maintenance of oral tolerance to beta-lactoglobulin in gnotobiotic mice. Clin Diagn Lab Immunol. 2003 Sep;10(5):787-92.

Pronina TS. Circadian and infradian rhythms of testosterone and aldosterone excretion in children. Probl Endokrinol. 1992 Sep-Oct;38(5):38-42.

Pronina TS. Circadian and infradian rhythms of testosterone and aldosterone excretion in children. Probl Endokrinol. 1992 Sep-Oct;38(5):38-42.

Protheroe WM, Captiotti ER, Newsom GH. Exploring the Universe. Columbus, OH: Merrill, 1989,

Prucksunand C, Indrasukhsri B, Leethochawalit M, Hungspreugs K. Phase II clinical trial on effect of the long turmeric (Curcuma longa Linn) on healing of peptic ulcer. Southeast Asian J Trop Med Public Health. 2001 Mar;32(1):208-15.

Pruthi S, Thapa MM. Infectious and inflammatory disorders. Magn Reson Imaging Clin N Am. 2009 Aug;17(3):423-38, v.

Purnima A, Koti BC, Tikare VP, Viswanathaswamy AH, Thippeswamy AH, Dabadi P. Evaluation of Analgesic and Antipyretic Activities of Centratherum anthelminticum (L) Kuntze Seed. Indian J Pharm Sci. 2009 Jul;71(4):461-4.

Puthoff H, Targ R, May E. Experimental Psi Research: Implication for Physics. AAAS Proceedings of the 1979 Symposium on the Role of Consciousness in the Physical World. 1981.

Puthoff H, Targ R. A Perceptual Channel for Information Transfer Over Kilometer distances: Historical Perspective and Recent Research. Proc. IEEE. 1976;64(3):329-254.

Qiblawi S, Al-Hazimi A, Al-Mogbel M, Hossain A, Bagchi D. Chemopreventive effects of cardamom (Elettaria cardamomum L.) on chemically induced skin carcinogenesis in Swiss albino mice. J Med Food. 2012 Jun;15(6):576-80. doi: 10.1089/jmf.2011.0266. Epub 2012 Mar 9. PMID: 22404574.

Qiblawi S, Dhanarasu S, Faris MA. Chemopreventive Effect of Cardamom (Elettaria cardamomum L.) Against Benzo(α)Pyrene-Induced Forestomach Papillomagenesis in Swiss Albino Mice. J Environ Pathol Toxicol Oncol. 2015;34(2):95-104. doi: 10.1615/jenvironpatholtoxicoloncol.2015010838.

Qin HL, Zheng JJ, Tong DN, Chen WX, Fan XB, Hang XM, Jiang YQ. Effect of Lactobacillus plantarum enteral feeding on the gut permeability and septic complications in the patients with acute pancreatitis. Eur J Clin Nutr. 2008 Jul;62(7):923-30.

Radin D. The Conscious Universe. San Francisco: HarperEdge, 1997.

Radon K, Danuser B, Iversen M, Jörres R, Monso E, Opravil U, Weber C, Donham KJ, Nowak D. Respiratory symptoms in European animal farmers. Eur Respir J. 2001 Apr;17(4):747-54.

Rafter J, Bennett M, Caderni G, Clune Y, Hughes R, Karlsson PC, Klinder A, O'Riordan M, O'Sullivan GC, Pool-Zobel B, Rechkemmer G, Roller M, Rowland I, Salvadori M, Thijs H, Van Loo J, Watzl B, Collins JK. Dietary synbiotics reduce cancer risk factors in polypectomized and colon cancer patients. Am J Clin Nutr. 2007 Feb;85(2):488-96.

Rahman MM, Bhattacharya A, Fernandes G. Docosahexaenoic acid is more potent inhibitor of osteoclast differentiation in RAW 264.7 cells than eicosapentaenoic acid. J Cell Physiol. 2008 Jan;214(1):201-9.

Raj L, Ide T, Gurkar AU, Foley M, Schenone M, Li X, Tolliday NJ, Golub TR, Carr SA, Shamji AF, Stern AM, Mandinova A, Schreiber SL, Lee SW. Selective killing of cancer cells by a small molecule targeting the stress response to ROS. Nature. 2011 Jul 13;475(7355):231-4.

Ramachandran C, Wilk B, Melnick SJ, Eliaz I. Synergistic Antioxidant and Anti-Inflammatory Effects between Modified Citrus Pectin and Honokiol. Evid Based Complement Alternat Med. 2017;2017:8379843. doi: 10.1155/2017/8379843.

Ramadan R, Tawdy A, Abdel Hay R, Rashed L, Tawfik D. The antioxidant role of paraoxonase 1 and vitamin E in three autoimmune diseases. Skin Pharmacol Physiol. 2013;26(1):2-7. doi: 10.1159/000342124.

Ramírez-Expósito MJ, Sánchez-López E, Cueto-Ureña C, Dueñas B, Carrera-González P, Navarro-Cecilia J, Mayas MD, Arias de Saavedra JM, Sánchez-Agesta R, Martínez-Martos JM. Circulating oxidative stress parameters in pre- and post-menopausal healthy women and in women suffering from breast cancer treated or not with neoadjuvant chemotherapy. Exp Gerontol. 2014 Jul 11. pii: S0531-5565(14)00211-3. doi: 10.1016/j.exger.2014.07.006.

Ramírez-Garza SL, Laveriano-Santos EP, Marhuenda-Muñoz M, et al. Health Effects of Resveratrol: Results from Human Intervention Trials. Nutrients. 2018;10(12):1892. Published 2018 Dec 3. doi:10.3390/nu10121892

Ramprasath VR, Awad AB. Role of Phytosterols in Cancer Prevention and Treatment. J AOAC Int. 2015 May-Jun;98(3):735-8. doi: 10.5740/jaoacint.SGERamprasath.

Rampton DS, Murdoch RD, Sladen GE. Rectal mucosal histamine release in ulcerative colitis. Clin Sci (Lond). 1980 Nov;59(5):389-91.

Rancé F, Kanny G, Dutau G, Moneret-Vautrin DA. Food allergens in children. Arch Pediatr. 1999;6(Suppl 1):61S-66S.

Rangavajhyala N, Shahani KM, Sridevi G, Srikumaran S. Nonlipopolysaccharide component(s) of Lactobacillus acidophilus stimulate(s) the production of interleukin-1 alpha and tumor necrosis factor-alpha by murine macrophages. Nutr Cancer. 1997;28(2):130-4.

Ranilla LG, Genovese MI, Lajolo FM. Polyphenols and antioxidant capacity of seed coat and cotyledon from Brazilian and Peruvian bean cultivars (Phaseolus vulgaris L.). J Agric Food Chem. 2007 Jan 10;55(1):90-8.

Ranjbaran Z, Keefer L, Stepanski E, Farhadi A, Keshavarzian A. The relevance of sleep abnormalities to chronic inflammatory conditions. Inflamm Res. 2007 Feb;56(2):51-7.

Rao S, Shenoy SD, Davis S, Nayak S. Detection of formaldehyde in textiles by chromotropic acid method. Indian Journal of Dermatology, Venereology and Leprology 70(6). 2004 Nov.

Rao SK, Rao PS, Rao BN. Preliminary investigation of the radiosensitizing activity of guduchi (Tinospora cordifolia) in tumor-bearing mice. Phytother Res. 2008 Nov;22(11):1482-9.

Rapin JR, Wiernsperger N. Possible links between intestinal permeablity and food processing: A potential therapeutic niche for glutamine. Clinics (Sao Paulo). 2010 Jun;65(6):635-43.

Rappoport J. Both sides of the pharmaceutical death coin. Townsend Letter for Doctors and Patients. 2006 Oct.

Rauha JP, Remes S, Heinonen M, Hopia A, Kähkönen M, Kujala T, Pihlaja K, Vuorela H, Vuorela P. Antimicrobial effects of Finnish plant extracts containing flavonoids and other phenolic compounds. Int J Food Microbiol. 2000 May 25;56(1):3-12.

Rauma A. Antioxidant status in vegetarians versus omnivores. Nutrition. 2003;16(2): 111-119.

Rautava S, Salminen S, Isolauri E. Specific probiotics in reducing the risk of acute infections in infancy—a randomised, double-blind, placebo-controlled study. Br J Nutr. 2009 Jun;101(11):1722-6.

Ravindra T, Lakshmi NK, Ahuja YR. Melatonin in pathogenesis and therapy of cancer. Indian J Med Sci. 2006 Dec;60(12):523-35.

Rayes N, Seehofer D, Hansen S, Boucsein K, Müller AR, Serke S, Bengmark S, Neuhaus P. Early enteral supply of lactobacillus and fiber versus selective bowel decontamination: a controlled trial in liver transplant recipients. Transplantation. 2002 Jul 15;74(1):123-7.

Rayes N, Seehofer D, Müller AR, Hansen S, Bengmark S, Neuhaus P. Influence of probiotics and fibre on the incidence of bacterial infections following major abdominal surgery - results of a prospective trial. Z Gastroenterol. 2002 Oct;40(10):869-76.

Raza S, Graham SM, Allen SJ, Sultana S, Cuevas L, Hart CA, Kaila M, Isolauri E, Saxelin M, Arvilommi H, et al. Lactobacillus GG in acute diarrhea. Indian Pediatr. 1995 Oct;32(10):1140-2.

Regel SJ, Negovetic S, Roosli M, Berdinas V, Schuderer J, Huss A, et al. UMTS base station-like exposure, well-being, and cognitive performance. Environ Health Perspect. 2006 Aug;114(8):1270-5.

Reger D, Goode S, Mercer E. Chemistry: Principles & Practice. Fort Worth, TX: Harcourt Brace, 1993.

Regis E. Virus Ground Zero. New York: Pocket, 1996.

Reha CM, Ebru A. Specific immunotherapy is effective in the prevention of new sensitivities. Allergol Immunopathol (Madr). 2007 Mar-Apr;35(2):44-51.

Rehm J, Taylor B, Mohapatra S, Irving H, Baliunas D, Patra J, Roerecke M. Alcohol as a risk factor for liver cirrhosis: a systematic review and meta-analysis. Drug Alcohol Rev. 2010 Jul;29(4):437-45.

Reichrath J. The challenge resulting from positive and negative effects of sunlight: how much solar UV exposure is appropriate to balance between risks of vitamin D deficiency and skin cancer? Prog Biophys Mol Biol. 2006 Sep;92(1):9-16.

Reichrath J. The challenge resulting from positive and negative effects of sunlight: how much solar UV exposure is appropriate to balance between risks of vitamin D deficiency and skin cancer? Prog Biophys Mol Biol. 2006 Sep;92(1):9-16.

Reid G, Beuerman D, Heinemann C, Bruce AW. Probiotic Lactobacillus dose required to restore and maintain a normal vaginal flora. FEMS Immunol Med Microbiol. 2001 Dec;32(1):37-41.

Reid G, Burton J, Hammond JA, Bruce AW. Nucleic acid-based diagnosis of bacterial vaginosis and improved management using probiotic lactobacilli. J Med Food. 2004 Summer;7(2):223-8.

Reid G, Charbonneau D, Erb J, Kochanowski B, Beuerman D, Poehner R, Bruce AW. Oral use of Lactobacillus rhamnosus GR-1 and L. fermentum RC-14 significantly alters vaginal flora: randomized, placebo-controlled trial in 64 healthy women. FEMS Immunol Med Microbiol. 2003 Mar 20;35(2):131-4.

Reid IR, Bolland MJ, Grey A. Effects of vitamin D supplements on bone mineral density: a systematic review and meta-analysis. Lancet. 2014 Jan 11;383(9912):146-55. doi: 10.1016/S0140-6736(13)61647-5.

Reiffenberger DH, Amundson LH. Fibromyalgia syndrome: a review. Am Fam Physician. 1996;53:1698-704.

Reilly T, Stevenson I. An investigation of the effects of negative air ions on responses to submaximal exercise at different times of day. J Hum Ergol. 1993 Jun;22(1):1-9.

Reilly T, Stevenson I. An investigation of the effects of negative air ions on responses to submaximal exercise at different times of day. J Hum Ergol. 1993 Jun;22(1):1-9.

Reis CE, Ribeiro DN, Costa NM, Bressan J, Alfenas RC, Mattes RD. Acute and second-meal effects of peanuts on glycaemic response and appetite in obese women with high type 2 diabetes risk: a randomised cross-over clinical trial. Br J Nutr. 2013 Jun;109(11):2015-23. doi: 10.1017/S0007114512004217.

Reiter RJ, Garcia JJ, Pie J. Oxidative toxicity in models of neurodegeneration: responses to melatonin. Restor Neurol Neurosci. 1998 Jun;12(2-3):135-42.

Reiter RJ, Tan DX, Korkmaz A, Erren TC, Piekarski C, Tamura H, Manchester LC. Light at night, chronodisruption, melatonin suppression, and cancer risk: a review. Crit Rev Oncog. 2007;13(4):303-28.

Reiter RJ, Tan DX, Manchester LC, Qi W. Biochemical reactivity of melatonin with reactive oxygen and nitrogen species: a review of the evidence. Cell Biochem Biophys. 2001;34(2):237-56.

Renkonen R, Renkonen J, Joenväärä S, Mattila P, Parviainen V, Toppila-Salmi S. Allergens are transported through the respiratory epithelium. Expert Rev Clin Immunol. 2010 Jan;6(1):55-9.

Renvert S, Lindahl C, Renvert H, Persson GR. Clinical and microbiological analysis of subjects treated with Brånemark or AstraTech implants: a 7-year follow-up study. Clin Oral Implants Res. 2008 Apr;19(4):342-7.

Retallack D. The Sound of Music and Plants. Marina Del Rey, CA: Devorss, 1973.

Reznik M, Sharif I, Ozuah PO. Rubbing ointments and asthma morbidity in adolescents. J Altern Complement Med. 2004 Dec;10(6):1097-9. Uu

Riccia DN, Bizzini F, Perilli MG, Polimeni A, Trinchieri V, Amicosante G, Cifone MG. Anti-inflammatory effects of Lactobacillus brevis (CD2) on periodontal disease. Oral Dis. 2007 Jul;13(4):376-85.

Riccioni G, D'Orazio N. The role of selenium, zinc and antioxidant vitamin supplementation in the treatment of bronchial asthma: adjuvant therapy or not? Expert Opin Investig Drugs. 2005 Sep;14(9):1145-55.

Richards DG, McMillin DL, Mein EA, Nelson CD. Colonic irrigations: a review of the historical controversy and the potential for adverse effects. J Altern Complement Med. 2006 May;12(4):389-93. '

Rimkiene S, Ragazinskiene O, Savickiene N. The cumulation of Wild pansy (Viola tricolor L.) accessions: the possibility of species preservation and usage in medicine. Medicina (Kaunas). 2003;39(4):411-6.

Rinne M, Kalliomaki M, Arvilommi H, Salminen S, Isolauri E. Effect of probiotics and breastfeeding on the bifidobacterium and lactobacillus/enterococcus microbiota and humoral immune responses. J Pediatr. 2005 Aug;147(2):186-91.

Rinne M, Kalliomaki M, Arvilommi H, Salminen S, Isolauri E. Effect of probiotics and breastfeeding on the bifidobacterium and lactobacillus/enterococcus microbiota and humoral immune responses. J Pediatr. 2005 Aug;147(2):186-91.

Rinne M, Kalliomäki M, Salminen S, Isolauri E. Probiotic intervention in the first months of life: short-term effects on gastrointestinal symptoms and long-term effects on gut microbiota. J Pediatr Gastroenterol Nutr. 2006 Aug;43(2):200-5.

Río ME, Zago Beatriz L, Garcia H, Winter L. The nutritional status change the effectiveness of a dietary supplement of lactic bacteria on the emerging of respiratory tract diseases in children. Arch Latinoam Nutr. 2002 Mar;52(1):29-34.

Riza E, Linos A, Petralias A, de Martinis L, Duntas L, Linos D. The effect of Greek herbal tea consumption on thyroid cancer: a case-control study. Eur J Public Health. 2015 Apr 4. pii: ckv063.

Rizzello CG, Mueller T, Coda R, Reipsch F, Nionelli L, Curiel JA, Gobbetti M. Synthesis of 2-methoxy benzoquinone and 2,6-dimethoxybenzoquinone by selected lactic acid bacteria during sourdough fermentation of wheat germ. Microb Cell Fact. 2013 Nov 11;12(1):105.

Rizzi M, Cravello B, Renò F. Textile industry manufacturing by-products induce human melanoma cell proliferation via ERK1/2 activation. Cell Prolif. 2014 Dec;47(6):578-86. doi: 10.1111/cpr.12132.

Robbins KS, Shin EC, Shewfelt RL, Eitenmiller RR, Pegg RB. Update on the Healthful Lipid Constituents of Tree Nuts. J Agric Food Chem. 2011 Oct 27.

Robert AM, Groult N, Six C, Robert L. The effect of procyanidolic oligomers on mesenchymal cells in culture II-Attachment of elastic fibers to the cells. Pathol Biol. 1990 Jun;38(6):601-7.

Robert AM, Robert L, Renard G. Protection of cornea against proteolytic damage. Experimental study of procyanidolic oligomers (PCO) on bovine cornea. J Fr Ophtalmol. 2002 Apr;25(4):351-5.

Robert AM, Tixier JM, Robert L, Legeais JM, Renard G. Effect of procyanidolic oligomers on the permeability of the blood-brain barrier. Pathol Biol. 2001 May;49(4):298-304.

Roberts JE. Light and immunomodulation. Ann N Y Acad Sci. 2000;917:435-45.

Robilliard DL, Archer SN, Arendt J, Lockley SW, Hack LM, English J, Leger D, Smits MG, Williams A, Skene DJ, Von Schantz M. The 3111 Clock gene polymorphism is not associated with sleep and circadian rhythmicity in phenotypically characterized human subjects. J Sleep Res. 2002 Dec;11(4):305-12.

Robinson L, Cherewatenko VS, Reeves S. Epicor: The Key to a Balanced Immune System. Sherman Oaks, CA: Health Point, 2009.

Robinson TN. Television viewing and childhood obesity. Pediatr Clin North Am. 2001 Aug;48(4):1017-25.

Rock CL, Flatt SW, Pakiz B, Quintana EL, Heath DD, Rana BK, Natarajan L. Effects of diet composition on weight loss, metabolic factors and biomarkers in a 1-year weight loss intervention in obese women examined by baseline insulin resistance status. Metabolism. 2016 Nov;65(11):1605-1613. doi: 10.1016/j.metabol.2016.07.008.

Rodermel SR, Smith-Sonneborn J. Age-correlated changes in expression of micronuclear damage and repair in Paramecium tetraurelia. Genetics. 1977 Oct;87(2):259-74.

Rodgers JT, Puigserver P. Fasting-dependent glucose and lipid metabolic response through hepatic sirtuin 1. Proc Natl Acad Sci USA. 2007 Jul 31;104(31):12861-6.

Rodgers KM, Udesky JO, Rudel RA, Brody JG. Environmental chemicals and breast cancer: An updated review of epidemiological literature informed by biological mechanisms. Environ Res. 2018;160:152-182. doi:10.1016/j.envres.2017.08.045

Rodrigues C, Milkovic L, Bujak IT, Tomljanovic M, Soveral G, Cipak Gasparovic A. Lipid Profile and Aquaporin Expression under Oxidative Stress in Breast cancer Cells of Different Malignancies. Oxid Med Cell Longev. 2019;2019:2061830. Published 2019 Jul 11. doi:10.1155/2019/2061830

Rodriguez E, Valbuena MC, Rey M, Porras de Quintana L. Causal agents of photoallergic contact dermatitis diagnosed in the national institute of dermatology of Colombia. Photodermatol Photoimmunol Photomed. 2006 Aug;22(4):189-92.

Rodriguez-Fragoso L, Reyes-Esparza J, Burchiel SW, Herrera-Ruiz D, Torres E. Risks and benefits of commonly used herbal medicines in Mexico. Toxicol Appl Pharmacol. 2008 Feb 15;227(1):125-35.

Rodríguez-Sánchez D, Silva-Platas C, Rojo RP, García N, Cisneros-Zevallos L, García-Rivas G, Hernández-Brenes C. Activity-guided identification of acetogenins as novel lipophilic antioxidants present in avocado pulp (Persea americana). J Chromatogr B Analyt Technol Biomed Life Sci. 2013 Oct 18;942-943C:37-45. doi:10.1016/j.jchromb.2013.10.013.

Roduit C, Scholtens S, de Jongste JC, Wijga AH, Gerritsen J, Postma DS, Brunekreef B, Hoekstra MO, Aalberse R, Smit HA. Asthma at 8 years of age in children born by caesarean section. Thorax. 2009 Feb;64(2):107-13.

Rohrmann S, Lukas Jung SU, Linseisen J, Pfau W. Dietary intake of meat and meat-derived heterocyclic aromatic amines and breast tissue DNA adducts. Mutagenesis. 2009 Mar;24(2):127-32. doi: 10.1093/mutage/gen058.

Roller M, Clune Y, Collins K, Rechkemmer G, Watzl B. Consumption of prebiotic inulin enriched with oligofructose in combination with the probiotics Lactobacillus rhamnosus and Bifidobacterium lactis has minor effects on selected immune parameters in polypectomised and colon cancer patients. Br J Nutr. 2007 Apr;97(4):676-84.

Rollier A. Le Pansement Solaire. Paris: Payot, 1916.

Rollison DE, Iannacone MR, Messina JL, Glass LF, Giuliano AR, Roetzheim RG, Cherpelis BS, Fenske NA, Jonathan KA, Sondak VK. Case-control study of smoking and non-melanoma skin cancer. Cancer Causes Control. 2011 Nov 19.

Romeo J, Wärnberg J, Nova E, Díaz LE, González-Gross M, Marcos A. Changes in the immune system after moderate beer consumption. Ann Nutr Metab. 2007;51(4):359-66.

Romieu I, Barraza-Villarreal A, Escamilla-Núñez C, Texcalac-Sangrador JL, Hernandez-Cadena L, Díaz-Sánchez D, De Batlle J, Del Rio-Navarro BE. Dietary intake, lung function and airway inflammation in Mexico City school children exposed to air pollutants. Respir Res. 2009 Dec 10;10:122.

Roncero-Ramos I, Mendiola-Lanao M, Pérez-Clavijo M, Delgado-Andrade C. Effect of different cooking methods on nutritional value and antioxidant activity of cultivated mushrooms. Int J Food Sci Nutr. 2017 May;68(3):287-297. doi: 10.1080/09637486.2016.1244662.

Rook GA, Hernandez-Pando R. Pathogenetic role, in human and murine tuberculosis, of changes in the peripheral metabolism of glucocorticoids and antiglucocorticoids. Psychoneuroendocrinology. 1997;22 Suppl 1:S109-13.

Ros E, Mataix J. Fatty acid composition of nuts—implications for cardiovascular health. Br J Nutr. 2006 Nov;96 Suppl 2:S29-35.

Ros E. Health benefits of nut consumption. Nutrients. 2010 Jul;2(7):652-82. doi: 10.3390/nu2070683.

Rosander A, Connolly E, Roos S. Removal of antibiotic resistance gene-carrying plasmids from Lactobacillus reuteri ATCC 55730 and characterization of the resulting daughter strain, L. reuteri DSM 17938. Appl Environ Microbiol. 2008 Oct;74(19):6032-40.

Rosenfeldt V, Benfeldt E, Valerius NH, Paerregaard A, Michaelsen KF. Effect of probiotics on gastrointestinal symptoms and small intestinal permeability in children with atopic dermatitis. J Pediatr. 2004 Nov;145(5):612-6.

Rosenfeldt V, Michaelsen KF, Jakobsen M, Larsen CN, Møller PL, Pedersen P, Tvede M, Weyrehter H, Valerius NH, Paerregaard A. Effect of probiotic Lactobacillus strains in young children hospitalized with acute diarrhea. Pediatr Infect Dis J. 2002 May;21(5):411-6.

Rosenkranz SK, Swain KE, Rosenkranz RR, Beckman B, Harms CA. Modifiable lifestyle factors impact airway health in non-asthmatic prepubescent boys but not girls. Pediatr Pulmonol. 2010 Dec 30.

Rosenlund H, Bergström A, Alm JS, Swartz J, Scheynius A, van Hage M, Johansen K, Brunekreef B, von Mutius E, Ege MJ, Riedler J, Braun-Fahrländer C, Waser M, Pershagen G; PARSIFAL Study Group. Allergic disease and atopic sensitization in children in relation to measles vaccination and measles infection. Pediatrics. 2009 Mar;123(3):771-8.

Rosenthal N, Blehar M (Eds.). Seasonal affective disorders and phototherapy. New York: Guildford Press, 1989.

Rosenthal N, Blehar M. Seasonal affective disorders and phototherapy. New York: Guildford Press, 1989.

Rossouw JE, Prentice RL, Manson JE, Wu L, Barad D, Barnabei VM, Ko M, LaCroix AZ, Margolis KL, Stefanick ML. Postmenopausal hormone therapy and risk of cardiovascular disease by age and years since menopause. JAMA. 2007 Apr 4;297(13):1465-77.

Rostand SG. Ultraviolet light may contribute to geographic and racial blood pressure differences. Hypertension. 1997 Aug;30(2 Pt 1):150-6.

Rostand SG. Ultraviolet light may contribute to geographic and racial blood pressure differences. Hypertension. 1997 Aug;30(2 Pt 1):150-6.

Rousseaux C, Thuru X, Gelot A, Barnich N, Neut C, Dubuquoy L, Dubuquoy C, Merour E, Geboes K, Chamaillard M, Ouwehand A, Leyer G, Carcano D, Colombel JF, Ardid D, Desreumaux P. Lactobacillus acidophilus modulates intestinal pain and induces opioid and cannabinoid receptors. Nat Med. 2007 Jan;13(1):35-7

Routasalo P, Isola A. The right to touch and be touched. Nurs Ethics. 1996 Jun;3(2):165-76.

Rowe A, Ramzan I. Are mould hepatotoxins responsible for kava hepatotoxicity? Phytother Res. 2012 Nov;26(11):1768-70. doi: 10.1002/ptr.4620.

Roy M, Kirschbaum C, Steptoe A. Intraindividual variation in recent stress exposure as a moderator of cortisol and testosterone levels. Ann Behav Med. 2003 Dec;26(3):194-200.

Royal Society of Canada A Review of the Potential Health Risks of Radiofrequency Fields from Wireless Telecommunica-tion Devices. Ottawa, Ontario: Royal Society of Canada. 1999.

Roybal K, Theobold D, Graham A, DiNieri JA, Russo SJ, Krishnan V, Chakravarty S, Peevey J, Oehrlein N, Birnbaum S, Vitaterna MH, Orsulak P, Takahashi JS, Nestler EJ, Carlezon WA Jr, McClung CA. Mania-like behavior induced by disruption of CLOCK. Proc Natl Acad Sci USA 2007;104(15):6406-6411.

Royer RJ, Schmidt CL. Evaluation of venotropic drugs by venous gas plethysmography. A study of procyanidolic oligomers Sem Hop. 1981 Dec 18-25;57(47-48):2009-13.

Rozycki VR, Baigorria CM, Freyre MR, Bernard CM, Zannier MS, Charpentier M. Nutrient content in vegetable species from the Argentine Chaco. Arch Latinoam Nutr. 1997 Sep;47(3):265-70.

Ruan H, Zhan YY, Hou J, Xu B, Chen B, Tian Y, Wu D, Zhao Y, Zhang Y, Chen X, Mi P, Zhang L, Zhang S, Wang X, Cao H, Zhang W, Wang H, Li H, Su Y, Zhang XK, Hu T. Berberine binds RXRα to suppress β-catenin signaling in colon cancer cells. Oncogene. 2017 Dec 14;36(50):6906-6918. doi: 10.1038/onc.2017.296.

Rubin E., Farber JL. Pathology. 3rd Ed. Philadelphia: Lippincott-Raven, 1999.

Rubin GJ, Hahn G, Everitt BS, Cleare AJ, Wessely S. Are some people sensitive to mobile phone signals? Within participants double blind randomised provocation study. BMJ. 2006 Apr 15;332(7546):886-91.

Rudel RA, Attfield KR, Schifano JN, Brody JG. Chemicals causing mammary gland tumors in animals signal new directions for epidemiology, chemicals testing, and risk assessment for breast cancer prevention. Cancer. 2007;109(12 Suppl):2635-2666. doi:10.1002/cncr.22653

Russ MJ, Clark WC, Cross LW, Kemperman I, Kakuma T, Harrison K. Pain and self-injury in borderline patients: sensory decision theory, coping strategies, and locus of control. Psychiatry Res. 1996 Jun 26;63(1):57-65.

Russell IJ. Advances in fibromyalgia: possible role for central neurochemicals. Am J Med Sci. 1998;315:377-84.

Russo PA, Halliday GM. Inhibition of nitric oxide and reactive oxygen species production improves the ability of a sunscreen to protect from sunburn, immunosuppression and photocarcinogenesis. Br J Dermatol. 2006 Aug;155(2):408-15.

Rynard PB, Palij B, Galloway CA, Roughley FR. Resperin inhalation treatment for chronic respiratory diseases. Can Fam Physician. 1968 Oct;14(10):70-1.

Rzeski W, Stepulak A, Szymański M, Sifringer M, Kaczor J, Wejksza K, Zdzisińska B, Kandefer-Szerszeń M. Betulinic acid decreases expression of bcl-2 and cyclin D1, inhibits proliferation, migration and induces apoptosis in cancer cells. Naunyn Schmiedebergs Arch Pharmacol. 2006 Oct;374(1):11-20.

Saarijarvi S, Lauerma H, Helenius H, Saarilehto S. Seasonal affective disorders among rural Finns and Lapps. Acta Psychiatr Scand. 1999 Feb;99(2):95-101.

Saavedra JM, Abi-Hanna A, Moore N, Yolken RH. Long-term consumption of infant formulas containing live probiotic bacteria: tolerance and safety. Am J Clin Nutr. 2004 Feb;79(2):261-7.

Saavedra JM, Bauman NA, Oung I, Perman JA, Yolken RH. Feeding of Bifidobacterium bifidum and Streptococcus thermophilus to infants in hospital for prevention of diarrhoea and shedding of rotavirus. Lancet. 1994 Oct 15;344(8929):1046-9.

Sabeena Farvin KH, Jacobsen C. Phenolic compounds and antioxidant activities of selected species of seaweeds from Danish coast. Food Chem. 2013 Jun 1;138(2-3):1670-81.

Saggioro A. Probiotics in the treatment of irritable bowel syndrome. J Clin Gastroenterol. 2004 Jul;38(6 Suppl):S104-6.

Sahagún-Flores JE, López-Peña LS, de la Cruz-Ramírez Jaimes J, García-Bravo MS, Peregrina-Gómez R, de Alba-García JE. Eradication of Helicobacter pylori: triple treatment scheme plus Lactobacillus vs. triple treatment alone. Cir Cir. 2007 Sep-Oct;75(5):333-6.

Sahakian NM, White SK, Park JH, Cox-Ganser JM, Kreiss K. Identification of mold and dampness-associated respiratory morbidity in 2 schools: comparison of questionnaire survey responses to national data. J Sch Health. 2008 Jan;78(1):32-7.

Sahar S, Sassone-Corsi P. Circadian clock and breast cancer: a molecular link. Cell Cycle. 2007 Jun 1;6(11):1329-31.

Sahin-Yilmaz A, Nocon CC, Corey JP. Immunoglobulin E-mediated food allergies among adults with allergic rhinitis. Otolaryngol Head Neck Surg. 2010 Sep;143(3):379-85.

Sahu N, Meena S, Shukla V, Chaturvedi P, Kumar B, Datta D, Arya KR. Extraction, fractionation and re-fractionation of Artemisia nilagirica for anticancer activity and HPLC-ESI-QTOF-MS/MS determination. J Ethnopharmacol. 2017 Nov 3. pii: S0378-8741(17)32820-9. doi: 10.1016/j.jep.2017.10.029.

Saini M, Goyal PK, Chaudhary G. Anti-tumor activity of Aloe vera against DMBA/croton oil-induced skin papillomagenesis in Swiss albino mice. J Environ Pathol Toxicol Oncol. 2010;29(2):127-35.

Sainte-Laudy J, Belon P. Analysis of immunosuppressive activity of serial dilutions of histamine on human basophil activation by flow cytometry. Inflam Rsrch. 1996 Suppl. 1: S33-S34.

Saito T, Abe D, Nogata Y. Polymethoxylated flavones potentiate the cytolytic activity of NK leukemia cell line KHYG-1 via enhanced expression of granzyme B. Biochem Biophys Res Commun. 2015 Jan 16;456(3):799-803. doi: 10.1016/j.bbrc.2014.12.027.

Saito Y, Ito S, Koltunow AM, Sakai H. Crystallization and preliminary X-ray analysis of geraniol dehydrogenase from Backhousia citriodora (lemon myrtle). Acta Crystallogr Sect F Struct Biol Cryst Commun. 2011 Jun 1;67(Pt 6):665-7.

Sakai T, Eskander RN, Guo Y, Kim KJ, Mefford J, Hopkins J, Bhatia NN, Zi X, Hoang BH. Flavokawain B, a kava chalcone, induces apoptosis in synovial sarcoma cell lines. J Orthop Res. 2012 Jul;30(7):1045-50. doi: 10.1002/jor.22050.

Sakao K, Vyas AR, Chinni S, Amjad AI, Parikh R, Singh SV. CXCR4 Is a Novel Target of Cancer Chemo-preventative Isothiocyanates in Prostate Cancer Cells. Cancer Prev Res (Phila). 2015 Feb 23. pii: can-prevres.0386.2014.

Sakhi AK, Russnes KM, Thoresen M, Bastani NE, Karlsen A, Smeland S, Blomhoff R. Pre-radiotherapy plasma carotenoids and markers of oxidative stress are associated with survival in head and neck squamous cell carcinoma patients: a prospective study. BMC Cancer. 2009 Dec 21;9:458. doi: 10.1186/1471-2407-9-458.

Sakulnarmrat K, Fenech M, Thomas P, Konczak I. Cytoprotective and pro-apoptotic activities of native Australian herbs polyphenolic-rich extracts. Food Chem. 2013 Jan 1;136(1):9-17. doi: 10.1016/j.foodchem.2012.07.089.

Salama OE, Naga RM. Cellular phones: are they detrimental? J Egypt Pub Hlth. 2004;79(3-4):197-223.

Salazar-Lindo E, Figueroa-Quintanilla D, Caciano MI, Reto-Valiente V, Chauviere G, Colin P; Lacteol Study Group. Effectiveness and safety of Lactobacillus LB in the treatment of mild acute diarrhea in children. J Pediatr Gastroenterol Nutr. 2007 May;44(5):571-6.

Salazar-Lindo E, Miranda-Langschwager P, Campos-Sanchez M, Chea-Woo E, Sack RB. Lactobacillus casei strain GG in the treatment of infants with acute watery diarrhea: a randomized, double-blind, placebo controlled clinical trial [ISRCTN67363048]. BMC Pediatr. 2004 Sep 2;4:18.

Salem N, Wegher B, Mena P, Uauy R. Arachidonic and docosahexaenoic acids are biosynthesized from their 18-carbon precursors in human infants. Proc Natl Acad Sci. 1996;93:49-54.

Salford LG, Brun AE, Eberhardt JL, Malmgren L, Persson BR. Nerve cell damage in mammalian brain after exposure to microwaves from GSM mobile phones. Environ Health Perspect. 2003 Jun;111(7):881-3; dis-cussion A408.

Salim AS. Sulfhydryl-containing agents in the treatment of gastric bleeding induced by nonsteroidal anti-inflammatory drugs. Can J Surg. 1993 Feb;36(1):53-8.

Salminen E, Elomaa I, Minkkinen J, Vapaatalo H, Salminen S. Preservation of intestinal integrity during radiotherapy using live Lactobacillus acidophilus cultures. Clin Radiol. 1988 Jul;39(4):435-7.

Salminen S, Isolauri E, Salminen E. Clinical uses of probiotics for stabilizing the gut mucosal barrier: successful strains and future challenges. Antonie Van Leeuwenhoek. 1996 Oct;70(2-4):347-58.

Salom IL, Silvis SE, Doscherholmen A. Effect of cimetidine on the absorption of vitamin B12. Scand J Gastroenterol. 1982;17:129-31.

Salvi SS, Barnes PJ. Chronic obstructive pulmonary disease in non-smokers. Lancet. 2009 Aug 29;374(9691):733-43.

Samanta M, Sarkar M, Ghosh P, Ghosh J, Sinha M, Chatterjee S. Prophylactic probiotics for prevention of necrotizing enterocolitis in very low birth weight newborns. J Trop Pediatr. 2009 Apr;55(2):128-31.

Sarah Janssen S, Solomon G, Schettler T. Chemical Contaminants and Human Disease: A Summary of Evidence. The Collaborative on Health and the Environment. healthandenvironment.org. Acc. 2020 Jul.

Saran S, Gopalan S, Krishna TP. Use of fermented foods to combat stunting and failure to thrive. Nutrition. 2002 May;18(5):393-6.

Saran, S., Gopalan, S. and Krishna, T. P. Use of fermented foods to combat stunting and failure to thrive. Nutrition. 2002;8:393-396.

Sarris J, Kavanagh DJ, Adams J, Bone K, Byrne G. Kava Anxiety Depression Spectrum Study (KADSS): a mixed methods RCT using an aqueous extract of Piper methysticum. Complement Ther Med. 2009 Jun;17(3):176-8. doi: 10.1016/j.ctim.2009.01.001.

Sarris J, Kavanagh DJ, Byrne G, Bone KM, Adams J, Deed G. The Kava Anxiety Depression Spectrum Study (KADSS): a randomized, placebo-controlled crossover trial using an aqueous extract of Piper methysticum. Psychopharmacology (Berl). 2009 Aug;205(3):399-407. doi: 10.1007/s00213-009-1549-9.

Sarris J, LaPorte E, Schweitzer I. Kava: a comprehensive review of efficacy, safety, and psychopharmacology. Aust N Z J Psychiatry. 2011 Jan;45(1):27-35. doi: 10.3109/00048674.2010.522554.

Sarris J, Scholey A, Schweitzer I, Bousman C, Laporte E, Ng C, Murray G, Stough C. The acute effects of kava and oxazepam on anxiety, mood, neurocognition; and genetic correlates: a randomized, placebo-controlled, double-blind study. Hum Psychopharmacol. 2012 May;27(3):262-9. doi: 10.1002/hup.2216.

Sarveiya V, Risk S, Benson HA. Liquid chromatographic assay for common sunscreen agents: application to in vivo assessment of skin penetration and systemic absorption in human volunteers. J Chromatogr B Analyt Technol Biomed Life Sci. 2004 Apr 25;803(2):225-31.

Sato TK, Yamada RG, Ukai H, Baggs JE, Miraglia LJ, Kobayashi TJ, Welsh DK, Kay SA, Ueda HR, Hogenesch JB. Feedback repression is required for mammalian circadian clock function. Nat Genet. 2006 Mar;38(3):312-9.

Satyanarayana S, Sushruta K, Sarma GS, Srinivas N, Subba Raju GV. Antioxidant activity of the aqueous extracts of spicy food additives – evaluation and comparison with ascorbic acid in in-vitro systems. J Herb Pharmacother. 2004;4(2):1-10.

Savino F, Pelle E, Palumeri E, Oggero R, Miniero R. Lactobacillus reuteri (American Type Culture Collection Strain 55730) versus simethicone in the treatment of infantile colic: a prospective randomized study. Pediatrics. 2007 Jan;119(1):e124-30.

Savitz DA. Epidemiologic studies of electric and magnetic fields and cancer: strategies for extending knowledge. Environ Health Perspect. 1993 Dec;101 Suppl 4:83-91.

Sazanova NE, Varnacheva LN, Novikova AV, Pletneva NB. Immunological aspects of food intolerance in children during first years of life. Pediatriia. 1992;(3):14-8.

Scadding G, Bjarnason I, Brostoff J, Levi AJ, Peters TJ. Intestinal permeability to 51Cr-labelled ethylenediaminetetraacetate in food-intolerant subjects. Digestion. 1989;42(2):104-9.

Scalabrin DM, Johnston WH, Hoffman DR, P'Pool VL, Harris CL, Mitmesser SH. Growth and tolerance of healthy term infants receiving hydrolyzed infant formulas supplemented with Lactobacillus rhamnosus GG: randomized, double-blind, controlled trial. Clin Pediatr (Phila). 2009 Sep;48(7):734-44.

Schaafsma G, Meuling WJ, van Dokkum W, Bouley C. Effects of a milk product, fermented by Lactobacillus acidophilus and with fructo-oligosaccharides added, on blood lipids in male volunteers. Eur J Clin Nutr. 1998 Jun;52(6):436-40.

Schäfer A, Kratky KW. The effect of colored illumination on heart rate variability. Forsch Komplementmed. 2006 Jun;13(3):167-73.

Schauenberg P, Paris F. Guide to Medicinal Plants. New Canaan, CT: Keats Publ, 1977.

Schauss AG, Wu X, Prior RL, Ou B, Huang D, Owens J, Agarwal A, Jensen GS, Hart AN, Shanbrom E. Antioxidant capacity and other bioactivities of the freeze-dried Amazonian palm berry, Euterpe oleraceae mart. (acai). J Agric Food Chem. 2006 Nov 1;54(22):8604-10.

Schempp H, Weiser D, Elstner EF. Biochemical model reactions indicative of inflammatory processes. Activities of extracts from Fraxinus excelsior and Populus tremula. Arzneimittelforschung. 2000 Apr;50(4):362-72.

Schiffrin EJ, Brassart D, Servin AL, Rochat F, Donnet-Hughes A. Immune modulation of blood leukocytes in humans by lactic acid bacteria: criteria for strain selection. Am J Clin Nutr. 1997 Aug;66(2):515S-520S.

Schillaci D, Arizza V, Dayton T, Camarda L, Di Stefano V. In vitro anti-biofilm activity of Boswellia spp. oleogum resin essential oils. Lett Appl Microbiol. 2008 Nov;47(5):433-8.

Schirber M. Earth as a Giant Pinball Machine. LiveScience. 2004; 19 Nov 19. http://www.livescience.com/ environment/041119_earth_layers.html. Acc. 2006 Nov.

Schirmacher A, Winters S, Fischer S, Goeke J, Galla HJ, Kullnick U, Ringelstein EB, Stögbauer F. Electromagnetic fields (1.8 GHz) increase the permeability to sucrose of the blood-brain barrier in vitro. Bioelectromagnetics. 2000 Jul;21(5):338-45.

Schlebusch KP, Maric-Oehler W, Popp FA. Biophotonics in the infrared spectral range reveal acupuncture meridian structure of the body. J Altern Complement Med. 2005 Feb;11(1):171-3.

Schlörmann W, Lamberty J, Lorkowski S, Ludwig D, Mothes H, Saupe C, Glei M. Chemopreventive potential of in vitro fermented nuts in LT97 colon adenoma and primary epithelial colon cells. Mol Carcinog. 2017 May;56(5):1461-1471. doi: 10.1002/mc.22606.

Schlumpf M, Cotton B, Conscience M, Haller V, Steinmann B, Lichtensteiger W. In vitro and in vivo estrogenicity of UV screens. Environ Health Perspect. 2001 Mar;109(3):239-44.

Schmid B, Kötter I, Heide L. Pharmacokinetics of salicin after oral administration of a standardised willow bark extract. Eur J Clin Pharmacol. 2001 Aug;57(5):387-91.

Schmidt C, Collette F, Cajochen C, Peigneux P. A time to think: circadian rhythms in human cognition. Cogn Neuropsychol. 2007 Oct;24(7):755-89.

Schmidt H, Quantum processes predicted? New Sci. 1969 Oct 16.

Schmitt B, Frölich L. Creative therapy options for patients with dementia – a systematic review. Fortschr Neurol Psychiatr. 2007 Dec;75(12):699-707.

Schmitt B, Frölich L. Creative therapy options for patients with dementia—a systematic review. Fortschr Neurol Psychiatr. 2007 Dec;75(12):699-707.

Schönfeld P. Phytanic Acid toxicity: implications for the permeability of the inner mitochondrial membrane to ions. Toxicol Mech Methods. 2004;14(1-2):47-52.

Schottner M, Gansser D, Spiteller G. Lignans from the roots of Urtica dioica and their metabolites bind to human sex hormone binding globulin (SHBG). Planta Med. 1997;65:529-532.

Schreiber, G.H., Swaen, G.M., Meijers, J.M.M., Slangen, J.J.M., and Sturmans, F. Cancer mortality and residence near electricity transmission equipment: A retrospective cohort study. Int. J. Epidemiol. 1993;22:9–15.

Schröder L, Koch J, Mahner S, Kost BP, Hofmann S, Jeschke U, Haumann J, Schmedt J, Richter DU. The Effects of Petroselinum Crispum on Estrogen Receptor-positive Benign and Malignant Mammary Cells (MCF12A/MCF7). Anticancer Res. 2017 Jan;37(1):95-102.

Schroecksnadel S, Jenny M, Fuchs D. Sensitivity to sulphite additives. Clin Exp Allergy. 2010 Apr;40(4):688-9.

Schulick P. Ginger: Common Spice & Wonder Drug. Brattleboro, VT: Herbal Free Perss, 1996.

Schulman G. A nexus of progression of chronic kidney disease: charcoal, tryptophan and profibrotic cytokines. Blood Purif. 2006;24(1):143-8.

Schulz TJ, Zarse K, Voigt A, Urban N, Birringer M, Ristow M. Glucose restriction extends Caenorhabditis elegans life span by inducing mitochondrial respiration and increasing oxidative stress. Cell Metab. 2007 Oct;6(4):280-93.

Schulz V, Hansel R, Tyler VE. Rational Phytotherapy. Berlin: Springer-Verlag; 1998.

Schumacher P. Biophysical Therapy Of Allergies. Stuttgart: Thieme, 2005.

Schütz K, Carle R, Schieber A. Taraxacum—a review on its phytochemical and pharmacological profile. J Ethnopharmacol. 2006 Oct 11;107(3):313-23.

Schüz J, Mann S. A discussion of potential exposure metrics for use in epidemiological studies on human exposure to radiowaves from mobile phone base stations. J Expo Anal Environ Epidemiol. 2000 Nov-Dec;10(6 Pt 1):600-5.

Schüz J, Mann S. A discussion of potential exposure metrics for use in epidemiological studies on human exposure to radiowaves from mobile phone base stations. J Expo Anal Environ Epidemiol. 2000 Nov-Dec;10(6 Pt 1):600-5.

Schwartz GG, Skinner HG. Vitamin D status and cancer: new insights. Curr Opin Clin Nutr Metab Care. 2007 Jan;10(1):6-11.

Schwartz S, De Mattei R, Brame E, Spottiswoode S. Infrared spectra alteration in water proximate to the palms of therapeutic practitioners. In: Wiener D, Nelson R (Eds.): Research in parapsychology 1986. Metu-chen, NJ: Scarecrow Press, 1987:24-29.

Schwelberger HG. Histamine intolerance: a metabolic disease? Inflamm Res. 2010 Mar;59 Suppl 2:S219-21.

Schwellenbach LJ, Olson KL. McConnell KJ, Stolepart RS, Nash JD, Merenich JA. The triglyceride-lowering effects of a modest dose of docosahexaenoic acid alone versus in combination with low dose eicosapentaenoic acid in patients with coronary artery disease and elevated triglycerides. J Am Coll Nutr. 2006;25(6):480-485.

Scott BO. The history of ultraviolet therapy. in Licht S. ed. Therapeutic Electricity and Ultraviolet Radiation. Phys Med Lib 4. Connecticut: Licht, 1967.

Scoville WB, Milner B. Loss of recent memory after bilateral hippocampal lesions. J Neurol Neurosurg Psychia-try. 1957;20:11-21.

Sealey-Voyksner JA, Khosla C, Voyksner RD, Jorgenson JW. Novel aspects of quantitation of immunogenic wheat gluten peptides by liquid chromatography-mass spectrometry. J Chromatogr A. 2010 Jun 18;1217(25):4167-83.

See D, Mason S, Roshan R. Increased tumor necrosis factor alpha (TNF-alpha) and natural killer cell (NK) function using an integrative approach in late stage cancers. Immunol Invest. 2002 May;31(2):137-53.

Sekiguchi I, Suzuki M, Izumi A, Aida I, Tamada T. (1990). The study on the immunological effect of sizofilan combined with radiotherapy in patients with uterine cervical cancer. Nippon Gan Chiryo Gakkai shi, 25(11), 2659-64.

Sekine K, Toida T, Saito M, Kuboyama M, Kawashima T, Hashimoto Y. A new morphologically character-ized cell wall preparation (whole peptidoglycan) from Bifidobacterium infantis with a higher efficacy on the regression of an established tumor in mice. Cancer Res. 1985 Mar;45(3):1300-7.

Semenza C. Retrieval pathways for common and proper names. Cortex. 2006 Aug;42(6):884-91.

Senekowitsch F, Endler PC, Pongratz W, Smith CW. Hormone effects by CD record /replay. FASEB J. 1995:A12025.

Sengupta A, Ghosh S, Bhattacharjee S. Allium vegetables in cancer prevention: an overview. Asian Pac J Cancer Prev. 2004 Jul-Sep;5(3):237-45.

Senior F. Fallout. New York Magazine. Fall: 2003.

Senna G, Gani F, Leo G, Schiappoli M. Alternative tests in the diagnosis of food allergies. Recenti Prog Med. 2002 May;93(5):327-34.

Seo K, Jung S, Park M, Song Y, Choung S. Effects of leucocyanidines on activities of metabolizing enzymes and antioxidant enzymes. Biol Pharm Bull. 2001 May;24(5):592-3.

Seo SW, Koo HN, An HJ, Kwon KB, Lim BC, Seo EA, Ryu DG, Moon G, Kim HY, Kim HM, Hong SH. Taraxacum officinale protects against cholecystokinin-induced acute pancreatitis in rats. World J Gas-troenterol. 2005 Jan 28;11(4):597-9.

Seppo L, Jauhiainen T, Poussa T, Korpela R. A fermented milk high in bioactive peptides has a blood pressure-lowering effect in hypertensive subjects. Am J Clin Nutr. 2003 Feb;77(2):326-30.

Serra A, Cocuzza S, Poli G, La Mantia I, Messina A, Pavone P. Otologic findings in children with gastroe-sophageal reflux. Int J Pediatr Otorhinolaryngol. 2007 Nov;71(11):1693-7. 2007 Aug 22.

Serway R. Physicis For Scientists & Engineers. Philadelphia: Harcourt Brace, 1992.

Sevar R. Audit of outcome in 455 consecutive patients treated with homeopathic medicines. Homeopathy. 2005 Oct;94(4):215-21.

Shahani KM, Friend BA. Properties of and prospects for cultured dairy foods. Soc Appl Bacteriol Symp Ser. 1983;11:257-69.

Shahani KM, Meshbesher BF, Mangalampalli V. Cultivate Health From Within. Danbury, CT: Vital Health Publ, 2005.

Shaheen S, Potts J, Gnatiuc L, Makowska J, Kowalski ML, Joos G, van Zele T, van Durme Y, De Rudder I, Wöhrl S, Godnic-Cvar J, Skadhauge L, Thomsen G, Zuberbier T, Bergmann KC, Heinzerling L, Gjomarkaj M, Bruno A, Pace E, Bonini S, Fokkens W, Weersink EJ, Loureiro C, Todo-Bom A, Villanueva CM, Sanjuas C, Zock JP, Janson C, Burney P; Selenium and Asthma Research Integration project; GA2LEN. The relation between paracetamol use and asthma: a GA2LEN European case-control study. Eur Respir J. 2008 Nov;32(5):1231-6.

Shaheen SO, Newson RB, Rayman MP, Wong AP, Tumilty MK, Phillips JM, Potts JF, Kelly FJ, White PT, Burney PG. Randomised, double blind, placebo-controlled trial of selenium supplementation in adult asthma. Thorax. 2007 Jun;62(6):483-90.

Shaik AA, Hermanson DL, Xing C. Identification of methysticin as a potent and non-toxic NF-kappaB inhibitor from kava, potentially responsible for kava's chemopreventive activity. Bioorg Med Chem Lett. 2009 Oct 1;19(19):5732-6. doi: 10.1016/j.bmcl.2009.08.003.

Shalev E, Battino S, Weiner E, Colodner R, Keness Y. Ingestion of yogurt containing Lactobacillus aci-dophilus compared with pasteurized yogurt as prophylaxis for recurrent Candidal vaginitis and bacte-rial vaginosis. Arch Fam Med. 1996 Nov-Dec;5(10):593-6.

Shamir R, Makhoul IR, Etzioni A, Shehadeh N. Evaluation of a diet containing probiotics and zinc for the treatment of mild diarrheal illness in children younger than one year of age. J Am Coll Nutr. 2005 Oct;24(5):370-5.

Shamsabadi FT, Khoddami A, Fard SG, Abdullah R, Othman HH, Mohamed S. Comparison of Tamoxifen with Edible Seaweed (Eucheuma cottonii L.) Extract in Suppressing Breast Tumor. Nutr Cancer. 2013 Feb;65(2):255-62.

Shan L, Li Y, Jiang H, Tao Y, Qian Z, Li L, Cai F, Ma L, Yu Y. Huaier Restrains Migratory Potential of Hepatocellular Carcinoma Cells Partially Through Decreased Yes-Associated Protein 1. J Cancer. 2017 Nov 6;8(19):4087-4097. doi: 10.7150/jca.21018.

Sharma NK, Dey S, Prasad R. In vitro antioxidant potential evaluation of Euphorbia hirta L. Pharmacologyonline. 2007;1:91–8.

Sharma P, McClees SF, Afaq F. Pomegranate for Prevention and Treatment of Cancer: An Update. Molecules. 2017 Jan 24;22(1):177. doi: 10.3390/molecules22010177.

Sharma P, Sharma BC, Puri V, Sarin SK. An open-label randomized controlled trial of lactulose and probiotics in the treatment of minimal hepatic encephalopathy. Eur J Gastroent Hepatol. 2008 Jun;20(6):506-11.

Sharma SC, Sharma S, Gulati OP. Pycnogenol inhibits the release of histamine from mast cells. Phytother Res. 2003 Jan;17(1):66-9.

Shawcross DL, Wright G, Olde Damink SW, Jalan R. Role of ammonia and inflammation in minimal hepatic encephalopathy. Metab Brain Dis. 2007 Mar;22(1):125-38.

Shea-Donohue T, Stiltz J, Zhao A, Notari L. Mast Cells. Curr Gastroenterol Rep. 2010 Aug 14.

Shearman LP, Zylka MJ, Weaver DR, Kolakowski LF Jr, Reppert SM. Two period homologs: circadian expression and photic regulation in the suprachiasmatic nuclei. Neuron. 1997 Dec;19(6):1261-9.

Sheih YH, Chiang BL, Wang LH, Liao CK, Gill HS. Systemic immunity-enhancing effects in healthy subjects following dietary consumption of the lactic acid bacterium Lactobacillus rhamnosus HN001. J Am Coll Nutr. 2001 Apr;20(2 Suppl):149-56.

Shen FY, Lee MS, Jung SK. Effectiveness of pharmacopuncture for asthma: a systematic review and meta-analysis. Evid Based Complement Alternat Med. 2011;2011. pii: 678176.

Shen YF, Goddard G. The short-term effects of acupuncture on myofascial pain patients after clenching. Pain Pract. 2007 Sep;7(3):256-64.

Shevelev IA, Kostelianetz NB, Kamenkovich VM, Sharaev GA. EEG alpha-wave in the visual cortex: check of the hypothesis of the scanning process. Int J Psychophysiol. 1991 Aug;11(2):195-201.

Shi S, Zhao Y, Zhou H, Zhang Y, Jiang X, Huang K. Identification of antioxidants from Taraxacum mongolicum by high-performance liquid chromatography-diode array detection-radical-scavenging detection-electrospray ionization mass spectrometry and nuclear magnetic resonance experiments. J Chromatogr A. 2008 Oct 31;1209(1-2):145-52

Shi S, Zhou H, Zhang Y, Huang K, Liu S. Chemical constituents from Neo-Taraxacum siphonathum. Zhongguo Zhong Yao Za Zhi. 2009 Apr;34(8):1002-4.

Shi SY, Zhou CX, Xu Y, Tao QF, Bai H, Lu FS, Lin WY, Chen HY, Zheng W, Wang LW, Wu YH, Zeng S, Huang KX, Zhao Y, Li XK, Qu J. Studies on chemical constituents from herbs of Taraxacum mongolicum. Zhongguo Zhong Yao Za Zhi. 2008 May;33(10):1147-57.

Shi YQ, He Q, Zhao YJ, Wang EH, Wu GP. Lectin microarrays differentiate carcinoma cells from reactive mesothelial cells in pleural effusions. Cytotechnology. 2013 May;65(3):355-62. doi: 10.1007/s10616-012-9474-x.

Shibata H, Nabe T, Yamamura H, Kohno S. l-Ephedrine is a major constituent of Mao-Bushi-Saishin-To, one of the formulas of Chinese medicine, which shows immediate inhibition after oral administration of passive cutaneous anaphylaxis in rats. Inflamm Res. 2000 Aug;49(8):398-403.

Shichinohe K, Shimizu M, Kurokawa K. Effect of M-711 on experimental asthma in rats. J Vet Med Sci. 1996 Jan;58(1):55-9.

Shimauchi H, Mayanagi G, Nakaya S, Minamibuchi M, Ito Y, Yamaki K, Hirata H. Improvement of periodontal condition by probiotics with Lactobacillus salivarius WB21: a randomized, double-blind, placebo-controlled study. J Clin Periodontol. 2008 Oct;35(10):897-905.

Shimizu K, Ogura H, Goto M, Asahara T, Nomoto K, Morotomi M, Matsushima A, Tasaki O, Fujita K, Hosotsubo H, Kuwagata Y, Tanaka H, Shimazu T, Sugimoto H. Synbiotics decrease the incidence of septic complications in patients with severe SIRS: a preliminary report. Dig Dis Sci. 2009 May;54(5):1071-8.

Shimizu Y, Teshima H, Chen JT, Fujimoto I, Hasumi K, Masubuchi K. [Augmentative effect of sizofiran on the immune functions of regional lymph nodes in patients with cervical cancer]. Nihon Sanka Fujinka Gakkai Zasshi. 1991 Jun;43(6):581-8.

Shimoi T, Ushiyama H, Kan K, Saito K, Kamata K, Hirokado M. Survey of glycoalkaloids content in the various potatoes. Shokuhin Eiseigaku Zasshi. 2007 Jun;48(3):77-82.

Shin A, Lee J, Lee J, Park MS, Park JW, Park SC, Oh JH, Kim J. Isoflavone and Soyfood Intake and Colorectal Cancer Risk: A Case-Control Study in Korea. PLoS One. 2015 Nov 17;10(11):e0143228. doi: 10.1371/journal.pone.0143228.

Shishodia S, Harikumar KB, Dass S, Ramawat KG, Aggarwal BB. The guggul for chronic diseases: ancient medicine, modern targets. Anticancer Res. 2008 Nov-Dec;28(6A):3647-64.

Shivers RR, Kavaliers M, Teskey GC, Prato FS, Pelletier RM. Magnetic resonance imaging temporarily alters blood-brain barrier permeability in the rat. Neurosci Lett. 1987 Apr 23;76(1):25-31.

Shivpuri DN, Menon MP, Parkash D. Preliminary studies in Tylophora indica in the treatment of asthma and allergic rhinitis. J Assoc Physicians India. 1968 Jan;16(1):9-15.

Shoaf K, Mulvey GL, Armstrong GD, Hutkins RW. Prebiotic galactooligosaccharides reduce adherence of enteropathogenic Escherichia coli to tissue culture cells. Infect Immun. 2006 Dec;74(12):6920-8.

Shupak NM, Prato FS, Thomas AW. Human exposure to a specific pulsed magnetic field: effects on thermal sensory and pain thresholds. Neurosci Lett. 2004 Jun 10;363(2):157-62.

Shutov AA, Panasiuk IIa. Efficacy of rehabilitation of patients with chronic primary low back pain at the spa Klyuchi using balneopelotherapy and transcranial electrostimulation. Vopr Kurortol Fizioter Lech Fiz Kult. 2007 Mar-Apr;(2):16-8.

Sicher F, Targ E, Moore D, Smith H. A Randomized Double-Blind Study of the Effect of Distant Healing in a Population With Advanced AIDS. Western Journal of Medicine. 1998;169 Dec::356-363.

Siegfried J. Electrostimulation and neurosurgical measures in cancer pain. Recent Results Cancer Res. 1988;108:28-32.

Sies H, Stahl W. Nutritional protection against skin damage from sunlight. Annu Rev Nutr. 2004;24:173-200.

Sigstedt SC, Hooten CJ, Callewaert MC, Jenkins AR, Romero AE, Pullin MJ, Kornienko A, Lowrey TK, Slambrouck SV, Steelant WF. Evaluation of aqueous extracts of Taraxacum officinale on growth and invasion of breast and prostate cancer cells. Int J Oncol. 2008 May;32(5):1085-90.

Sikdar S, Kumar Saha S, Rahman Khuda-Bukhsh A. Relative Apoptosis-inducing Potential of Homeopathic Condurango 6C and 30C in H460 Lung Cancer Cells In vitro: -Apoptosis-induction by homeopathic Condurango in H460 cells. J Pharmacopuncture. 2014 Mar;17(1):59-69. doi: 10.3831/KPI.2014.17.008.

Silman AJ, MacGregor AJ, Thomson W, Holligan S, Carthy D, Farhan A, Ollier WE. Twin concordance rates for rheumatoid arthritis: results from a nationwide study. Br J Rheumatol. 1993 Oct;32(10):903-7.

Silva MF, Kamphorst AO, Hayashi EA, Bellio M, Carvalho CR, Faria AM, Sabino KC, Coelho MG, Nobrega A, Tavares D, Silva AC. Innate profiles of cytokines implicated on oral tolerance correlate with low- or high-suppression of humoral response. Immunology. 2010 Jul;130(3):447-57.

Silva MR, Dias G, Ferreira CL, Franceschini SC, Costa NM. Growth of preschool children was improved when fed an iron-fortified fermented milk beverage supplemented with Lactobacillus acidophilus. Nutr Res. 2008 Apr;28(4):226-32.

Simenhoff ML, Dunn SR, Zollner GP, Fitzpatrick ME, Emery SM, Sandine WE, Ayres JW. Biomodulation of the toxic and nutritional effects of small bowel bacterial overgrowth in end-stage kidney disease using freeze-dried Lactobacillus acidophilus. Miner Electrolyte Metab. 1996;22(1-3):92-6.

Simeone D, Miele E, Boccia G, Marino A, Troncone R, Staiano A. Prevalence of atopy in children with chronic constipation. Arch Dis Child. 2008 Dec;93(12):1044-7.

Simon S. World Health Organization Says Processed Meat Causes Cancer. 10/26/15. Accessed Jan 24, 2016.

Simons FER. What's in a name? The allergic rhinitis-asthma connection. Clin Exp All Rev. 2003;3:9-17.

Simopoulos AP. Essential fatty acids in health and chronic disease. Am J Clin Nutr. 1999 Sep;70(3 Suppl):560S-569S.

Simpson A, Tan VY, Winn J, Svensén M, Bishop CM, Heckerman DE, Buchan I, Custovic A. Beyond atopy: multiple patterns of sensitization in relation to asthma in a birth cohort study. Am J Respir Crit Care Med. 2010 Jun 1;181(11):1200-6.

Singer P, Shapiro H, Theilla M, Anbar R, Singer J, Cohen J. Anti-inflammatory properties of omega-3 fatty acids in critical illness: novel mechanisms and an integrative perspective. Intensive Care Med. 2008 Sep;34(9):1580-92.

Singh BB, Khorsan R, Vinjamury SP, Der-Martirosian C, Kizhakkeveettil A, Anderson TM. Herbal treatments of asthma: a systematic review. J Asthma. 2007 Nov;44(9):685-98.

Singh KB, Hahm ER, Alumkal JJ, Foley LM, Hitchens TK, Shiva SS, Parikh RA, Jacobs BL, Singh SV. Reversal of the Warburg phenomenon in chemoprevention of prostate cancer by sulforaphane. Carcinogenesis. 2019 Dec 31;40(12):1545-1556. doi: 10.1093/carcin/bgz155.

Singh O, Ali M, Husain SS. Phytochemical investigation and antifungal activity of the seeds of Centratherum anthelminticum Kuntze. Acta Pol Pharm. 2012 Nov-Dec;69(6):1183-7.

Singh S, Khajuria A, Taneja SC, Johri RK, Singh J, Qazi GN. Boswellic acids: A leukotriene inhibitor also effective through topical application in inflammatory disorders. Phytomedicine. 2008 Jun;15(6-7):400-7.

Singh V, Jain NK. Asthma as a cause for, rather than a result of, gastroesophageal reflux. J Asthma. 1983;20(4):241-3. 3.

Sinn DH, Song JH, Kim HJ, Lee JH, Son HJ, Chang DK, Kim YH, Kim JJ, Rhee JC, Rhee PL. Therapeutic effect of Lactobacillus acidophilus-SDC 2012, 2013 in patients with irritable bowel syndrome. Dig Dis Sci. 2008 Oct;53(10):2714-8.

Sita-Lumsden A, Lapthorn G, Swaminathan R, Milburn HJ. Reactivation of tuberculosis and vitamin D deficiency: the contribution of diet and exposure to sunlight. Thorax. 2007 Nov;62(11):1003-7.

Sita-Lumsden A, Lapthorn G, Swaminathan R, Milburn HJ. Reactivation of tuberculosis and vitamin D deficiency: the contribution of diet and exposure to sunlight. Thorax. 2007 Nov;62(11):1003-7.

SK. Oleuropein reduces free fatty acid-induced lipogenesis via lowered extracellular signal-regulated kinase activation in hepatocytes. Nutr Res. 2012 Oct;32(10):778-86.

Skovbjerg S, Roos K, Holm SE, Grahn Håkansson E, Nowrouzian F, Ivarsson M, Adlerberth I, Wold AE. Spray bacteriotherapy decreases middle ear fluid in children with secretory otitis media. Arch Dis Child. 2009 Feb;94(2):92-8.

Skwerer RG, Jacobsen FM, Duncan CC, Kelly KA, Sack DA, Tamarkin L, Gaist PA, Kasper S, Rosenthal NE. Neurobiology of Seasonal Affective Disorder and Phototherapy. J Biolog Rhyth. 1988;3(2):135-154.

Skwerer RG, Jacobsen FM, Duncan CC, Kelly KA, Sack DA, Tamarkin L, Gaist PA, Kasper S, Rosenthal NE. Neurobiology of Seasonal Affective Disorder and Phototherapy. J Biolog Rhyth. 1988;3(2):135-154.

Slezakova S, Ruda-Kucerova J. Anticancer Activity of Artemisinin and its Derivatives. Anticancer Res. 2017 Nov;37(11):5995-6003.

Sliva D. Ganoderma lucidum (Reishi) in cancer treatment. Integr Cancer Ther. 2003 Dec;2(4):358-64.

Sloan F and Gelband (ed). Cancer Control Opportunities in Low- and Middle-Income Countries. Committee on Cancer Control in Low- and Middle-Income Countries. 2007.

Smeester L, Fry RC. Long-Term Health Effects and Underlying Biological Mechanisms of Developmental Exposure to Arsenic. Curr Environ Health Rep. 2018 Feb 6. doi: 10.1007/s40572-018-0184-1.

Smith CW. Coherence in living biological systems. Neural Network World. 1994:4(3):379-388.

Smith J. Genetic Roulette: The Documented Health Risks of Genetically Engineered Foods. White River Jct, Vermont: Chelsea Green, 2007.

Smith K, Warholak T, Armstrong E, Leib M, Rehfeld R, Malone D. Evaluation of risk factors and health outcomes among persons with asthma. J Asthma. 2009 Apr;46(3):234-7.

Smith LJ, Holbrook JT, Wise R, Blumenthal M, Dozor AJ, Mastronarde J, Williams L; American Lung Association Asthma Clinical Research Centers. Dietary intake of soy genistein is associated with lung function in patients with asthma. J Asthma. 2004;41(8):833-43.

Smith MJ. Effect of Magnetic Fields on Enzyme Reactivity. In Barnothy M.(ed.), Biological Effects of Magnetic Fields. New York: Plenum Press, 1969.

Smith-Sonneborn J. DNA repair and longevity assurance in Paramecium tetraurelia. Science. 1979 Mar 16;203(4385):1115-7.

Smith-Spangler C, Brandeau ML, Hunter GE, Bavinger JC, Pearson M, Eschbach PJ, Sundaram V, Liu H, Schirmer P, Stave C, Olkin I, Bravata DM. Are organic foods safer or healthier than conventional alternatives?: a systematic review. Ann Intern Med. 2012 Sep 4;157(5):348-66. doi: 10.7326/0003-4819-157-5-201209040-00007.

Smits MG, Williams A, Skene DJ, Von Schantz M. The 3111 Clock gene polymorphism is not associated with sleep and circadian rhythmicity in phenotypically characterized human subjects. J Sleep Res. 2002 Dec;11(4):305-12.

Snow WB. The Therapeutics of Radiant Light and Heat and Convective Heat. NY: Sci Auth Publ, 1909.

Snyder K. Researchers Produce Firsts with Bursts of Light: Team generates most energetic terahertz pulses yet, observes useful optical phenomena. Press Release: Brookhaven National Laboratory. 2007 July 24.

Snyder K. Researchers Produce Firsts with Bursts of Light: Team generates most energetic terahertz pulses yet, observes useful optical phenomena. Press Release: Brookhaven National Laboratory. 2007 July 24.

Sofic E, Denisova N, Youdim K, Vatrenjak-Velagic V, De Filippo C, Mehmedagic A, Causevic A, Cao G, Joseph JA, Prior RL. Antioxidant and pro-oxidant capacity of catecholamines and related compounds. Effects of hydrogen peroxide on glutathione and sphingomyelinase activity in pheochromocytoma PC12 cells: potential relevance to age-related diseases. J Neural Transm. 2001;108(5):541-57.

Soga K, Teruya F, Tateno H, Hirabayashi J, Yamamoto K. Terminal N -acetylgalactosamine-specific leguminous lectin from Wisteria japonica as a probe for human lung squamous cell carcinoma. PLoS One. 2013 Dec 13;8(12):e83886. doi: 10.1371/journal.pone.0083886.

Soica CM, Dehelean CA, Peev C, Aluas M, Zupkó I, Kása P Jr, Alexa E. Physico-chemical comparison of betulinic acid, betulin and birch bark extract and in vitro investigation of their cytotoxic effects towards skin epidermoid carcinoma (A431), breast carcinoma (MCF7) and cervix adenocarcinoma (HeLa) cell lines. Nat Prod Res. 2012;26(10):968-74.

Soleo L, Colosio C, Alinovi R, Guarneri D, Russo A, Lovreglio P, Vimercati L, Birindelli S, Cortesi I, Flore C, Carta P, Colombi A, Parrinello G, Ambrosi L. Immunologic effects of exposure to low levels of inorganic mercury. Med Lav. 2002 May-Jun;93(3):225-32.

Soler M, Chandra S, Ruiz D, Davidson E, Hendrickson D, Christou G. A third isolated oxidation state for the Mn12 family of single molecule magnets. ChemComm; 2000; Nov 22.

Solomons NW, Guerrero AM, Torun B. Effective in vivo hydrolysis of milk lactose by beta-galactosidases in the presence of solid foods. Am J Clin Nutr. 1985 Feb;41(2):222-7.

Sompamit K, Kukongviriyapan U, Nakmareong S, Pannangpetch P, Kukongviriyapan V. Curcumin improves vascular function and alleviates oxidative stress in non-lethal lipopolysaccharide-induced endotoxaemia in mice. Eur J Pharmacol. 2009 Aug 15;616(1-3):192-9.

Song X, Li Y, Zhang H, Yang Q. The anticancer effect of Huaier (Review). Oncol Rep. 2015 Jul;34(1):12-21. doi: 10.3892/or.2015.3950.

Sonibare MA, Gbile ZO. Ethnobotanical survey of anti-asthmatic plants in South Western Nigeria. Afr J Tradit Complement Altern Med. 2008 Jun 18;5(4):340-5.

Sontag SJ, O'Connell S, Khandelwal S, Greenlee H, Schnell T, Nemchausky B, Chejfec G, Miller T, Seidel J, Sonnenberg A. Asthmatics with gastroesophageal reflux: long term results of a randomized trial of medical and surgical antireflux therapies. Am J Gastroenterol. 2003 May;98(5):987-99.

Soriano-Hernandez AD, Madrigal-Perez DG, Galvan-Salazar HR, Arreola-Cruz A, Briseño-Gomez L, Guzmán-Esquivel J, Dobrovinskaya O, Lara-Esqueda A, Rodríguez-Sanchez IP, Baltazar-Rodriguez LM, Espinoza-Gomez F, Martinez-Fierro ML, de-Leon-Zaragoza L, Olmedo-Buenrostro BA, Delgado-Enciso I. The protective effect of peanut, walnut, and almond consumption on the development of breast cancer. Gynecol Obstet Invest. 2015;80(2):89-92. doi: 10.1159/000369997.

Sosa M, Saavedra P, Valero C, Guañabens N, Nogués X, del Pino-Montes J, Mosquera J, Alegre J, Gómez-Alonso C, Muñoz-Torres M, Quesada M, Pérez-Cano R, Jódar E, Torrijos A, Lozano-Tonkin C, Díaz-Curiel M; GIUMO Study Group. Inhaled steroids do not decrease bone mineral density but increase risk of fractures: data from the GIUMO Study Group. J Clin Densitom. 2006 Apr-Jun;9(2):154-8.

Soyka F, Edmonds A. The Ion Effect: How Air Electricity Rules your Life and Health. Bantam, New York: Bantam, 1978.

Spanagel R, Rosenwasser AM, Schumann G, Sarkar DK. Alcohol consumption and the body's biological clock. Alcohol Clin Exp Res. 2005 Aug;29(8):1550-7.

Speed Of Light May Not Be Constant, Physicist Suggests. Science Daily. 1999 Oct 6. www.sciencedaily.com/releases/1999/10/991005114024.htm. Accessed: 2007 June.

Speed Of Light May Not Be Constant, Physicist Suggests. Science Daily. 1999 Oct 6. www.sciencedaily.com/releases/1999/10/991005114024.htm. Accessed: 2007 June.

Spence A. Basic Human Anatomy. Menlo Park, CA: Benjamin/Commings, 1986.

Spence S. Scientists tie walnuts to gene expressions related to breast cancer. Marshall University School of Medicine. Thursday, March 28, 2019.

Spencer FA, Goldberg RJ, Becker RC, Gore JM. Seasonal distribution of acute myocardial infarction in the second National Registry of Myocardial Infarction. J Am Coll Cardiol. 1998 May;31(6):1226-33.

Spiller G. The Super Pyramid. New York: HRS Press, 1993.

Sporik R, Squillace SP, Ingram JM, Rakes G, Honsinger RW, Platts-Mills TA. Mite, cat, and cockroach exposure, allergen sensitisation, and asthma in children: a case-control study of three schools. Thorax. 1999 Aug;54(8):675-80.

Squire LR, Zola-Morgan S. The medial temporal lobe memory system. Science. 1991;253(5026):1380-1386.

St Hilaire MA, Gronfier C, Zeitzer JM, Klerman EB. A physiologically based mathematical model of melatonin including ocular light suppression and interactions with the circadian pacemaker. J Pineal Res. 2007 Oct;43(3):294-304.

St Hilaire MA, Klerman EB, Khalsa SB, Wright KP Jr, Czeisler CA, Kronauer RE. Addition of a non-photic component to a light-based mathematical model of the human circadian pacemaker. J Theor Biol. 2007 Aug 21;247(4):583-99.

Stach A, Emberlin J, Smith M, Adams-Groom B, Myszkowska D. Factors that determine the severity of Betula spp. pollen seasons in Poland (Poznań and Krakow) and the United Kingdom (Worcester and London). Int J Biometeorol. 2008 Mar;52(4):311-21.

Stachowska E, Dolegowska B, Chlubek D, Wesolowska T, Ciechanowski K, Gutowski P, Szumilowicz H, Turowski R. Dietary trans fatty acids and composition of human atheromatous plaques. Eur J Nutr. 2004 Oct;43(5):313-8.

Stadlbauer V, Mookerjee RP, Hodges S, Wright GA, Davies NA, Jalan R. Effect of probiotic treatment on deranged neutrophil function and cytokine responses in patients with compensated alcoholic cirrhosis. J Hepatol. 2008 Jun;48(6):945-51.

Stahl SM. Selective histamine H1 antagonism: novel hypnotic and pharmacologic actions challenge classical notions of antihistamines. CNS Spectr. 2008 Dec;13(12):1027-38.

Stahl W, Heinrich U, Wiseman S, Eichler O, Sies H, Tronnier H. Dietary tomato paste protects against ultraviolet light-induced erythema in humans. J Nutr. 2001 May;131(5):1449-51.

Stamatakis E, Rogers K, Ding D, Berrigan D, Chau J, Hamer M, Bauman A. All-cause mortality effects of replacing sedentary time with physical activity and sleeping using an isotemporal substitution model: a prospective study of 201,129 mid-aged and older adults. Int J Behav Nutr Phys Act. 2015 Sep 30;12:121. doi: 10.1186/s12966-015-0280-7.

Stancioiu F, Mihai D, Papadakis GZ, Tsatsakis A, Spandidos DA, Badiu C. Treatment for benign thyroid nodules with a combination of natural extracts. Mol Med Rep. 2019 Sep;20(3):2332-2338. doi: 10.3892/mmr.2019.10453.

Staples JA, Ponsonby AL, Lim LL, McMichael AJ. Ecologic analysis of some immune-related disorders, including type 1 diabetes, in Australia: latitude, regional ultraviolet radiation, and disease prevalence. Environ Health Perspect. 2003 Apr;111(4):518-23.

State Pharmacopoeia Commission of The People's Republic of China. Pharmacopoeia of the People's Republic of China. Beijing: Chemical Industry Press; 2005.

Steck B. Effects of optical radiation on man. Light Resch Techn. 1982;14:130-141.

Steely AM, Willoughby JA Sr, Sundar SN, Aivaliotis VI, Firestone GL. Artemisinin disrupts androgen responsiveness of human prostate cancer cells by stimulating the 26S proteasome-mediated degradation of the androgen receptor protein. Anticancer Drugs. 2017 Oct;28(9):1018-1031. doi: 10.1097/CAD.0000000000000547.

Steenland K, Zhao L, Winquist A. A cohort incidence study of workers exposed to perfluorooctanoic acid (PFOA). Occup Environ Med. 2015;72(5):373-380. doi:10.1136/oemed-2014-102364

Steevens J, Schouten LJ, Goldbohm RA, van den Brandt PA. Vegetables and fruits consumption and risk of esophageal and gastric cancer subtypes in the Netherlands Cohort Study. Int J Cancer. 2011;129:2681–2693.

Steinman HA, Le Roux M, Potter PC. Sulphur dioxide sensitivity in South African asthmatic children. S Afr Med J. 1993 Jun;83(6):387-90.

Stenberg JA, Hambäck PA, Ericson L. Herbivore-induced "rent rise" in the host plant may drive a diet breadth enlargement in the tenant. Ecology. 2008 Jan;89(1):126-33.

Stengler M. The Natural Physician's Healing Therapies. Stamford, CT: Bottom Line Books, 2008.

Stensrud T, Carlsen KH. Can one single test protocol for provoking exercise-induced bronchoconstriction also be used for assessing aerobic capacity? Clin Respir J. 2008 Jan;2(1):47-53.

Stephenson R. Circadian rhythms and sleep-related breathing disorders. Sleep Med. 2007 Sep;8(6):681-7.

Steurer-Stey C, Russi EW, Steurer J: Complementary and alternative medicine in asthma: do they work? Swiss Med Wkly. 2002, 132:338-344.

Stoebner-Delbarre A, Thezenas S, Kuntz C, Nguyen C, Giordanella JP, Sancho-Garnier H, Guillot B; Le Groupe EPI-CES. Sun exposure and sun protection behavior and attitudes among the French population. Ann Dermatol Venereol. 2005 Aug-Sep;132(8-9 Pt 1):652-7.

Stoebner-Delbarre A, Thezenas S, Kuntz C, Nguyen C, Giordanella JP, Sancho-Garnier H, Guillot B; Le Groupe EPI-CES. Sun exposure and sun protection behavior and attitudes among the French population. Ann Dermatol Venereol. 2005 Aug-Sep;132(8-9 Pt 1):652-7.

Stojanovic MP, Abdi S. Spinal cord stimulation. Pain Physician. 2002 Apr;5(2):156-66.

Størdal K, Johannesdottir GB, Bentsen BS, Knudsen PK, Carlsen KC, Closs O, Handeland M, Holm HK, Sandvik L. Acid suppression does not change respiratory symptoms in children with asthma and gastro-oesophageal reflux disease. Arch Dis Child. 2005 Sep;90(9):956-60.

Stoupel E, Babayev E, Mustafa F, Abramson E, Israelevich P, Sulkes J. Acute myocardial infarction occurrence: environmental links - Baku 2003-2005 data. Med Sci Monit. 2007 Aug;13(8):BR175-9.

Stoupel E, Kalediene R, Petrauskiene J, Gaizauskiene A, Israelevich P, Abramson E, Sulkes J. Monthly number of newborns and environmental physical activity. Medicina Kaunas. 2006;42(3):238-41.

Stoupel E, Monselise Y, Lahav J. Changes in autoimmune markers of the anti-cardiolipin syndrome on days of extreme geomagnetic activity. J Basic Clin Physiol Pharmacol. 2006;17(4):269-78.

Stoupel E, Frimer H, Appelman Z, Ben-Neriah Z, Dar H, Fejgin MD, Gershoni-Baruch R, Manor E, Barkai G, Shalev S, Gelman-Kohan Z, Reish O, Lev D, Davidov B, Goldman B, Shohat M. Chromosome aberration and environmental physical activity: Down syndrome and solar and cosmic ray activity, Israel, 1990-2000. Int J Biometeorol. 2005 Sep;50(1):1-5.

Stout NL, Baima J, Swisher AK, Winters-Stone KM, Welsh J. A Systematic Review of Exercise Systematic Reviews in the Cancer Literature (2005-2017). PM R. 2017 Sep;9(9S2):S347-S384. doi: 10.1016/j.pmrj.2017.07.074.

Strange BA, Dolan RJ. Anterior medial temporal lobe in human cognition: memory for fear and the unexpected. Cognit Neuropsychiatry. 2006 May;11(3):198-218.

Streitberger K, Ezzo J, Schneider A. Acupuncture for nausea and vomiting: an update of clinical and experimental studies. Auton Neurosci. 2006 Oct 30;129(1-2):107-17.

Strinnholm A, Brulin C, Lindh V. Experiences of double-blind, placebo-controlled food challenges (DBPCFC): a qualitative analysis of mothers' experiences. J Child Health Care. 2010 Jun;14(2):179-88.

Stull DE, Schaefer M, Crespi S, Sandor DW. Relative strength of relationships of nasal congestion and ocular symptoms with sleep, mood and productivity. Curr Med Res Opin. 2009 Jul;25(7):1785-92.

Sturtzel B, Mikulits C, Gisinger C, Elmadfa I. Use of fiber instead of laxative treatment in a geriatric hospital to improve the wellbeing of seniors. J Nutr Health Aging. 2009 Feb;13(2):136-9.

Su P, Henriksson A, Tandianus JE, Park JH, Foong F, Dunn NW. Detection and quantification of Bifidobacterium lactis LAFTI B94 in human faecal samples from a consumption trial. FEMS Microbiol Lett. 2005 Mar 1;244(1):99-103.

Su X, Tamimi RM, Collins LC, Baer HJ, Cho E, Sampson L, Willett WC, Schnitt SJ, Connolly JL, Rosner BA, Colditz GA. Intake of fiber and nuts during adolescence and incidence of proliferative benign breast disease. Cancer CausesControl. 2010 Jul;21(7):1033-46. doi: 10.1007/s10552-010-9532-7.

Sugarman E. Warning, The Electricity Around You May be Hazardous To Your Health. NY: Sim & Schuster, 1992.

Sugawara G, Nagino M, Nishio H, Ebata T, Takagi K, Asahara T, Nomoto K, Nimura Y. Perioperative synbiotic treatment to prevent postoperative infectious complications in biliary cancer surgery: a randomized controlled trial. Ann Surg. 2006 Nov;244(5):706-14.

Sugimachi K, Maehara Y, Ogawa M, Kakegawa T, Tomita M. Dose intensity of uracil and tegafur in postoperative chemotherapy for patients with poorly differentiated gastric cancer. Cancer Chemother Pharmacol. 1997;40(3):233-8.

Sullivan A, Barkholt L, Nord CE. Lactobacillus acidophilus, Bifidobacterium lactis and Lactobacillus F19 prevent antibiotic-associated ecological disturbances of Bacteroides fragilis in the intestine. J Antimicrob Chemother. 2003 Aug;52(2):308-11.

Sulman FG. Migraine and headache due to weather and allied causes and its specific treatment. Ups J Med Sci Suppl. 1980;31:41-4.

Sumantran VN, Kulkarni AA, Harsulkar A, Wele A, Koppikar SJ, Chandwaskar R, Gaire V, Dalvi M, Wagh UV. Hyaluronidase and collagenase inhibitory activities of the herbal formulation Triphala guggulu. J Biosci. 2007 Jun;32(4):755-61.

Sun Y, Tan YJ, Lu ZZ, Li BB, Sun CH, Li T, Zhao LL, Liu Z, Zhang GM, Yao JC, Li J. Arctigenin Inhibits Liver Cancer Tumorigenesis by Inhibiting Gankyrin Expression via C/EBPα and PPARα. Front Pharmacol. 2018 Mar 27;9:268. doi: 10.3389/fphar.2018.00268.

Sun Y, Wang W, Tong Y. Berberine Inhibits Proliferative Ability of Breast cancer Cells by Reducing Metadherin. Med Sci Monit. 2019 Nov 28;25:9058-9066. doi: 10.12659/MSM.914486.

Sun ZL, Dong JL, Wu J. Juglanin induces apoptosis and autophagy in human breast cancer progression via ROS/JNK promotion. Biomed Pharmacother. 2017 Jan;85:303-312. doi: 10.1016/j.biopha.2016.11.030.

Sung JH, Lee JO, Son JK, Park NS, Kim MR, Kim JG, Moon DC. Cytotoxic constituents from Solidago virga-aurea var. gigantea MIQ. Arch Pharm Res. 1999 Dec;22(6):633-7.

Suppes P, Han B, Epelboim J, Lu ZL. Invariance of brain-wave representations of simple visual images and their names. Proceedings of the National Academy of Sciences Psychology-BS. 1999;96(25):14658-14663.

Suppes P, Han B, Epelboim J, Lu ZL. Invariance of brain-wave representations of simple visual images and their names. Proc Natl Acad Sci Psych-BS. 1999;96(25):14658-14663.

Susanti S, Iwasaki H, Inafuku M, Taira N, Oku H. Mechanism of arctigenin-mediated specific cytotoxicity against human lung adenocarcinoma cell lines. Phytomedicine. 2013 Sep 7. doi:pii: S0944-7113(13)00285-7.

Susanti S, Iwasaki H, Itokazu Y, Nago M, Taira N, Saitoh S, Oku H. Tumor specific cytotoxicity of arctigenin isolated from herbal plant Arctium lappa L. J Nat Med. 2012 Oct;66(4):614-21. doi: 10.1007/s11418-012-0628-0.

Suzuki Y, Kondo K, Ichise H, Tsukamoto Y, Urano T, Umemura K. Dietary supplementation with fermented soybeans suppresses intimal thickening. Nutrition. 2003 Mar;19(3):261-4.

Svendsen AJ, Holm NV, Kyvik K, et al. Relative importance of genetic effects in rheumatoid arthritis: historical cohort study of Danish nationwide twin population. BMJ 2002;324(7332): 264-266.

Sweeney B, Vora M, Ulbricht C, Basch E. Evidence-based systematic review of dandelion (Taraxacum officinale) by natural standard research collaboration. J Herb Pharmacother. 2005;5(1):79-93.

Swett. JA. A Treatise on Disease of the Chest. New York, 1852.

Swiderska-Kiełbik S, Krakowiak A, Wiszniewska M, Dudek W, Walusiak-Skorupa J, Krawczyk-Szulc P, Michowicz A, Pałczyński C. Health hazards associated with occupational exposure to birds. Med Pr. 2010;61(2):213-22.

Swislocki A, Orth M, Bales M, Weisshaupt J, West C, Edrington J, Cooper B, Saputo L, Islas M, Miaskowski C. A randomized clinical trial of the effectiveness of photon stimulation on pain, sensation, and quality of life in patients with diabetic peripheral neuropathy. J Pain Symptom Manage. 2010 Jan;39(1):88-99. Epub 2009 Nov 5.

Swislocki A, Orth M, Bales M, Weisshaupt J, West C, Edrington J, Cooper B, Saputo L, Islas M, Miaskowski C. A randomized clinical trial of the effectiveness of photon stimulation on pain, sensation, and quality of life in patients with diabetic peripheral neuropathy. J Pain Symptom Manage. 2010 Jan;39(1):88-99. Epub 2009 Nov 5.

Szyf M, McGowan P, Meaney MJ. The social environment and the epigenome. Environ Mol Mutagen. 2008 Jan;49(1):46-60.

Szymański H, Chmielarczyk A, Strus M, Pejcz J, Jawień M, Kochan P, Heczko PB. Colonisation of the gastrointestinal tract by probiotic L. rhamnosus strains in acute diarrhoea in children. Dig Liver Dis. 2006 Dec;38 Suppl 2:S274-6.

Szymański H, Pejcz J, Jawień M, Chmielarczyk A, Strus M, Heczko PB. Treatment of acute infectious diarrhoea in infants and children with a mixture of three Lactobacillus rhamnosus strains—a randomized, double-blind, placebo-controlled trial. Aliment Pharmacol Ther. 2006 Jan 15;23(2):247-53.

Tahvanainen K, Nino J, Halonen P, Kuusela T, Alanko T, Laitinen T, Lansimies E, Hietanen M, Lindholm H. Effects of cellular phone use on ear canal temperature measured by NTC thermistors. Clin Physiol Funct Imaging. 2007 May;27(3):162-72.

Taka T, Huang L, Wongnoppavich A, Tam-Chang SW, Lee TR, Tuntiwechapikul W. Telomere shortening and cell senescence induced by perylene derivatives in A549 human lung cancer cells. Bioorg Med Chem. 2012 Dec 23. doi:pii: S0968-0896(12)00991-1.

Takada Y, Ichikawa H, Badmaev V, Aggarwal BB. Acetyl-11-keto-beta-boswellic acid potentiates apoptosis, inhibits invasion, and abolishes osteoclastogenesis by suppressing NF-kappa B and NF-kappa B-regulated gene expression. J Immunol. 2006 Mar 1;176(5):3127-40.

Takagi A, Ikemura H, Matsuzaki T, Sato M, Nomoto K, Morotomi M, Yokokura T. Relationship between the in vitro response of dendritic cells to Lactobacillus and prevention of tumorigenesis in the mouse. J Gastroenterol. 2008;43(9):661-9.

Takahashi N, Eisenhuth G, Lee I, Schachtele C, Laible N, Binion S. Nonspecific antibacterial factors in milk from cows immunized with human oral bacterial pathogens. J Dairy Sci. 1992 Jul;75(7):1810-20.

Takaku, Takeshi; Kimura, Yoshiyuki; Okuda, Hiromichi. 2001. Isolation of an antitumor compound from Agaricus blazei Murill and its mechanism of action. Journal of Nutrition, 131(5), 1409-1413.

Takasaki M, Konoshima T, Tokuda H, Masuda K, Arai Y, Shiojima K, Ageta H. Anti-carcinogenic activity of Taraxacum plant. I. Biol Pharm Bull. 1999 Jun;22(6):602-5.

Takaya Y, Tasaka H, Chiba T, Uwai K, Tanitsu M, Kim HS, Wataya Y, Miura M, Takeshita M, Oshima Y. New type of febrifugine analogues, bearing a quinolizidine moiety, show potent antimalarial activity against Plasmodium malaria parasite. J Med Chem. 1999 Aug 12;42(16):3163-6.

Takeda K, Okumura K. Effects of a fermented milk drink containing Lactobacillus casei strain Shirota on the human NK-cell activity. J Nutr. 2007 Mar;137(3 Suppl 2):791S-3S.

Takeda K, Suzuki T, Shimada SI, Shida K, Nanno M, Okumura K. Interleukin-12 is involved in the enhancement of human natural killer cell activity by Lactobacillus casei Shirota. Clin Exp Immunol. 2006 Oct;146(1):109-15.

Tamaoki J, Chiyotani A, Sakai A, Takemura H, Konno K. Effect of menthol vapour on airway hyperresponsiveness in patients with mild asthma. Respir Med. 1995 Aug;89(7):503-4.

Tan DX, Manchester LC, Reiter RJ, Qi WB, Karbownik M, Calvo JR. Significance of melatonin in antioxidative defense system: reactions and products. Biol Signals Recept. 2000 May-Aug;9(3-4):137-59.

Tan KW, Cooney J, Jensen D, Li Y, Paxton JW, Birch NP, Scheepens A. Hop-derived prenylflavonoids are substrates and inhibitors of the efflux transporter breast cancer resistance protein (BCRP/ABCG2). Mol Nutr Food Res. 2014 Nov;58(11):2099-110. doi: 10.1002/mnfr.201400288.

Tan KW, Killeen DP, Li Y, Paxton JW, Birch NP, Scheepens A. Dietary polyacetylenes of the falcarinol type are inhibitors of breast cancer resistance protein (BCRP/ABCG2). Eur J Pharmacol. 2014 Jan 15;723:346-52. doi: 10.1016/j.ejphar.2013.11.005.

Tanagho EA. Principles and indications of electrostimulation of the urinary bladder. Urologe A. 1990 Jul;29(4):185-90.

Tang G, Serfaty-Lacrosniere C, Camilo ME, Russell RM. Gastric acidity influences the blood response to a beta-carotene dose in humans. Am J Clin Nutr. 1996;64:622-6.

Tang Y, Li X, Liu Z, Simoneau AR, Xie J, Zi X. Flavokawain B, a kava chalcone, induces apoptosis via upregulation of death-receptor 5 and Bim expression in androgen receptor negative, hormonal refractory prostate cancer cell lines and reduces tumor growth. Int J Cancer. 2010 Oct 15;127(8):1758-68. doi: 10.1002/ijc.25210.

Tang Y, Simoneau AR, Xie J, Shahandeh B, Zi X. Effects of the kava chalcone flavokawain A differ in bladder cancer cells with wild-type versus mutant p53. Cancer Prev Res (Phila). 2008 Nov;1(6):439-51. doi: 10.1158/1940-6207.CAPR-08-0165.

Taniguchi C, Homma M, Takano O, Hirano T, Oka K, Aoyagi Y, Niitsuma T, Hayashi T. Pharmacological effects of urinary products obtained after treatment with saiboku-to, a herbal medicine for bronchial asthma, on type IV allergic reaction. Planta Med. 2000 Oct;66(7):607-11.

Taoka S, Padmakumar R, Grissom C, Banerjee R. Magnetic Field Effects on Coenzyme B-12 Dependent Enzymes: Validation of Ethanolamine Ammonia Lyase Results and Extension to Human Methylmalonyl CoA Mutase. Bioelectromagnetics. 1997;18: 506-513.

Tapiero H, Ba GN, Couvreur P, Tew KD. Polyunsaturated fatty acids (PUFA) and eicosanoids in human health and pathologies. Biomed Pharmacother. 2002 Jul;56(5):215-22.

405

Tapsell LC, Hemphill I, Cobiac L, Patch CS, Sullivan DR, Fenech M, Roodenrys S, Keogh JB, Clifton PM, Williams PG, Fazio VA, Inge KE. Health benefits of herbs and spices: the past, the present, the future. Med J Aust. 2006 Aug 21;185(4 Suppl):S4-24.

Taraban M, Leshina T, Anderson M, Grissom C. Magnetic Field Dependence and the Role of electron spin in Heme Enzymes: Horseradish Peroxidase. J. Am. Chem. Soc. 1997;119: 5768-5769.

Targ R, Puthoff H. Information transfer under conditions of sensory shielding. Nature. 1975;251:602-607.

Tárraga López PJ, Albero JS, Rodríguez-Montes JA. Primary and secondary prevention of colorectal cancer. Clin Med Insights Gastroenterol. 2014 Jul 14;7:33-46. doi: 10.4137/CGast.S14039. eCollection 2014.

Taskinen H, Kyyrönen P, Hemminki K. Effects of ultrasound, shortwaves, and physical exertion on pregnancy outcome in physiotherapists. J Epidemiol Community Health. 1990 Sep;44(3):196-201.

Tasli L, Mat C, De Simone C, Yazici H. Lactobacilli lozenges in the management of oral ulcers of Behçet's syndrome. Clin Exp Rheumatol. 2006 Sep-Oct;24(5 Suppl 42):S83-6.

Taussig SJ, Batkin S. Bromelain, the enzyme complex of pineapple (Ananas comosus) and its clinical application. An update. J Ethnopharmacol. 1988 Feb-Mar;22(2):191-203.

Tavil B, Koksal E, Yalcin SS, Uckan D. Pretransplant nutritional habits and clinical outcome in children undergoing hematopoietic stem cell transplant. Exp Clin Transplant. 2012 Feb;10(1):55-61.

Tayarani-Najaran Z, Makki FS, Alamolhodaei NS, Mojarrab M, Emami SA. Cytotoxic and apoptotic effects of Artemisia biennis Willd. on K562 and HL-60 cell lines. Iran J Basic Med Sci. 2017 Feb;20(2):166-171. doi: 10.22038/ijbms.2017.8242.

Taylor RB, Lindquist N, Kubanek J, Hay ME. Intraspecific variation in palatability and defensive chemistry of brown seaweeds: effects on herbivore fitness. Oecologia. 2003 Aug;136(3):412-23.

Taylor SL, Kaur M, LoSicco K, Willard J, Camacho F, O'Rourke KS, Feldman SR. Pilot study of the effect of ultraviolet light on pain and mood in fibromyalgia syndrome. J Altern Complement Med. 2009 Jan;15(1):15-23.

Tayyem RF, Bawadi HA, Shehadah I, Agraib LM, Al-Awwad NJ, Heath DD, Bani-Hani KE. Consumption of Whole Grains, Refined Cereals, and Legumes and Its Association With Colorectal Cancer Among Jordanians. Integr Cancer Ther. 2015 Dec 1. pii: 1534735415620010.

Teitelbaum J. From Fatigue to Fantastic. New York: Avery, 2001.

Teschke R, Lebot V. Proposal for a kava quality standardization code. Food Chem Toxicol. 2011 Oct;49(10):2503-16. doi: 10.1016/j.fct.2011.06.075.

Teschke R, Sarris J, Lebot V. Contaminant hepatotoxins as culprits for kava hepatotoxicity–fact or fiction? Phytother Res. 2013 Mar;27(3):472-4. doi: 10.1002/ptr.4729.

Teschke R, Sarris J, Schweitzer I. Kava hepatotoxicity in traditional and modern use: the presumed Pacific kava paradox hypothesis revisited. Br J Clin Pharmacol. 2012 Feb;73(2):170-4. doi: 10.1111/j.1365-2125.2011.04070.x.

Tesse R, Schieck M, Kabesch M. Asthma and endocrine disorders: Shared mechanisms and genetic pleiotropy. Mol Cell Endocrinol. 2010 Dec 4. [ahead of print].

Tevini M, ed. UV-B Radiation and Ozone Depletion: Effects on humans, animals, plants, microorganisms and materials. Boca Raton: Lewis Pub, 1993.

Thafeni MA, Sayed Y, Motadi LR. Euphorbia mauritanica and Kedrostis hirtella extracts can induce antiproliferative activities in lung cancer cells. Mol Biol Rep. 2012;39(12):10785-10794. doi:10.1007/s11033-012-1972-6

Thaker JP, Patel MB, Jongnarangsin K, Liepa VV, Thakur RK. Electromagnetic interference with pacemakers caused by portable media players. Heart Rhythm. 2008 Apr;5(4):538-44.

Thakkar K, Boatright RO, Gilger MA, El-Serag HB. Gastroesophageal reflux and asthma in children: a systematic review. Pediatrics. 2010 Apr;125(4):e925-30. 2010 Mar 29.

Thakkar RR, Garrison MM, Christakis DA. A systematic review for the effects of television viewing by infants and preschoolers. Pediatrics. 2006 Nov;118(5):2025-31.

Thampithak A, Jaisin Y, Meesarapee B, Chongthammakun S, Piyachaturawat P, Govitrapong P, Supavilai P, Sanvarinda Y. Transcriptional regulation of iNOS and COX-2 by a novel compound from Curcuma comosa in lipopolysaccharide-induced microglial activation. Neurosci Lett. 2009 Sep 22;462(2):171-5.

Thaut MH. The future of music in therapy and medicine. Ann N Y Acad Sci. 2005 Dec;1060:303-8.

The Guardian. Exposure to small particle air pollution: mapped by city. Accessed May 4, 2016.

The Nutrition Source. Harvard School of Public Health. Acc. Nov. 10, 2011. Harvard.edu

The Timechart Company. Timetables of Medicine. New York: Black Dog & Leventhal, 2000.

Theofilopoulos AN, Kono DH: The genes of systemic autoimmunity. Proc Assoc Am Physicians. 1999;111(3): 228-240.

Thibault H, Aubert-Jacquin C, Goulet O. Effects of long-term consumption of a fermented infant formula (with Bifidobacterium breve c50 and Streptococcus thermophilus 065) on acute diarrhea in healthy infants. J Pediatr Gastroenterol Nutr. 2004 Aug;39(2):147-52.

Thie J. Touch for Health. Marina del Rey, CA: Devorss Publications, 1973-1994.

Thiruvengadam KV, Haranath K, Sudarsan S, Sekar TS, Rajagopal KR, Zacharian MG, Devarajan TV. Tylophora indica in bronchial asthma (a controlled comparison with a standard anti-asthmatic drug). J Indian Med Assoc. 1978 Oct 1;71(7):172-6.

Thomas M. Are breathing exercises an effective strategy for people with asthma? Nurs Times. 2009 Mar 17-23;105(10):22-7.

Thomas MK, Lloyd-Jones DM, Thadhani RI, Shaw AC, Deraska DJ, Finkelstein JS, et al. Hypovitaminosis D in Medical Inpatients. NEJM. 1998 March 19;338(12):777-783.

Thomas Y, Litime H, Benveniste J. Modulation of human neutrophil activation by "electronic" phorbol myristate acetate (PMA). FASEB Jnl. 1996;10: A1479.

Thomas Y, Schiff M, Belkadi L, Jurgens P, Kahhak L, Benveniste J. Activation of human neutrophils by electronically transmitted phorbol-myristate acetate. Med Hypoth. 2000;54: 33-39.

Thomas Y, Schiff M, Litime M, Belkadi L, Benveniste J. Direct transmission to cells of a molecular signal (phorbol myristate acetate, PMA) via an electronic device. FASEB Jnl. 1995;9: A227.

Thomas, R.G., Gebhardt, S.E. 2008. Nutritive value of pomegranate fruit and juice. Maryland Dietetic Association Annual Meeting, USDA-ARS. 2008 April 11.

Thomas-Anterion C, Jacquin K, Laurent B. Differential mechanisms of impairment of remote memory in Alzheimer's and frontotemporal dementia. Dement Geriatr Cogn Disord. 2000 Mar-Apr;11(2):100-6.

Thompson T, Lee AR, Grace T. Gluten contamination of grains, seeds, and flours in the United States: a pilot study. J Am Diet Assoc. 2010 Jun;110(6):937-40.

Tian FS, Zhang HR, Li WD, Qiao P, Duan HB, Jia CX. Study on acupuncture treatment of diabetic neurogenic bladder. Zhongguo Zhen Jiu. 2007 Jul;27(7):485-7.

Tierra L. The Herbs of Life. Freedom, CA: Crossing Press, 1992.

Tierra M. The Way of Herbs. New York: Pocket Books, 1990.

Tietze LF, Stewart SG, Polomska ME, Modi A, Zeeck A. Towards a total synthesis of the new anticancer agent mensacarcin: synthesis of the carbocyclic core. Chemistry. 2004 Oct 11;10(20):5233-42.

Timofeev I, Steriade M. Low-frequency rhythms in the thalamus of intact-cortex and decorticated cats. J Neurophysiol. 1996 Dec;76(6):4152-68.

Ting W, Schultz K, Cac NN, Peterson M, Walling HW. Tanning bed exposure increases the risk of malignant melanoma. Int J Dermatol. 2007 Dec;46(12):1253-7.

Tisserand R. The Art of Aromatherapy. New York: Inner Traditions, 1979.

Tiwari M. Ayurveda: A Life of Balance. Rochester, VT: Healing Arts, 1995.

Tlaskalová-Hogenová H, Stepánková R, Hudcovic T, Tucková L, Cukrowska B, Lodinová-Zádníková R, Kozáková H, Rossmann P, Bártová J, Sokol D, Funda DP, Borovská D, Reháková Z, Sinkora J, Hofman J, Drastich P, Kokesová A. Commensal bacteria (normal microflora), mucosal immunity and chronic inflammatory and autoimmune diseases. Immunol Lett. 2004 May 15;93(2-3):97-108.

Todd GR, Acerini CL, Ross-Russell R, Zahra S, Warner JT, McCance D. Survey of adrenal crisis associated with inhaled corticosteroids in the United Kingdom. Arch Dis Child. 2002 Dec;87(6):457-61.

Tomasek L, Rogel A, Tirmarche M, Mitton N, Laurier D. Lung cancer in French and Czech uranium miners: Radon-associated risk at low exposure rates and modifying effects of time since exposure and age at exposure. Radiat Res. 2008 Feb;169(2):125-37.

Tomasek L, Rogel A, Tirmarche M, Mitton N, Laurier D. Lung cancer in French and Czech uranium miners: Radon-associated risk at low exposure rates and modifying effects of time since exposure and age at exposure. Radiat Res. 2008 Feb;169(2):125-37.

Tonkal AM, Morsy TA. An update review on Commiphora molmol and related species. J Egypt Soc Parasitol. 2008 Dec;38(3):763-96.

Toomer G. Ptolemy: The Dictionary of Scientific Biography. New York: Gale Cengage, 1970.

Topçu G, Erenler R, Cakmak O, Johansson CB, Celik C, Chai HB, Pezzuto JM. Diterpenes from the berries of Juniperus excelsa. Phytochemistry. 1999 Apr;50(7):1195-9.

Tormo Carnicer R, Infante Piña D, Rosselló Mayans E, Bartolomé Comas R. Intake of fermented milk containing Lactobacillus casei DN-114 001 and its effect on gut flora. An Pediatr. 2006 Nov;65(5):448-53.

Torres-Sánchez L, López-Carrillo L, López-Cervantes M, Rueda-Neria C, Wolff MS. Food sources of phytoestrogens and breast cancer risk in Mexican women. Nutr Cancer. 2000;37(2):134-9.

Touhami M, Boudraa G, Mary JY, Soltana R, Desjeux JF. Clinical consequences of replacing milk with yogurt in persistent infantile diarrhea. Ann Pediatr. 1992 Feb;39(2):79-86.

Towle A. Modern Biology. Austin: Harcourt Brace, 1993.

Traber MG, Elsner A, Brigelius-Flohé R. Synthetic as compared with natural vitamin E is preferentially excreted as alpha-CEHC in human urine: studies using deuterated alpha-tocopheryl acetates. FEBS Lett. 1998 Oct 16;437(1-2):145-8.

Trenev N. Probiotics: Nature's Internal Healers. New York: Avery, 1998.

Triglia A, La Malfa G, Musumeci F, Leonardi C, Scordino A. Delayed luminescence as an indicator of tomato fruit quality. J Food Sci. 1998;63:512-515.

Tripkovic L, Lambert H, Hart K, Smith CP, Bucca G, Penson S, Chope G, Hyppönen E, Berry J, Vieth R, Lanham-New S. Comparison of vitamin D2 and vitamin D3 supplementation in raising serum 25-hydroxyvitamin D status: a systematic review and meta-analysis. Am J Clin Nutr. 2012 Jun;95(6):1357-64.

Trivedi B. Magnetic Map" Found to Guide Animal Migration. Natl Geogr Today. 2001 Oct 12.

Trois L, Cardoso EM, Miura E. Use of probiotics in HIV-infected children: a randomized double-blind controlled study. J Trop Pediatr. 2008 Feb;54(1):19-24.

Trojanová I, Rada V, Kokoska L, Vlková E. The bifidogenic effect of Taraxacum officinale root. Fitoterapia. 2004 Dec;75(7-8):760-3.

Trombete, F., Porto, Y., Freitas Silva, O., Pereira, R., Direito, G., Saldanha, T. and Fraga, M. (2017), Efficacy of Ozone Treatment on Mycotoxins and Fungal Reduction in Artificially Contaminated Soft Wheat Grains. Journal of Food Processing and Preservation, 41: e12927. doi:10.1111/jfpp.12927

Tronina T, Bartmańska A, Filip-Psurska B, Wietrzyk J, Popłoński J, Huszcza E. Fungal metabolites of xanthohumol with potent antiproliferative activity on human cancer cell lines in vitro. Bioorg Med Chem. 2013 Apr 1;21(7):2001-6. doi: 10.1016/j.bmc.2013.01.026.

Trout L, King M, Feng W, Inglis SK, Ballard ST. Inhibition of airway liquid secretion and its effect on the physical properties of airway mucus. Am J Physiol. 1998 Feb;274(2 Pt 1):L258-63.

Tsai JC, Tsai S, Chang WC. Comparison of two Chinese medical herbs, Huangbai and Qianniuzi, on influence of short circuit current across the rat intestinal epithelia. J Ethnopharmacol. 2004 Jul;93(1):21-5.

Tsang KW, Lam CL, Yan C, Mak JC, Ooi GC, Ho JC, Lam B, Man R, Sham JS, Lam WK. Coriolus versicolor polysaccharide peptide slows progression of advanced non-small cell lung cancer. Respir Med. 2003 Jun;97(6):618-24.

Tsinkalovsky O, Smaaland R, Rosenlund B, Sothern RB, Hirt A, Steine S, Badiee A, Abrahamsen JF, Eiken HG, Laerum OD. Circadian variations in clock gene expression of human bone marrow CD34+ cells. J Biol Rhythms. 2007 Apr;22(2):140-50.

Tsong T. Deciphering the language of cells. Trends in Biochem Sci. 1989;14: 89-92.

Tsuchiya J, Barreto R, Okura R, Kawakita S, Fesce E, Marotta F. Single-blind follow-up study on the effectiveness of a symbiotic preparation in irritable bowel syndrome. Chin J Dig Dis. 2004;5(4):169-74.

Tsuei JJ, Lam Jr. F, Zhao Z. Studies in Bioenergetic Correlations-Bioenergetic Regulatory Measurement Instruments and Devices. Am J Acupunct. 1988;16:345-9.

Tsuei JJ, Lehman CW, Lam F, Jr, Zhu D. A food allergy study utilizing the EAV acupuncture technique. Am J Acupunct. 1984;12:105-16.

Tu QQ, Zheng RY, Li J, Hu L, Chang YX, Li L, Li MH, Wang RY, Huang DD, Wu MC, Hu HP, Chen L, Wang HY. Palmitic acid induces autophagy in hepatocytes via JNK2 activation. Acta Pharmacol Sin. 2014 Apr;35(4):504-12. doi: 10.1038/aps.2013.170.

Tubelius P, Stan V, Zachrisson A. Increasing work-place healthiness with the probiotic Lactobacillus reuteri: a randomised, double-blind placebo-controlled study. Environ Health. 2005 Nov 7;4:25.

Tucker KL, Olson B, Bakun P, Dallal GE, Selhub J, Rosenberg IH. Breakfast cereal fortified with folic acid, vitamin B-6, and vitamin B-12 increases vitamin concentrations and reduces homocysteine concentrations: a randomized trial. Am J Clin Nutr. 2004 May;79(5):805-11.

Tulk HM, Robinson LE. Modifying the n-6/n-3 polyunsaturated fatty acid ratio of a high-saturated fat challenge does not acutely attenuate postprandial changes in inflammatory markers in men with metabolic syndrome. Metabolism. 2009 Jul 20.

Tunnicliffe WS, Burge PS, Ayres JG. Effect of domestic concentrations of nitrogen dioxide on airway responses to inhaled allergen in asthmatic patients. Lancet. 1994 Dec 24-31;344(8939-8940):1733-6.

Tunnicliffe WS, Fletcher TJ, Hammond K, Roberts K, Custovic A, Simpson A, Woodcock A, Ayres JG. Sensitivity and exposure to indoor allergens in adults with differing asthma severity. Eur Respir J. 1999 Mar;13(3):654-9.

Tuomilehto J, Lindström J, Hyyrynen J, Korpela R, Karhunen ML, Mikkola L, Jauhiainen T, Seppo L, Nissinen A. Effect of ingesting sour milk fermented using Lactobacillus helveticus bacteria producing tripeptides on blood pressure in subjects with mild hypertension. J Hum Hypertens. 2004 Nov;18(11):795-802.

Turchet P, Laurenzano M, Auboiron S, Antoine JM. Effect of fermented milk containing the probiotic Lactobacillus casei DN-114001 on winter infections in free-living elderly subjects: a randomised, controlled pilot study. J Nutr Health Aging. 2003;7(2):75-7.

Tursi A, Brandimarte G, Giorgetti GM, Elisei W. Mesalazine and/or Lactobacillus casei in maintaining long-term remission of symptomatic uncomplicated diverticular disease of the colon. Hepatogastroenterology. 2008 May-Jun;55(84):916-20.

Twardowski P, Kanaya N, Frankel P, Synold T, Ruel C, Pal SK, Junqueira M, Prajapati M, Moore T, Tryon P, Chen S. A phase I trial of mushroom powder in patients with biochemically recurrent prostate cancer: Roles of cytokines and myeloid-derived suppressor cells for Agaricus bisporus-induced prostate-specific antigen responses. Cancer. 2015 Sep 1;121(17):2942-50. doi: 10.1002/cncr.29421.

Twetman S, Derawi B, Keller M, Ekstrand K, Yucel-Lindberg T, Stecksen-Blicks C. Short-term effect of chewing gums containing probiotic Lactobacillus reuteri on the levels of inflammatory mediators in gingival crevicular fluid. Acta Odontol Scand. 2009 Feb;67(1):19-24.

U.S. Department of Health and Human Services. The Health Consequences of Smoking—50 Years of Progress. A Report of the Surgeon General. Atlanta: U.S. Department of Health and Human Services, Centers for Disease Control and Prevention, National Center for Chronic Disease Prevention and Health Promotion, Office on Smoking and Health, 2014. Accessed 2020 Sep 21.

U.S. Food and Drug Administration Guidance for Industry Botanical Drug Products. CfDEaR. 2000

UC San Diego News Center. Pancreatic Cancer Risk Linked to Weak Sunlight. April 29, 2015.

Uddenfeldt M, Janson C, Lampa E, Leander M, Norbäck D, Larsson L, Rask-Andersen A. High BMI is related to higher incidence of asthma, while a fish and fruit diet is related to a lower- Results from a long-term follow-up study of three age groups in Sweden. Respir Med. 2010 Jul;104(7):972-80.

Udermann H, Fischer G. Studies on the influence of positive or negative small ions on the catechol amine content in the brain of the mouse following shorttime or prolonged exposure. Zentralbl Bakteriol Mikro-biol Hyg. 1982 Apr;176(1):72-8.

Udupa AL, Udupa SL, Guruswamy MN. The possible site of anti-asthmatic action of Tylophora asthmatica on pituitary-adrenal axis in albino rats. Planta Med. 1991 Oct;57(5):409-13.

Ueno H, Yoshioka K, Matsumoto T. Usefulness of the skin index in predicting the outcome of oral challenges in children. J Investig Allergol Clin Immunol. 2007;17(4):207-10.

Ueno M, Adachi A, Fukumoto T, Nishitani N, Fujiwara N, Matsuo H, Kohno K, Morita E. Analysis of causative allergen of the patient with baker's asthma and wheat-dependent exercise-induced anaphylaxis (WDEIA). Arerugi. 2010 May;59(5):552-7.

Uesato S, Yamashita H, Maeda R, Hirata Y, Yamamoto M, Matsue S, Nagaoka Y, Shibano M, Taniguchi M, Baba K, Ju-ichi M. Synergistic antitumor effect of a combination of paclitaxel and carboplatin with nobiletin from Citrus depressa on lung cancer cell lines. Planta Med. 2014 Apr;80(6):452-7. doi: 10.1055/s-0034-1368321.

Ukabam SO, Mann RJ, Cooper BT. Small intestinal permeability to sugars in patients with atopic eczema. Br J Dermatol. 1984 Jun;110(6):649-52.

Ulett G. Electroacupuncture: mechanisms and clinical application. Biological Psychiatry. 1998;44(2):129-138.

Ulrich RS, Simons RF, Losito BD, Fiorito E, Miles MA, Zelson M. Stress recovery during exposure to natural and urban environments. J Envir Psychol. 1991;11:201-30.

Ulrich RS. Aesthetic and affective response to natural environment. In Altman, I. and Wohlwill, J. F. (eds) Human Behaviour and Environment: Advances in Theory and Research. Volume 6: Behaviour and the Natural Envi-ronment. New York: Plenum Press: 1983:85-125.

Ulrich RS. Influences of passive experiences with plants on individual wellbeing and health. In Relf, D. (ed) The Role of Horticulture in Human Well-Being and Social Development: A National Symposium. Portland: Tim-ber Press, Portland. 1992:93 -105.

Ulrich RS. Natural versus urban scenes: some psychophysiological effects. Environment and Behaviour. 1981:523-556.

Ulrich RS. View through window may influence recovery from surgery. Science. 1984;224:420 - 421.

Ulrich RS. Visual landscapes and psychological well being. Landscape Research. 1979;4:17-23.

Une S, Nonaka K, Akiyama J. Lectin Isolated from Japanese Red Sword Beans (Canavalia gladiata) as a Potential Cancer Chemopreventive Agent. J Food Sci. 2018 Feb 13. doi: 10.1111/1750-3841.14057.

Unger RH. Leptin physiology: a second look. Regul Pept. 2000 Aug 25;92(1-3):87-95.

United States Department of Agriculture. Agricultural Research Service. National Nutrient Database for Standard Reference Release 28. ndb.nal.usda.gov/ndb/nutrients/index. Accessed Feb 15, 2016.

United States Government Accountability Office. Report to Congressional Committees. Formaldehyde in Textiles. August 2010 GAO-10-875.

University of Birmingham. Exposure to particulate air pollutants associated with numerous cancers. Public Release: 29-Apr-2016

Upadhyay AK, Kumar K, Kumar A, Mishra HS. Tinospora cordifolia (Willd.) Hook. f. and Thoms. (Guduchi) - validation of the Ayurvedic pharmacology through experimental and clinical studies. Int J Ayurveda Res. 2010 Apr;1(2):112-21.

Urata Y, Yoshida S, Irie Y, Tanigawa T, Amayasu H, Nakabayashi M, Akahori K. Treatment of asthma patients with herbal medicine TJ-96: a randomized controlled trial. Respir Med. 2002 Jun;96(6):469-74.

Urbaniak C, Cummins J, Brackstone M, Macklaim JM, Gloor GB, Baban CK, Scott L, O'Hanlon DM, Burton JP, Francis KP, Tangney M, Reid G. Microbiota of human breast tissue. Appl Environ Micro-biol. 2014 May;80(10):3007-14. doi: 10.1128/AEM.00242-14.

Urbaniak C, Gloor GB, Brackstone M, Scott L, Tangney M, Reid G. The Microbiota of Breast Tissue and Its Association with Breast cancer. and Its Association with Breast cancer. and Its Association with Breast cancer. Appl Environ Microbiol. 2016 Jul 29;82(16):5039-48. doi: 10.1128/AEM.01235-16.

Vakil JR, Shahani KM. Carbohydrate metabolism of lactic acid cultures. V. Lactobionate and gluconate metabolism of Streptococcus lactis UN. J Dairy Sci. 1969 Dec;52(12):1928-34.

Valeur N, Engel P, Carbajal N, Connolly E, Ladefoged K. Colonization and immunomodulation by Lactobacillus reuteri ATCC 55730 in the human gastrointestinal tract. Appl Environ Microbiol. 2004 Feb;70(2):1176-81.

Vallance A. Can biological activity be maintained at ultra-high dilution? An overview of homeopathy, evidence, and Bayesian philosophy. J Altern Complement Med. 1998 Spring;4(1):49-76.

van Baarlen P, Troost FJ, van Hemert S, van der Meer C, de Vos WM, de Groot PJ, Hooiveld GJ, Brummer RJ, Kleerebezem M. Differential NF-kappaB pathways induction by Lactobacillus plantarum in the duodenum of healthy humans correlating with immune tolerance. Proc Natl Acad Sci U S A. 2009 Feb 17;106(7):2371-6

van Beelen VA, Roeleveld J, Mooibroek H, Sijtsma L, Bino RJ, Bosch D, Rietjens IM, Alink GM. A comparative study on the effect of algal and fish oil on viability and cell proliferation of Caco-2 cells. Food Chem Toxicol. 2007 May;45(5):716-24.

Van Cauter E, Leproult R, Plat L. Age-related changes in slow wave sleep and REM sleep and relationship with growth hormone and cortisol levels in healthy men. JAMA. 2000 Aug 16;284(7):861-8.

Van Cauter E. Slow wave sleep and release of growth hormone. JAMA. 2000 Dec 6;284(21):2717-8.

van den Brandt PA, Schouten LJ. Relationship of tree nut, peanut and peanut butter intake with total and cause-specific mortality: a cohort study and meta-analysis. Int J Epidemiol. 2015 Jun;44(3):1038-49.

van den Heuvel EG, Schoterman MH, Muijs T. Transgalactooligosaccharides stimulate calcium absorption in postmenopausal women. J Nutr. 2000 Dec;130(12):2938-42.

van Elburg RM, Uil JJ, de Monchy JG, Heymans HS. Intestinal permeability in pediatric gastroenterology. Scand J Gastroenterol Suppl. 1992;194:19-24.

van Huisstede A, Braunstahl GJ. Obesity and asthma: co-morbidity or causal relationship? Monaldi Arch Chest Dis. 2010 Sep;73(3):116-23.

van Zwol A, Moll HA, Fetter WP, van Elburg RM. Glutamine-enriched enteral nutrition in very low birthweight infants and allergic and infectious diseases at 6 years of age. Paediatr Perinat Epidemiol. 2011 Jan;25(1):60-6.

Vanduchova A, Anzenbacher P, Anzenbacherova E. Isothiocyanate from Broccoli, Sulforaphane, and Its Properties. J Med Food. 2019 Feb;22(2):121-126. doi: 10.1089/jmf.2018.0024.

VanHaitsma TA, Mickleborough T, Stager JM, Koceja DM, Lindley MR, Chapman R. Comparative effects of caffeine and albuterol on the bronchoconstrictor response to exercise in asthmatic athletes. Int J Sports Med. 2010 Apr;31(4):231-6.

Vanto T, Helppilä S, Juntunen-Backman K, Kalimo K, Klemola T, Korpela R, Koskinen P. Prediction of the development of tolerance to milk in children with cow's milk hypersensitivity. J Pediatr. 2004 Feb;144(2):218-22.

Vaquero JM, Gallego MC. Sunspot numbers can detect pandemic influenza A: the use of different sunspot numbers. Med Hypotheses. 2007;68(5):1189-90.

Vargas C, Bustos P, Diaz PV, Amigo H, Rona RJ. Childhood environment and atopic conditions, with emphasis on asthma in a Chilean agricultural area. J Asthma. 2008 Jan-Feb;45(1):73-8.

Vargha-Khadem F, Polkey CE. A review of cognitive outcome after hemidecortication in humans. Adv Exp Med Biol. 1992;325:137-51.

Varonier HS, de Haller J, Schopfer C. Prevalence of allergies in children and adolescents. Helv Paediat Acta. 1984;39:129-136.

Varraso R, Fung TT, Barr RG, Hu FB, Willett W, Camargo CA Jr. Prospective study of dietary patterns and chronic obstructive pulmonary disease among US women. Am J Clin Nutr. 2007 Aug;86(2):488-95.

Varraso R, Fung TT, Hu FB, Willett W, Camargo CA. Prospective study of dietary patterns and chronic obstructive pulmonary disease among US men. Thorax. 2007 Sep;62(9):786-91. 2007 May 15.

Vauthier JM, Lluch A, Lecomte E, Artur Y, Herbeth B. Family resemblance in energy and macronutrient intakes: the Stanislas Family Study. Int J Epidemiol.1996 Oct;25(5):1030-7.

Vaziri F, Najarpeerayeh S, Alebouyeh M, Molaei M, Maghsudi N, Zali MR. Determination of Helicobacter pylori CagA EPIYA types in Iranian isolates with different gastroduodenal disorders. Infect Genet Evol. 2013 Apr 6.

Vempati R, Bijlani RL, Deepak KK. The efficacy of a comprehensive lifestyle modification programme based on yoga in the management of bronchial asthma: a randomized controlled trial. BMC Pulm Med. 2009 Jul 30;9:37.

Vena JE, Graham S, Hellmann R, Swanson M, Brasure J. Use of electric blankets and risk of postmenopausal breast cancer. Am J Epidemiol. 1991 Jul 15;134(2):180-5.

Venil N. Sumantran and Girish Tillu, "Cancer, Inflammation, and Insights from Ayurveda," Evidence-Based Complementary and Alternative Medicine, vol. 2012, Article ID 306346, 11 pages, 2012. doi:10.1155/2012/306346.

Venkatachalam KV. Human 3'-phosphoadenosine 5'-phosphosulfate (PAPS) synthase: biochemistry, molecular biology and genetic deficiency. IUBMB Life. 2003 Jan;55(1):1-11.

Venkatesan N, Punithavathi D, Babu M. Protection from acute and chronic lung diseases by curcumin. Adv Exp Med Biol. 2007;595:379-405.

Venter C, Meyer R. Session 1: Allergic disease: The challenges of managing food hypersensitivity. Proc Nutr Soc. 2010 Feb;69(1):11-24.

Ventura MT, Polimeno L, Amoruso AC, Gatti F, Annoscia E, Marinaro M, Di Leo E, Matino MG, Buquicchio R, Bonini S, Tursi A, Francavilla A. Intestinal permeability in patients with adverse reactions to food. Dig Liver Dis. 2006 Oct;38(10):732-6.

Venturi A, Gionchetti P, Rizzello F, Johansson R, Zucconi E, Brigidi P, Matteuzzi D, Campieri M. Impact on the composition of the faecal flora by a new probiotic preparation: preliminary data on maintenance treatment of patients with ulcerative colitis. Aliment Pharmacol Ther. 1999 Aug;13(8):1103-8.

Verhasselt V. Oral tolerance in neonates: from basics to potential prevention of allergic disease. Mucosal Immunol. 2010 Jul;3(4):326-33.

Vescelius E. Music and Health. New York: Goodyear Book Shop, 1918.

Vgontzas AN. The diagnosis and treatment of chronic insomnia in adults. Sleep. 2005 Sep 1;28(9):1047-8.

Vidgren HM, Agren JJ, Schwab U, Rissanen T, Hanninen O, Uusitupa MI. Incorporation of n-3 fatty acids into plasma lipid fractions, and erythrocyte membranes and platelets during dietary supplementation with fish, fish oil, and docosahexaenoic acid-rich oil among healthy young men. Lipids. 1997 Jul;32(7):697-705.

Vierling-Claassen D, Siekmeier P, Stufflebeam S, Kopell N. Modeling GABA alterations in schizophrenia: a link between impaired inhibition and altered gamma and beta range auditory entrainment. J Neurophysiol. 2008 May;99(5):2656-71.

Vigny P, Duquesne M. On the fluorescence properties of nucleotides and polynucleotides at room temperature. In. Birks J (ed.). Excited states of biological molecules. London-NY: J Wiley, 1976:167-177.

Vila R, Mundina M, Tomi F, Furlán R, Zacchino S, Casanova J, Cañigueral S. Composition and antifungal activity of the essential oil of Solidago chilensis. Planta Med. 2002 Feb;68(2):164-7.

Villani S. Impact of media on children and adolescents: a 10-year review of the research. J Am Acad Child Adolesc Psychiatry. 2001 Apr;40(4):392-401.

Villarruel G, Rubio DM, Lopez F, Cintioni J, Gurevech R, Romero G, Vandenplas Y. Saccharomyces boulardii in acute childhood diarrhoea: a randomized, placebo-controlled study. Acta Paediatr. 2007 Apr;96(4):538-41.

Viner RM, Cole TJ. Television viewing in early childhood predicts adult body mass index. J Pediatr. 2005 Oct;147(4):429-35.

Vinson JA, Proch J, Bose P. MegaNatural((R)) Gold Grapeseed Extract: In Vitro Antioxidant and In Vivo Human Supplementation Studies. J Med Food. 2001 Spring;4(1):17-26.

Viola AU, James LM, Schlangen LJ, Dijk DJ. Blue-enriched white light in the workplace improves self-reported alertness, performance and sleep quality. Scand J Work Environ Hlth. 2008 Aug;34(4):297-306.

Visness CM, London SJ, Daniels JL, Kaufman JS, Yeatts KB, Siega-Riz AM, Calatroni A, Zeldin DC. Association of childhood obesity with atopic and nonatopic asthma: results from the National Health and Nutrition Examination Survey 1999-2006. J Asthma. 2010 Sep;47(7):822-9.

Vivatvakin B, Kowitdamrong E. Randomized control trial of live Lactobacillus acidophilus plus Bifidobacterium infantis in treatment of infantile acute watery diarrhea. J Med Assoc Thai. 2006 Sep;89 Suppl 3:S126-33.

Voicekovska JG, Orlikov GA, Karpov IuG, Teibe U, Ivanov AD, Baidekalne I, Voicehovskis NV, Maulins E. External respiration function and quality of life in patients with bronchial asthma in correction of selenium deficiency. Ter Arkh. 2007;79(8):38-41.

Voïtsekhovskaia IuG, Skesters A, Orlikov GA, Silova AA, Rusakova NE, Larmane LT, Karpov IuG, Ivanov AD, Maulins E. Assessment of some oxidative stress parameters in bronchial asthma patients beyond add-on selenium supplementation. Biomed Khim. 2007 Sep-Oct;53(5):577-84.

Vojdani A. Antibodies as predictors of complex autoimmune diseases. Int J Immunopathol Pharmacol. 2008 Apr-Jun;21(2):267-78.

Volkmann H, Dannberg G, Kuhnert H, Heinke M. Therapeutic value of trans-esophageal electrostimulation in tachycardic arrhythmias. Z Kardiol. 1991 Jun;80(6):382-8.

von Hagens C, Walter-Sack I, Goeckenjan M, et al. Long-term add-on therapy (compassionate use) with oral artesunate in patients with metastatic breast cancer after participating in a phase I study (ARTIC M33/2). Phytomedicine. 2019;54:140-148. doi:10.1016/j.phymed.2018.09.178

von Kruedener S, Schneider W, Elstner EF. A combination of Populus tremula, Solidago virgaurea and Fraxinus excelsior as an anti-inflammatory and antirheumatic drug. A short review. Arzneimittelforschung. 1995 Feb;45(2):169-71.

von Schantz M, Archer SN. Clocks, genes and sleep. J R Soc Med. 2003 Oct;96(10):486-9.

411

Vuksan V, Whitham D, Sievenpiper JL, Jenkins AL, Rogovik AL, Bazinet RP, Vidgen E, Hanna A. Supplementation of conventional therapy with the novel grain Salba (Salvia hispanica L.) improves major and emerging cardiovascular risk factors in type 2 diabetes: results of a randomized controlled trial. Diabetes Care. 2007 Nov;30(11):2804-10.

Vulevic J, Drakoularakou A, Yaqoob P, Tzortzis G and Gibson GR; Modulation of the fecal microflora profile and immune function by a novel trans-galactooligosaccharide mixture (B-GOS) in healthy elderly volunteers. Am J Clin Nutr. 1988 88;1438-1446.

Vyas A, Syeda K, Ahmad A, Padhye S, Sarkar FH. Perspectives on medicinal properties of mangiferin. Mini Rev Med Chem. 2012 May 1;12(5):412-25.

Wachiuli M, Koyama M, Utsuyama M, Bittman BB, Kitagawa M, Hirokawa K. Recreational music-making modulates natural killer cell activity, cytokines, and mood states in corporate employees. Med Sci Monit. 2007 Feb;13(2):CR57-70.

Wada S. Cancer Preventive Effects of Vitamin E. Curr Pharm Biotechnol. 2011 Apr 5. Ju J, Picinich SC, Yang Z, Zhao Y, Suh N, Kong AN, Yang CS. Cancer-preventive activities of tocopherols and tocotrienols. Carcinogenesis. 2010 Apr;31(4):533-42.

Wahler D, Gronover CS, Richter C, Foucu F, Twyman RM, Moerschbacher BM, Fischer R, Muth J, Prufer D. Polyphenoloxidase silencing affects latex coagulation in Taraxacum spp. Plant Physiol. 2009 Jul 15.

Walch JM, Rabin BS, Day R, Williams JN, Choi K, Kang JD. The effect of sunlight on postoperative analgesic medication use: a prospective study of patients undergoing spinal surgery. Psychosom Med. 2005 Jan-Feb;67(1):156-63.

Walders-Abramson N, Wamboldt FS, Curran-Everett D, Zhang L. Encouraging physical activity in pediatric asthma: a case-control study of the wonders of walking (WOW) program. Pediatr Pulmonol. 2009 Sep;44(9):909-16.

Walker M. The Power of Color. New Delhi: B. Jain Publishers. 2002.

Walker S, Wing A. Allergies in children. J Fam Health Care. 2010;20(1):24-6.

Walker WA. Antigen absorption from the small intestine and gastrointestinal disease. Pediatr Clin North Am. 1975 Nov;22(4):731-46.

Walker WA. Antigen handling by the small intestine. Clin Gastroenterol. 1986 Jan;15(1):1-20.

Walle UK, Walle T. Transport of the cooked-food mutagen 2-amino-1-methyl-6-phenylimidazo- 4,5-b pyridine (PhIP) across the human intestinal Caco-2 cell monolayer: role of efflux pumps. Carcinogenesis. 1999 Nov;20(11):2153-7.

Walsh MG. Toxocara infection and diminished lung function in a nationally representative sample from the United States population. Int J Parasitol. 2010 Nov 8.

Walsh SJ, Rau LM: Autoimmune diseases: a leading cause of death among young and middle-aged women in the United States. Am J Public Health 2000, 90(9): 1463-1466.

Wang CZ, Anderson S, DU W, He TC, Yuan CS. Red ginseng and cancer treatment. Chin J Nat Med. 2016 Jan;14(1):7-16. doi: 10.3724/SP.J.1009.2016.00007. PMID: 26850342.

Wang G, Liu CT, Wang ZL, Yan CL, Luo FM, Wang L, Li TQ. Effects of Astragalus membranaceus in promoting T-helper cell type 1 polarization and interferon-gamma production by up-regulating T-bet expression in patients with asthma. Chin J Integr Med. 2006 Dec;12(4):262-7.

Wang H, Chang B, Wang B. The effect of herbal medicine including astragalus membranaceus (fisch) bge, codonpsis pilosula and glycyrrhiza uralensis fisch on airway responsiveness. Zhonghua Jie He He Hu Xi Za Zhi. 1998 May;21(5):287-8.

Wang H, Zhang H, Tang L, Chen H, Wu C, Zhao M, Yang Y, Chen X, Liu G. Resveratrol inhibits TGF-β1-induced epithelial-to-mesenchymal transition and suppresses lung cancer invasion and metastasis. Toxicology. 2012 Nov 9.

Wang J, Dong B, Tan Y, Yu S, Bao YX. A study on the immunomodulation of polysaccharopeptide through the TLR4-TIRAP/MAL-MyD88 signaling pathway in PBMCs from breast cancer patients. Immunopharmacol Immunotoxicol. 2013 Aug;35(4):497-504. doi: 10.3109/08923973.2013.805764.

Wang JL, Shaw NS, Kao MD. Magnesium deficiency and its lack of association with asthma in Taiwanese elementary school children. Asia Pac J Clin Nutr. 2007;16 Suppl 2:579-84.

Wang JS, Hung WP. The effects of a swimming intervention for children with asthma. Respirology. 2009 Aug;14(6):838-42.

Wang KS, Li J, Wang Z, Mi C, Ma J, Piao LX, Xu GH, Li X, Jin X. Artemisinin inhibits inflammatory response via regulating NF-κB and MAPK signaling pathways. Immunopharmacol Immunotoxicol. 2017 Feb;39(1):28-36. doi: 10.1080/08923973.2016.1267744.

Wang KY, Li SN, Liu CS, Perng DS, Su YC, Wu DC, Jan CM, Lai CH, Wang TN, Wang WM. Effects of ingesting Lactobacillus- and Bifidobacterium-containing yogurt in subjects with colonized Helicobacter pylori. Am J Clin Nutr. 2004 Sep;80(3):737-41.

Wang L, Li B, Pan MX, Mo XF, Chen YM, Zhang CX. Specific carotenoid intake inversely associated with breast cancer among Chinese women. Br J Nutr. 2014 May;111(9):1686-95. doi: 10.1017/S000711451300411X.

Wang N, Wang ZY, Mo SL, Loo TY, Wang DM, Luo HB, Yang DP, Chen YL, Shen JG, Chen JP. Ellagic acid, a phenolic compound, exerts anti-angiogenesis effects via VEGFR-2 signaling pathway in breast cancer. Breast cancer Res Treat. 2012 Feb 21.

Wang P, Solorzano W, Diaz T, Magyar CE, Henning SM, Vadgama JV. Arctigenin inhibits prostate tumor cell growth in vitro and in vivo. Clin Nutr Exp. 2017 Jun;13:1-11. doi: 10.1016/j.yclnex.2017.04.001.

Wang QZ, Chen XP, Huang JP, Jiang XW. [Effects of Couplet Medicines (Astragalus Membranaceus and Jiaozhen) on Intestinal Barrier in Postoperative Colorectal Cancer Patients]. Zhongguo Zhong Xi Yi Jie He Za Zhi. 2015 Nov;35(11):1307-12. Chinese. PMID: 26775475.

Wang R, Jiang C, Lei Z, Yin K. The role of different therapeutic courses in treating 47 cases of rheumatoid arthritis with acupuncture. J Tradit Chin Med. 2007 Jun;27(2):103-5.

Wang R, Paul VJ, Luesch H. Seaweed extracts and unsaturated fatty acid constituents from the green alga Ulva lactuca as activators of the cytoprotective Nrf2-ARE pathway. Free Radic Biol Med. 2013 Apr;57:141-53.

Wang S, Dunlap TL, Howell CE, Mbachu OC, Rue EA, Phansalkar R, Chen SN, Pauli GF, Dietz BM, Bolton JL. Hop (Humulus lupulus L.) Extract and 6-Prenylnaringenin Induce P450 1A1 Catalyzed Estrogen 2-Hydroxylation. Chem Res Toxicol. 2016 Jul 18;29(7):1142-50. doi: 10.1021/acs.chemrestox.6b00112.

Wang X, Govind S, Sajankila SP, Mi L, Roy R, Chung FL. Phenethyl isothiocyanate sensitizes human cervical cancer cells to apoptosis induced by cisplatin. Mol Nutr Food Res. 2011 Oct;55(10):1572-81.

Wang X, Liu JZ, Hu JX, Wu H, Li YL, Chen HL, Bai H, Hai CX. ROS-activated p38 MAPK/ERK-Akt cascade plays a central role in palmitic acid-stimulated hepatocyte proliferation. Free Radic Biol Med. 2011 Jul 15;51(2):539-51. doi: 10.1016/j.freeradbiomed.2011.04.019.

Wang XY, Shi X, He L. Effect of electroacupuncture on gastrointestinal dynamics in acute pancreatitis patients and its mechanism. Zhen Ci Yan Jiu. 2007;32(3):199-202.

Wang Y, Gapstur SM, Gaudet MM, Furtado JD, Campos H, McCullough ML. Plasma carotenoids and breast cancer risk in the Cancer Prevention Study II Nutrition Cohort. Cancer Causes Control. 2015 Sep;26(9):1233-44. doi: 10.1007/s10552-015-0614-4.

Wang Y, Kloog I, Coull BA, Kosheleva A, Zanobetti A, Schwartz JD. Estimating Causal Effects of Long-Term PM(2.5) Exposure on Mortality in New Jersey. Environ Health Perspect. 2016 Apr 15.

Wang Y, Wei S, Wang J, Fang Q, Chai Q. Phenethyl isothiocyanate inhibits growth of human chronic myeloid leukemia K562 cells via reactive oxygen species generation and caspases. Mol Med Rep. 2014 Jul;10(1):543-9. doi:

Wang Y, Zhang S. Berberine suppresses growth and metastasis of endometrial cancer cells via miR-101/COX-2. Biomed Pharmacother. 2018 Jul;103:1287-1293. doi: 10.1016/j.biopha.2018.04.161.

Wang YH, Yang CP, Ku MS, Sun HL, Lue KH. Efficacy of nasal irrigation in the treatment of acute sinusitis in children. Int J Pediatr Otorhinolaryngol. 2009 Dec;73(12):1696-701. 2009 Sep 27.

Wang YM, Huan GX. Utilization of Classical Formulas. Beijing, China: Chinese Medicine and Pharmacology Publishing Co, 1998.

Wang Z, Loo WT, Wang N, Chow LW, Wang D, Han F, Zheng X, Chen JP. Effect of Sanguisorba officinalis L on breast cancer growth and angiogenesis. Expert Opin Ther Targets. 2012 Feb 9.

Wang Z, Wang C, Wu Z, Xue J, Shen B, Zuo W, Wang Z, Wang SL. Artesunate Suppresses Growth of Prostatic Cancer Cells through Inhibiting Androgen Receptor. Biol Pharm Bull. 2017;40(4):479-485. doi: 10.1248/bpb.b16-00908.

Waring G, Levy D. Challenging adverse reactions in children with food allergies. Paediatr Nurs. 2010 Jul;22(6):16-22.

Waterman E, Lockwood B. Active components and clinical applications of olive oil. Altern Med Rev. 2007 Dec;12(4):331-42.

Watkins BA, Hannon K, Ferruzzi M, Li Y. Dietary PUFA and flavonoids as deterrents for environmental pollutants. J Nutr Biochem. 2007 Mar;18(3):196-205.

Watson J. Oxidants, antioxidants and the current incurability of metastatic cancers. Open Biol. 2013 Jan 8;3(1):120144.

Watson R. Preedy VR. Botanical Medicine in Clinical Practice. Oxfordshire: CABI, 2008.

Watve MG, Tickoo R, Jog MM, Bhole BD. How many antibiotics are produced by the genus Streptomyces? Arch Microbiol. 2001 Nov;176(5):386-90.

Watzl B, Bub A, Blockhaus M, Herbert BM, Lührmann PM, Neuhäuser-Berthold M, Rechkemmer G. Prolonged tomato juice consumption has no effect on cell-mediated immunity of well-nourished elderly men and women. J Nutr. 2000 Jul;130(7):1719-23.

Wayne R. Chemistry of the Atmospheres. Oxford Press, 1991.

Weaver J, Astumian R. The response of living cells to very weak electric fields: the thermal noise limit. Science. 1990;247: 459-462.

Weaver J, Astumian R. The response of living cells to very weak electric fields: the thermal noise limit. Science. 1990;247: 459-462.

Webster D, Taschereau P, Belland RJ, Sand C, Rennie RP. Antifungal activity of medicinal plant extracts; preliminary screening studies. J Ethnopharmacol. 2008 Jan 4;115(1):140-6.

Wee K, Rogers T, Altan BS, Hackney SA, Hamm C. Engineering and medical applications of diatoms. J Nanosci Nanotechnol. 2005 Jan;5(1):88-91.

Weekes DJ. The treatment of aphthous stomatitis with Lactobacillus tablets. NY State J Med. 1958 Aug 15;58(16):2672-3.

Wegrowski J, Robert AM, Moczar M. The effect of procyanidolic oligomers on the composition of normal and hypercholesterolemic rabbit aortas. Biochem Pharmacol. 1984 Nov 1;33(21):3491-7.

Wei A, Shibamoto T. Antioxidant activities and volatile constituents of various essential oils. J Agric Food Chem. 2007 Mar 7;55(5):1737-42.

Wei J, Liu M, Liu H, Wang F, Zhang Y, Han L, Lin X. Oleanolic acid arrests cell cycle and induces apoptosis via ROS-mediated mitochondrial depolarization and lysosomal membrane permeabilization in human pancreatic cancer cells. J Appl Toxicol. 2013 Aug;33(8):756-65. doi: 10.1002/jat.2725.

Weinberger P, Measures M. The effect of two audible sound frequencies on the germination and growth of a spring and winter wheat. Can. J. Bot. 1968;46(9):1151-1158.

Weiner MA. Secrets of Fijian Medicine. Berkeley, CA: Univ. of Calif., 1969.

Weinert D, Waterhouse J. The circadian rhythm of core temperature: effects of physical activity and aging. Physiol Behav. 2007 Feb 28;90(2-3):246-56.

Weisgerber M, Webber K, Meurer J, Danduran M, Berger S, Flores G. Moderate and vigorous exercise programs in children with asthma: safety, parental satisfaction, and asthma outcomes. Pediatr Pulmonol. 2008 Dec;43(12):1175-82.

Weiss RF. Herbal Medicine. Gothenburg, Sweden: Beaconsfield, 1988.

Weizman Z, Asli G, Alsheikh A. Effect of a probiotic infant formula on infections in child care centers: comparison of two probiotic agents. Pediatrics. 2005 Jan;115(1):5-9.

Weng CJ, Yen GC. The in vitro and in vivo experimental evidences disclose the chemopreventive effects of Ganoderma lucidum on cancer invasion and metastasis. Clin Exp Metastasis. 2010 May;27(5):361-9. doi: 10.1007/s10585-010-9334-z.

Weng CJ, Yen GC. The in vitro and in vivo experimental evidences disclose the chemopreventive effects of Ganoderma lucidum on cancer invasion and metastasis. Clin Exp Metastasis. 2010 May;27(5):361-9. doi: 10.1007/s10585-010-9334-z.

Wenus C, Goll R, Loken EB, Biong AS, Halvorsen DS, Florholmen J. Prevention of antibiotic-associated diarrhoea by a fermented probiotic milk drink. Eur J Clin Nutr. 2008 Feb;62(2):299-301.

Werbach M. Nutritional Influences on Illness. Tarzana, CA: Third Line Press, 1996.

Wertheimer N, Leeper E. Electrical wiring configurations and childhood cancer. Am J Epidemiol. 1979 Mar;109(3):273-84.

Wesa KM, Cunningham-Rundles S, Klimek VM, Vertosick E, Coleton MI, Yeung KS, Lin H, Nimer S, Cassileth BR. Maitake mushroom extract in myelodysplastic syndromes (MDS): a phase II study. Cancer Immunol Immunother. 2015 Feb;64(2):237-47. doi: 10.1007/s00262-014-1628-6.

West P. Surf Your Biowaves. London: Quantum, 1999.

West R. Risk of death in meat and non-meat eaters. BMJ. 1994 Oct 8;309(6959):955.

Wetterberg L. Light and biological rhythms. J Intern Med. 1994 Jan;235(1):5-19.

Weyandt TB, Schrader SM, Turner TW, Simon SD. Semen analysis of military personnel associated with military duty assignments. Reprod Toxicol. 1996 Nov-Dec;10(6):521-8.

Weyandt TB, Schrader SM, Turner TW, Simon SD. Semen analysis of military personnel associated with military duty assignments. Reprod Toxicol. 1996 Nov-Dec;10(6):521-8.

Wharton B, Bishop N. Rickets. Lancet. 2003 Oct 25;362(9393):1389-400.

Wheeler JG, Bogle ML, Shema SJ, Shirrell MA, Stine KC, Pittler AJ, Burks AW, Helm RM. Impact of dietary yogurt on immune function. Am J Med Sci. 1997 Feb;313(2):120-3.

White AR, Rampes H, Ernst E. Acupuncture for smoking cessation. Cochrane Database Syst Rev. 2002;(2):CD000009.

White J, Krippner S (eds). Future Science: Life Energies & the Physics of Paranormal Phenomena. Garden City: Anchor, 1977.

White LB, Foster S. The Herbal Drugstore. Emmaus, PA: Rodale, 2000.

White S. The Unity of the Self. Cambridge: MIT Press, 1991.

Whitfield KE, Wiggins SA, Belue R, Brandon DT. Genetic and environmental influences on forced expiratory volume in African Americans: the Carolina African-American Twin Study of Aging. Ethn Dis. 2004 Spring;14(2):206-11.

Whittaker E. History of the Theories of Aether and Electricity. New York: Nelson LTD, 1953.

WHO. Guidelines for Drinking-water Quality. 2nd ed, vol. 2. Geneva: World Health Organization. 1996.

WHO. How trace elements in water contribute to health. WHO Chronicle. 1978;32: 382-385.

REFERENCES AND BIBLIOGRAPHY

Whorwell PJ, Altringer L, Morel J, Bond Y, Charbonneau D, O'Mahony L, Kiely B, Shanahan F, Quigley EM. Efficacy of an encapsulated probiotic Bifidobacterium infantis 35624 in women with irritable bowel syndrome. Am J Gastroenterol. 2006 Jul;101(7):1581-90.

Wichmann HE. Diesel exhaust particles. Inhal Toxicol. 2007;19 Suppl 1:241-4.

Widdicombe JG, Ernst E. Clinical cough V: complementary and alternative medicine: therapy of cough. Handb Exp Pharmacol. 2009;(187):321-42.

Wildt S, Munck LK, Vinter-Jensen L, Hanse BF, Nordgaard-Lassen I, Christensen S, Avnstroem S, Rasmussen SN, Rumessen JJ. Probiotic treatment of collagenous colitis: a randomized, double-blind, placebo-controlled trial with Lactobacillus acidophilus and Bifidobacterium animalis subsp. Lactis. Inflamm Bowel Dis. 2006 May;12(5):395-401.

Wilen J, Hornsten R, Sandstrom M, Bjerle P, Wiklund U, Stensson O, Lyskov E, Mild KH. Electromagnetic field exposure and health among RF plastic sealer operators. Bioelectromag. 2004 Jan;25(1):5-15.

Wilkens H, Wilkens JH, Uffmann J, Bövers J, Fröhlich JC, Fabel H. Effect of the platelet-activating factor antagonist BN 52063 on exertional asthma. Pneumologie. 1990 Feb;44 Suppl 1:347-8.

Willard T, Jones K. Reishi Mushroom: Herb of Spiritual Potency and Medical Wonder. Issaquah, Washington: Sylvan Press, 1990.

Willard T. Edible and Medicinal Plants of the Rocky Mountains and Neighbouring Territories. Calgary: 1992.

Willemsen LE, Koetsier MA, Balvers M, Beermann C, Stahl B, van Tol EA. Polyunsaturated fatty acids support epithelial barrier integrity and reduce IL-4 mediated permeability in vitro. Eur J Nutr. 2008 Jun;47(4):183-91.

Williams AB, Yu C, Tashima K, Burgess J, Danvers K. Evaluation of two self-care treatments for prevention of vaginal candidiasis in women with HIV. J Assoc Nurses AIDS Care. 2001 Jul-Aug;12(4):51-7.

Williams DM. Considerations in the long-term management of asthma in ambulatory patients. AM J Health Sits Pham. 2006;63:S14-21.

Williams MC, Lecluyse K, Rock-Faucheux A. Effective interventions for reading disability. J Am Optom Assoc. 1992 Jun;63(6):411-7.

Williams SP, Nowicki MO, Liu F, Press R, Godlewski J, Abdel-Rasoul M, Kaur B, Fernandez SA, Chiocca EA, Lawler SE. Indirubins decrease glioma invasion by blocking migratory phenotypes in both the tumor and stromal endothelial cell compartments. Cancer Res. 2011 Aug 15;71(16):5374-80.

Wilson D, Evans M, Guthrie N, Sharma P, Baisley J, Schonlau F, Burki C. A randomized, double-blind, placebo-controlled exploratory study to evaluate the potential of pycnogenol for improving allergic rhinitis symptoms. Phytother Res. 2010 Aug;24(8):1115-9.

Wilson L. Nutritional Balancing and Hair Mineral Analysis. Prescott, AZ: LD Wilson, 1998.

Wilson MK, Baguley BC, Wall C, Jameson MB, Findlay MP. Review of high-dose intravenous vitamin C as an anticancer agent. Asia Pac J Clin Oncol. 2014 Mar;10(1):22-37. doi: 10.1111/ajco.12173.

Wilson NM, Charette L, Thomson AH, Silverman M. Gastro-oesophageal reflux and childhood asthma: the acid test. Thorax. 1985 Aug;40(8):592-7.

Winchester AM. Biology and its Relation to Mankind. New York: Van Nostrand Reinhold, 1969.

Wiseman H. Vitamin D is a membrane antioxidant. Ability to inhibit iron-dependent lipid peroxidation in liposomes compared to cholesterol, ergosterol and tamoxifen and relevance to anticancer action. FEBS Lett. 1993 Jul 12;326(1-3):285-8.

Witsell DL, Garrett CG, Yarbrough WG, Dorrestein SP, Drake AF, Weissler MC. Effect of Lactobacillus acidophilus on antibiotic-associated gastrointestinal morbidity: a prospective randomized trial. J Otolaryngol. 1995 Aug;24(4):230-3.

Wittenberg JS. The Rebellious Body. New York: Insight, 1996.

Wolpowitz D, Gilchrest BA. The vitamin D questions: how much do you need and how should you get it? J Am Acad Dermatol 2006;54:301-17.

Wolverton BC. How to grow fresh air: 50 houseplants that purify your home or office. New York: Penguin, 1997.

Wong CK, Bao YX, Wong EL, Leung PC, Fung KP, Lam CW. Immunomodulatory activities of Yunzhi and Danshen in post-treatment breast cancer patients. Am J Chin Med. 2005;33(3):381-95.

Wong CM, et al. Cancer Mortality Risks from Long-term Exposure to Ambient Fine Particle. Cancer Epidemiol Biomarkers Prev May 2016 25; 839. doi: 10.1158/1055-9965.EPI-15-0626

Wong WM, Lai KC, Lam KF, Hui WM, Hu WH, Lam CL, Xia HH, Huang JQ, Chan CK, Lam SK, Wong BC. Prevalence, clinical spectrum and health care utilization of gastro-oesophageal reflux disease in a Chinese population: a population-based study. Aliment Pharmacol Ther. 2003 Sep 15;18(6):595-604.

Wood M. The Book of Herbal Wisdom. Berkeley, CA: North Atlantic, 1997.

Wood RA, Kraynak J. Food Allergies for Dummies. Hoboken, NJ: Wiley Publ, 2007.

World Health Organization. Q&A on the carcinogenicity of the consumption of red meat and processed meat. www.who.int/features/qa/cancer-red-meat/en/. 26 Oct. 2015. Accessed October 18, 2020.

World Health Organization: 2014 Air Pollution Ranking. May 16, 2015.

Wouters EF, Reynaert NL, Dentener MA, Vernooy JH. Systemic and local inflammation in asthma and chronic obstructive pulmonary disease: is there a connection? Proc Am Thorac Soc. 2009 Dec;6(8):638-47.

WP6 ECRHS II FINAL REPORT European Community Respiratory Health Survey II Final Report of Work Package 6: PM 2.5 assessment in 21 European Cities of ECRHS II. May 2004.

Wright GR, Howieson S, McSharry C, McMahon AD, Chaudhuri R, Thompson J, Donnelly I, Brooks RG, Lawson A, Jolly L, McAlpine L, King EM, Chapman MD, Wood S, Thomson NC. Effect of improved home ventilation on asthma control and house dust mite allergen levels. Allergy. 2009 Nov;64(11):1671-80.

Wright ME, Michaud DS, Pietinen P, Taylor PR, Virtamo J, Albanes D. Estimated urine pH and bladder cancer risk in a cohort of male smokers (Finland). Cancer Causes Control. 2005 Nov;16(9):1117-23. doi: 10.1007/s10552-005-0348-9. PMID: 16184478.

Wu B, Yu J, Wang Y. Effect of Chinese herbs for tonifying Shen on balance of Th1 /Th2 in children with asthma in remission stage. Zhongguo Zhong Xi Yi Jie He Za Zhi. 2007 Feb;27(2):120-2.

Wu JG, Kan YJ, Wu YB, Yi J, Chen TQ, Wu JZ. Hepatoprotective effect of ganoderma triterpenoids against oxidative damage induced by tert-butyl hydroperoxide in human hepatic HepG2 cells. Pharm Biol. 2016;54(5):919-29. doi: 10.3109/13880209.2015.1091481.

Wu Q, Wu K, Ye Y, Dong X, Zhang J. Quorum sensing and its roles in pathogenesis among animal-associated pathogens—a review. Wei Sheng Wu Xue Bao. 2009 Jul 4;49(7):853-8.

Wyart C, Webster WW, Chen JH, Wilson SR, McClary A, Khan RM, Sobel N. Smelling a single component of male sweat alters levels of cortisol in women. J Neurosci. 2007 Feb 7;27(6):1261-5.

Xi L, Han DM, Lü XF, Zhang L. Psychological characteristics in patients with allergic rhinitis and its associated factors analysis.. Zhonghua Er Bi Yan Hou Tou Jing Wai Ke Za Zhi. 2009 Dec;44(12):985-8.

Xiao P, Kubo H, Ohsawa M, Higashiyama K, Nagase H, Yan YN, Li JS, Kamei J, Ohmiya S. kappa-Opioid receptor-mediated antinociceptive effects of stereoisomers and derivatives of (+)-matrine in mice. Planta Med. 1999 Apr;65(3):230-3.

Xiao SD, Zhang DZ, Lu H, Jiang SH, Liu HY, Wang GS, Xu GM, Zhang ZB, Lin GJ, Wang GL. Multicenter, randomized, controlled trial of heat-killed Lactobacillus acidophilus LB in patients with chronic diarrhea. Adv Ther. 2003 Sep-Oct;20(5):253-60.

Xie JY, Dong JC, Gong ZH. Effects on herba epimedii and radix Astragali on tumor necrosis factor-alpha and nuclear factor-kappa B in asthmatic rats. Zhongguo Zhong Xi Yi Jie He Za Zhi. 2006 Aug;26(8):723-7.

Xu T, Beelman RB, Lambert JD. The cancer preventive effects of edible mushrooms. Anticancer Agents Med Chem. 2012 Dec;12(10):1255-63.

Xu X, Cheng Y, Li S, Zhu Y, Xu X, Zheng X, Mao Q, Xie L. Dietary carrot consumption and prostate cancer. Eur J Nutr. 2014 Dec;53(8):1615-23. doi: 10.1007/s00394-014-0667-2

Xu X, Zhang D, Zhang H, Wolters PJ, Killeen NP, Sullivan BM, Locksley RM, Lowell CA, Caughey GH. Neutrophil histamine contributes to inflammation in mycoplasma pneumonia. J Exp Med. 2006 Dec 25;203(13):2907-17.

Xu Z, Zheng G, Wang Y, Zhang C, Yu J, Teng F, Lv H, Cheng X. Aqueous Huaier Extract Suppresses Gastric Cancer Metastasis and Epithelial to Mesenchymal Transition by Targeting Twist. J Cancer. 2017 Oct 19;8(18):3876-3886. doi: 10.7150/jca.20380.

Yadav H, Jain S, Sinha PR. Antidiabetic effect of probiotic dahl containing Lactobacillus acidophilus and Lactobacillus casei in high fructose fed rats. Nutrition. 2007 Jan;23(1):62-8.

Yadav RK, Ray RB, Vempati R, Bijlani RL. Effect of a comprehensive yoga-based lifestyle modification program on lipid peroxidation. Indian J Physiol Pharmacol. 2005 Jul-Sep;49(3):358-62.

Yadav VS, Mishra KP, Singh DP, Mehrotra S, Singh VK. Immunomodulatory effects of curcumin. Immunopharmacol Immunotoxicol. 2005;27(3):485-97.

Yadzir ZH, Misnan R, Abdullah N, Bakhtiar F, Arip M, Murad S. Identification of Ige-binding proteins of raw and cooked extracts of Loligo edulis (white squid). Southeast Asian J Trop Med Public Health. 2010 May;41(3):653-9.

Yamamoto K, Noda K, Hatae M, Kudo T, Hasegawa K, Nishimura R, Honjo H, Yajima A, Sato S, Mizutani K, Yakushiji M, Terashima Y, Ochiai K, Sasaki H, Ozaki M. (2001). Effects of concomitant use of doxifluridine, radiotherapy and immunotherapy in patients with advanced cervical cancer. Oncology Reports, 8(2), 273-277.

Yamamura S, Morishima H, Kumano-go T, Suganuma N, Matsumoto H, Adachi H, Sigedo Y, Mikami A, Kai T, Masuyama A, Takano T, Sugita Y, Takeda M. The effect of Lactobacillus helveticus fermented milk on sleep and health perception in elderly subjects. Eur J Clin Nutr. 2009 Jan;63(1):100-5.

Yamaoka Y. Solid cell nest (SCN) of the human thyroid gland. Acta Pathol Jpn. 1973 Aug;23(3):493-506.

Yan B, Peng ZY. Honokiol induces cell cycle arrest and apoptosis in human gastric carcinoma MGC-803 cell line. Int J Clin Exp Med. 2015 Apr 15;8(4):5454-61.

Yan YF, Wei YY, Chen YH, Chen MM. Effect of acupuncture on rehabilitation training of child's autism. Zhongguo Zhen Jiu. 2007 Jul;27(7):503-5.

Yang A, Zhao Y, Wang Y, Zha X, Zhao Y, Tu P, Hu Z. Huaier suppresses proliferative potential of prostate cancer PC3 cells via downregulation of Lamin B1 and induction of autophagy. Oncol Rep. 2018 Apr 5. doi: 10.3892/or.2018.6358.

Yang AL, Hu ZD, Tu PF. Research progress on anti-tumor effect of Huaier. Zhongguo Zhong Yao Za Zhi. 2015 Dec;40(24):4805-10.

Yang CS, Wang X, Lu G, Picinich SC: Cancer prevention by tea: animal studies, molecular mechanisms and human relevance. Nat Rev Cancer2009, 9(6):429–439.

Yang D, Li S, Wang H, Li X, Liu S, Han W, Hao J, Zhang H. Prevention of postoperative recurrence of bladder cancer: a clinical study. Zhonghua Wai Ke Za Zhi. 1999 Aug;37(8):464-5.

Yang DA, Li SQ, Li XT. [Prophylactic effects of zhuling and BCG on postoperative recurrence of bladder cancer]. Zhonghua Wai Ke Za Zhi. 1994 Jul;32(7):433-4.

Yang G, Li X, Li X, Wang L, Li J, Song X, Chen J, Guo Y, Sun X, Wang S, Zhang Z, Zhou X, Liu J. Traditional chinese medicine in cancer care: a review of case series published in the chinese literature. Evid Based Complement Alternat Med. 2012;2012:751046.

Yang HQ, Xie SS, Hu XL, Chen L, Li H. Appearance of human meridian-like structure and acupoints and its time correlation by infrared thermal imaging. Am J Chin Med. 2007;35(2):231-40.

Yang M, Kenfield SA, Van Blarigan EL, Batista JL, Sesso HD, Ma J, Stampfer MJ, Chavarro JE. Dietary patterns after prostate cancer diagnosis in relation to disease-specific and total mortality. Cancer Prev Res (Phila). 2015 Jun;8(6):545-51. doi: 10.1158/1940-6207.CAPR-14-0442.

Yang Z. Are peanut allergies a concern for using peanut-based formulated foods in developing countries? Food Nutr Bull. 2010 Jun;31(2 Suppl):S147-53.

Yasuda T, Takeyama Y, Ueda T, Shinzeki M, Sawa H, Nakajima T, Kuroda Y. Breakdown of Intestinal Mucosa Via Accelerated Apoptosis Increases Intestinal Permeability in Experimental Severe Acute Pancreatitis. J Surg Res. 2006 Apr 4.

Yeager RL, Oleske DA, Sanders RA, Watkins JB 3rd, Eells JT, Henshel DS. Melatonin as a principal component of red light therapy. Med Hypotheses. 2007;69(2):372-6.

Yeager S. The Doctor's Book of Food Remedies. Emmaus, PA: Rodale Press, 1998.

Yeh CC, Lin CC, Wang SD, Chen YS, Su BH, Kao ST. Protective and anti-inflammatory effect of a traditional Chinese medicine, Xia-Bai-San, by modulating lung local cytokine in a murine model of acute lung injury. Int Immunopharmacol. 2006 Sep;6(9):1506-14.

Yennurajalingam S, Tannir NM, Williams JL, Lu Z, Hess KR, Frisbee-Hume S, House HL, Lim ZD, Lim KH, Lopez G, Reddy A, Azhar A, Wong A, Patel SM, Kuban DA, Kaseb AO, Cohen L, Bruera E. A Double-Blind, Randomized, Placebo-Controlled Trial of Panax Ginseng for Cancer-Related Fatigue in Patients With Advanced Cancer. J Natl Compr Canc Netw. 2017 Sep;15(9):1111-1120. doi: 10.6004/jnccn.2017.0149..

Yoo YB, Park KS, Kim JB, Kang HJ, Yang JH, Lee EK, Kim HY. Xanthohumol inhibits cellular proliferation in a breast cancer cell line (MDA-MB231) through an intrinsic mitochondrial-dependent pathway. Indian J Cancer. 2014 Oct-Dec;51(4):518-23. doi: 10.4103/0019-509X.175328.

Yoon HE, Kim SA, Choi HS, Ahn MY, Yoon JH, Ahn SG. Inhibition of Plk1 and Pin1 by 5'-nitro-indirubinoxime suppresses human lung cancer cells. Cancer Lett. 2012 Mar;316(1):97-104.

Yoshida T, Saeki T, Aoyama Y, Okudaira T, Okada T, Funasaka S. (1997). Treatment of head and neck cancers with BRMs. Biotherapy, 10(2), 115-120.

Yoshigai E, Machida T, Okuyama T, et al. Citrus nobiletin suppresses inducible nitric oxide synthase gene expression in interleukin-1β-treated hepatocytes. Biochem Biophys Res Commun. 2013;439(1):54-59. doi:10.1016/j.bbrc.2013.08.029

Yu CH, Kan SF, Shu CH, Lu TJ, Sun-Hwang L, Wang PS. Inhibitory mechanisms of Agaricus blazei Murill on the growth of prostate cancer in vitro and in vivo. J Nutr Biochem. 2009 Oct;20(10):753-64. doi: 10.1016/j.jnutbio.2008.07.004.

Yu K, Deng SL, Sun TC, Li YY, Liu YX. Melatonin Regulates the Synthesis of Steroid Hormones on Male Reproduction: A Review. Molecules. 2018 Feb 17;23(2). pii: E447. doi: 10.3390/molecules23020447.

Yu L, Zhang Y, Chen C, Cui HF, Yan XK. Meta-analysis on randomized controlled clinical trials of acupuncture for asthma. Zhongguo Zhen Jiu. 2010 Sep;30(9):787-92.

Yu XM, Zhu GM, Chen YL, Fang M, Chen YN. Systematic assessment of acupuncture for treatment of herpes zoster in domestic clinical studies. Zhongguo Zhen Jiu. 2007 Jul;27(7):536-40.

Yuan H, Lu X, Ma Q, Li D, Xu G, Piao G. Flavonoids from Artemisia sacrorum Ledeb. and their cytotoxic activities against human cancer cell lines. Exp Ther Med. 2016 Sep;12(3):1873-1878.

Yuan JM, Stepanov I, Murphy SE, Wang R, Allen S, Jensen J, Strayer L, Adams-Haduch J, Upadhyaya P, Le C, Kurzer MS, Nelson HH, Yu MC, Hatsukami D, Hecht SS. Clinical Trial of 2-Phenethyl Isothiocyanate as an Inhibitor of Metabolic Activation of a Tobacco-Specific Lung Carcinogen in Cigarette Smokers. Cancer Prev Res (Phila). 2016 May;9(5):396-405. doi: 10.1158/1940-6207.CAPR-15-0380.

417

Yue GG, Fung KP, Tse GM, Leung PC, Lau CB. Comparative studies of various ganoderma species and their different parts with regard to their antitumor and immunomodulating activities in vitro. J Altern Complement Med. 2006 Oct;12(8):777-89.

Yue GG, Fung KP, Tse GM, Leung PC, Lau CB. Comparative studies of various ganoderma species and their different parts with regard to their antitumor and immunomodulating activities in vitro. J Altern Complement Med. 2006 Oct;12(8):777-89.

Yusakul G, Kitirattrakarn W, Tanwanichkul N, Tanaka H, Putalun W. Development and Application of an Enzyme-linked Immunosorbent Assay for Specific Detection of Mangiferin Content in Various Cultivars of Mangifera indica Leaves Using Anti-mangiferin Polyclonal Antibody. J Food Sci. 2012 Apr;77(4):C414-C419.

Yusoff NA, Hampton SM, Dickerson JW, Morgan JB. The effects of exclusion of dietary egg and milk in the management of asthmatic children: a pilot study. J R Soc Promot Health. 2004 Mar;124(2):74-80.

Zaets VN, Karpov PA, Smertenko PS, Blium IaB. Molecular mechanisms of the repair of UV-induced DNA damages in plants. Tsitol Genet. 2006 Sep-Oct;40(5):40-68.

Zamora-Ros R, Agudo A, Luján-Barroso L, Romieu I, Ferrari P, Knaze V, Bueno-de-Mesquita HB, Leenders M, Travis RC, Navarro C, Sánchez-Cantalejo E, Slimani N, Scalbert A, Fedirko V, Hjartåker A, Engeset D, Skeie G, Boeing H, Förster J, Li K, Teucher B, Agnoli C, Tumino R, Mattiello A, Saieva C, Johansson I, Stenling R, Redondo ML, Wallström P, Ericson U, Khaw KT, Mulligan AA, Trichopoulou A, Dilis V, Katsoulis M, Peeters PH, Igali L, Tjønneland A, Halkjær J, Touillaud M, Perquier F, Fagherazzi G, Amiano P, Ardanaz E, Bredsdorff L, Overvad K, Ricceri F, Riboli E, González CA. Dietary flavonoid and lignan intake and gastric adenocarcinoma risk in the European Prospective Investigation into Cancer and Nutrition (EPIC) study. Am J Clin Nutr. 2012 Dec;96(6):1398-408.

Zarate G, Gonzalez S, Chaia AP. Assessing survival of dairy propionibacteria in gastrointestinal conditions and adherence to intestinal epithelia. Centro de Referencia para Lactobacilos-CONICET. Tucuman, Argentina: Humana Press. 2004.

Zarkadas M, Scott FW, Salminen J, Ham Pong A. Common Allergenic Foods and Their Labelling in Canada. Can J Allerg Clin Immun. 1999; 4:118-141.

Zeng J, Li YQ, Zuo XL, Zhen YB, Yang J, Liu CH. Clinical trial: effect of active lactic acid bacteria on mucosal barrier function in patients with diarrhoea-predominant irritable bowel syndrome. Aliment Pharmacol Ther. 2008 Oct 15;28(8):994-1002.

Zhai QL, Hu XD, Xiao J, Yu DQ. [Astragalus polysaccharide may increase sensitivity of cervical cancer HeLa cells to cisplatin by regulating cell autophagy]. Zhongguo Zhong Yao Za Zhi. 2018 Feb;43(4):805-812. Chinese. doi: 10.19540/j.cnki.cjcmm.20171113.018.

Zhang C, Popp, F., Bischof, M.(eds.). Electromagnetic standing waves as background of acupuncture system. Current Development in Biophysics - the Stage from an Ugly Duckling to a Beautiful Swan. Hangzhou: Hangzhou Univer-sity Press, 1996.

Zhang CS, Yang AW, Zhang AL, Fu WB, Thien FU, Lewith G, Xue CC. Ear-acupressure for allergic rhinitis: a systematic review. Clin Otolaryngol. 2010 Feb;35(1):6-12.

Zhang D, Ke L, Ni Z, Chen Y, Zhang LH, Zhu SH, Li CJ, Shang L, Liang J, Shi YQ. Berberine... Helicobacter pylori eradication... trial. Medicine (Baltimore). 2017 Aug;96(32):e7697. doi: 10.1097/MD.0000000000007697.

Zhang DF, Sun BB, Yue YY, Zhou QJ, Du AF. Anticoccidial activity of traditional Chinese herbal Dichroa febrifuga Lour. extract against Eimeria tenella infection in chickens. Parasitol Res. 2012 Aug 17.

Zhang J, Liu L, Chen F. Production and characterization of exopolysaccharides from Chlorella zofingiensis and Chlorella vulgaris with anti-colorectal cancer activity. Int J Biol Macromol. 2019 Aug 1;134:976-983. doi: 10.1016/j.ijbiomac.2019.05.117.

Zhang RL, Luo WD, Bi TN, Zhou SK. Evaluation of antioxidant and immunity-enhancing activities of Sargassum pallidum aqueous extract in gastric cancer rats. Molecules. 2012 Jul 11;17(7):8419-29.

Zhang S, Sugawara Y, Chen S, Beelman RB, Tsuduki T, Tomata Y, Matsuyama S, Tsuji I. Mushroom consumption and incident risk of prostate cancer in Japan: A pooled analysis of the Miyagi Cohort Study and the Ohsaki Cohort Study. Int J Cancer. 2019 Sep 4. doi: 10.1002/ijc.32591.

Zhang T, Srivastava K, Wen MC, Yang N, Cao J, Busse P, Birmingham N, Goldfarb J, Li XM. Pharmacology and immunological actions of a herbal medicine ASHMI on allergic asthma. Phytother Res. 2010 Jul;24(7):1047-55.

Zhang X, Zheng L, Sun Y, Wang T, Wang B. Tangeretin enhances radiosensitivity and inhibits the radiation-induced epithelial-mesenchymal transition of gastric cancer cells. Oncol Rep. 2015 Jul;34(1):302-10. doi: 10.3892/or.2015.3982.

Zhang Y, Wang XQ, Liu H, Liu J, Hou W, Lin HS. [A multicenter, large-sample, randomized clinical trial on improving the median survival time of advanced non-small cell lung cancer by combination of Ginseng Rg3 and chemotherapy]. Zhonghua Zhong Liu Za Zhi. 2018 Apr 23;40(4):295-299. Chinese. doi: 10.3760/cma.j.issn.0253-3766.2018.04.011.

Zhang Y, Zhang M, Jiang Y, Li X, He Y, Zeng P, Guo Z, Chang Y, Luo H, Liu Y, Hao C, Wang H, Zhang G, Zhang L. Lentinan as an immunotherapeutic for treating lung cancer: a review of 12 years clinical studies in China. J Cancer Res Clin Oncol. 2018 Nov;144(11):2177-2186. doi: 10.1007/s00432-018-2718-1.

Zhang Z, Teruya K, Eto H, Shirahata S. Induction of Apoptosis by Low-Molecular-Weight Fucoidan through Calcium- and Caspase-Dependent Mitochondrial Pathways in MDA-MB-231 Breast cancer Cells. Biosci Biotechnol Biochem. 2013;77(2):235-42.

Zhang Z, Wang CZ, Wen XD, Shoyama Y, Yuan CS. Role of saffron and its constituents on cancer chemo-prevention. Pharm Biol. 2013 Jul;51(7):920-4. doi: 10.3109/13880209.2013.771190.

Zhao CX. [Effect of Dichroa febrifuga L. on chloroquinsensible and chloroquinresistant malaria parasites]. J Tongji Med Univ. 1986;6(2):112-5.

Zhao F, Wang L, Liu K. In vitro anti-inflammatory effects of arctigenin, a lignan from Arctium lappa L., through inhibition on iNOS pathway. J Ethnopharmacol. 2009 Apr 21;122(3):457-62. doi:10.1016/j.jep.2009.01.038.

Zhao FD, Dong JC, Xie JY. Effects of Chinese herbs for replenishing shen and strengthening qi on some indexes of neuro-endocrino-immune network in asthmatic rats. Zhongguo Zhong Xi Yi Jie He Za Zhi. 2007 Aug;27(8):715-9.

Zhao HY, Wang HJ, Lu Z, Xu SZ. Intestinal microflora in patients with liver cirrhosis. Chin J Dig Dis. 2004;5(2):64-7.

Zhao J, Bai J, Shen K, Xiang L, Huang S, Chen A, Huang Y, Wang J, Ye R. Self-reported prevalence of childhood allergic diseases in three cities of China: a multicenter study. BMC Public Health. 2010 Sep 13;10:551.

Zhao L, Ni Y, Ma X, Zhao A, Bao Y, Liu J, Chen T, Xie G, Panee J, Su M, Yu H, Wang C, Hu C, Jia W, Jia W. A panel of free fatty acid ratios to predict the development of metabolic abnormalities in healthy obese individuals. Sci Rep. 2016 Jun 27;6:28418. doi: 10.1038/srep28418.

Zhao-Wilson X. What Dose of Resveratrol Should Humans Take? Life Extens. 2007 Mar.

Zheng M. Experimental study of 472 herbs with antiviral action against the herpes simplex virus. Zhong Xi Yi Jie He Za Zhi. 1990 Jan;10(1):39-41, 6.

Zheng Yan Zhao, Li Liang, Xiaoqing Fan, Zhonghua Yu, Arland T Hotchkiss, Barry J Wilk, Isaac Eliaz. The role of modified citrus pectin as an effective chelator of lead in children hospitalized with toxic lead levels. Alternative Therapies in Health and Medicine 2008, 14 (4): 34-8

Zhong K, Tong L, Liu L, Zhou X, Liu X, Zhang Q, Zhou S. Immunoregulatory and antitumor activity of schizophyllan under ultrasonic treatment. Int J Biol Macromol. 2015 Sep;80:302-8. doi: 10.1016/j.ijbiomac.2015.06.052.

Zhou Q, Zhang B, Verne GN. Intestinal membrane permeability and hypersensitivity in the irritable bowel syndrome. Pain. 2009 Nov;146(1-2):41-6.

Zhou R, Chen H, Chen J, Chen X, Wen Y, Xu L. Extract from Astragalus membranaceus inhibit breast cancer cells proliferation via PI3K/AKT/mTOR signaling pathway. BMC Complement Altern Med. 2018 Mar 9;18(1):83. doi: 10.1186/s12906-018-2148-2. PMID: 29523109; PMCID: PMC5845298.

Zhou Y, Wang X, Zhang J, He A, Wang YL, Han K, Su Y, Yin J, Lv X, Hu H. Artesunate suppresses the viability and mobility of prostate cancer cells through UCA1, the sponge of miR-184. Oncotarget. 2017 Mar 14;8(11):18260-18270. doi: 10.18632/oncotarget.15353.

Zhu HH, Chen YP, Yu JE, Wu M, Li Z. Therapeutic effect of Xincang Decoction on chronic airway in-flammation in children with bronchial asthma in remission stage. Zhong Xi Yi Jie He Xue Bao. 2005 Jan;3(1):23-7.

Zhu S, Chandrashekar G, Meng L, Robinson K, Chatterji D. Febrifugine analogue compounds: synthesis and antimalarial evaluation. Bioorg Med Chem. 2012 Jan 15;20(2):927-32.

Ziaei Kajbaf T, Asar S, Alipoor MR. Relationship between obesity and asthma symptoms among children in Ahvaz, Iran:A cross sectional study. Ital J Pediatr. 2011 Jan 6;37(1):1.

Ziemniak W. Efficacy of Helicobacter pylori eradication taking into account its resistance to antibiotics. J Physiol Pharmacol. 2006 Sep;57 Suppl 3:123-41.

Zimecki M. The lunar cycle: effects on human and animal behavior and physiology. Postepy Hig Med Dosw. 2006;60:1-7.

Ziment I. Alternative therapies for asthma. Curr Opin Pulm Med. 1997 Jan;3(1):61-71.

Zimmerman FJ, Christakis DA. Children's television viewing and cognitive outcomes: a longitudinal analysis of national data. Arch Pediatr Adolesc Med. 2005 Jul;159(7):619-25.

Zizza, C. The nutrient content of the Italian food supply 1961-1992. Euro J Clin Nutr. 1997;51: 259-265.

Żołnierczyk AK, Mączka WK, Grabarczyk M, Wińska K, Woźniak E, Anioł M. Isoxanthohumol--Biologically active hop flavonoid. Fitoterapia. 2015 Jun;103:71-82. doi: 10.1016/j.fitote.2015.03.007.

Zwolińska-Wcisło M, Brzozowski T, Mach T, Budak A, Trojanowska D, Konturek PC, Pajdo R, Droz-dowicz D, Kwiecień S. Are probiotics effective in the treatment of fungal colonization of the gastro-intestinal tract? Experimental and clinical studies. J Physiol Pharmacol. 2006 Nov;57 Suppl 9:35-49.

Index

(Herbs, foods and other natural solutions are too numerous to index)

cholinesterase, 43

chronic lymphocytic leukemia, 66, 230

cilia, 65, 66, 282

circulation, 20

Clostridium perfringens, 265

colon, 294, 295

colon cancer, 21, 51, 54, 55, 68, 111, 119, 125, 127, 128, 134, 138, 141, 143, 152, 153, 170, 171, 172, 175, 179, 180, 190, 193, 194, 201, 202, 229, 230, 232, 234, 235, 236, 237, 238, 243, 249, 255, 260, 261, 265, 266, 268, 271, 274, 285, 322, 340, 341, 359, 362, 371, 372, 385, 390, 393, 394

colorectal cancer, 54, 55, 112, 127, 131, 133, 140, 143, 149, 152, 153, 171, 176, 177, 178, 179, 194, 196, 223, 227, 230, 232, 235, 247, 256, 257, 258, 263, 268, 270, 293, 309, 329, 332, 338, 341, 355, 356, 357, 358, 366, 367, 372, 380, 406

congenital defects, 94

COPD, 67

cortisol, 17, 27, 100, 296, 297, 299, 309

cosmic rays, 88, 89

C-reactive protein (CRP), 29, 266

cryptoxanthins, 114

cyclic peroxides, 6

diazinon, 43

DNA

DNA damage, 114

duodenal cancers, 53

endometrial cancer, 96

endotoxins, 21, 33, 50, 58, 291, 294

Enterococcus faecium, 293

extremely high frequencies (EHF), 95

extremely low frequencies (ELF), 90, 94, 95

fiber, 96, 126, 128, 129, 130, 138, 139, 142, 143, 144, 145, 146, 152, 167, 177, 178, 186, 189, 195, 196, 207, 265, 293, 294, 303, 315, 322, 356, 366, 391, 403, 404

formaldehyde, 20, 40, 45, 61, 65, 82, 124, 304

fragrances, 303, 307

frequency, 90, 91, 94, 95, 106, 107

gallbladder cancer, 112

gamma rays, 88, 89, 90

gamma-glutamyl transpeptidase (GGT), 292

gastric cancer, 31, 52, 53, 54, 127, 138, 140, 157, 158, 161, 184, 185, 195, 196, 218, 232, 239, 245, 257, 265, 319, 330, 338, 340, 344, 365, 366, 370, 378, 383, 403, 404, 418

glioma, 99, 100, 101, 103, 351, 415

glutathione peroxidase, 5, 29, 30, 281, 282

glutathione reductase, 5, 30, 282

granulomas, 65

GSM phone frequency, 95

H. pylori, 32, 52, 53, 54, 158, 159, 184, 239

head and neck cancer, 244

head and neck cancers, 68

headaches, 97, 106

high-voltage lines, 91

Hodgkin lymphoma, 112

Hodgkin's disease, 51, 91

homosalate, 71

hydroperoxides, 5, 6, 7, 37, 205, 281, 282

hydroxyl radical, 66

hypervitaminosis-D, 288

imidacloprid, 43, 48

immunosuppression, 30, 46, 114

incandescent light, 87

interleukin, 46, 265, 293, 296

intestinal cancer, 21

inulin, 265

www.ingramcontent.com/pod-product-compliance
Lightning Source LLC
Chambersburg PA
CBHW050642270326
41927CB00012B/2837